Color Atlas of Oral Diseases

Contents

Preface

This atlas gives examples of oral diseases and those lesions in the wide range of systemic disorders that have oral manifestations. It differs from other atlases by the inclusion of a wide range of the more obvious extraoral manifestations and of some disorders of the teeth and hard tissues. It is intended primarily as a pictorial diagnostic aid, both for dentists and physicians, with text that provides a concise synopsis of stomatology. We have added very recent references for most topics, mainly where there are new developments, reviews or points of controversy.

The atlas covers clinical diagnostic features and includes some radiographs, but excludes laboratory tests and does not attempt to discuss management. Neither have we attempted to cover orthodontics, oral surgery or periodontology, as they are dealt with elsewhere.

It is impossible to organize the illustrations in a format that will please all and we have therefore elected to conform fairly closely to the World Health Organization International Classification of Diseases (ICD). This, like any system, cannot suit all needs but it does have the advantage of having received WHO acceptance. We have varied the system where we felt it absolutely necessary.

The illustrations are almost exclusively from our collection in the University Department of Oral Medicine, Surgery and Pathology at Bristol. We are indebted to former and present members of the Department who have contributed to the collection, particularly to the late Professor A I Darling; to Professors J Fletcher and A K Adatia; to Drs S R Porter and J Luker; and to Mr R G Smith. We are also grateful to Professor D K Mason, under whose care some of the patients were seen in Glasgow. A few slides are from other collections: Dr G Laskaris (Athens) has kindly helped with Figures 1.94, 1.95, 1.104, 12.76, 12.77 and 14.58; our colleagues, O Almeida, D Berry, M Griffiths, S Mutlu, F Nally, S Prime, J Ross, J Shepherd and A S Young have also helped with single contributions.

Most of the illustrations have not previously been published. For those that have, we are indebted to Professor R A Cawson as co-author of some publications; to the editors of the *British Dental Journal*; *Journal of Oral Pathology*; *Oral Surgery, Oral Medicine and Oral Pathology*; *Dental Update* and *Hospital Update*; and to publishers Churchill Livingstone; Heinemann Medical; Oxford University Press and John Wright for permission to reproduce some of the slides from our collection. We wish to acknowledge any other source whom we may have unwittingly omitted.

We are also grateful to Dr J W Eveson, who joined the Department after this project was started, and who has helped with constructive comments and our further education; to Ni Fathers and Derek Coles, for help with technical aspects related to the illustrations; and to Connie Blake, for typing the manuscript.

CS
SF

1

Infectious and parasitic diseases

TUBERCULOSIS

Figure 1.1 Tuberculosis is usually caused by *Mycobacterium tuberculosis*, although atypical mycobacteria may be implicated, particularly in immunocompromised patients. Oral lesions of tuberculosis are rare. The most common is a painless, irregular ulcer of the dorsum of the tongue, secondary to pulmonary tuberculosis. Typically the edge of the ulcer is undermined. Tuberculosis can be spread by the respiratory route.

Figure 1.2 The most common form of skin tuberculosis is lupus vulgaris. Lesions appear most frequently on the head and neck, rarely intraorally.

Figure 1.3 Lupus vulgaris begins as multiple red lesions, from their appearance called 'apple-jelly nodules'. The lesions ulcerate and scar.

Figure 1.4 Tuberculous cervical lymphadenitis is uncommon but may be seen particularly in Asian patients and may be caused by *Mycobacterium tuberculosis* or *M bovis*. The site of entry of the organism is usually the tonsils and, in some cases, *M scrofulaceum* or *M kansasii* may be implicated.

Figure 1.5 Tuberculous lymphadenitis caseates and discharges through multiple fistulae (scrofula), with scars on healing.

Figure 1.6 Haematogenous spread of tuberculosis is usually to vertebrae or long bones – rarely to the jaw, as here.

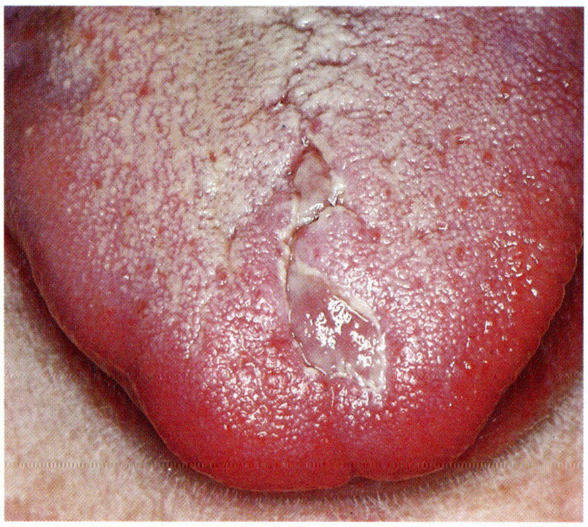

1.1

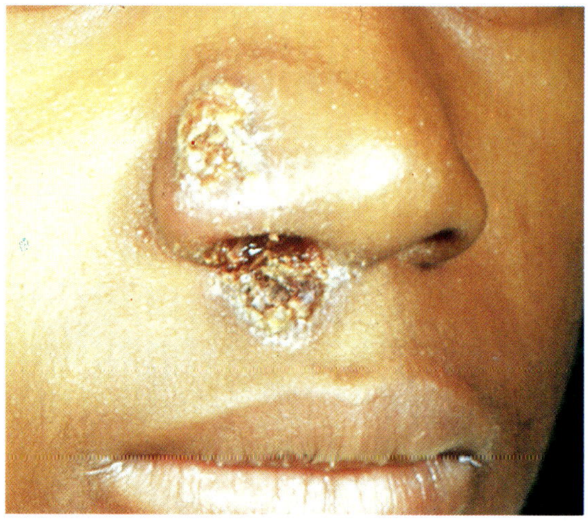

1.2

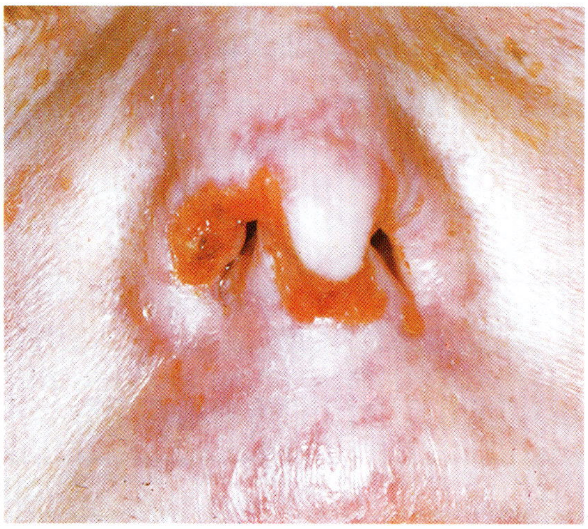

1.3

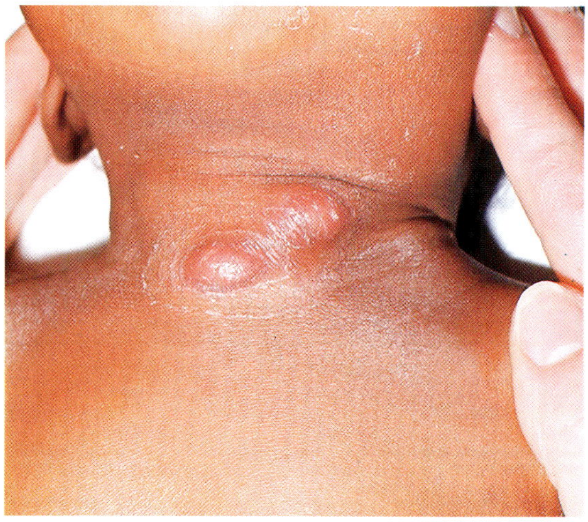

1.4

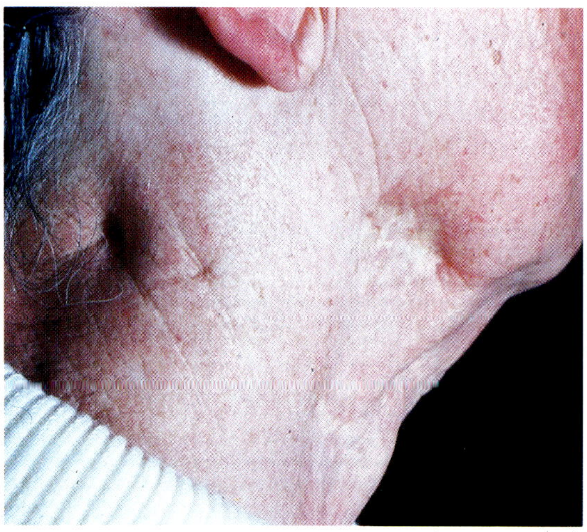

1.5

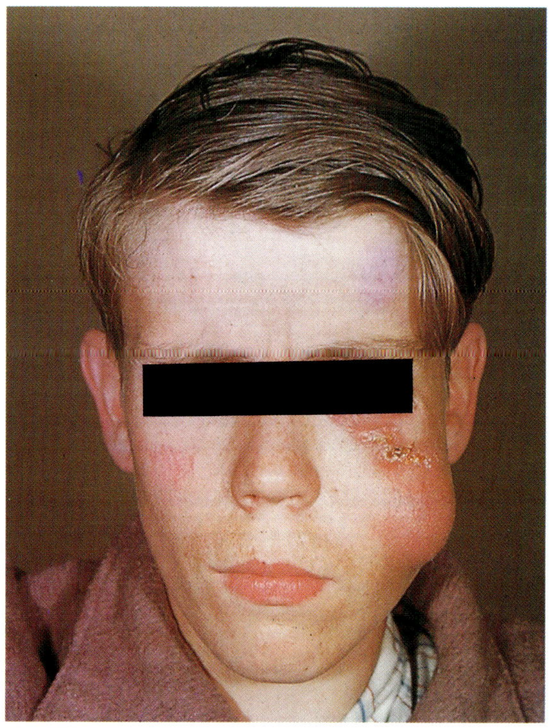

1.6

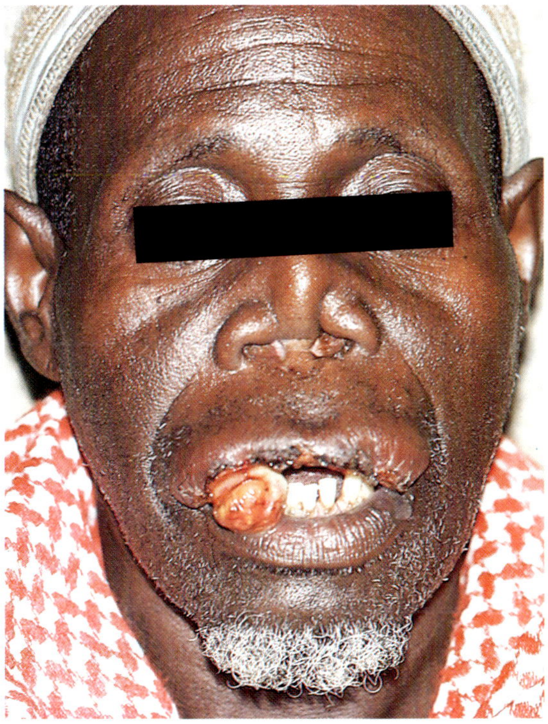

1.7

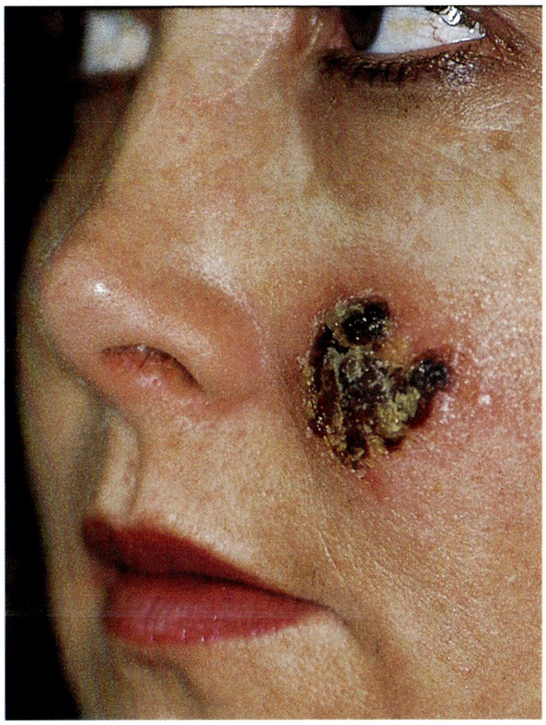

1.8

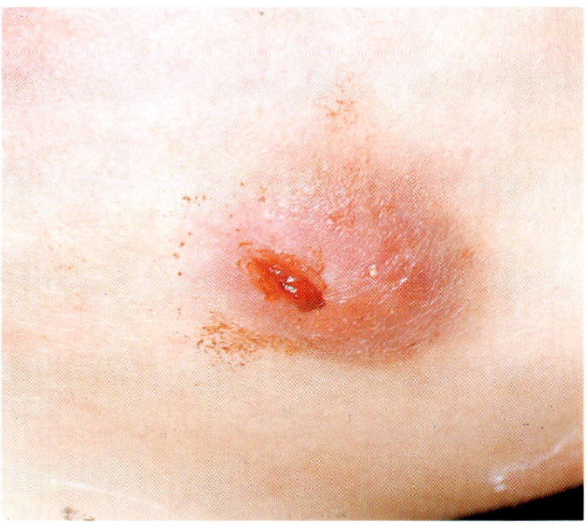

1.9

LEPROSY

Figure 1.7 Lepromatous leprosy, caused by *Mycobacterium leprae*, can produce widespread lesions, sometimes involving the mouth. Nodules can involve the lips or gingiva and elsewhere. The palate may necrose. The classic neural form of leprosy causes thickening of the greater auricular nerve and there may be cranial nerve lesions.

ANTHRAX

Figure 1.8 Cutaneous anthrax presents as a black eschar at the site of inoculation (malignant pustule).

ACTINOMYCOSIS

Figure 1.9 Cervicofacial actinomycosis is more common than thoracic or abdominal actinomycosis. *Actinomyces israelii* is a common oral commensal but rarely causes disease. Trauma, such as jaw fracture or tooth extraction, appears to initiate infection, which usually presents on the skin of the upper neck, typically just below or over the angle of the mandible. The lesion appears as a purplish firm swelling that enlarges and may eventually discharge through multiple sinuses, although this classical presentation is now uncommon.

UVULITIS

Figure 1.10 Uvulitis is a rare, potentially serious, infection. *Haemophilus influenzae* type b, may cause uvulitis in isolation or associated with epiglottitis and/or bacteraemia. Group A streptococci may cause uvulitis. The uvula is often more oedematous than shown here and the airway may be threatened. There may be palatal petechiae.

VACCINIA

Figure 1.11 Auto-inoculation of vaccinia virus from a vaccination site can produce single or multiple vaccinial lesions, with central scab and pronounced erythema and oedema.

Figure 1.12 Although vaccinia was extremely rare, it could affect the tongue or lip. Occasionally, in young children especially, vaccinial lesions were disseminated widely by auto-inoculation. Vaccination is no longer necessary, since smallpox has been eradicated.

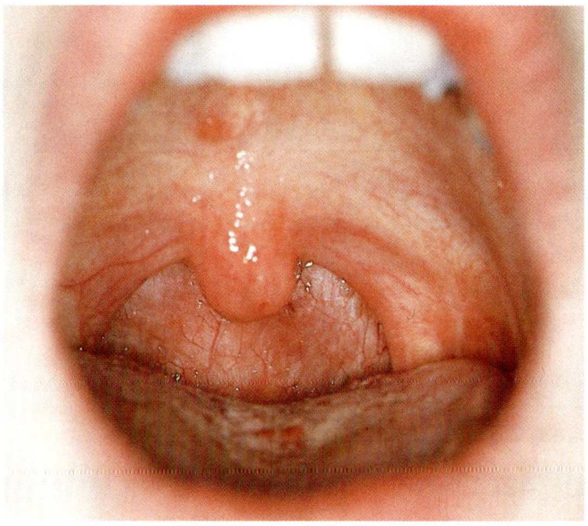

1.10

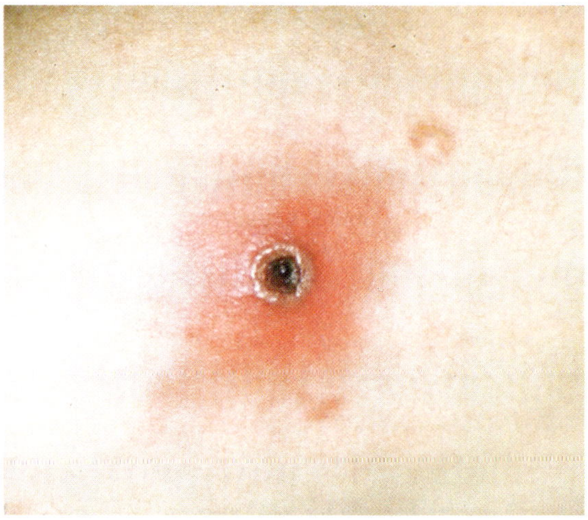

1.11

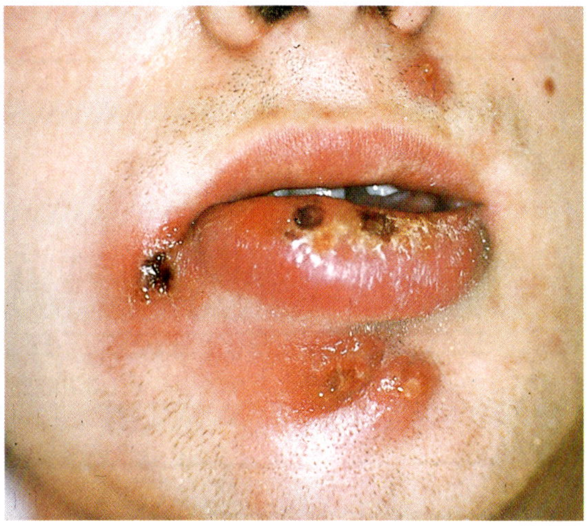

1.12

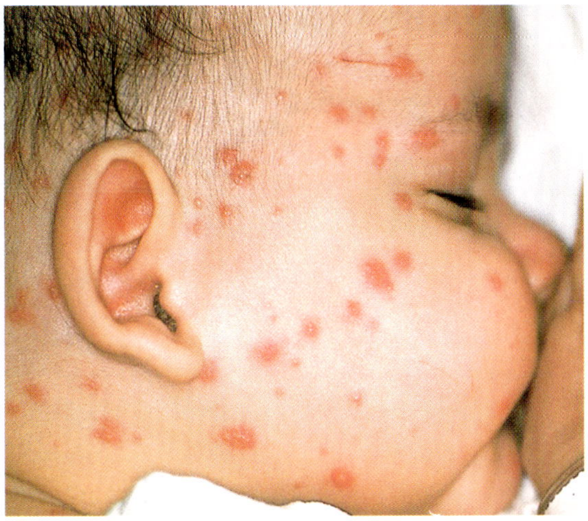

1.13

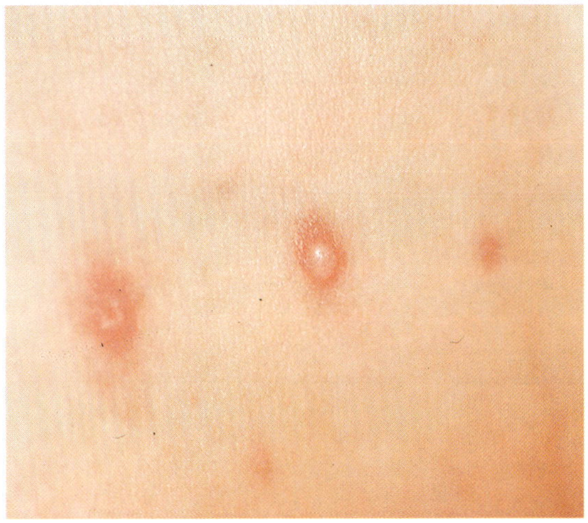

1.14

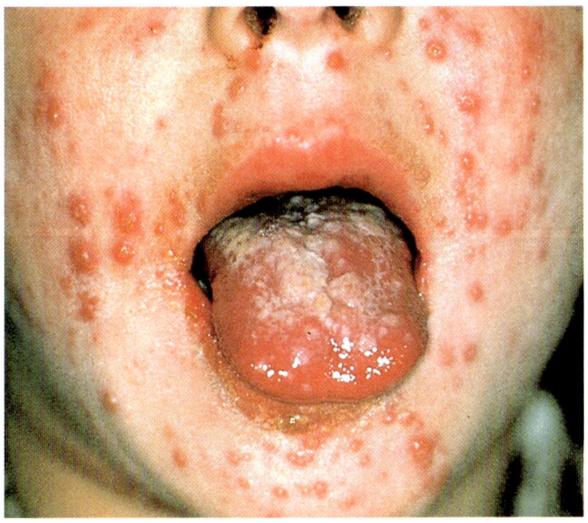

1.15

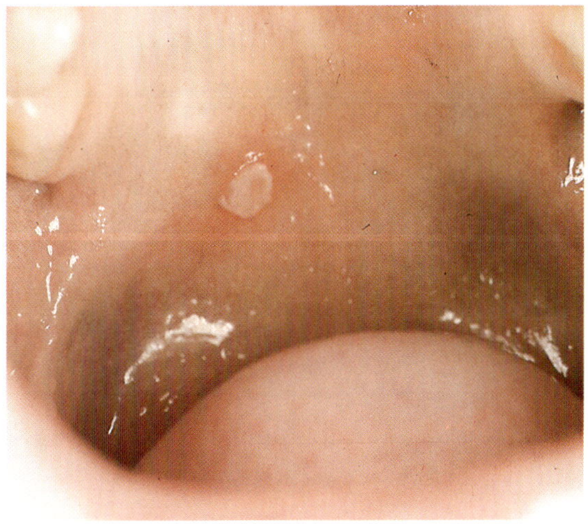

1.16

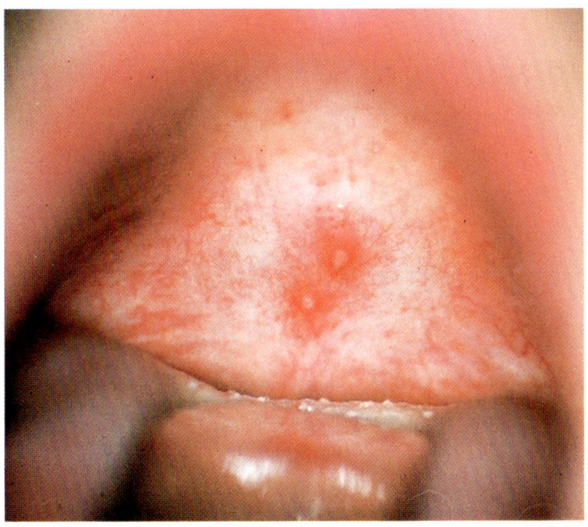

1.17

VARICELLA (*Chickenpox*)

Figure 1.13 Varicella is a highly contagious infection caused by the varicella-zoster virus (VZV). After an incubation period of 2–3 weeks, a variably dense rash appears, concentrated mainly on the trunk and head and neck.

Figure 1.14 The typical rash goes through macular, papular, vesicular and pustular stages before crusting.

Figure 1.15 The rash crops in waves over 2–4 days, so that lesions at different stages are typically seen.

Figure 1.16 The oral mucosa is commonly involved but there may be isolated lesions only. Vesicles appear, especially in the palate, and then rupture.

Figure 1.17 Ruptured oral vesicles produce painful round or ovoid ulcers with an inflammatory halo.

HERPES ZOSTER (*Shingles*)

Figure 1.18 Herpes zoster is caused by reactivation of VZV latent in dorsal root ganglia and, rarely, by reinfection. Zoster typically affects the elderly and those with cellular immune defects, and causes pain and a rash restricted to a dermatome (the mandibular division of the trigeminal nerve, in this case). Healing is usually uneventful, but there may be bone necrosis, tooth loss or hypoplasia of developing teeth.

Figure 1.19 Ipsilateral oral ulceration in the distribution of the mandibular division of the trigeminal nerve, in the same patient as shown in Figure 1.18. Mandibular and maxillary zoster may simulate toothache – the pain may precede the rash.

Figure 1.20 Zoster of the maxillary division of the trigeminal nerve causes a rash and periorbital oedema but the eye is not involved. The rash of zoster resembles that of varicella and occasionally pocks are seen beyond the affected dermatome (note lesions on forehead). Occasionally, oral lesions appear in the absence of a rash.

Figure 1.21 Ipsilateral oral ulceration in maxillary zoster.

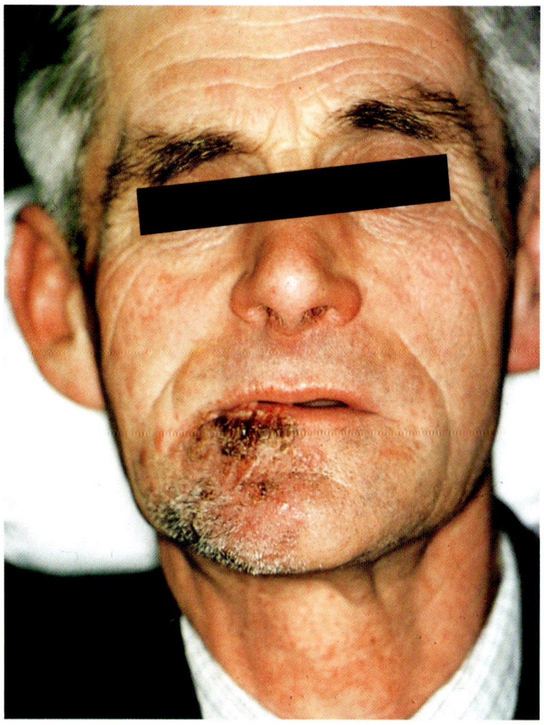

1.18

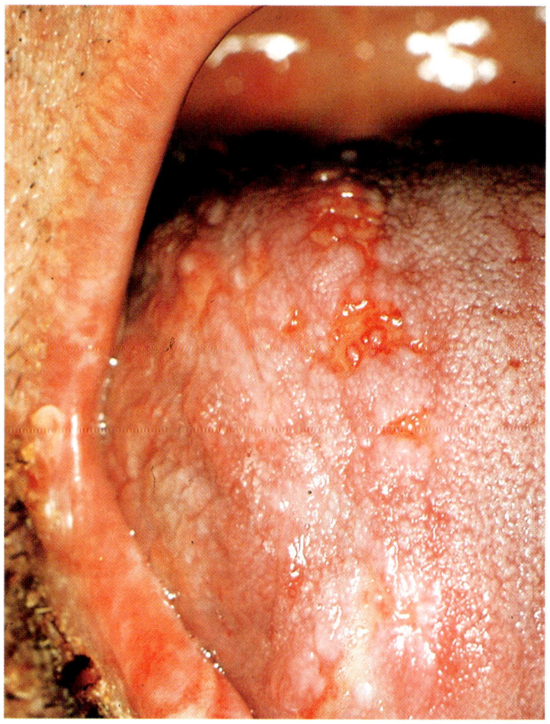

1.19

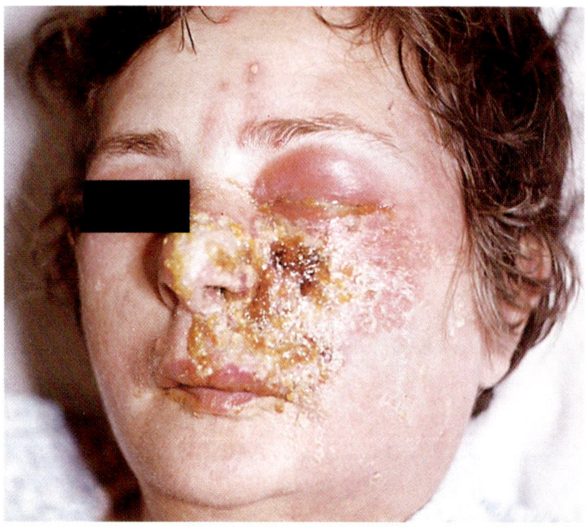

1.20

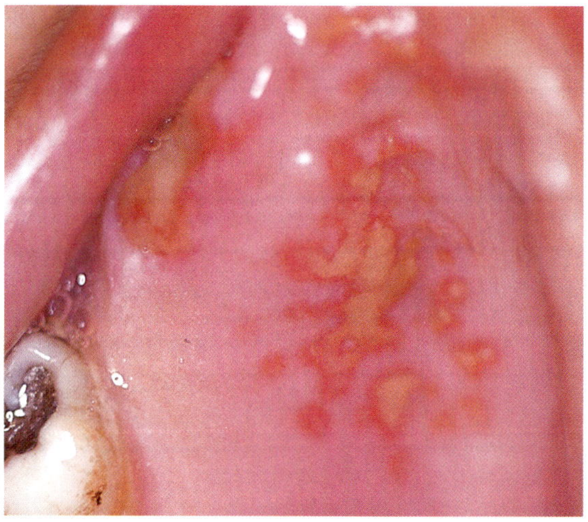

1.21

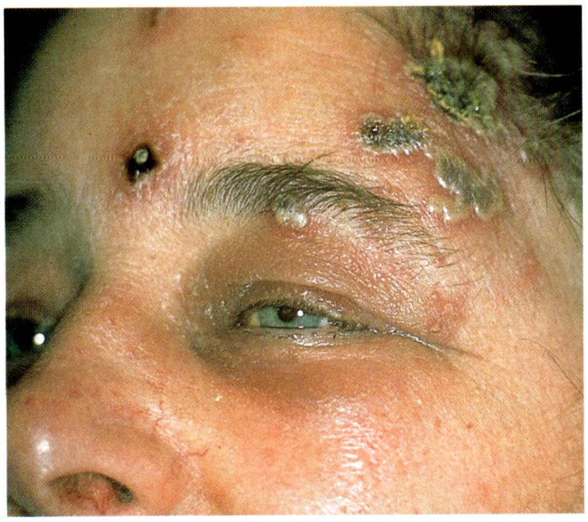

1.22

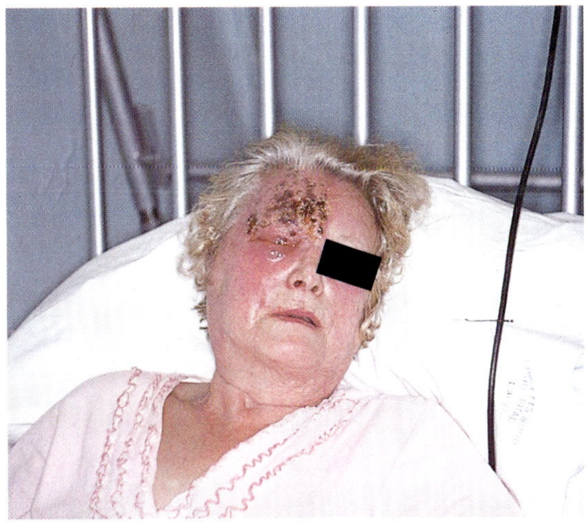

1.23

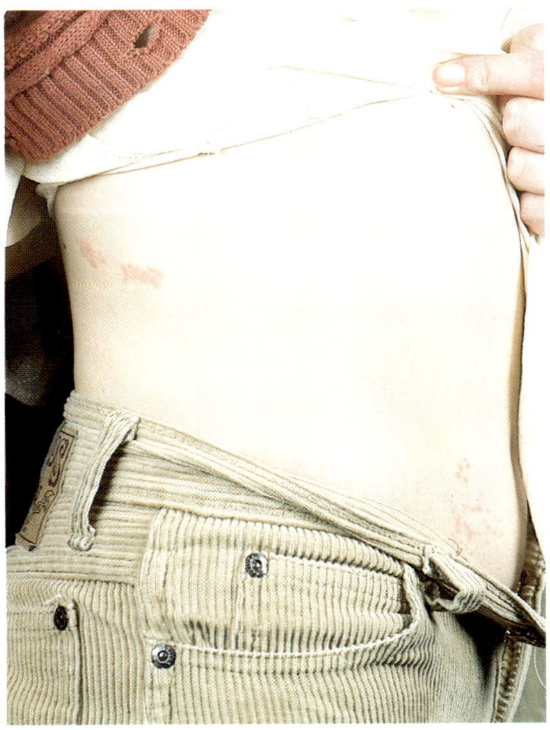

1.24

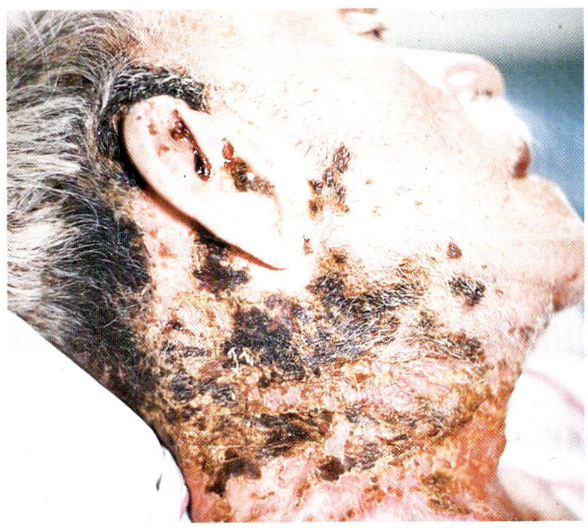

1.25

Figure 1.22 Zoster of the ophthalmic division of the trigeminal nerve does threaten sight, with the possibility of corneal ulceration, or panophthalmitis.

Figure 1.23 Ophthalmic zoster also produces chemosis and periorbital oedema which may become bilateral. Involvement of the central nervous system is common when zoster affects cranial nerves, and meningeal signs and symptoms are frequent.

Figure 1.24 Zoster more typically affects thoracic dermatomes. It has a bimodal distribution affecting a group of young adults who appear perfectly healthy otherwise, and also the elderly.

Figure 1.25 Occasionally, cervical dermatomes are affected, as here.

HERPES ZOSTER *(continued)*

Figure 1.26 There is an increased prevalence of zoster in persons with immunocompromised cellular immunity, including those with HIV infection, malignancy, and following bone marrow transplants. This patient, with Hodgkin's lymphoma, has sciatic zoster. Radiotherapy and chemotherapy also reactivate VZV.

Figure 1.27 Zoster may leave sequelae such as scarring (here from mandibular zoster) and post-herpetic neuralgia. Tissue destruction and severe post-herpetic neuralgia are more common in those who are immunocompromised. Infection of zoster lesions with *Staphylococcus aureus* can lead to a form of impetigo with delayed healing, greater scarring of the zoster lesions and dissemination of the bacterial lesions.

ZOSTER (*Ramsay-Hunt syndrome*)

Figure 1.28 Although zoster almost invariably affects sensory nerves, motor nerves may be involved occasionally. In Ramsay-Hunt syndrome, zoster of the geniculate ganglion of the facial nerve can cause ipsilateral lower motor neurone facial palsy, as here, with ipsilateral pharyngeal ulceration.

Figure 1.29 A rash may be seen in the external ear, in the distribution of a sensory branch of the facial nerve.

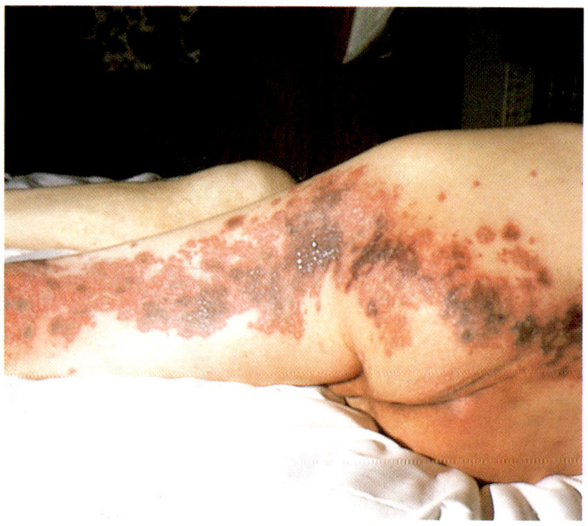

1.26

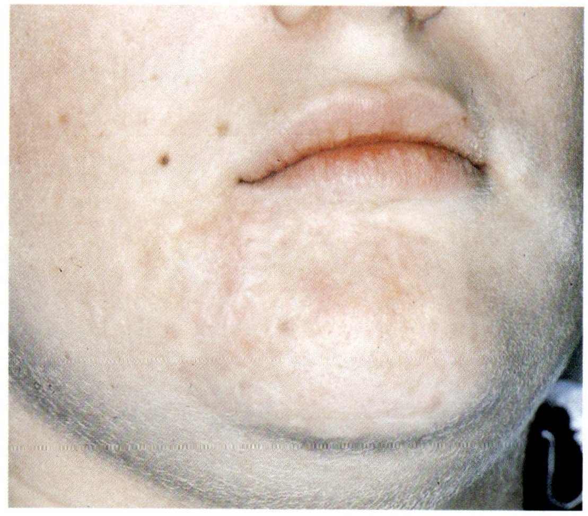

1.27

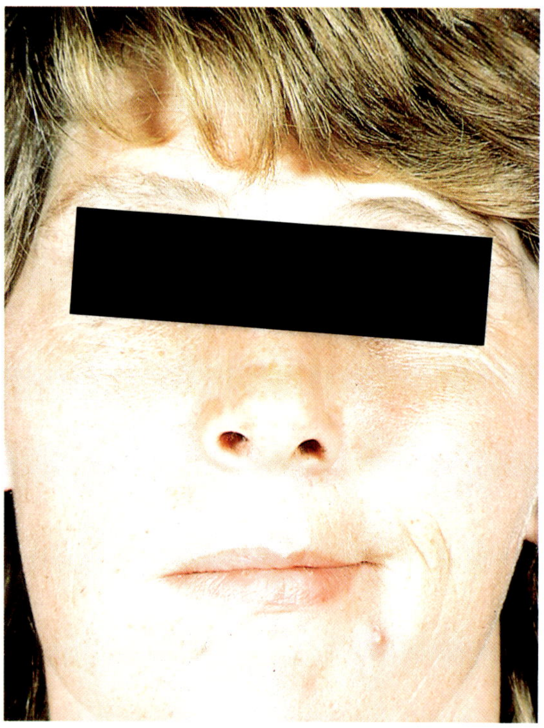

1.28

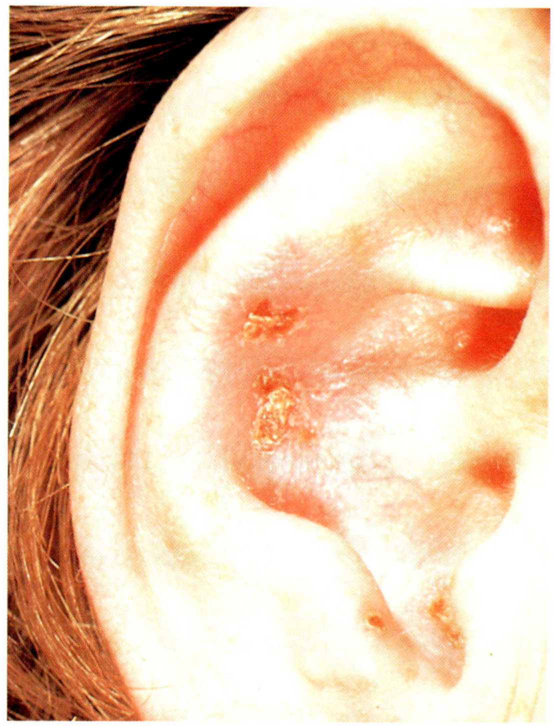

1.29

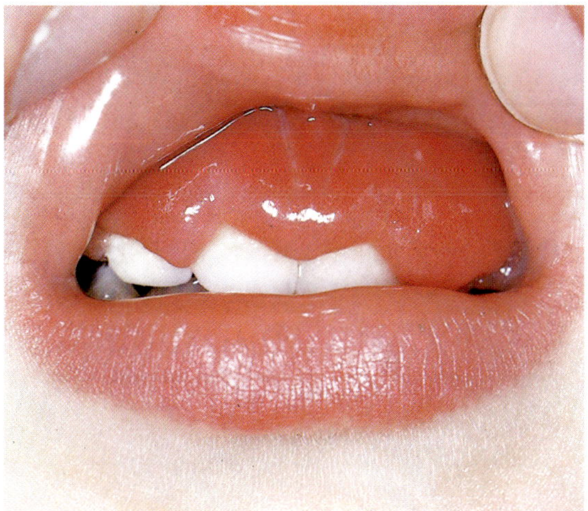

1.30

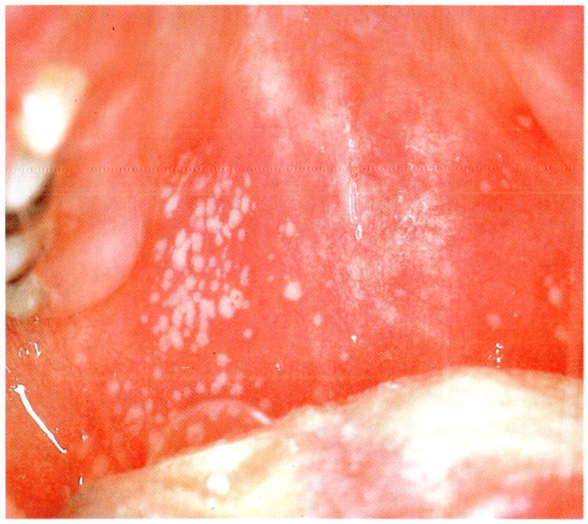

1.31

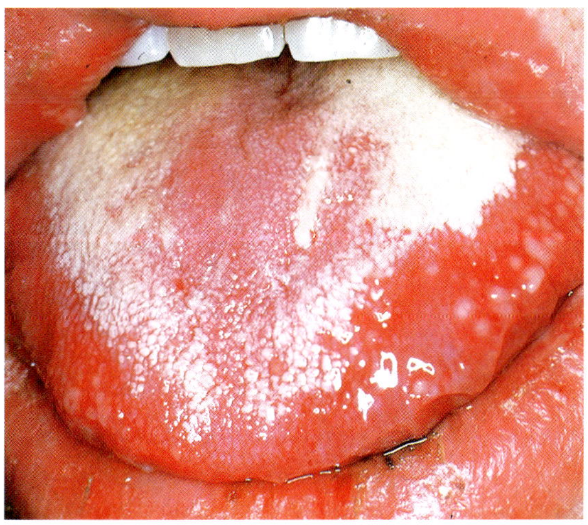

1.32

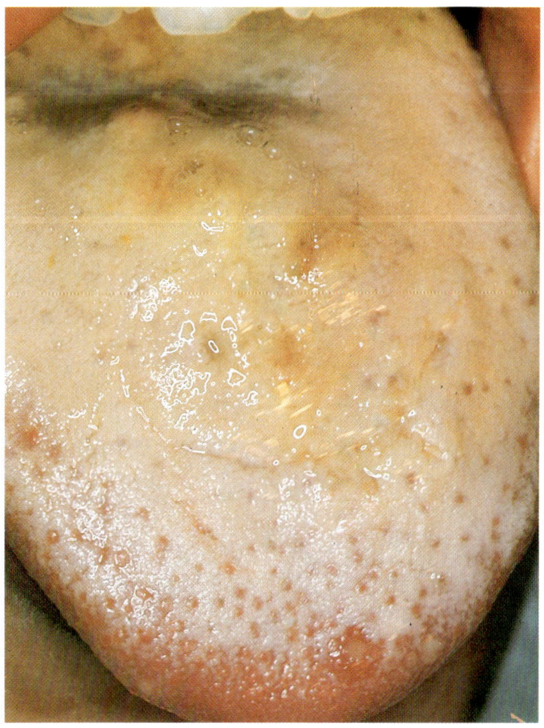

1.33

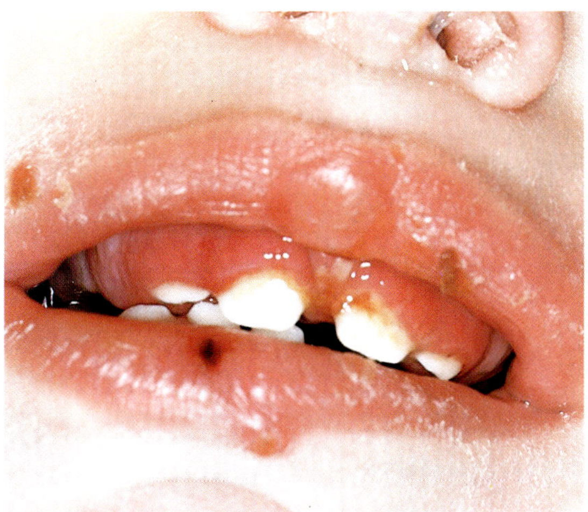

1.34

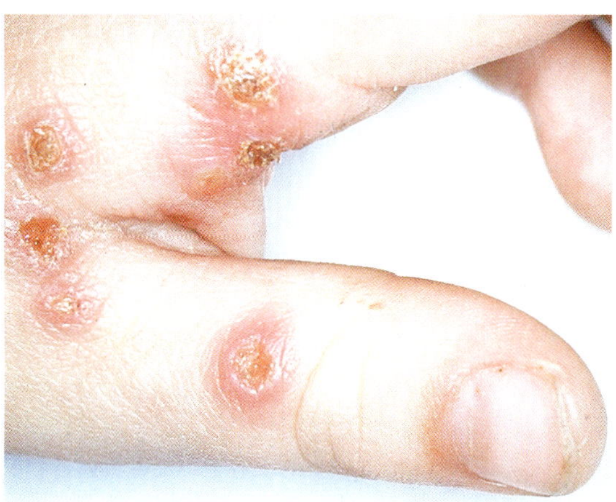

1.35

HERPES SIMPLEX INFECTIONS

Figure 1.30 After an incubation period of approximately 6–7 days, gingival oedema, erythema and ulceration are a prominent feature of primary infection with herpes simplex virus (HSV), usually caused by HSV1.

Figure 1.31 Widespread vesicles break down to leave pin-point ulcers that enlarge and fuse to produce irregular painful oral ulcers.

Figure 1.32 Typically a childhood infection between ages 2–4 years, an increasing number of adults are now affected and HSV2 is sometimes implicated.

Figure 1.33 Affected patients, especially adults, can be severely ill, with malaise, fever and cervical lymph node enlargement. The tongue is often coated and there is halitosis. Rarely, acute ulcerative gingivitis follows.

Figures 1.34 and 1.35 The saliva is heavily infected with HSV which may cause lip and skin lesions and is a source for cross-infection.

Rare complications of HSV infection include encephalitis and mononeuropathies.

HERPES SIMPLEX INFECTIONS *(continued)*

Figure 1.36 Primary infection of the finger can cause a painful whitlow. This is an occupational hazard for non-immune dental, medical or paramedical personnel.

RECURRENT HERPES SIMPLEX INFECTION

Figure 1.37 Reactivation of HSV latent in the trigeminal ganglion – for example, by fever, sunlight, trauma or immuno-suppression – produces herpes labialis. It presents as macules that rapidly become papular and vesicular, typically at the mucocutaneous junction of the lip. Some 6–14 per cent of the population have recurrent HSV infections.

Figures 1.38 and 1.39 Lesions then become pustular, scab and heal without scarring.

Figure 1.40 Any mucocutaneous site can be affected, including the anterior nares.

Figure 1.41 Herpes simplex infection can occasionally recur at sites other than mucocutaneous junctions and can simulate zoster.

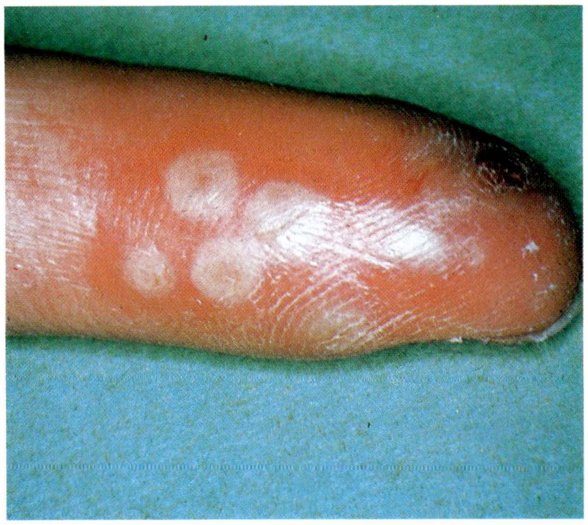

1.36

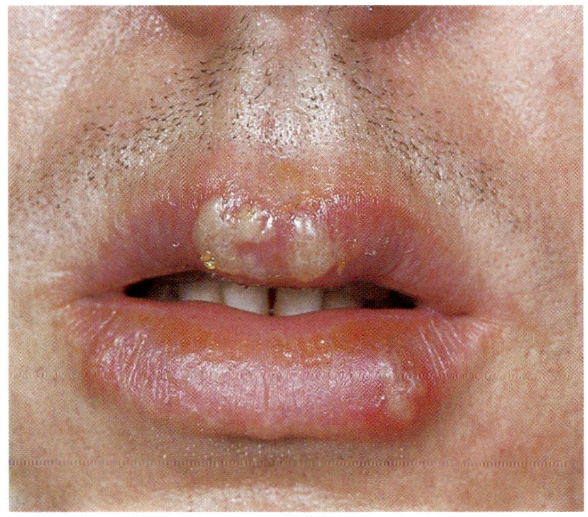

1.37

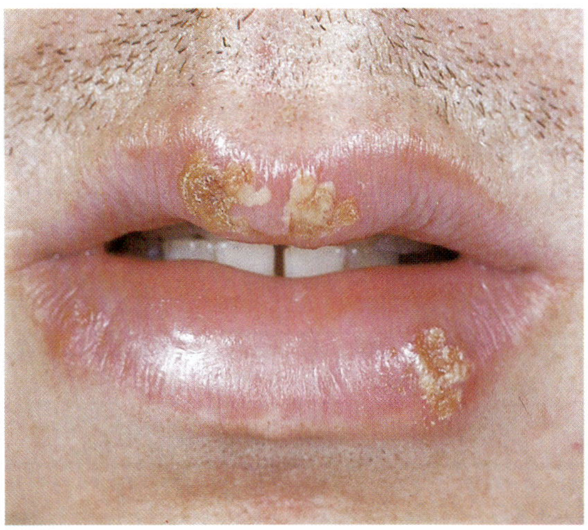

1.38

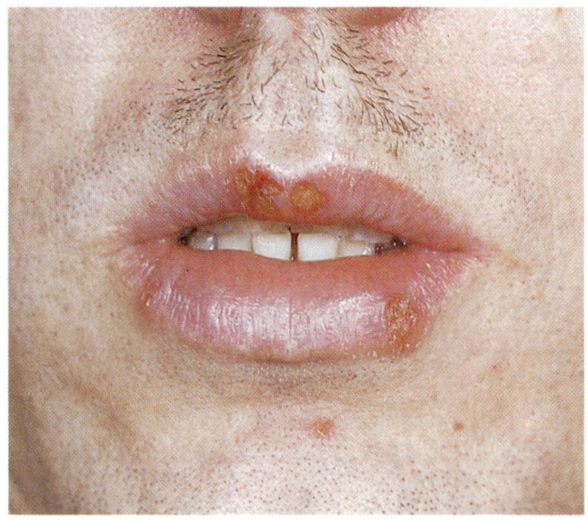

1.39

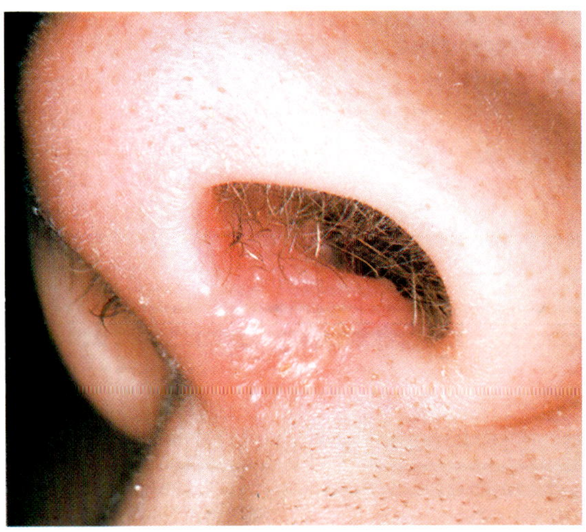

1.40

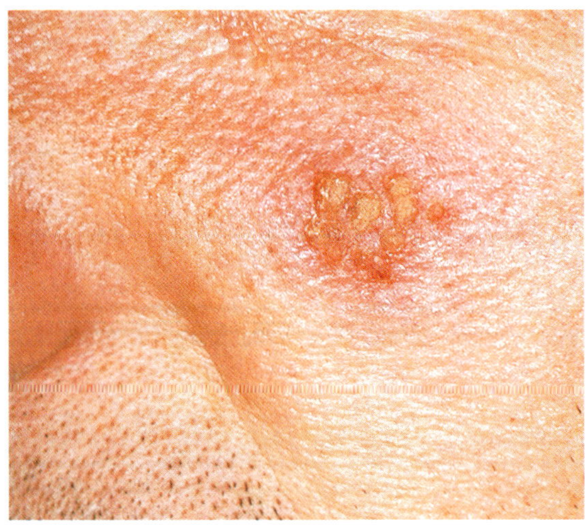

1.41

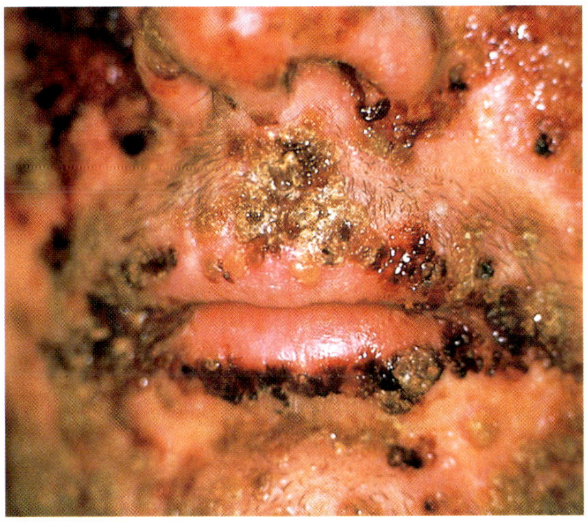

1.42

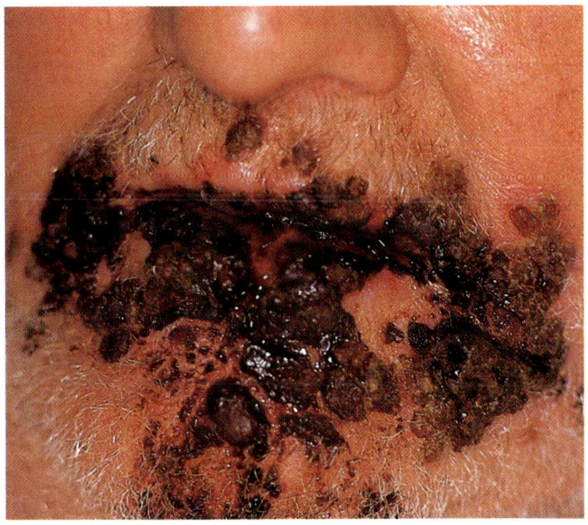

1.43

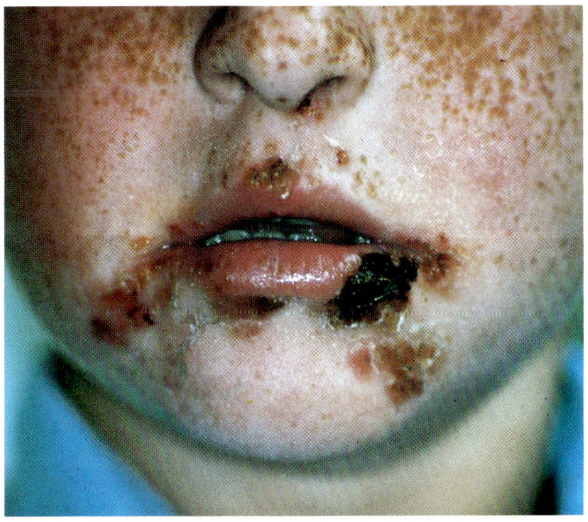

1.44

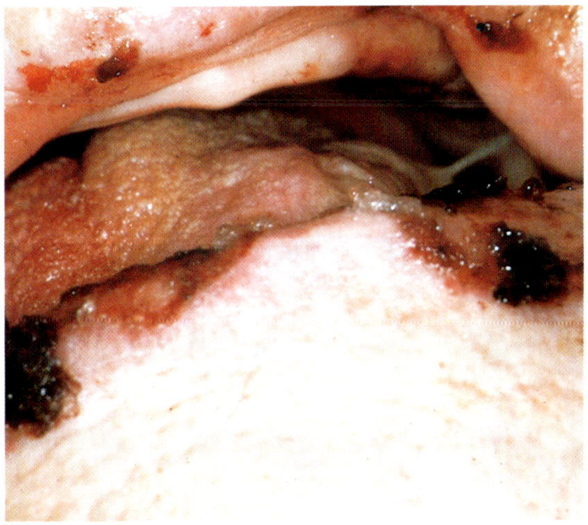

1.45

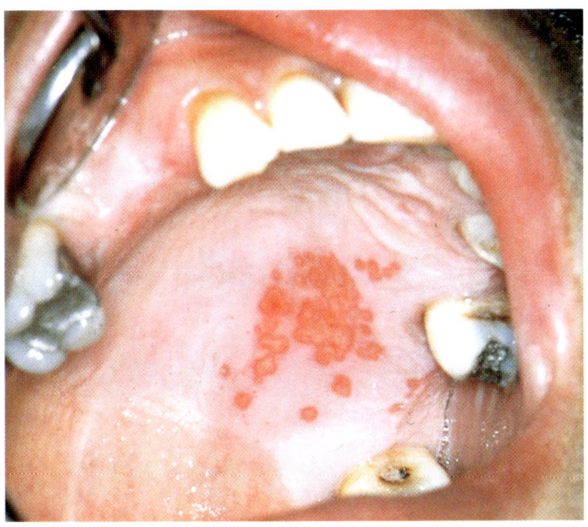

1.46

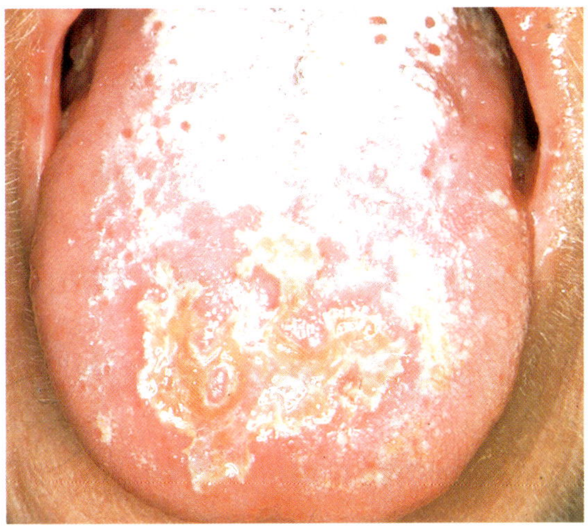

1.47

ECZEMA HERPETICUM

Figure 1.42 Eczema, other diseases of the skin, and the use of topical corticosteroids, predispose to disseminated herpetic lesions (eczema herpeticum, Kaposi's varicelliform eruption). Skin lesions in otherwise healthy patients are rare but a macular, vesicular or purpuric rash may be seen.

HERPES LABIALIS

Figure 1.43 Lesions eventually heal after crusting. Widespread lesions can affect debilitated patients, such as this man recovering from pneumonia.

Figure 1.44 Patients with T cell immune defects, such as this boy, are predisposed to recurrent herpes.

Figure 1.45 Haemorrhage into lesions produces a deceptive appearance in a leukaemic or other patient with thrombocytopenia.

RECURRENT INTRAORAL HERPES

Figure 1.46 Herpes simplex infection due to reactivation of latent HSV is rare intraorally, but may follow the trauma of a local anaesthetic injection, as here, or may be seen in immunocompromised patients. Recurrent intraoral herpes in normal patients tends to affect the hard palate or gingiva and heals within 1–2 weeks.

Figure 1.47 Immunocompromised patients may develop chronic, often dendritic, ulcers from HSV reactivation. Clinical diagnosis tends to underestimate the frequency of these lesions. The ulcers affect any site in the mouth. This is a patient with lymphoid leukaemia.

MEASLES (*Rubeola*)

Figure 1.48 Measles is an acute contagious infection with a paramyxovirus. The incubation period of 7–10 days is followed by fever, rhinitis, cough, conjunctivitis (coryza) and then a red maculopapular rash.

Figure 1.49 The rash appears initially on the forehead and behind the ears, and spreads over the whole body.

Figure 1.50 The rash is less immediately obvious in a dark-skinned patient.

Figure 1.51 Conjunctivitis in measles.

Figure 1.52 Koplik's spots – small, whitish, necrotic lesions, said to resemble grains of salt – are found in the buccal mucosa and occasionally also in the conjunctiva or genitalia. These spots precede the rash by 1–2 days and are pathognomonic.

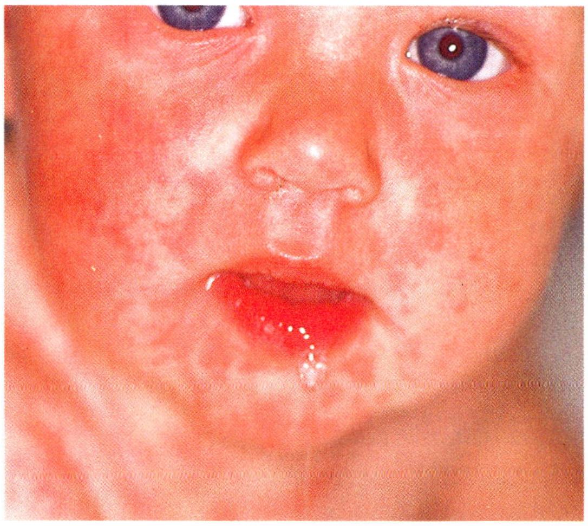

1.48

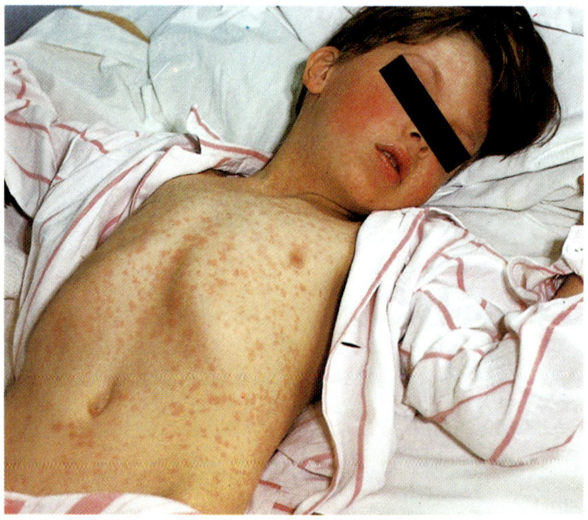

1.49

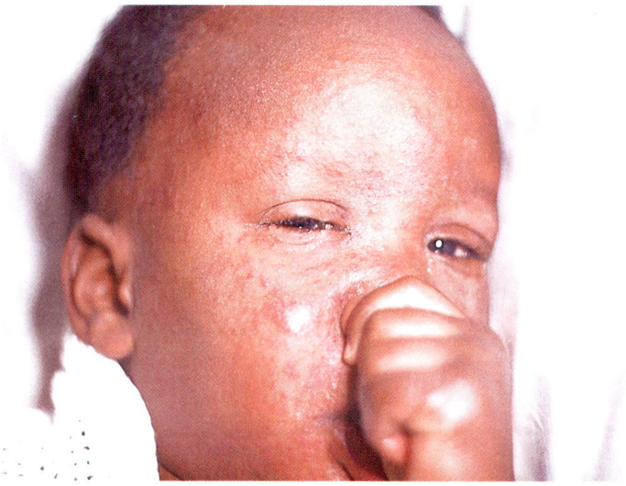

1.50

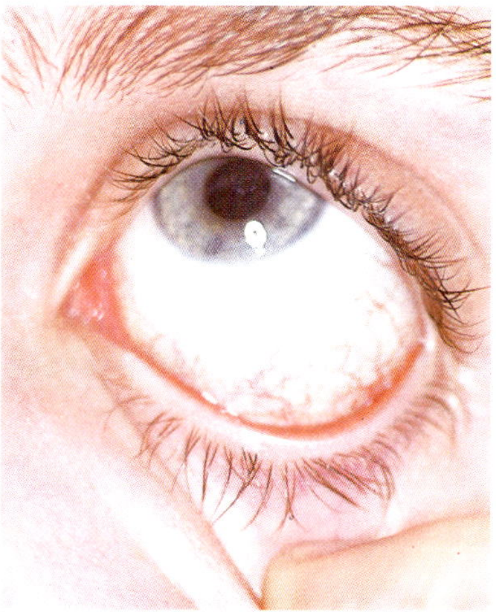

1.51

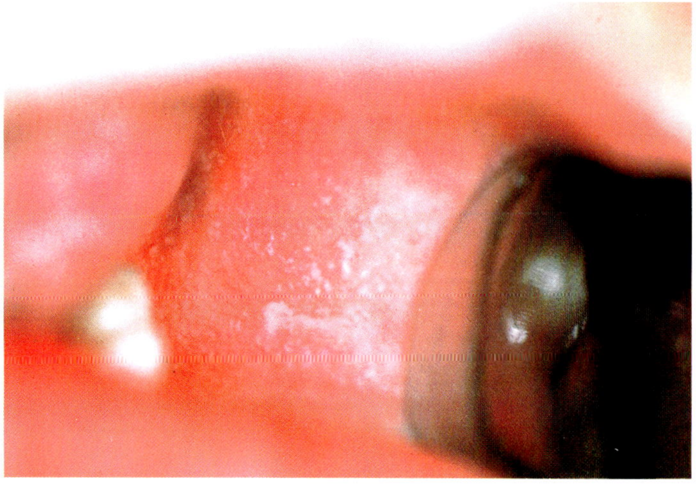

1.52

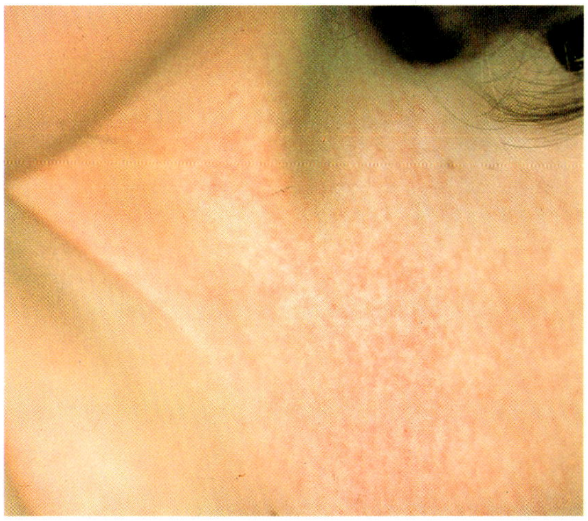

1.53

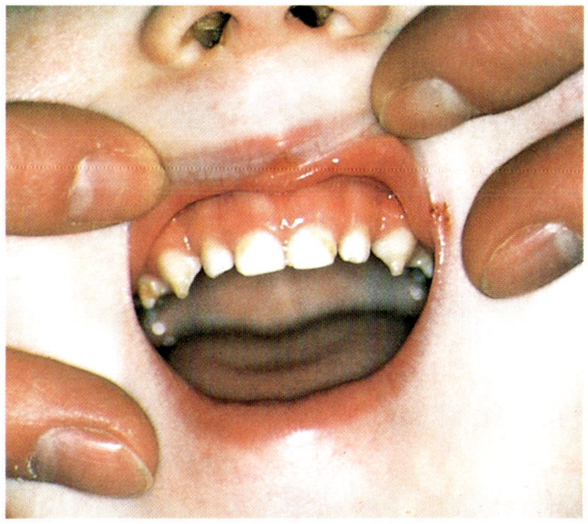

1.54

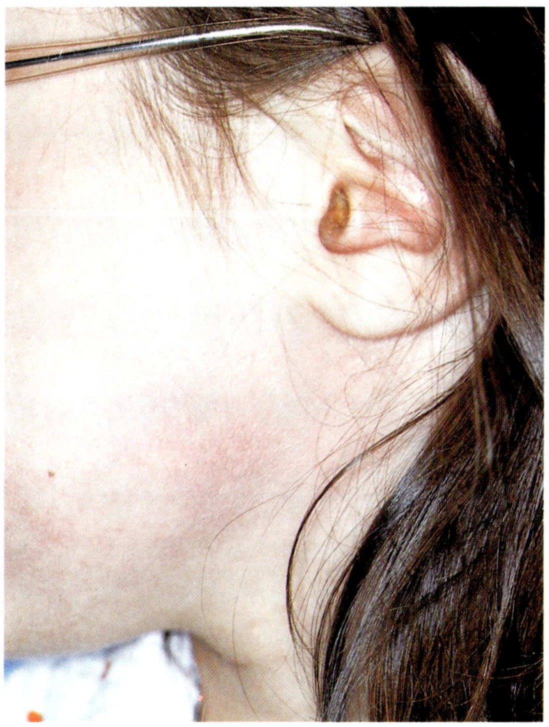

1.55

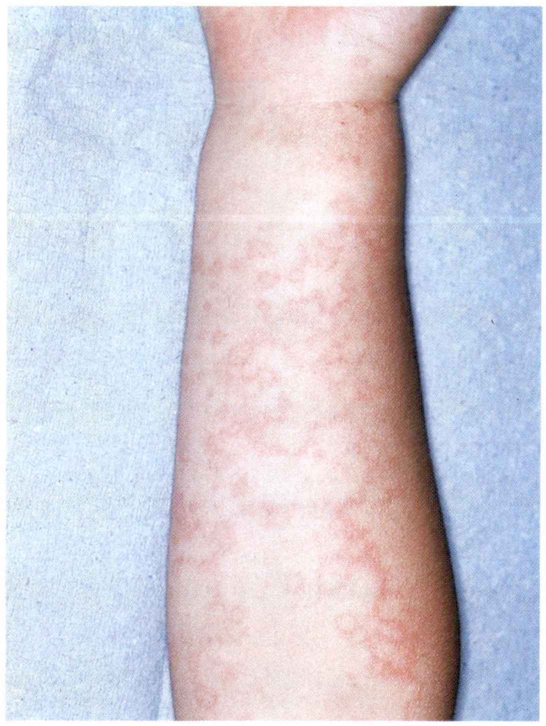

1.56

RUBELLA
(*German measles*)

Figure 1.53 Rubella is a togavirus infection with an incubation period of 2–3 weeks, followed by mild fever, mild conjunctivitis, a diffuse maculopapular rash and lymphadenopathy. Some enteroviruses, especially echovirus type 9, may cause a similar rash. There are no specific manifestations but there may be oral petechiae, known as Forcheimer's spots.

Figure 1.54 Maternal infection during the first trimester of pregnancy may lead to congenital rubella, causing mental handicap, deafness, blindness and cardiac defects, depending on the timing of the intrauterine infection. Congenital rubella may cause hypoplasia of the deciduous dentition. Similar defects may be found in other intrauterine infections, such as toxoplasmosis, cytomegalovirus, herpes simplex and Coxsackie B.

PARVOVIRUS INFECTION

Figure 1.55 Parvovirus is a DNA virus that may cause an acute febrile illness with rash that produces a 'slapped cheek' appearance on the face (Fifth disease or erythema infectiosum).

Figure 1.56 Pharyngitis, conjunctivitis, lymph node enlargement, splenomegaly and polyarthritis may occasionally be seen, especially in adults. The exanthem typically evolves into a reticular configuration as shown.

Parvovirus infection may occasionally precipitate aplastic crises, especially in those with sickle cell anaemia.

ACQUIRED IMMUNE DEFICIENCY SYNDROME (*AIDS, HIV-related disease*)

Figure 1.57 Infection with human immunodeficiency viruses (HIV) may cause an initial glandular fever-like illness but may be asymptomatic. The incubation period may extend over five or more years. Oral candidosis, especially thrush, is seen in over 60 per cent of AIDS patients, often as an early manifestation. It is the most common oral feature of HIV-related disease and may be a predictor of other opportunistic infections and of oesophageal thrush.

Figure 1.58 Other types of oral candidosis may be seen, including angular stomatitis. In healthy persons this is usually a local infection, emanating from a reservoir of candida beneath an upper denture.

Figure 1.59 Kaposi's sarcoma is a feature, especially in male homosexuals with AIDS, but may be seen occasionally in other groups of immuno-compromised patients. Oral lesions are macules or nodules, red to purple in colour, and most common in the palate.

Figure 1.60 Leukoplakia of the tongue antedates clinical AIDS in some patients. This lesion is not known to be premalignant but it is a predictor of bad prognosis.

Figure 1.61 The leukoplakia may be corrugated (or 'hairy') and usually affects the lateral margins of the tongue. Flat white lesions may be seen on the tongue in about one-third of cases. Hairy leukoplakia may be associated with Epstein-Barr virus and may resolve with antivirals such as acyclovir.

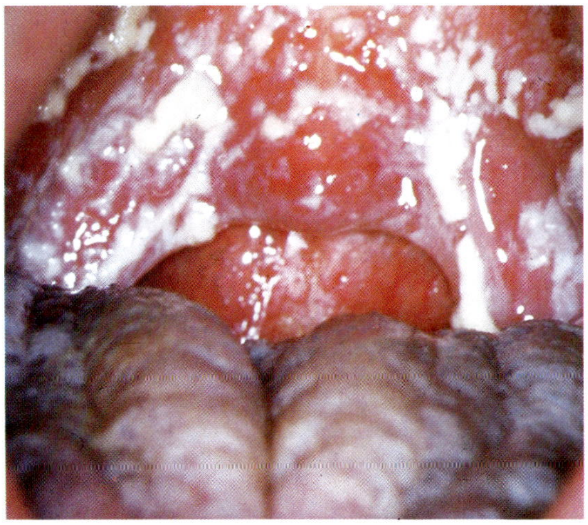

1.57

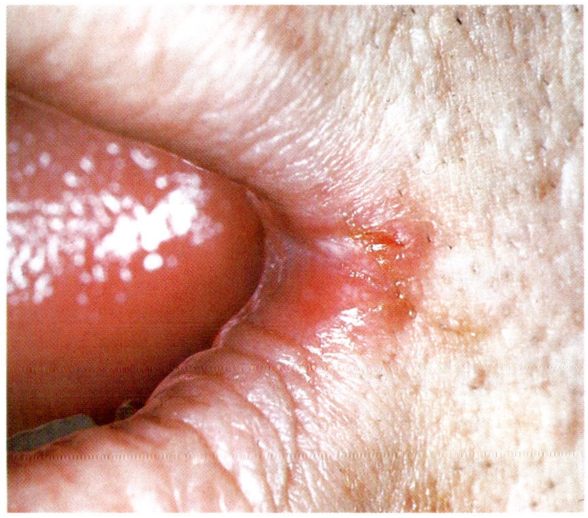

1.58

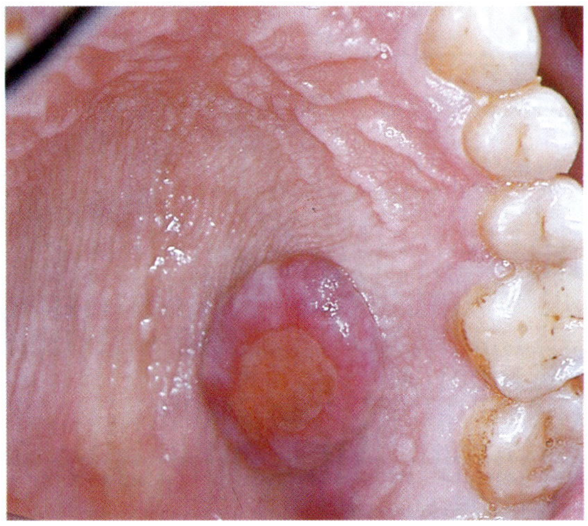

1.59

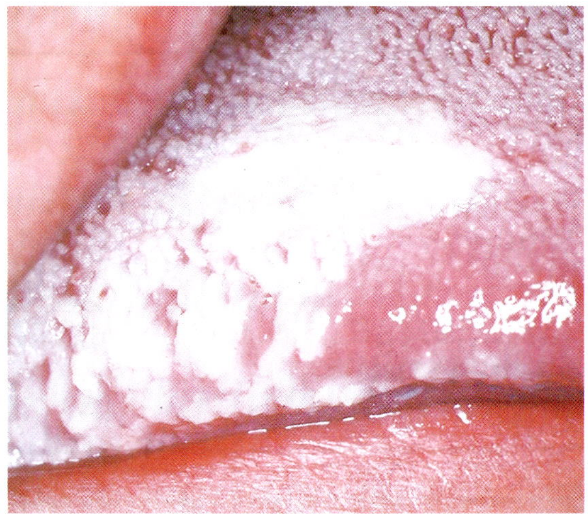

1.60

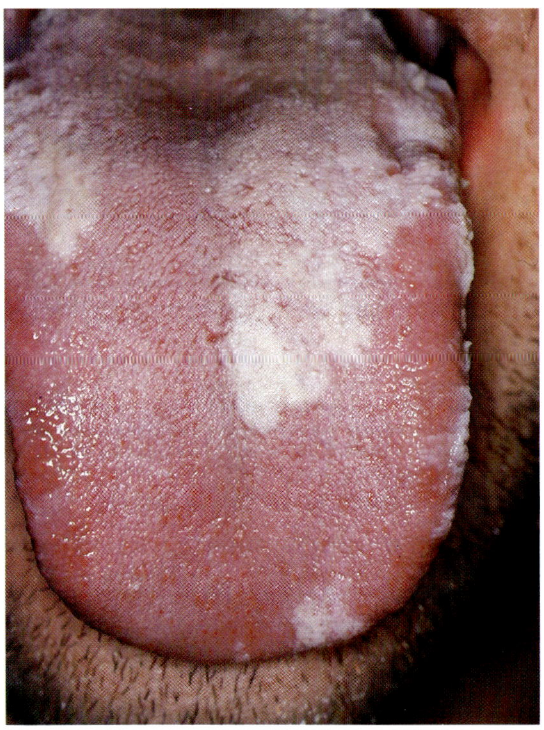

1.61

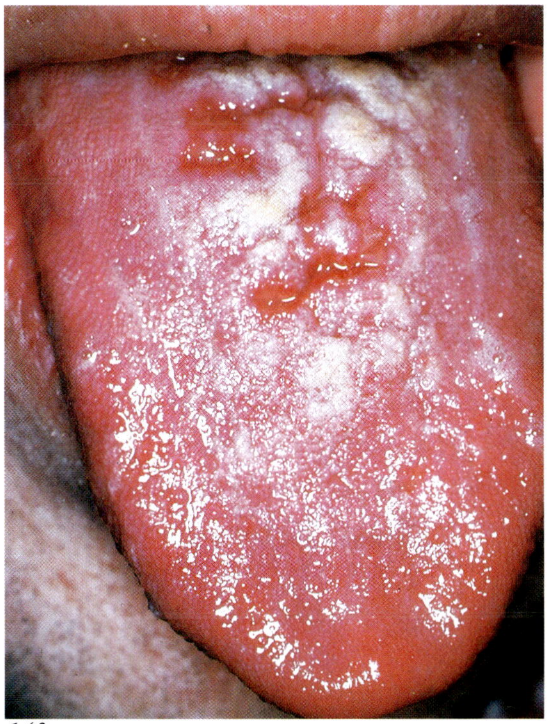
1.62

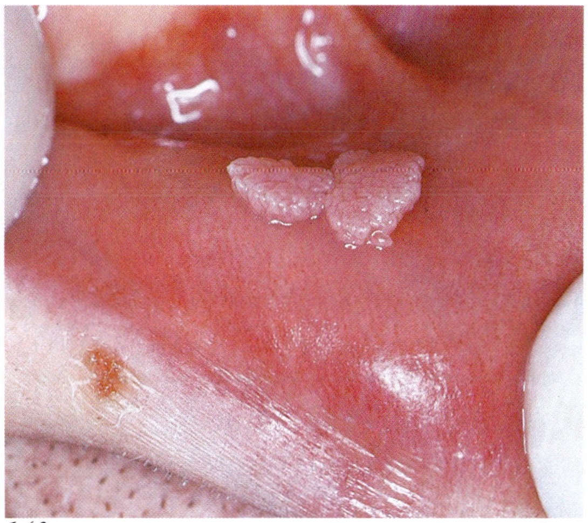
1.63

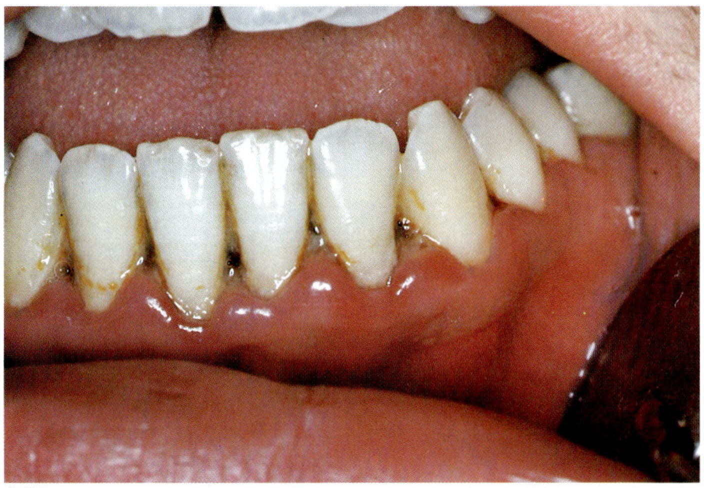
1.64

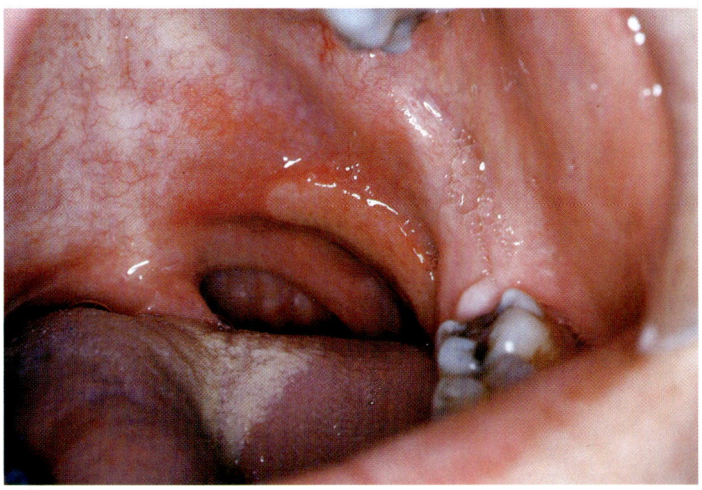
1.65

Figure 1.62 Recurrent herpes simplex infection may be intraoral in AIDS. This AIDS patient has a dendritic ulcer in the midline dorsum of the tongue.

Figure 1.63 Other viral infections, including human papillomavirus (HPV) infections and, in particular, genital warts (condyloma acuminata), may be seen in the mouth. This patient also has a healing lesion of herpes labialis.

Figure 1.64 Ulcerative gingivitis, and destructive periodontitis appear to be features of HIV infection. The condition is sometimes termed HIV-associated gingivitis (HIV-G) or periodontitis (HIV-P).

Figure 1.65 Aphthous-type ulcers, especially of the major type, may appear in AIDS. Mouth ulcers are also occasionally caused by opportunistic pathogens such as herpes viruses, mycobacteria and rarely by histoplasma or cryptococcus.

Other oral or perioral lesions in HIV infection include cervical lymph node enlargement, lymphomas (particularly non-Hodgkin's lymphomas), possibly squamous cell carcinoma, petechiae, cranial neuropathies and parotitis – possibly caused by cytomegalovirus (CMV). Intrauterine infection may cause facial dysmorphogenesis and a fetal AIDS syndrome.

MUMPS

Figure 1.66 Mumps is an acute viral infection that predominantly affects the major salivary glands. The parotid glands are usually affected and there is tender swelling with trismus. This may be unilateral, as here on the patient's right side, but is more frequently bilateral. The usual causal agent is a paramyxovirus but some Coxsackie, echo-, and other viruses occasionally cause similar features.

Figure 1.67 The incubation period of 2–3 weeks is followed by fever, malaise and sialadenitis, which can affect not only the parotids but also the submandibular glands, as here. Pancreatitis, oöphoritis and orchitis are less common features.

Figure 1.68 The most obvious intraoral feature is swelling and redness at the duct orifice of the affected gland (papillitis), in this case of the parotid.

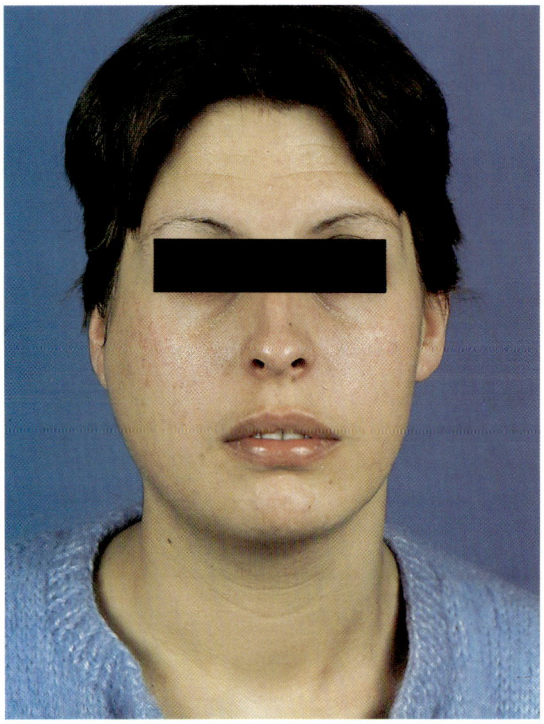

1.66

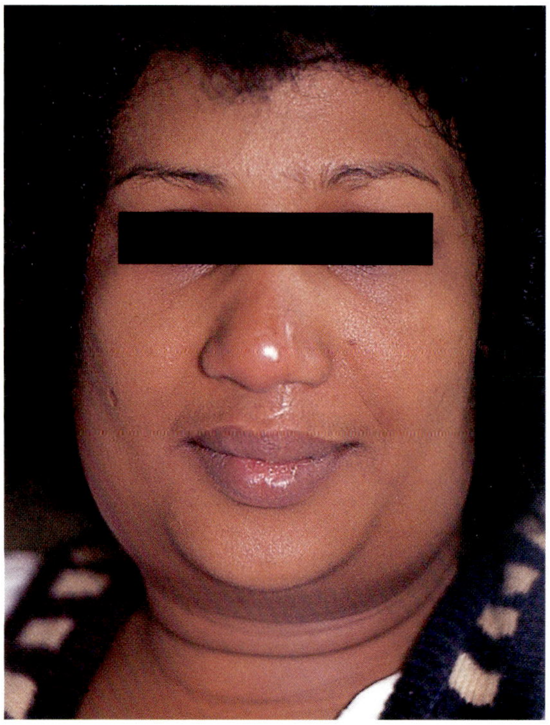

1.67

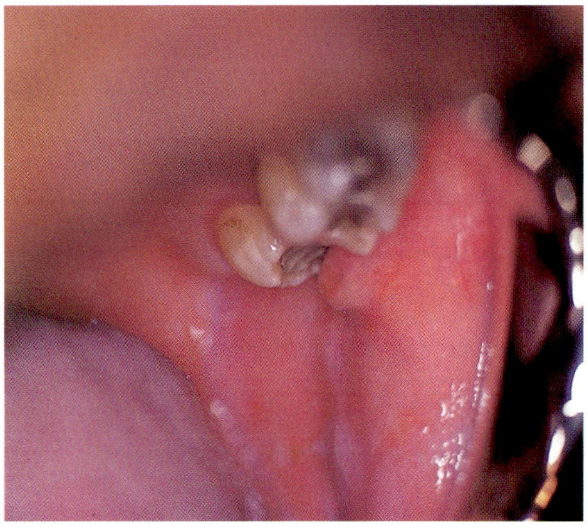

1.68

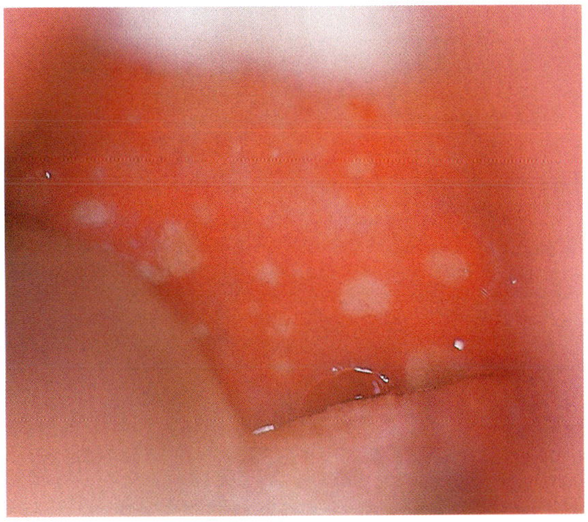

1.69

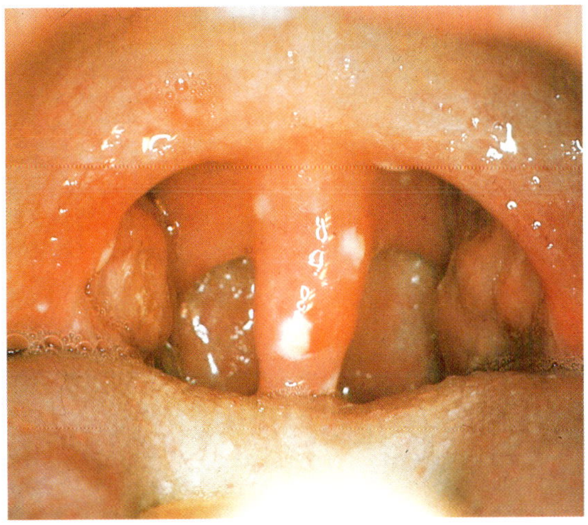

1.70

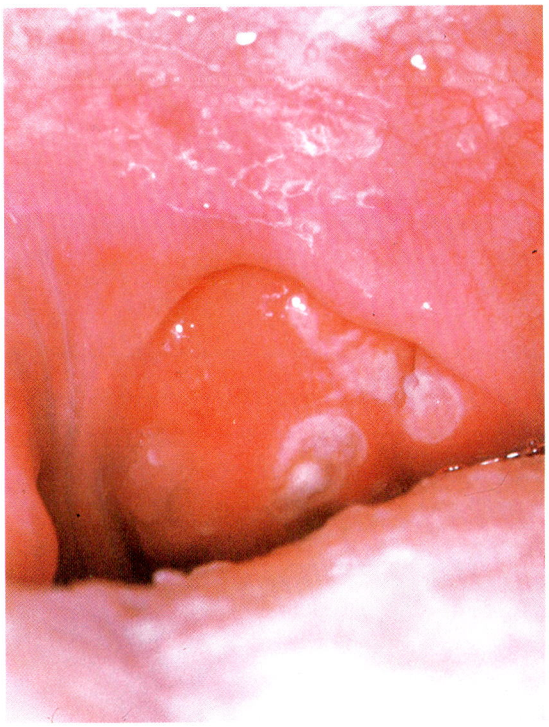

1.71

HERPANGINA

Figure 1.69 Herpangina, a Coxsackie virus infection, presents with fever, malaise, headache, and a sore throat caused by an ulcerating vesicular eruption in the oropharynx.

Figure 1.70 Vesicles rupture to leave painful, shallow, round ulcers, mainly on the fauces and soft palate. Ulcers heal spontaneously in 7–10 days.

Figure 1.71 Herpangina is usually caused by Coxsackie viruses A1–A6, A8, A10, A12 or A22, but similar syndromes can be caused by other viruses, especially Coxsackie B and echoviruses.

Lesions resembling Koplik's spots may be seen in echovirus 9 infections, along with a rash and aseptic meningitis. Faucial ulcers, sometimes with a rash and aseptic meningitis, are characteristics of echovirus 16 infection, of which this may be an example.

HAND, FOOT AND MOUTH DISEASE (*Vesicular stomatitis with exanthem*)

Figure 1.72 This Coxsackie virus infection produces small painful vesicles surrounded by an inflammatory halo especially on the dorsum and lateral aspect of the fingers and toes. The infection has an incubation period of up to a week. Coxsackie virus A16 is usually implicated, but A5, A7, A9 and A10 or viruses of the B9 group or other enteroviruses may be responsible.

Figure 1.73 A rash is not always present or may affect more proximal parts of the limbs or buttocks. The vesicles usually heal spontaneously in about 1 week. Reports of other systemic manifestations such as encephalitis are very rare, except in enterovirus 71 infection.

Figure 1.74 Oral lesions are non-specific, usually affecting the tongue or buccal mucosa. Ulcers are shallow, painful and very small, surrounded by an inflammatory halo.

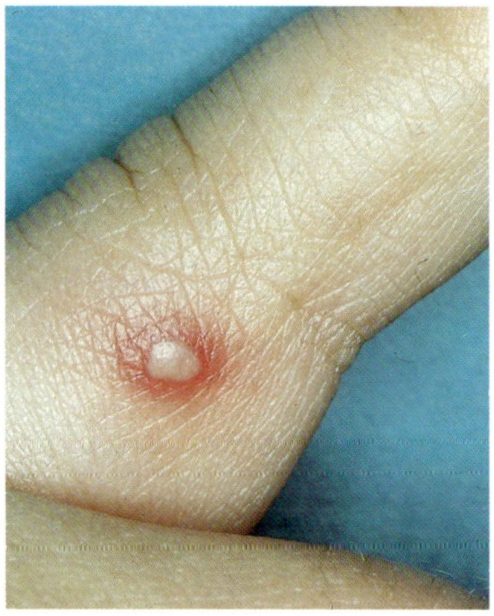

1.72

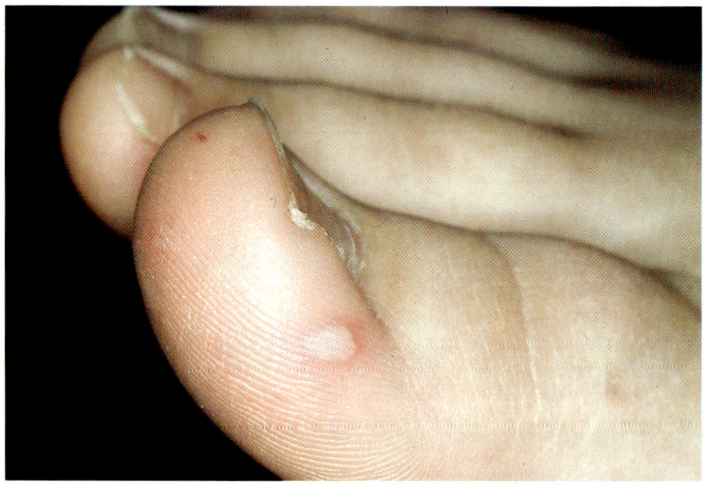

1.73

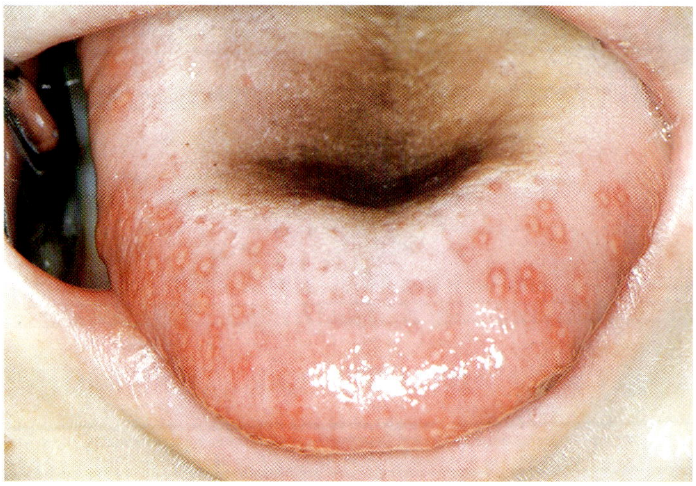

1.74

LYMPHONODULAR PHARYNGITIS

Figure 1.75 Lymphonodular pharyngitis is an acute Coxsackie infection associated with strain A10. Similar to herpangina, lymphonodular pharyngitis presents with fever and multiple small (2–5 mm) yellowish papules on the soft palate and oropharynx.

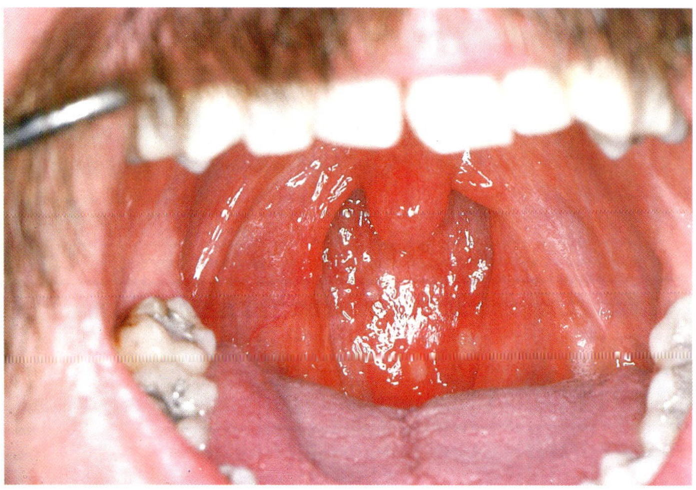

1.75

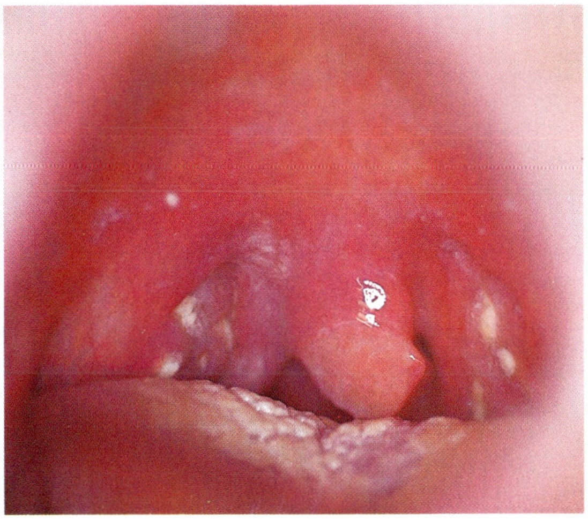

1.76

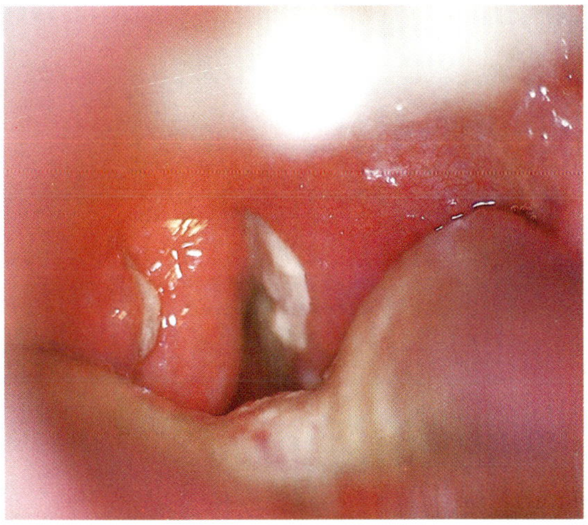

1.77

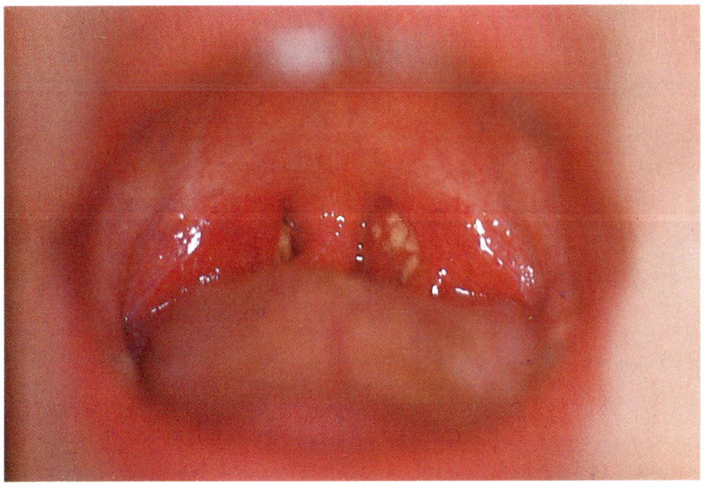

1.78

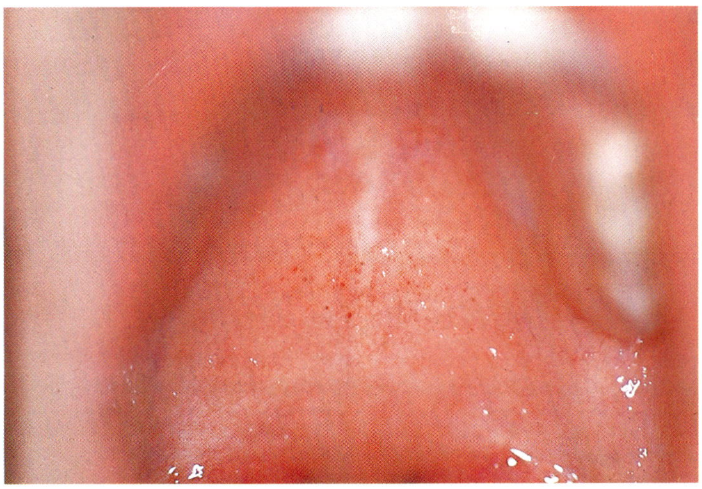

1.79

INFECTIOUS MONONUCLEOSIS (*Paul-Bunnell positive glandular fever*)

Figure 1.76 Infectious mononucleosis (IM) is caused by Epstein-Barr virus (EBV). More common in teenagers and young adults, the incubation of 30–50 days is followed by fever, sore throat and lymph node enlargement. Mouth ulcers may be seen, as here on the uvula, together with faucial oedema and tonsillar exudate. The white lesion on the soft palate is thrush. A rare presentation of IM is an isolated lower motor neurone facial palsy.

Figure 1.77 Faucial oedema and a thick yellow to white tonsillar exudate are typical of IM, although diphtheria may also produce a tonsillar pseudomembrane. There is severe dysphagia.

Figure 1.78 The faucial oedema can, rarely, obstruct the airway.

Figure 1.79 Palatal petechiae, especially at the junction of the hard and soft palate, are almost pathognomonic of IM but can be seen in other infections such as HIV.

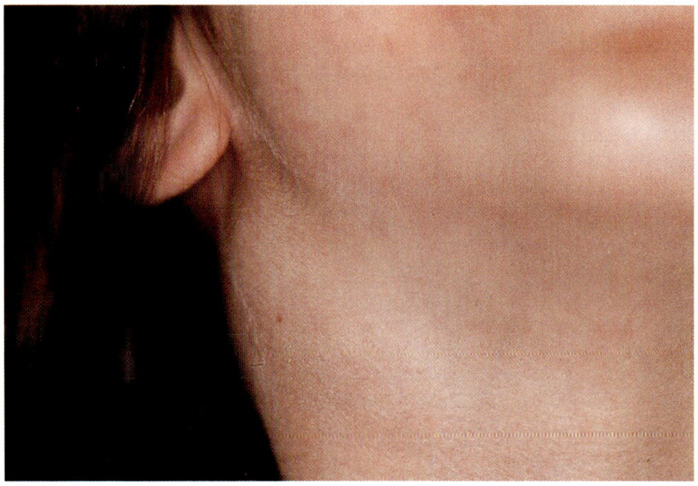

1.80

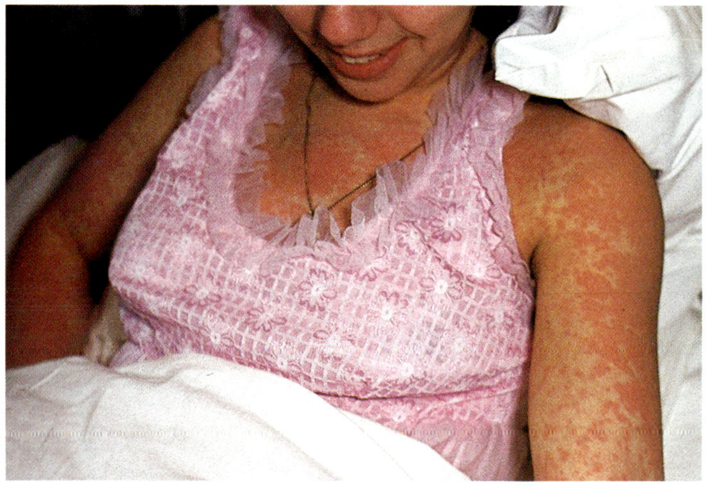

1.81

INFECTIOUS MONONUCLEOSIS

(continued)

Figure 1.80 Palatal petechiae may also be seen in HIV infection or rubella, but a glandular fever type of illness in young adults is still usually caused by IM. Generalized lymph node enlargement is present. The degree of cervical lymphadenopathy can be seen here.

Figure 1.81 A feature that may suggest IM is the occurrence of a rash if the patient is given ampicillin or amoxycillin (this may also be seen in lymphoid leukaemias). A few patients develop a maculopapular rash even if not taking synthetic penicillins.

Figure 1.82 The rash is often morbilliform and does not represent penicillin allergy. EBV may also cause persistent malaise, and has associations with Duncan's disease (X-linked lymphoproliferative syndrome), and Burkitt's lymphoma and other neoplasms (page 46).

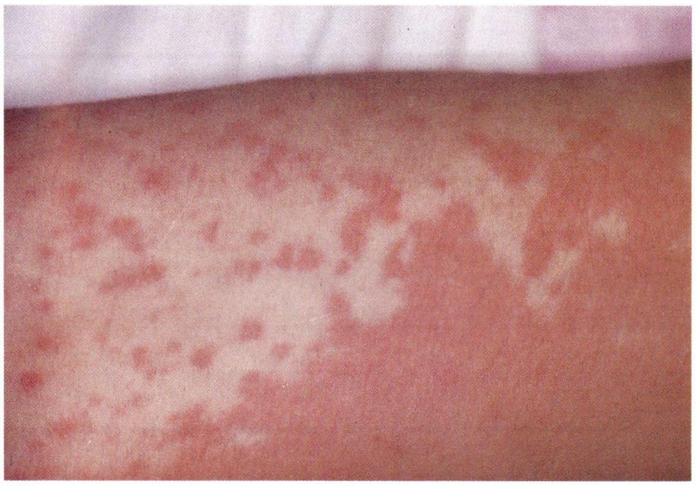

1.82

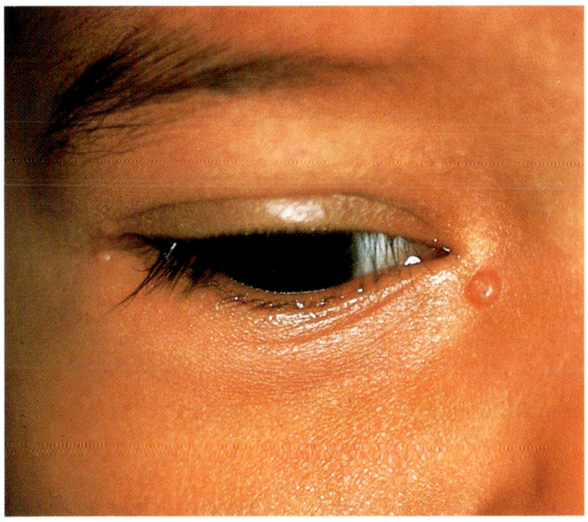

1.83

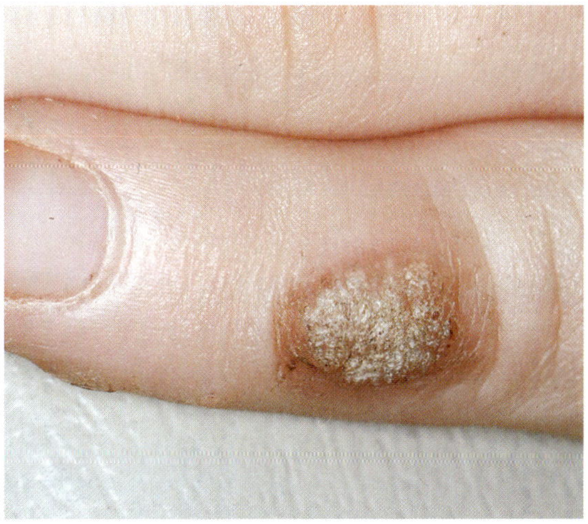

1.84

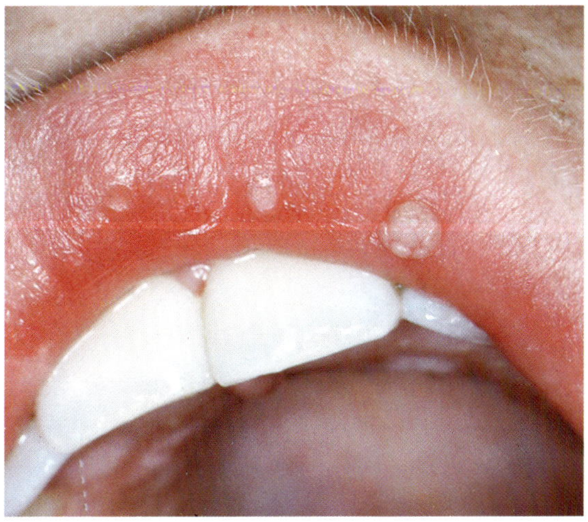

1.85

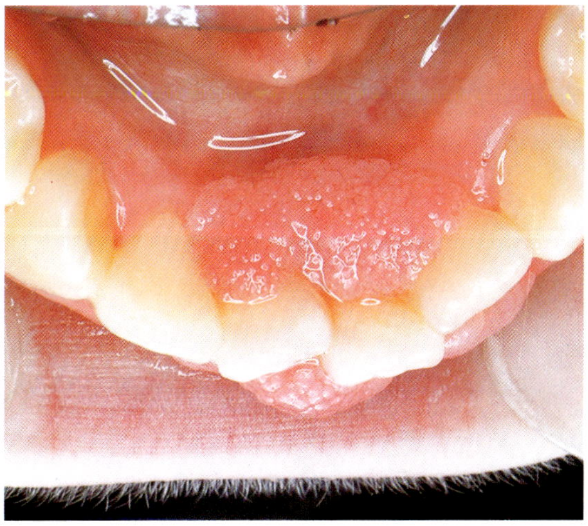

1.86

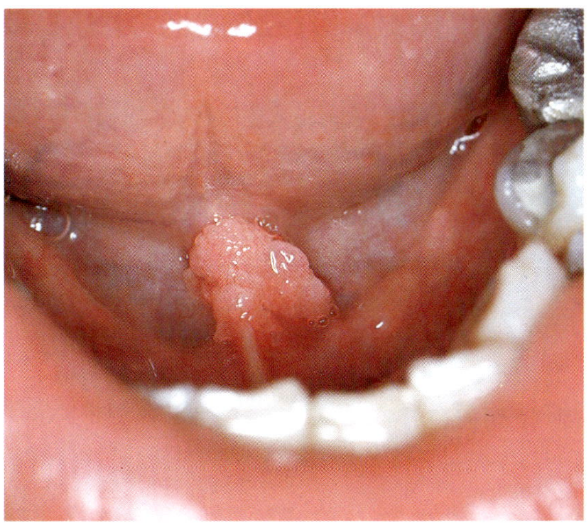

1.87

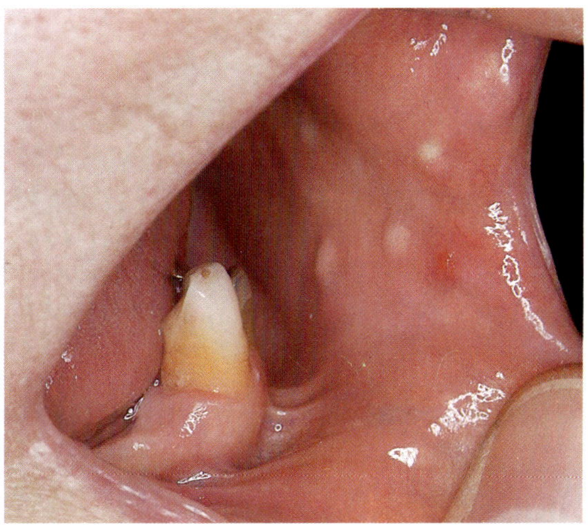

1.88

MOLLUSCUM CONTAGIOSUM

Figure 1.83 Molluscum contagiosum is a pox virus infection producing characteristic umbilicated non-tender papules, typically on the skin of male children. Oral lesions are very rare.

HUMAN PAPILLOMAVIRUS INFECTIONS

Figure 1.84 Human papillomavirus infections (HPV) cause both verruca vulgaris (common wart), as shown here, condyloma acuminatum (genital wart) and papilloma.

Figure 1.85 Infection of the oral regions by contact spread can lead to warts, especially on the lips or tongue.

Figure 1.86 Papillomas are most common on the palate or gingiva. The cauliflower-like appearance is obvious but indistinguishable from a wart.

Figure 1.87 Condyloma acuminatum (genital wart) is caused by HPV. It usually results from orogenital contact and appears as a cauliflower-like lump, mainly in the anterior mouth. The lesions are increasingly common, especially in sexually-active patients and as a complication of AIDS.

Figure 1.88 Focal epithelial hyperplasia (Heck's disease) is an HPV-13 or HPV-32 infection most frequent in Eskimos and North American Indians. Multiple painless, sessile, soft papules, generally whitish in colour, are found, usually in the buccal or lower labial mucosa.

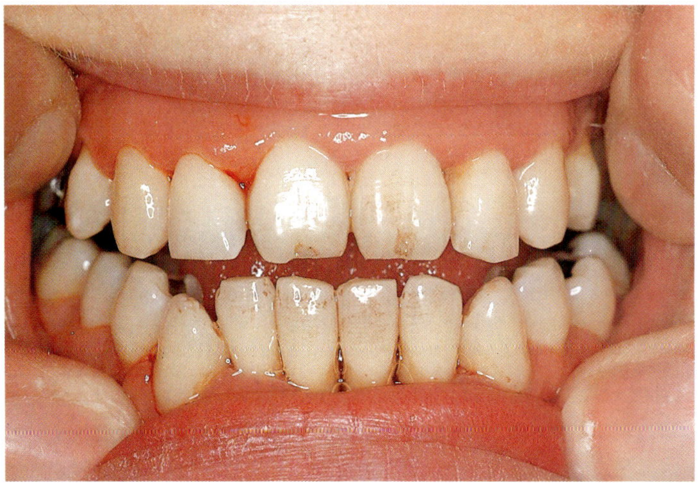

1.89

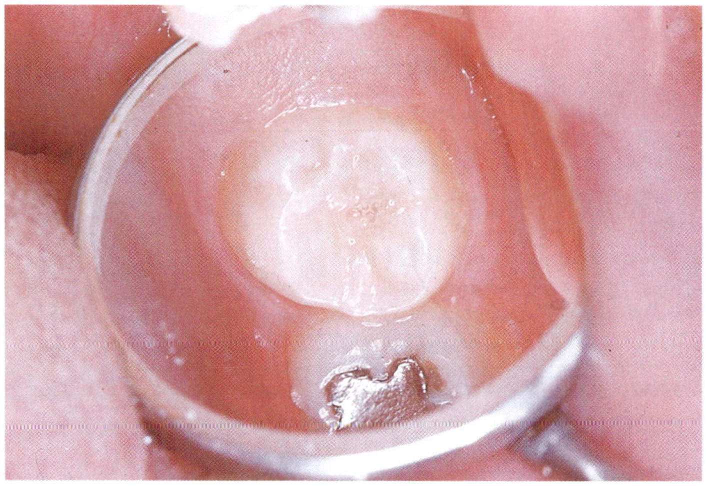

1.90

CONGENITAL SYPHILIS

Figure 1.89 Congenital syphilis is rare. *Treponema pallidum*, the causal bacterium of this sexually-transmitted disease, crosses the placenta only after the fifth month and then can produce dental defects, typically Hutchinson's incisors, as shown here. The teeth have a barrel-shape, often with a notched incisal edge. Dysplastic permanent incisors, along with nerve deafness and interstitial keratitis, are combined in Hutchinson's triad.

Figures 1.90 and 1.91 The molars may be hypoplastic (Moon's molars or mulberry molars).

Figure 1.92 Other stigmata include scarring at the commissures (rhagades or Parrot's furrows), high-arched palate and a saddle-shaped nose, as shown here.

Figure 1.93 Frontal and parietal bossing (nodular focal osteoperiostitis of the frontal and parietal bones called Parrot's nodes) may be seen, and mental handicap is common.

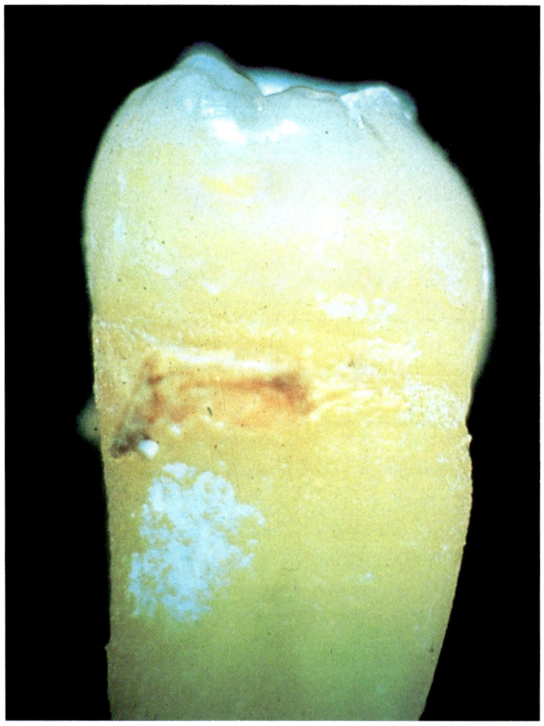

1.91

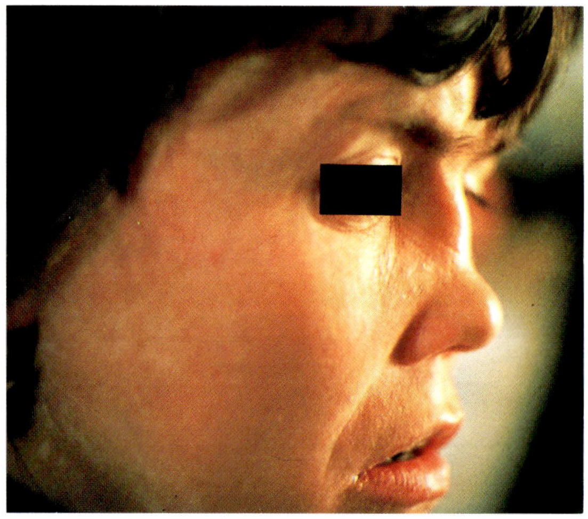

1.92

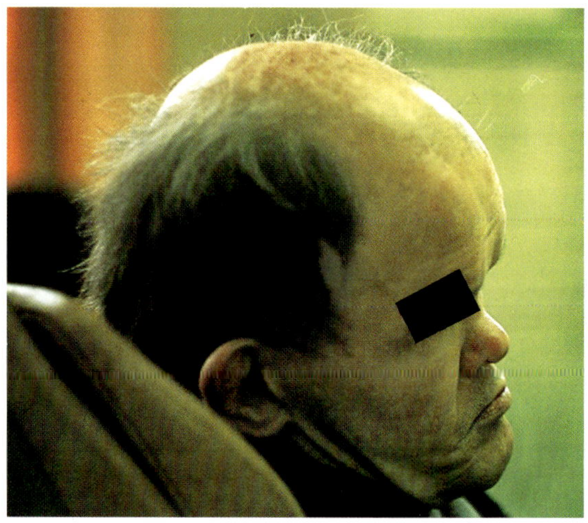

1.93

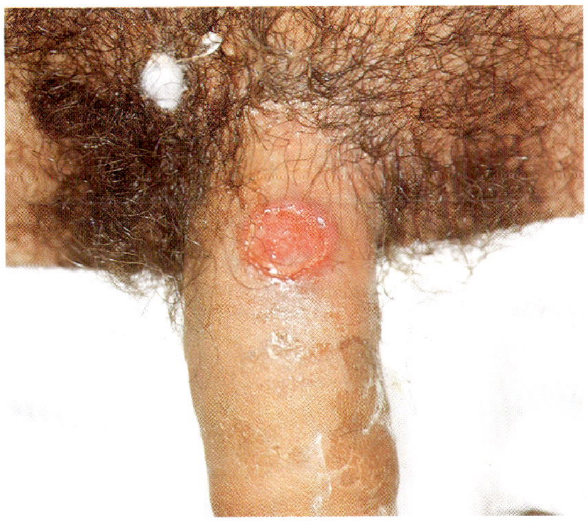

1.94

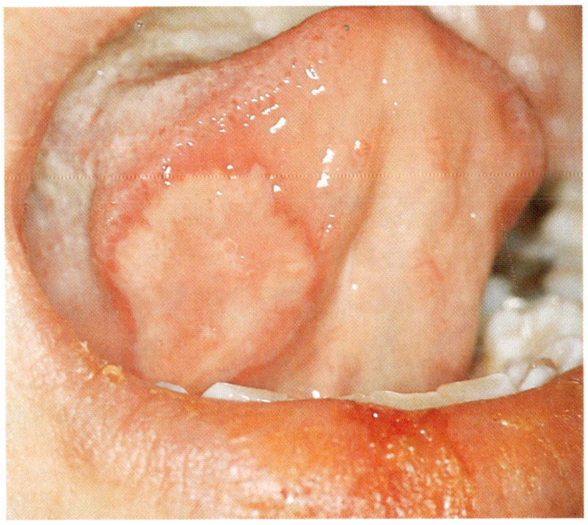

1.95

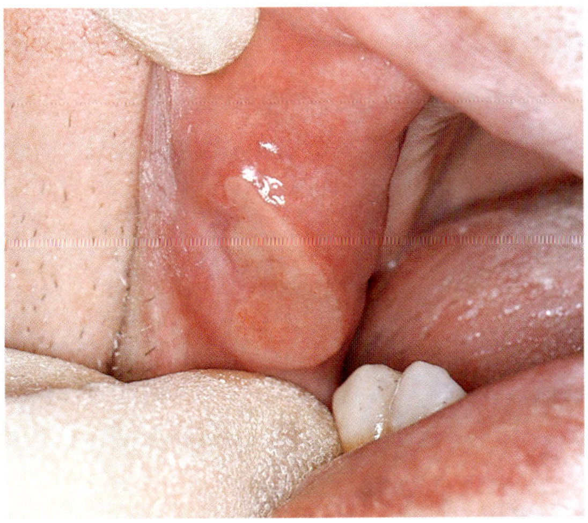

1.96

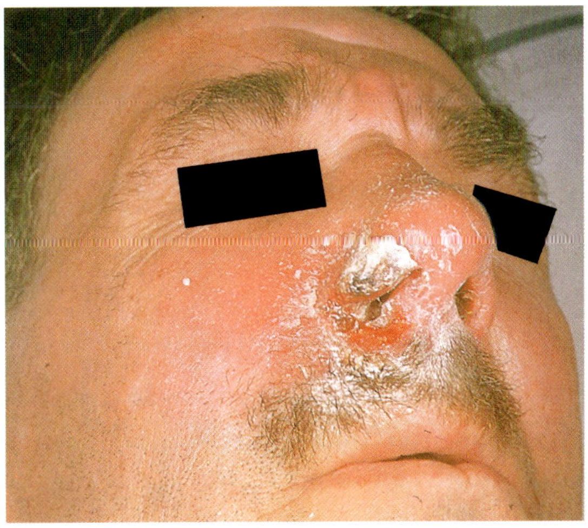

1.97

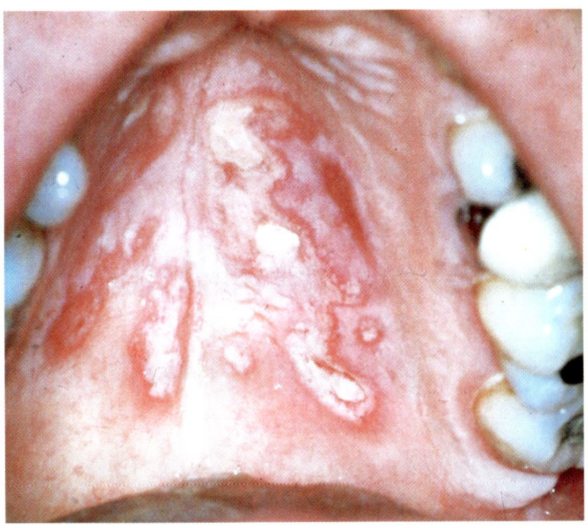

1.98

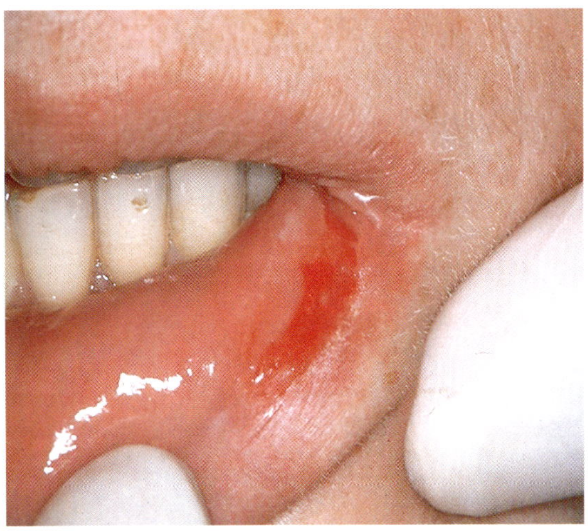

1.99

PRIMARY SYPHILIS

Figure 1.94 The incubation period of acquired syphilis is 10–90 days and the primary lesion (chancre) is usually seen in the anogenital region.

Figure 1.95 Oral chancres (hard or Hunterian chancre) begin as a papule which becomes a painless, hard-based ulcer with regional lymph node enlargement.

Figure 1.96 The chancre, which is usually on the lip, tongue or palate, heals in a few weeks but the patient remains infected and infectious.

Figure 1.97 Chancre on nose.

SECONDARY SYPHILIS

Figure 1.98 Some 6–8 weeks after primary infection, the patient develops non-specific general symptoms, such as fever and malaise, with generalized lymph node enlargement. Rashes are common – typically a macular rash on the palms and soles – but are extremely variable. Flat, painless, oval or round patches (mucous patches) or ulcers (snailtrack ulcers) may appear in the mouth, as in this patient, or on the genital mucosae.

Figure 1.99 Lesions at the commissure (split papules) are not uncommon. Oral lesions are highly infectious.

TERTIARY SYPHILIS

Figure 1.100 Tertiary, or late, syphilis appears 4–8 years after infection and may cause mucocutaneous, cardiovascular and/or neurological disease (involvement of the cardiovascular or nervous system has been called quarternary syphilis). Meningovascular syphilis, general paresis and tabes dorsalis are the main syndromes of neurosyphilis. Bilateral ptosis in this man causes the typical compensatory wrinkled brow.

Figure 1.101 Gumma is a painless nodule that undergoes necrosis, forming a punched-out ulcer that eventually heals with scarring. The site of predilection in the mouth is the hard palate, but lesions may affect the tongue or other sites. Any organ may be affected.

Figure 1.102 Atrophy of the papillae of the dorsum of the tongue produces, with endarteritis, an atrophic glossitis which leads to leukoplakia with a high premalignant potential.

Figure 1.103 Syphilitic osteitis is a rare complication.

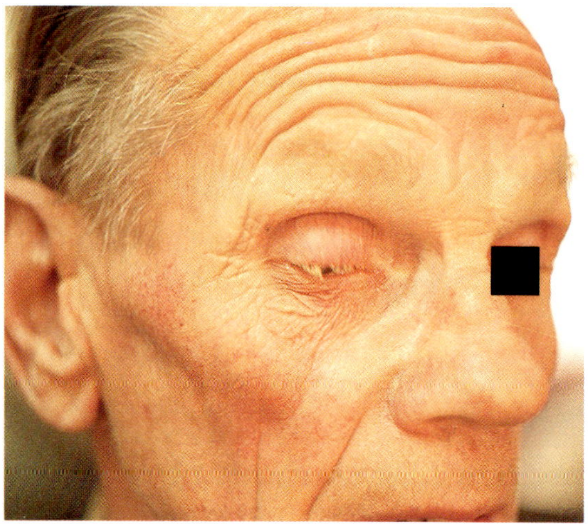

1.100

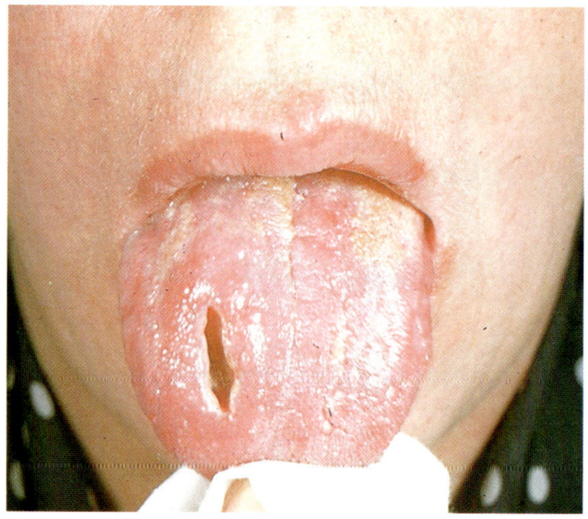

1.101

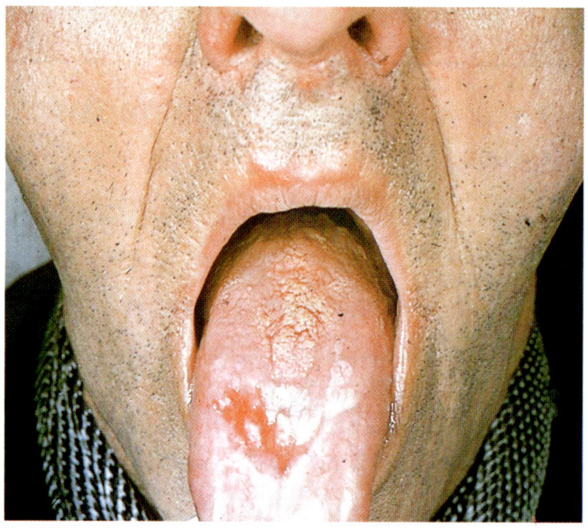

1.102

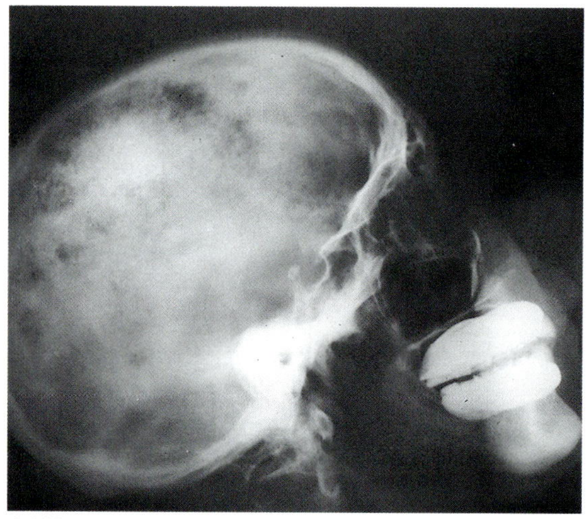

1.103

LEISHMANIASIS (*Mucocutaneous leishmaniasis: espundia*)

Figure 1.104 The protozoa *Leishmania brasiliensis* is found mainly in South America. A sandfly bite transmits infection and this usually heals although, in some, there is later metastasis to the mucocutaneous junctions of the mouth or nose. The palate is frequently affected and ulcerates. Leishmaniasis may also be found around the Mediterranean (*L donovanii* or *L tropica*).

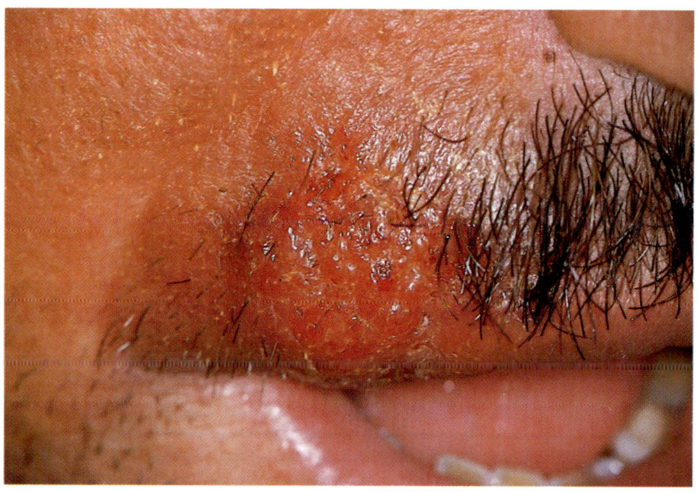

1.104

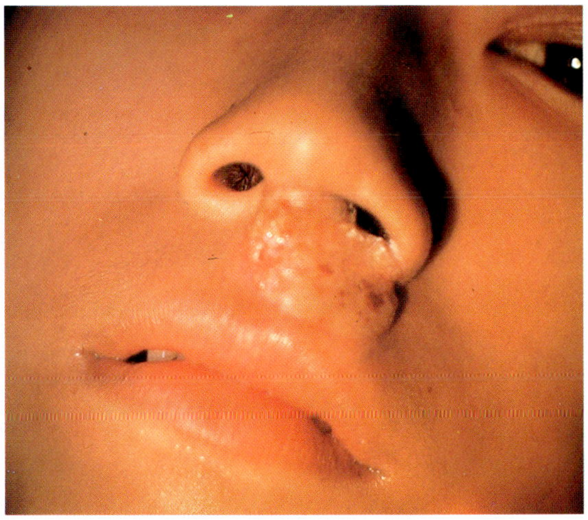

1.105

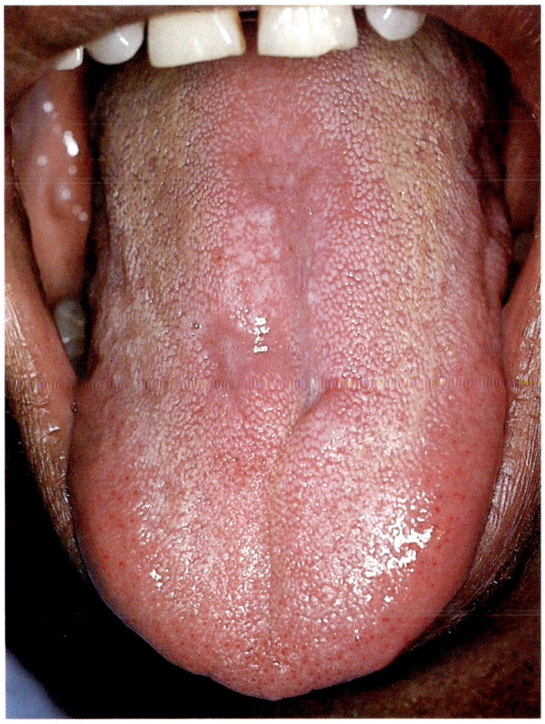

1.106

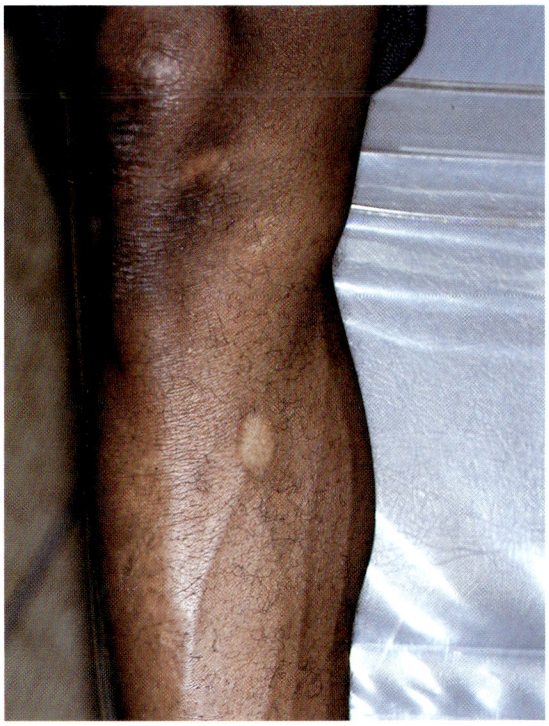

1.107

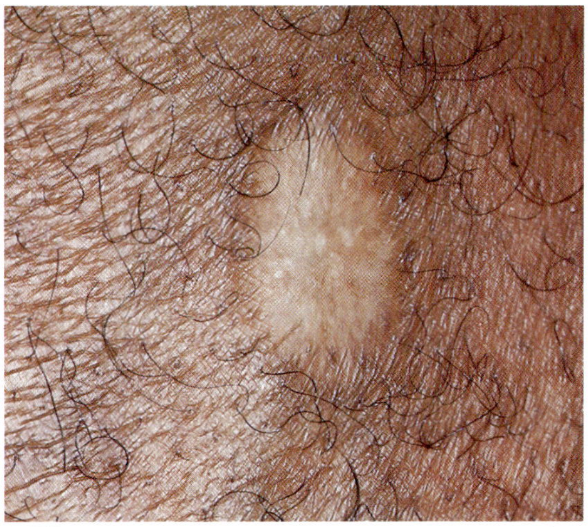

1.108

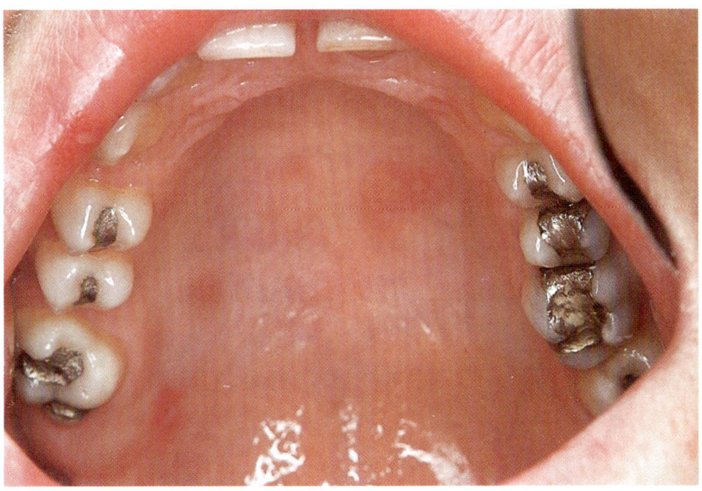

1.109

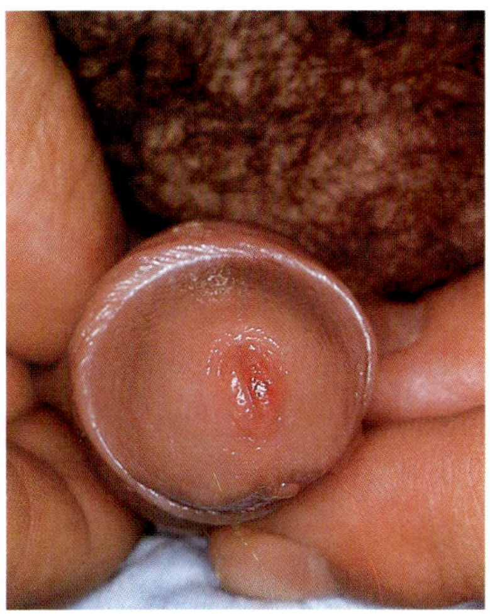

1.110

YAWS

Figure 1.105 Non-venereal syphilis, yaws and pinta (the 'endemic' treponematoses) follow a course not dissimilar from syphilis, with primary, secondary and tertiary stages. Yaws, caused by *Treponema pertenue* is seen predominantly in Equatorial regions. The primary lesion (mother yaw) is usually a single, painless papule that appears after 3–6 weeks and ulcerates.

Figure 1.106 After a secondary stage with lesions similar to the primary lesions, late lesions present as gummas, especially on the lower extremities. This is a gumma on the tongue which has healed following treatment. Mucosal lesions are extremely rare.

Figures 1.107 and 1.108 The skin may heal with 'tissue paper' scarring and depigmentation.

REITER'S SYNDROME

Figure 1.109 Reiter's syndrome is a disease predominantly of young males and may follow gonorrhoea, chlamydia, or enteric infection with salmonellae, shigella, or yersinia. Features include urethritis, uveitis or conjunctivitis, polyarthritis, macular or vesicular lesions of the palms and soles (keratoderma blenorrhagica) and red lesions, sometimes with a whitish border or superficial painful erosions in the mouth.

Figure 1.110 Mucocutaneous lesions are found in over half the patients but are typically painless initially. The urethritis, as here, may follow mouth lesions and there may be circinate balanitis.

ACUTE NECROTIZING ULCERATIVE GINGIVITIS (*Vincent's disease*)

Figure 1.111 Chiefly affecting young adults, acute ulcerative gingivitis (acute necrotizing gingivitis, AUG, ANG, ANUG) is associated with proliferation of *Borrelia vincentii*, fusiform bacilli, and other anaerobes. Ulceration of the interdental papillae is the typical feature of this condition, which is predisposed by smoking, respiratory infections, poor oral hygiene and immune defects. HIV infection is now a recognized predisposing factor in some patients.

Figure 1.112 Painful gingival ulceration occasionally spreads from the papillae to the gingival margins, with sialorrhoea, halitosis and pronounced tendency to gingival bleeding.

Figure 1.113 Gingival bleeding can be profuse and the patient may have malaise, low fever and regional lymph node enlargement. This patient had primary herpetic stomatitis (note ulcer in upper vestibule) complicated by ANUG.

CANCRUM ORIS (*Noma*)

Figure 1.114 Although usually a trivial illness in healthy persons, ANUG in malnourished, debilitated, or immunocompromised patients may extend, as here, onto the oral mucosa and skin with gangrenous necrosis (cancrum oris, noma). Anaerobes, particularly bacteroides species, have been implicated, and the condition is especially seen in malnourished patients from the Third World.

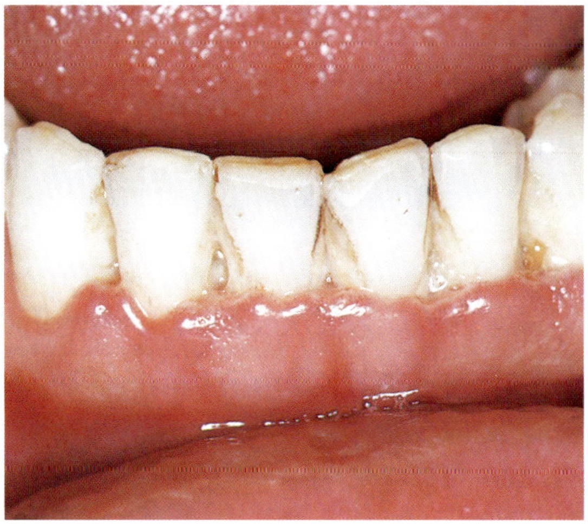

1.111

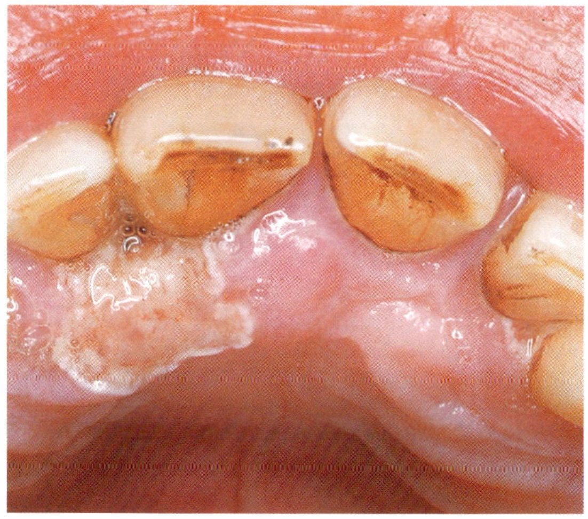

1.112

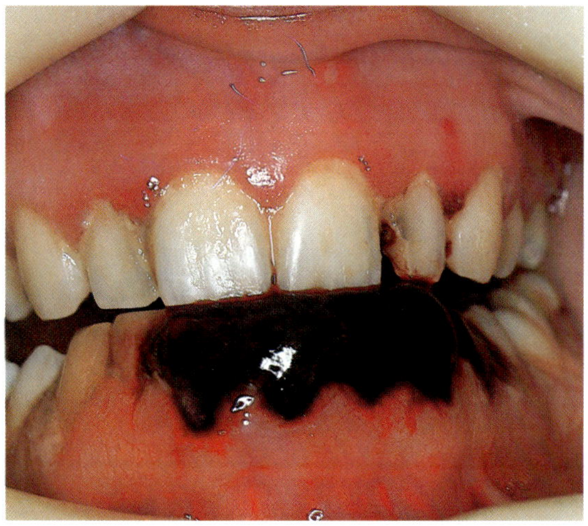

1.113

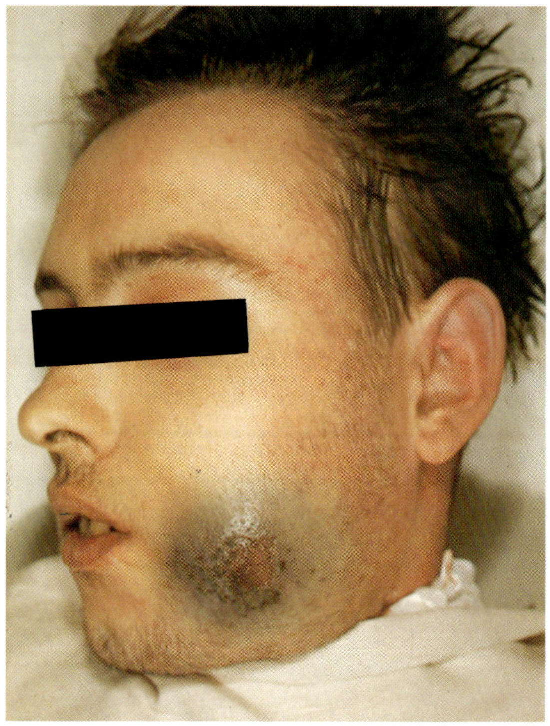

1.114

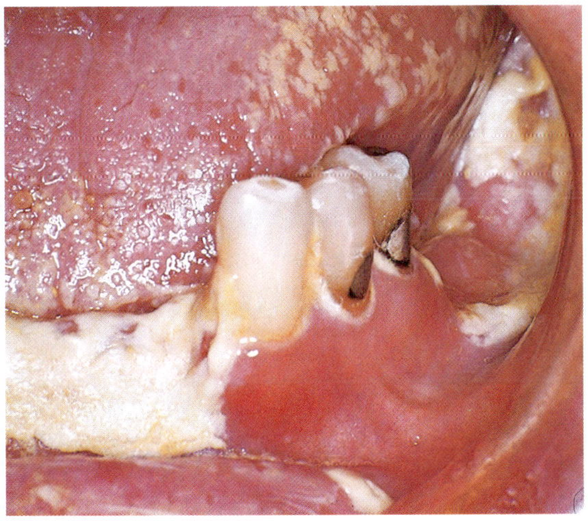

1.115

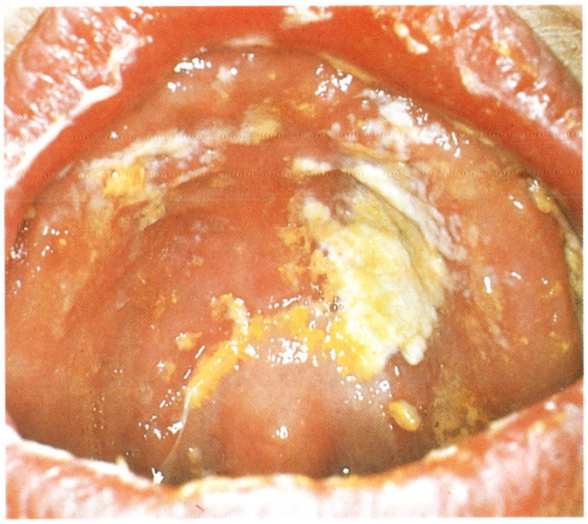

1.116

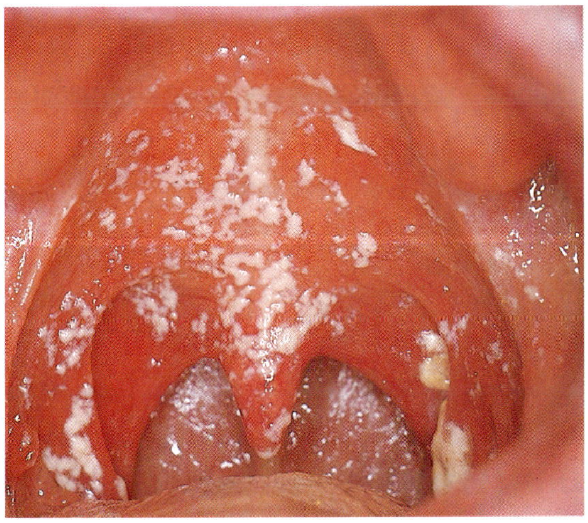

1.117

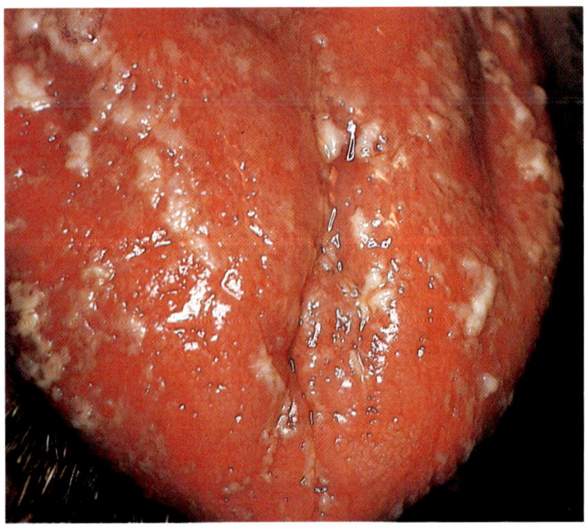

1.118

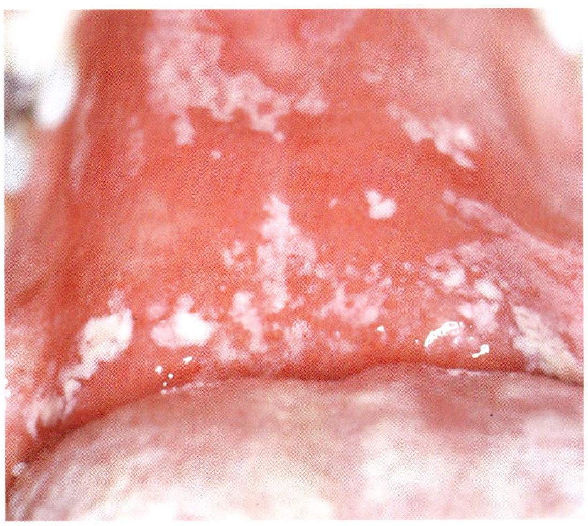

1.119

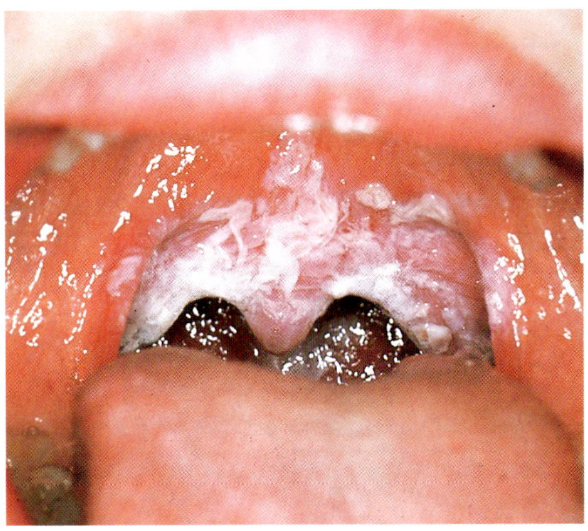

1.120

ACUTE CANDIDOSIS
(*Thrush, candidiasis, acute pseudomembranous candidosis, moniliasis*)

Figure 1.115 Candida species are common oral commensals. *Candida albicans* is the most common and virulent species, which can act as an opportunistic pathogen, causing thrush.

Figure 1.116 Thrush appears as white flecks or plaques, which are easily removed with gauze to leave an erythematous base. Apart from neonates, who have no immunity to candida species, thrush indicates an immunocompromised patient, as here, or a local disturbance in oral flora, such as that caused by xerostomia, antibiotic treatment or topical corticosteroids.

Figure 1.117 Thrush can affect any oral site, typically the palate or upper buccal vestibule posteriorly. The yellow colour is caused by amphotericin.

Figure 1.118 Thrush is a feature in many immune defects, especially leukaemia, as here, and particularly where there has also been radiotherapy affecting the mouth and salivary glands.

In severely immunocompromised patients, there may also be other fungal infections, such as aspergillus, mucor or trichosporon species.

Figure 1.119 Thrush in a male homosexual, intravenous drug abuser or in other high-risk patients is an early feature of AIDS or related disease. Orogenital and anogenital transmission of candida is also possible.

Figure 1.120 Local causes of thrush should always be excluded. The use of corticosteroid inhalers, as here, may produce faucial and oropharyngeal thrush.

ACUTE ATROPHIC CANDIDOSIS (*Antibiotic sore tongue*)

Figure 1.121 Broad spectrum antimicrobials such as tetracycline or ampicillin, and corticosteroids, predispose to an acute atrophic candidosis that causes soreness or a burning sensation, especially of the tongue.

CHRONIC ATROPHIC CANDIDOSIS (*Denture-induced stomatitis*)

Figure 1.122 Chronic atrophic candidosis is common beneath complete upper dentures, especially in the elderly. Although termed denture sore mouth, it is usually asymptomatic. Characteristically the erythema is limited to the denture-bearing area. It is rare below lower dentures. Occasionally the lesion is complicated by the development of papillary hyperplasia (see page 146).

Figure 1.123 Patients with denture stomatitis are usually otherwise healthy. The lesion is caused by candida proliferating on the denture surface, especially when it is worn during sleep. Inadequate dentures predispose to the lesion in some patients.

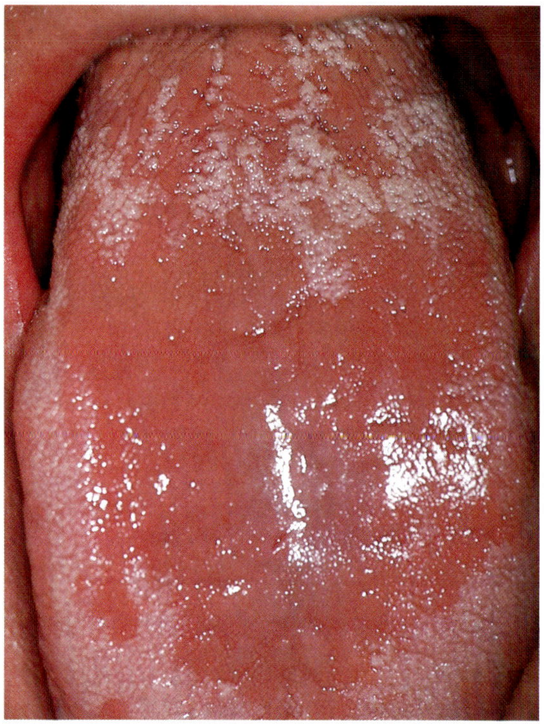

1.121

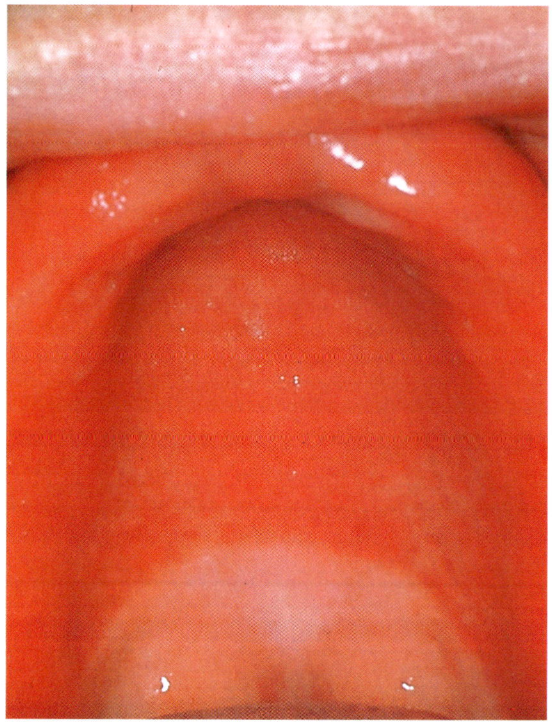

1.122

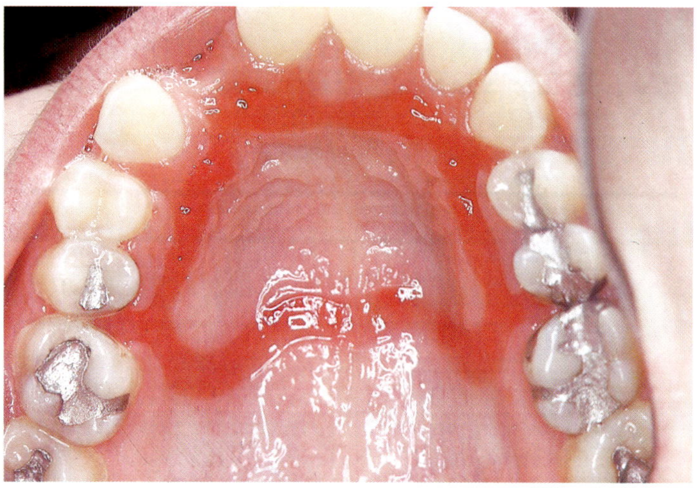

1.123

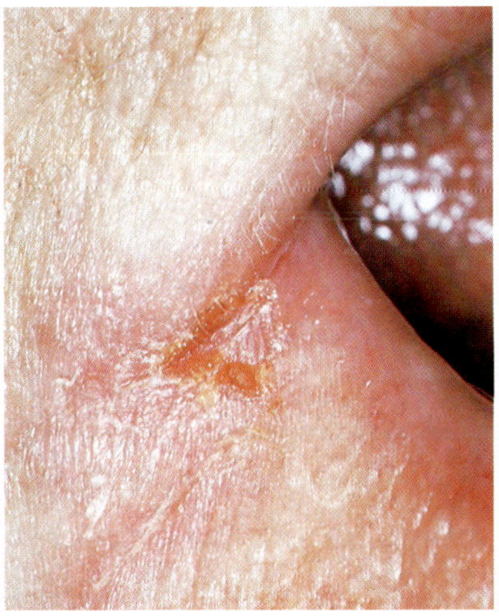

1.124

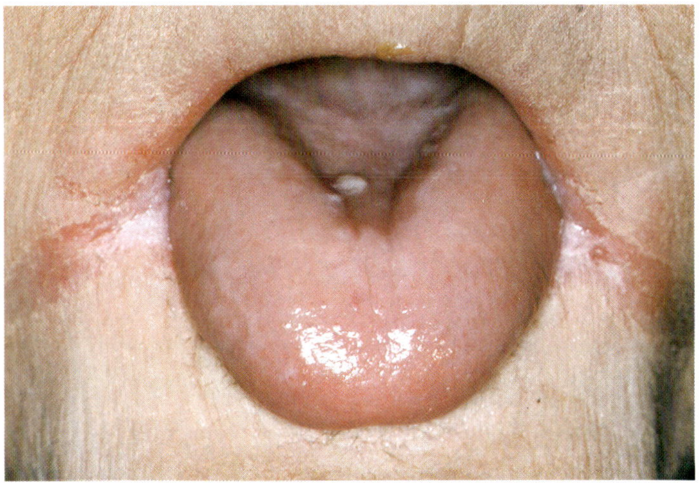

1.125

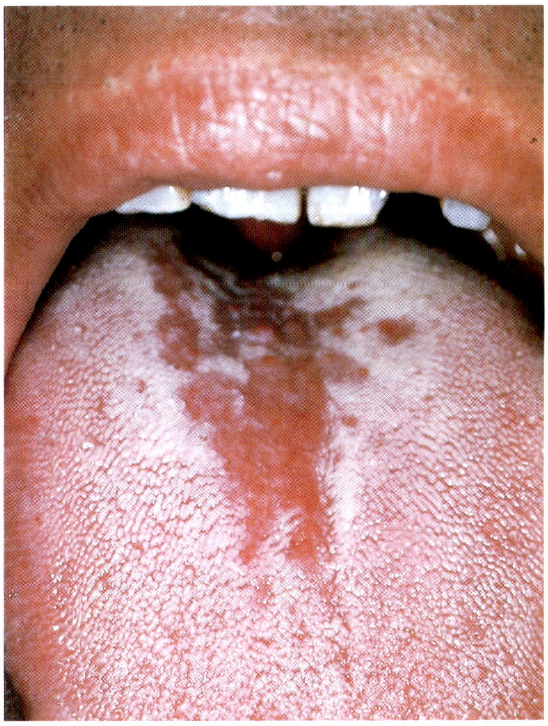

1.126

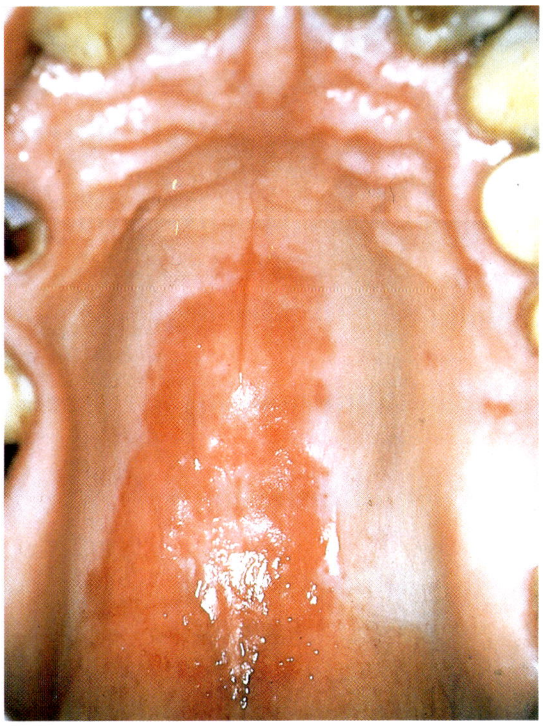

1.127

ANGULAR STOMATITIS
(*Angular cheilitis, cheilosis, perleche*)

Figure 1.124 Denture stomatitis may predispose to angular stomatitis, which is bilateral and produces erythema, fissuring or ulceration which can be painful and disfiguring.

Figure 1.125 Rarely, angular stomatitis is a manifestation of iron deficiency, as here, or of vitamin deficiency – when there may also be glossitis and mouth ulcers – or of an immune defect. Although *Candida albicans* is the prevalent organism, *Staphylococcus aureus* and other microorganisms may sometimes be isolated.

MEDIAN RHOMBOID GLOSSITIS

Figure 1.126 Median rhomboid glossitis, although originally thought to be a developmental lesion, is rarely seen in children and may be chronic focal candidosis. It is a fairly common lesion and is predisposed by diabetes, cigarette smoking and the wearing of dentures. See also page 153.

MULTIFOCAL CHRONIC CANDIDOSIS

Figure 1.127 Focal chronic candidosis may occur in apposition to the tongue lesion – the 'kissing lesion'.

Multifocal chronic candidosis may appear as red, white or mixed lesions and is usually seen in smokers.

CANDIDAL LEUKOPLAKIA

Figure 1.128 Chronic hyperplastic candidosis, or candidal leukoplakia, is a firm white adherent plaque, usually seen inside the commissures or on the tongue. These leukoplakias have a higher premalignant potential than many forms of keratosis.

Figure 1.129 Candidal leukoplakia may be a speckled red and white lesion. HIV infection or deficiencies of haematinics may underlie chronic candidosis.

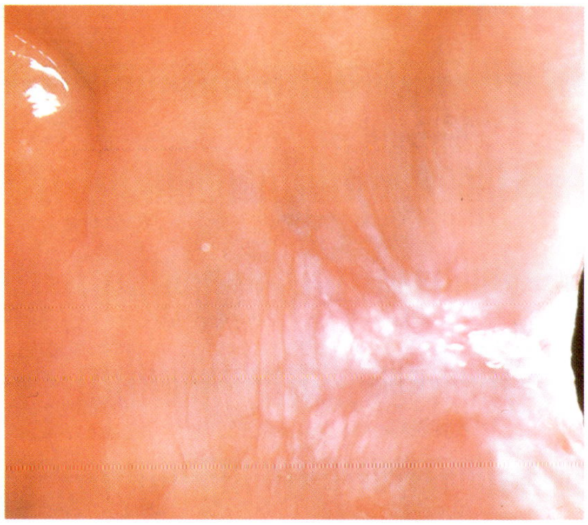

1.128

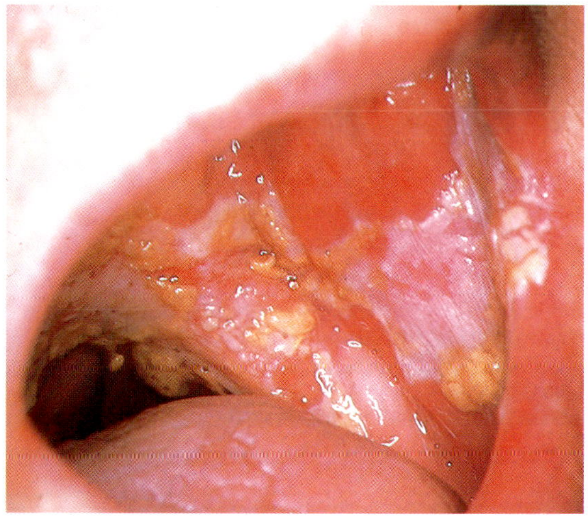

1.129

CHRONIC MUCOCUTANEOUS CANDIDOSIS

Figure 1.130 Chronic mucocutaneous candidosis (CMC) is a heterogeneous group of syndromes characterized by cutaneous, oral and other mucosal candidosis, usually from early life. Early lesions are of thrush, as here in a patient with one variant (candidosis-endocrinopathy syndrome: Wells' type 3 CMC) that also includes hypoparathyroidism (note dental defects) and often hypo-adrenocorticism, hypothyroidism and diabetes mellitus. *Candida albicans* is the usual cause of candidosis but *C tropicalis, C parapsilosis, C guilliermondii* and *C krusei* may also be implicated.

Figure 1.131 Enamel hypoplasia, and gingival erythema, caused by candidosis and poor oral hygiene (showing the same patient as in Figure 1.130, at a later age).

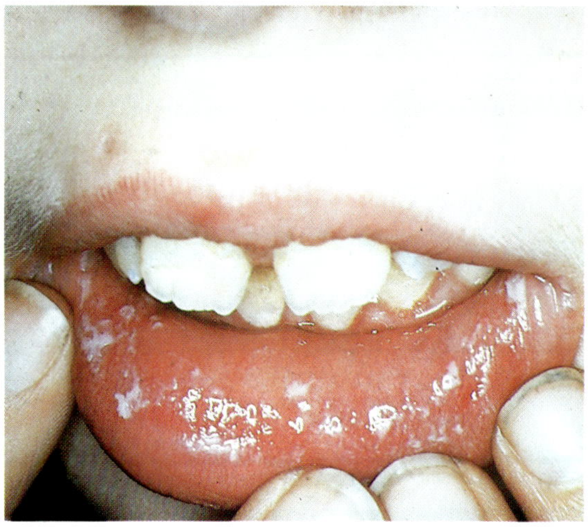

1.130

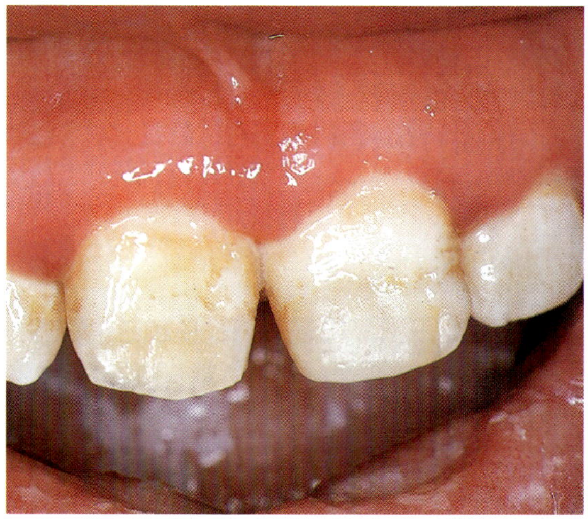

1.131

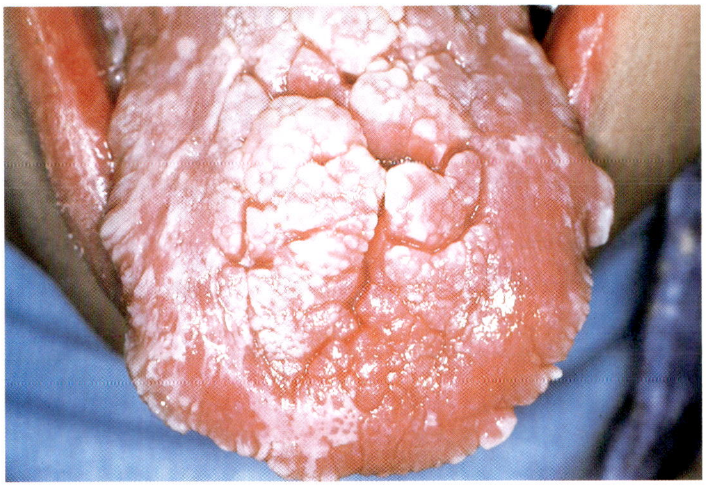

1.132

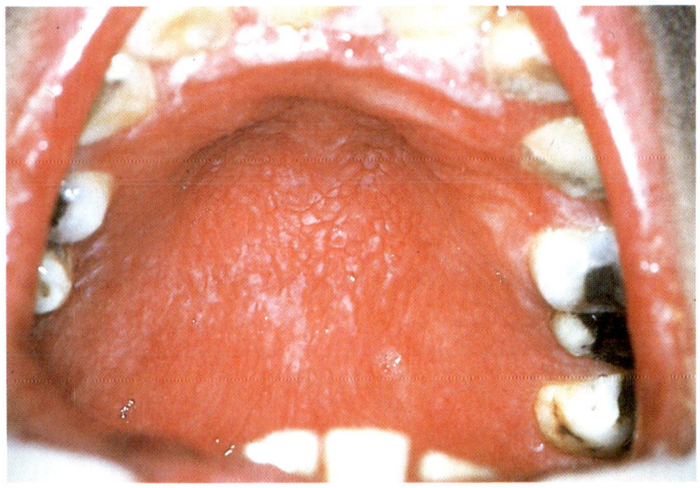

1.133

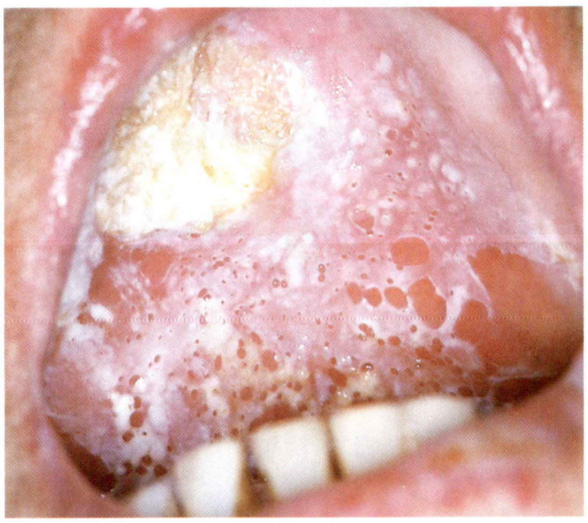

1.134

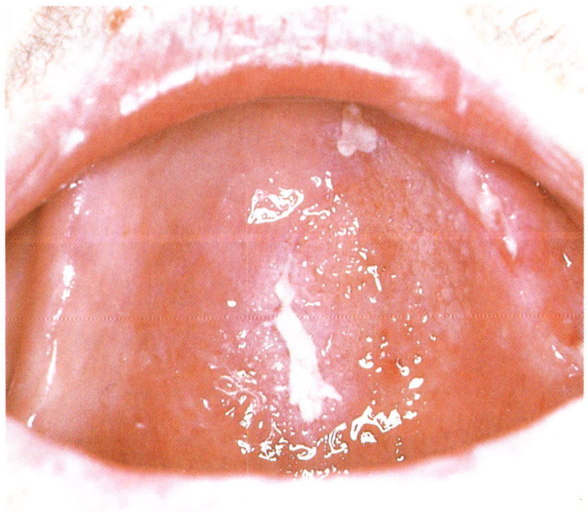

1.135

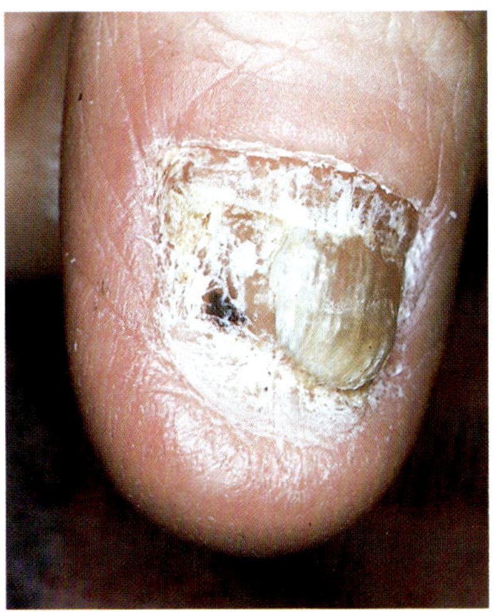

1.136

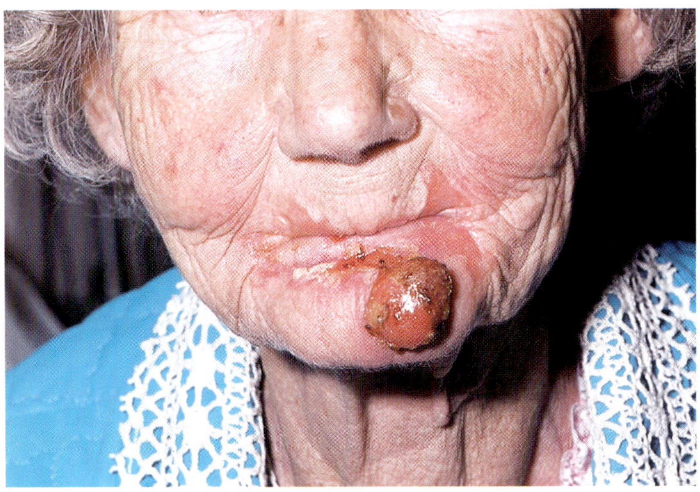

1.137

Figure 1.132 The white plaques eventually become widespread, thick and adherent and the tongue fissured.

Figure 1.133 Chronic mucocutaneous candidosis extends over the palate and into the oropharynx.

Figure 1.134 This patient had late onset CMC. Chronic oral candidosis is often associated with malignant thymoma in this type.

Figure 1.135 Showing the same patient as in Figure 1.134, after antifungal treatment.

Figure 1.136 In CMC, the nails are usually involved, but both cutaneous and nail involvement vary in severity.

Figure 1.137 Granulomas may be seen in one variant of CMC (type 2). These patients also have chronic oral candidosis, and candidosis may affect the larynx and eyes. Type 1 CMC has a familial pattern and early onset.

HISTOPLASMOSIS

Figure 1.138 Oral lesions appear as mucosal nodules or non-specific indurated ulcers. There may be associated low-grade fever, lymphadenopathy and hepatosplenomegaly. Rare in Europe, oral histoplasmosis may be seen in immunocompromised patients.

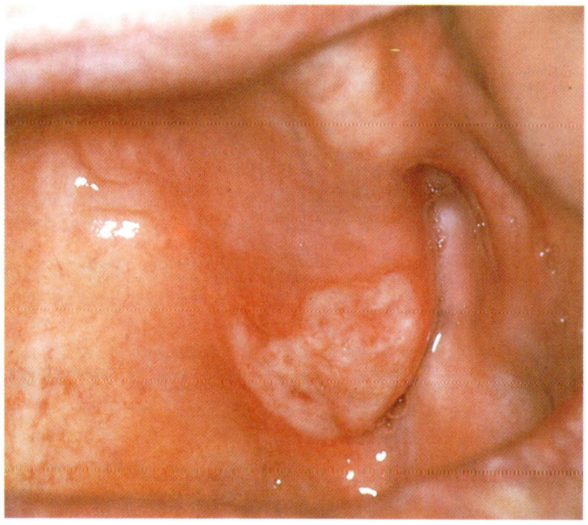

1.138

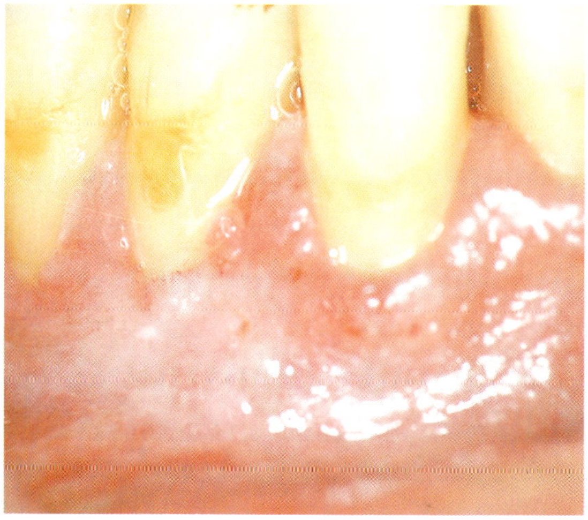

1.139

BLASTOMYCOSES

Figure 1.139 North American blastomycosis (Gilchrist's disease) is a rare fungal disease. Caused by *Blastomyces dermatidis*, it affects mainly the lungs and skin. Nearly 25 per cent have oral or nasal lesions – usually an ulcer with a warty surface which may simulate a neoplasm.

Figure 1.140 The oral lesions of South American blastomycosis (paracoccidioidomycosis, Lutz's disease) are similar to those of the North American form of this fungal disease. The causal organism, *Paracoccidioides brasiliensis*, may enter the body through the lungs or periodontium and cause granulomatous or ulcerative lesions and lymphadenopathy.

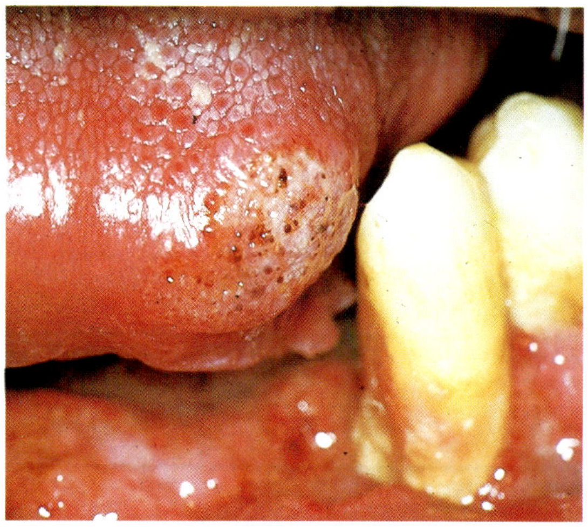

1.140

MUCORMYCOSIS (*Phycomycosis: zygomycosis*)

Figure 1.141 Despite the fact that Rhizopus, Mucor and Absidia are fungi ubiquitous in decaying vegetation and some sugary foods, infection is rare and seen almost exclusively in immunocompromised patients. Nasal and paranasal sinus mucormycosis is seen in poorly-controlled diabetics, and in particular presents resembling sinusitis. However, it may invade orbit, frontal lobe, palate and elsewhere.

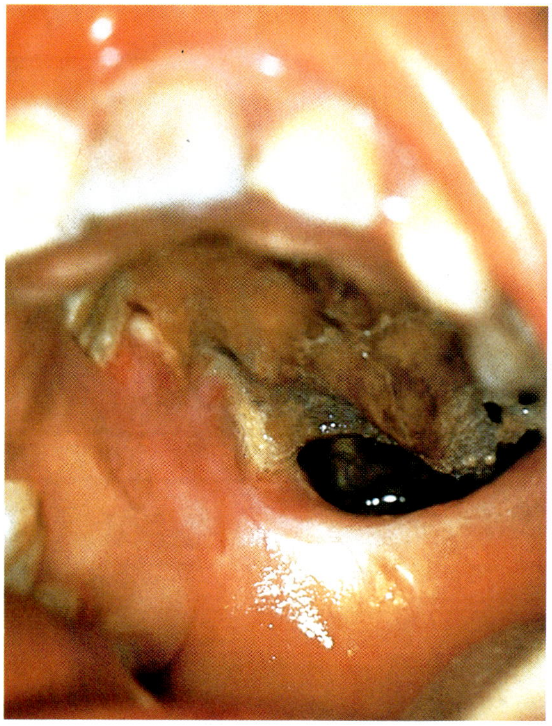

1.141

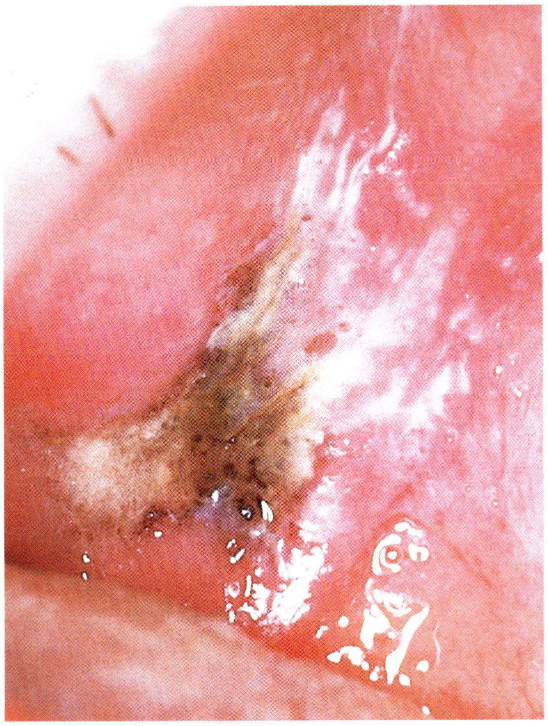

1.142

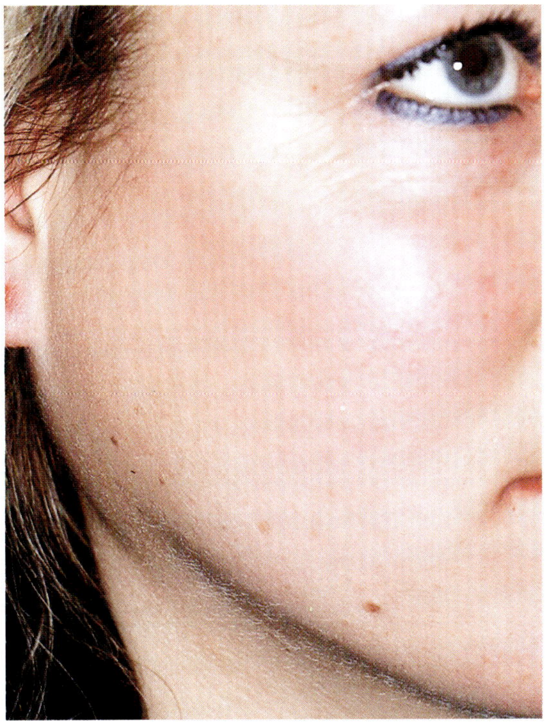

1.143

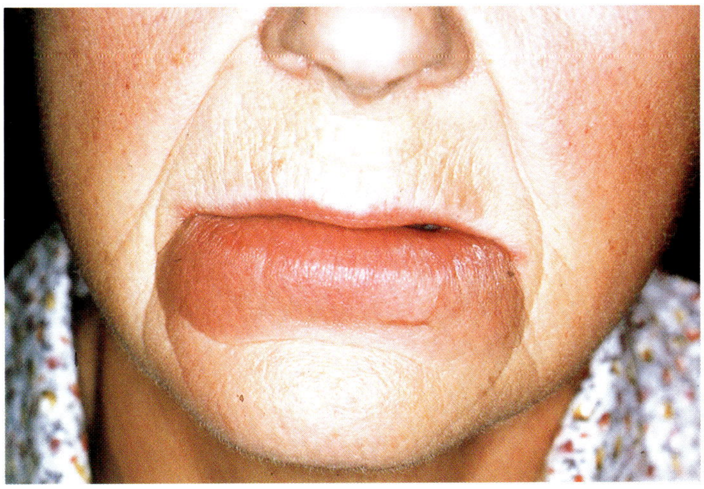

1.144

ASPERGILLOSIS

Figure 1.142 Infection with aspergillus species, usually *Aspergillus fumigatus*, but also *A flavus* and *A niger*, can present in several ways. The most serious is systemic aspergillosis, or respiratory tract aspergillus infection in immunocompromised patients. In aspergillus sinusitis, there are normally non-invasive fungus balls, but infection of the antrum may rarely invade the palate, orbit or brain. This child received a bone marrow transplant, and was immunosuppressed with cyclosporin and anti-lymphocyte sera. It has been reported that antral aspergillosis can be precipitated by overfilling maxillary root canals with endodontic material containing zinc oxide and paraformaldehyde.

SARCOIDOSIS
(*Boeck's sarcoid*)

Figure 1.143 Sarcoidosis is a multi-system non-caseating granulomatous condition of unknown aetiology that affects mainly the lungs, lymph nodes and eyes but seldom produces oral lesions. The salivary glands may be affected, as here, with firm, painless swelling and xerostomia and, rarely, with fever, uveitis, and facial palsy (Heerfordt's syndrome, uveoparotid fever).

Figure 1.144 Chronic swelling of the lip may be a feature of sarcoidosis and difficult to differentiate from oral Crohn's disease and variants thereof, such as Melkersson-Rosenthal syndrome and cheilitis granulomatosa.

SARCOIDOSIS (*continued*)

Figure 1.145 Obvious oral lesions are uncommon but include red nodules which may affect any oral site, including the gingiva. The tongue is rarely involved.

Figure 1.146 Red nodules of sarcoid in the palate. Palatal biopsy even from an apparently normal palate may show granulomas in sarcoidosis.

Figure 1.147 Lupus pernio large, persistent, red or violaceous infiltrations of the skin – is a typical feature of chronic sarcoidosis, and may be associated with pulmonary fibrosis.

Figure 1.148 Multiple small, purple-brown dermal macules, papules or nodules are common in early active sarcoidosis but may be transient. Arthropathy is a prominent early feature, associated with fever and erythema nodosum. Chronic periarticular swelling affects the fingers and toes especially and there may be bony changes.

Sarcoidosis may be rarely associated with primary biliary cirrhosis, Crohn's disease, coeliac disease or amyloidosis, and some patients develop lymphomas. It is as yet unclear which, if any, of these associations are true overlap syndromes.

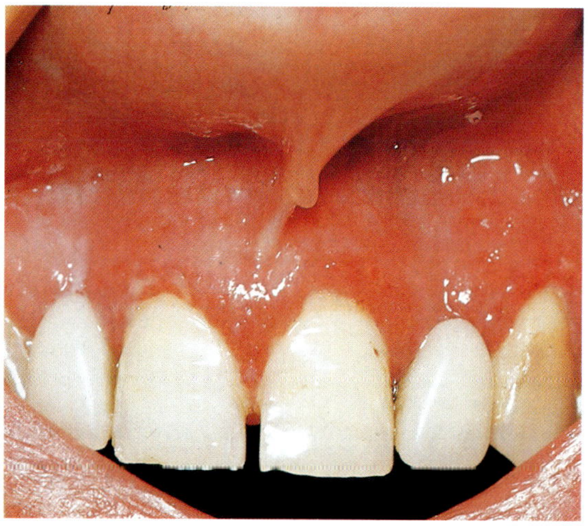

1.145

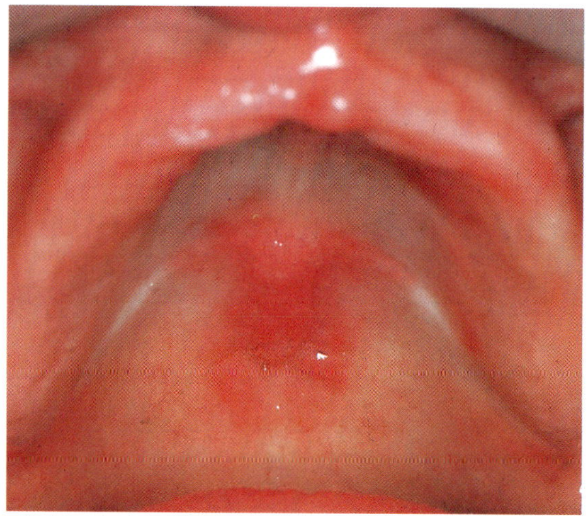

1.146

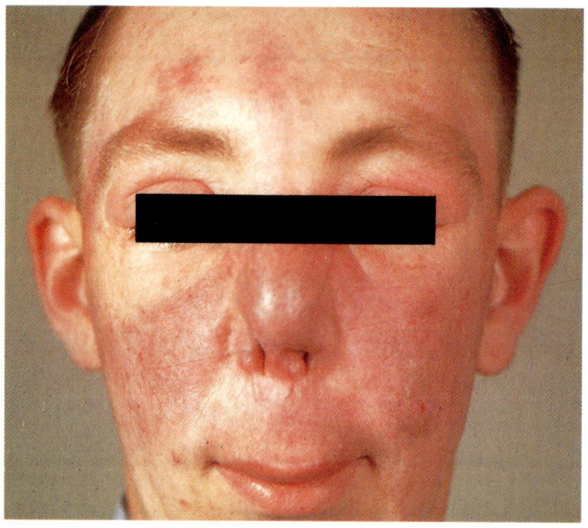

1.147

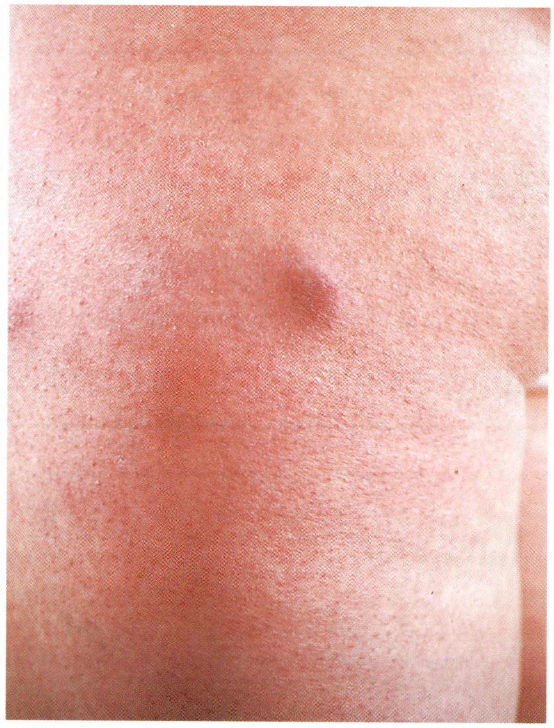

1.148

2

Neoplasms and hamartomas

CARCINOMA OF LIP

Figures 2.1 and 2.2 Oral carcinoma accounts for less than 3 per cent of cancer deaths in Western countries but in some Third World countries, particularly parts of India, oral cancer accounts for more than one third of admissions to cancer hospitals. Most oral malignant neoplasms are squamous cell carcinomas. Patients with carcinoma of the lip tend to present early and the prognosis is usually good. Oral carcinoma in this site is seen especially in male Caucasians living in sunny climes. Predisposing factors include chronic sun exposure, possibly smoking, and immunosuppression. The total incidence is decreasing.

Early carcinoma presents, as shown here, with an asymptomatic red or white lesion, small indurated lump, or erosion which crusts.

Figure 2.3 Typically located at the mucocutaneous junction, the neoplasm spreads within the vermilion and on to the skin.

Figure 2.4 An extreme example, showing a deep ulcer with an irregular surface and rolled edges. Metastasis is primarily to submental and submandibular lymph nodes.

CARCINOMA OF TONGUE

Figure 2.5 The tongue is the most common intraoral site of carcinoma. Most are on the lateral margin extending on to the ventrum. Tobacco or alcohol use and infections such as tertiary syphilis and chronic candidosis are predisposing factors. There also may be an increased prevalence in AIDS. There is an excess of oropharyngeal cancer in textile workers. The incidence of tongue cancer is now increasing.

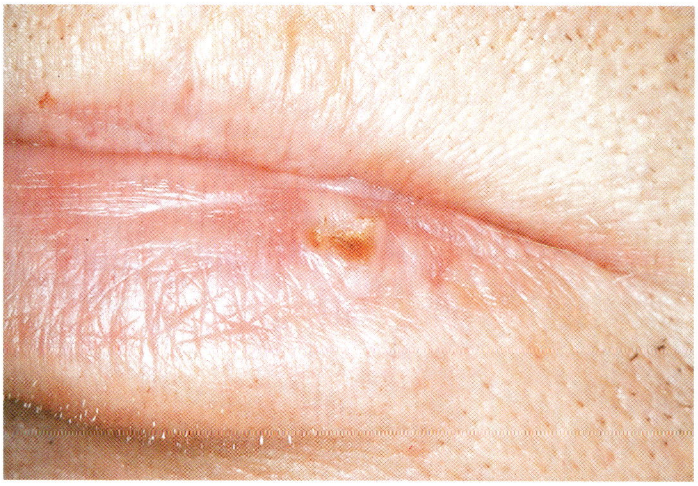

2.1

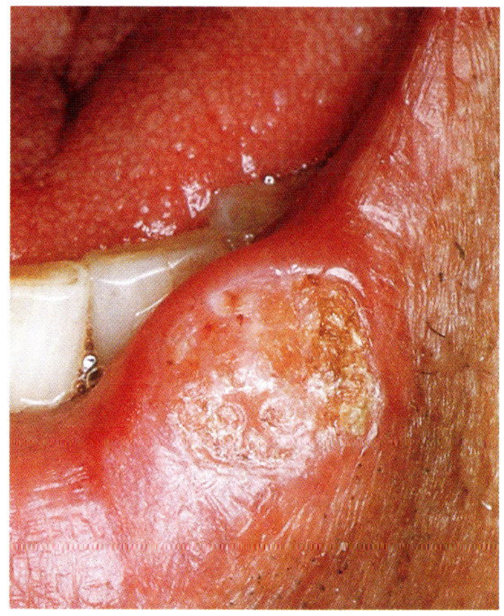

2.2

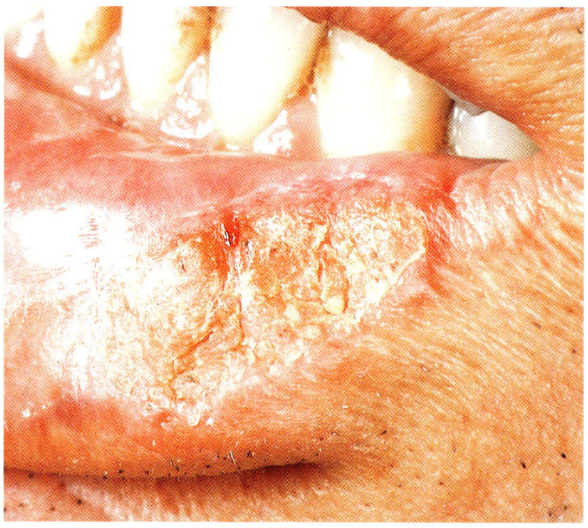

2.3

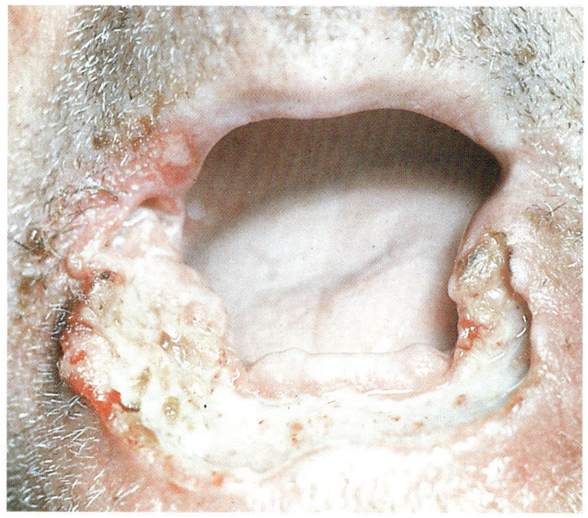

2.4

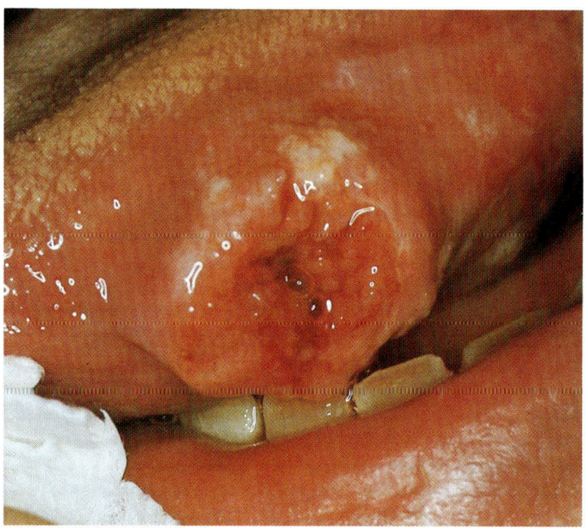

2.5

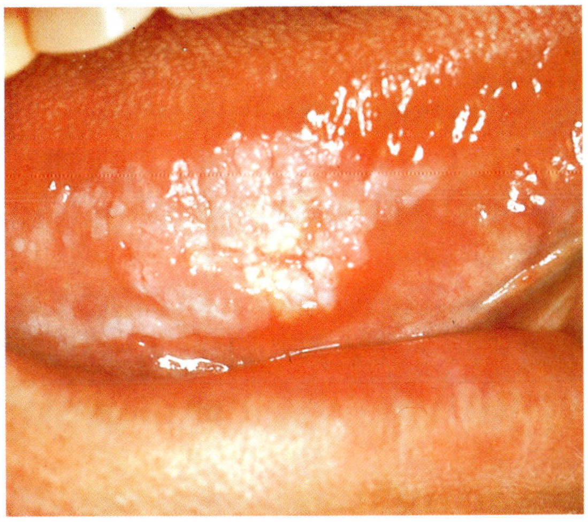

2.6

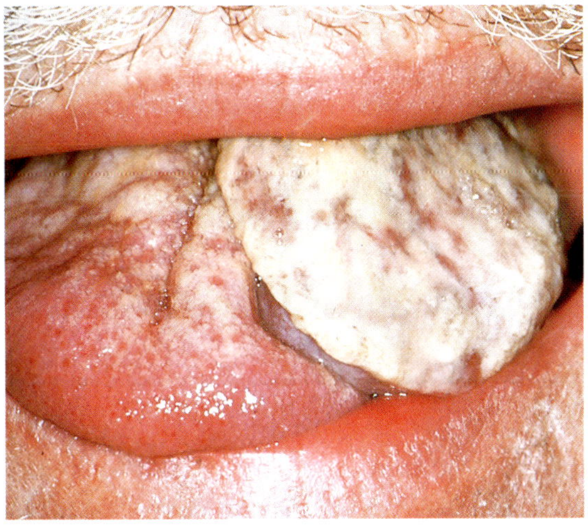

2.7

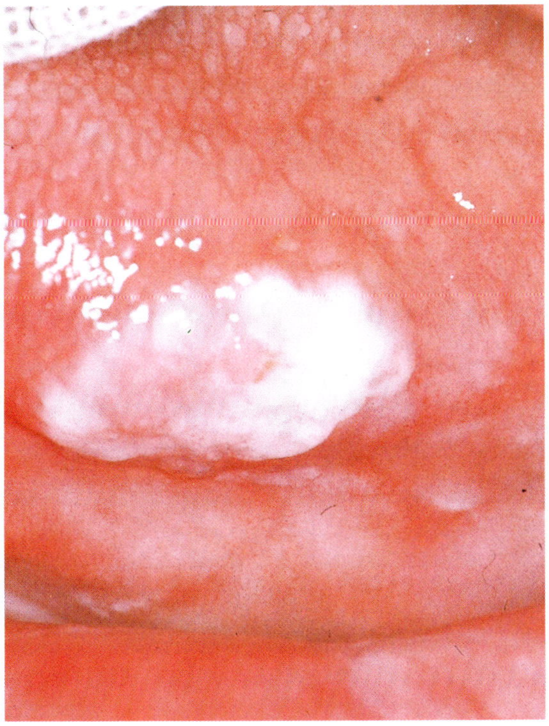

2.8

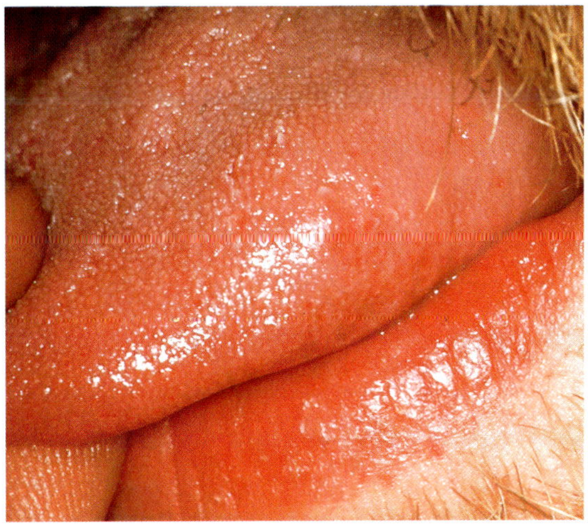

2.9

Figure 2.6 A lesion predominantly of elderly males, carcinoma presents as a red or white lesion, nodule, erosion or, as here, an ulcer. The lesion is indurated, usually sited on the posterolateral margin, and often associated with enlarged submandibular or jugulodigastric lymph nodes, sometimes bilaterally. The tumour tends to metastasize early and the patients present late.

Figure 2.7 Rarely the carcinoma is exophytic and extends on to the dorsum of the tongue.

Figure 2.8 Carcinoma may present as, or in, a white lesion. Leukoplakia of the floor of the mouth/ventrum of tongue may have a high premalignant potential – the so-called 'sublingual keratosis' (see page 143).

SARCOMA OF TONGUE

Figure 2.9 Apart from carcinoma, malignant oral soft tissue lesions are rare. They include melanoma, Kaposi's sarcoma, fibrosarcoma, malignant fibrous histiocytoma, lymphoproliferative disorders, soft tissue metastases and others. In most malignant neoplasms, the clinical features are insufficiently specific to give a reliable diagnosis. Biopsy is invariably indicated.

CARCINOMA OF GINGIVA

Figure 2.10 Carcinoma of the gingiva is rare. It may present as a lump or as a more obvious vegetating mass.

Figure 2.11 Suspicious red lesions, white lesions, ulcers or a mixed lesions, as here, should be biopsied to exclude carcinoma. Tobacco-chewing predisposes to carcinoma of the gingiva, buccal mucosa and the floor of the mouth.

CARCINOMA OF ALVEOLAR RIDGE

Figure 2.12 Carcinoma of lower alveolus: the variation in the clinical appearance of carcinomas is illustrated in Figures 2.12–15. In this instance, there is an obvious malignant ulcer with rolled edges and a red base, within an area of keratosis. There is an association between carcinoma, in the floor of the mouth, and cirrhosis.

Figure 2.13 A vegetating mass extending from the lower alveolus on to the floor of the mouth.

Figure 2.14 A carcinoma on the alveolus, but more aggressive in appearance and extending on to buccal mucosa.

Figure 2.15 Carcinoma of upper alveolus: the speckled appearance of the exophytic mass is a common finding in oral carcinoma. This is an oral squamous cell carcinoma but occasionally an antral carcinoma invades the alveolus or palate to present in a similar manner.

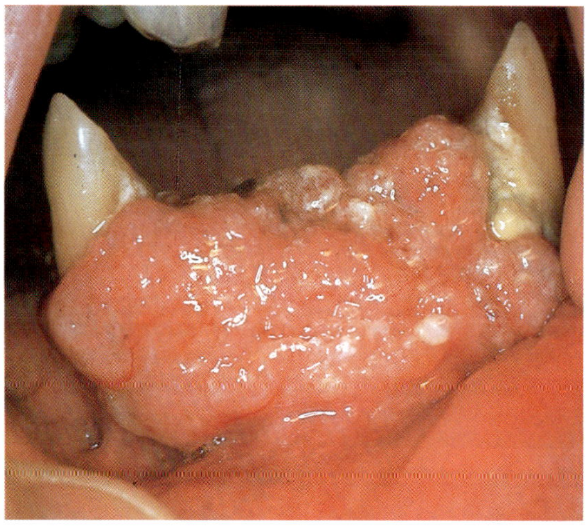

2.10

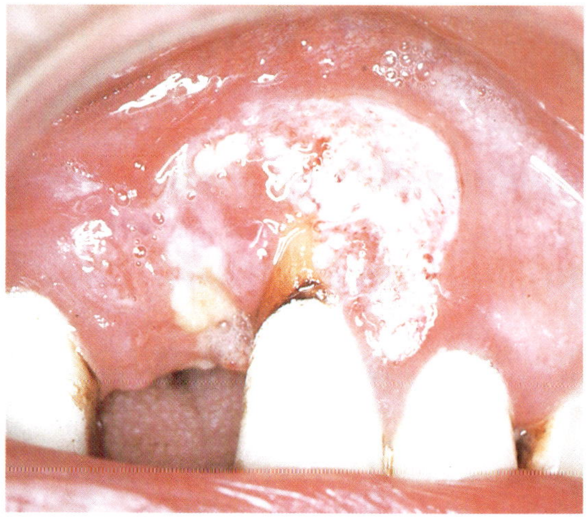

2.11

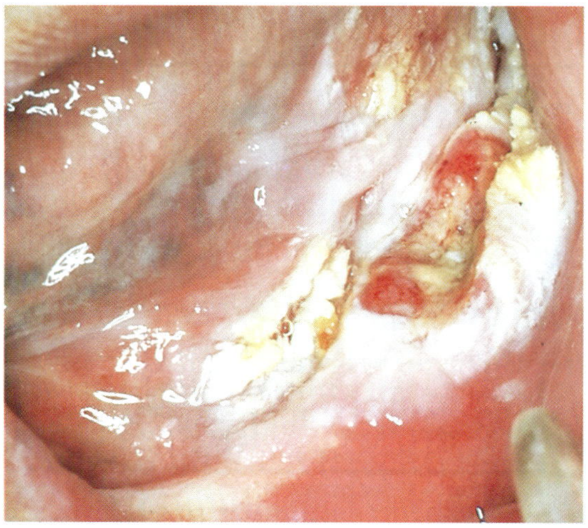

2.12

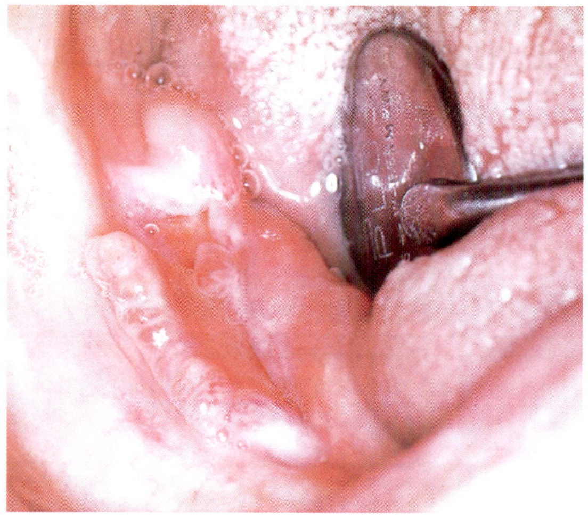

2.13

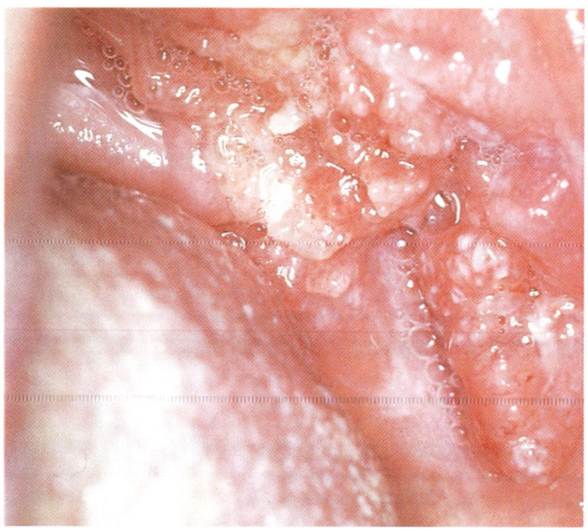

2.14

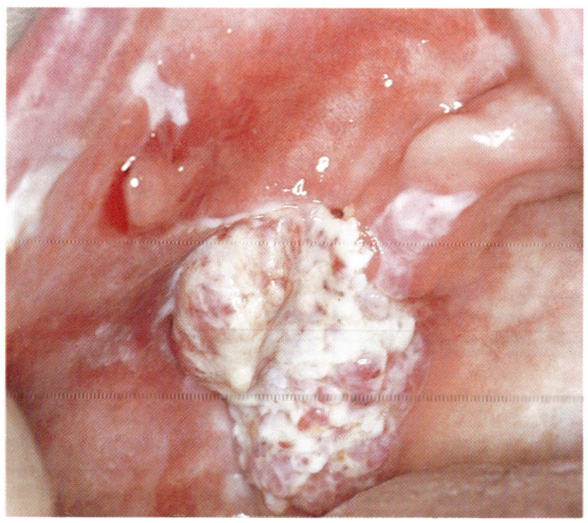

2.15

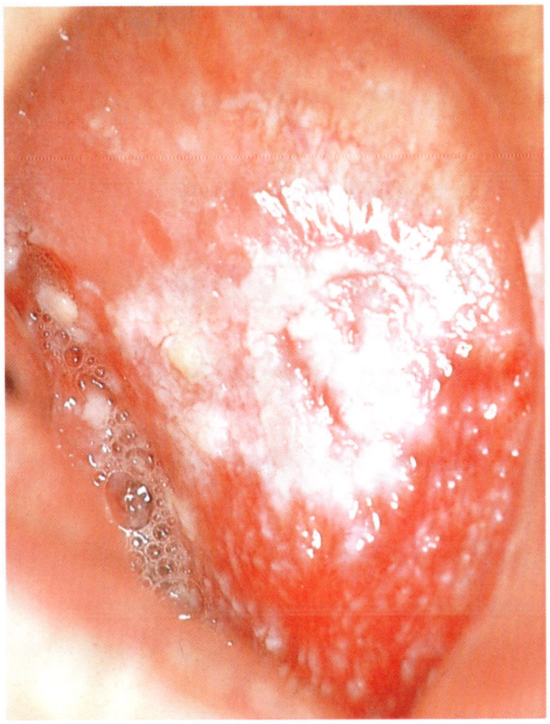

2.16

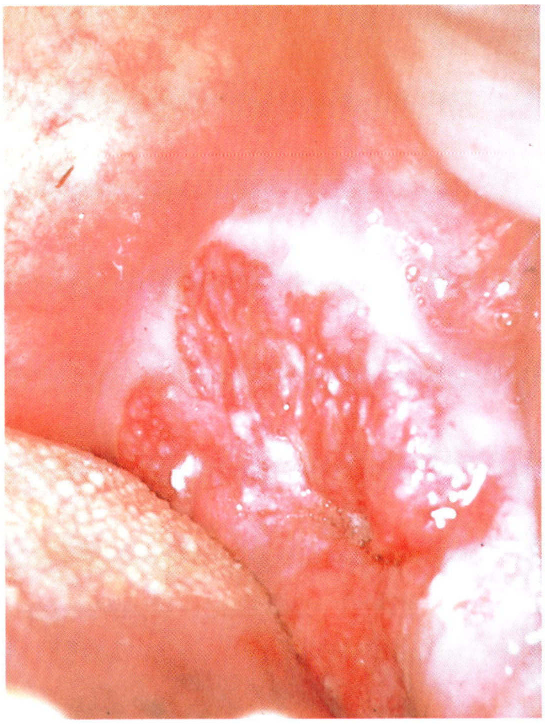

2.17

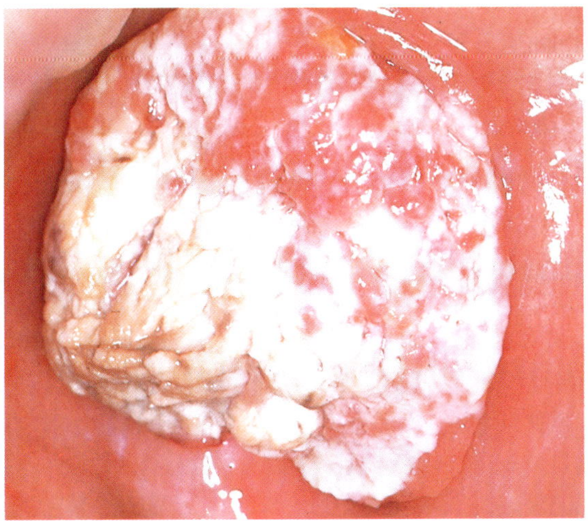

2.18

CARCINOMA OF BUCCAL MUCOSA

Figure 2.16 This particular example is diffuse rather than exophytic and has red (erythroplasia) and white (leukoplakia) components. Erythroplasia is often highly dysplastic or malignant (see page 144). Habits such as snuff-taking or tobacco-chewing (including the use of smokeless tobacco) may predispose to buccal carcinoma.

Figure 2.17 An ulcerated exophytic malignant ulcer.

Figure 2.18 Verrucous carcinoma is a variant of squamous cell carcinoma which is predominantly exophytic, slow-growing, and of relatively good prognosis. Most common in elderly males, typically it affects the buccal mucosa and has a pebbly surface, as here. A clinically similar condition, verrucous hyperplasia, is probably a variant.

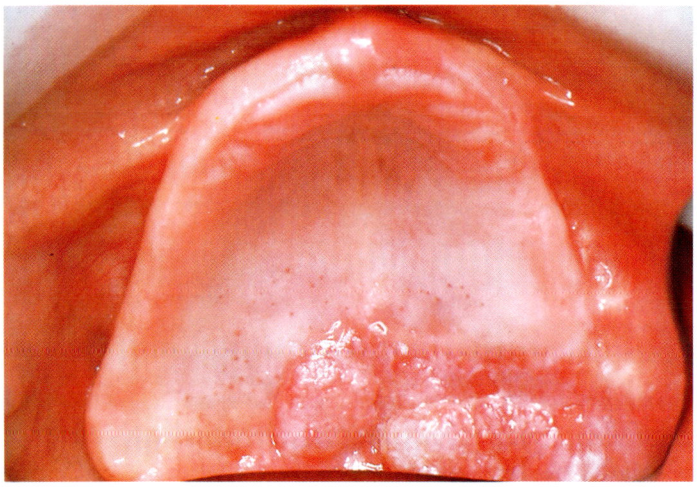

2.19

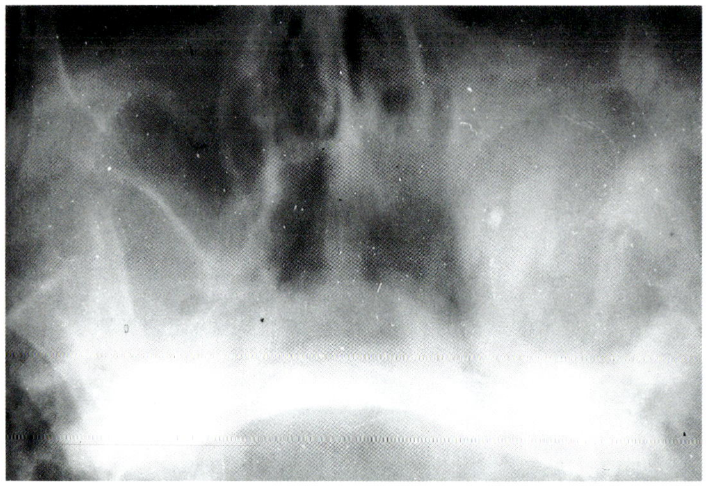

2.20

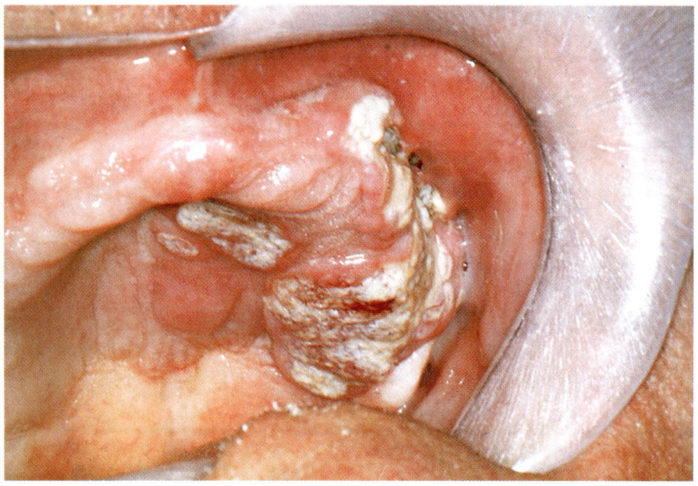

2.21

CARCINOMA OF PALATE

Figure 2.19 Palatal carcinoma is very rare in the West, but is fairly common in parts of the world where reverse cigarette smoking is practised.

CARCINOMA OF ANTRUM

Figure 2.20 Carcinoma of the maxillary antrum is a rare neoplasm, found especially in those who work with wood, for example, in the furniture industry, and in those who work in the shoe and boot industry. Snuff use also appears to predispose to antral carcinoma. Initially asymptomatic, antral carcinoma eventually invades the palate, nose or orbit. Occipitomental radiography shows opacity and invasion with loss of the bony walls of the antrum.

Figure 2.21 Antral carcinoma often presents clinically as a swelling in the palate or alveolus, usually in the premolar/molar region. The swelling may ulcerate, as here.

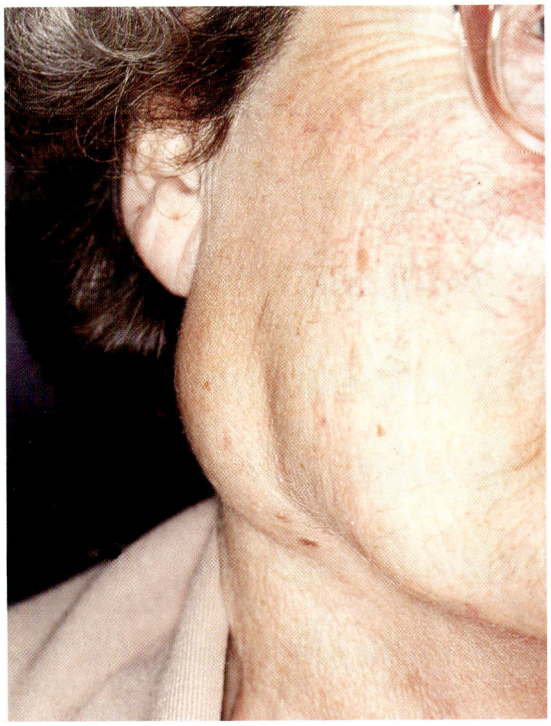

2.22

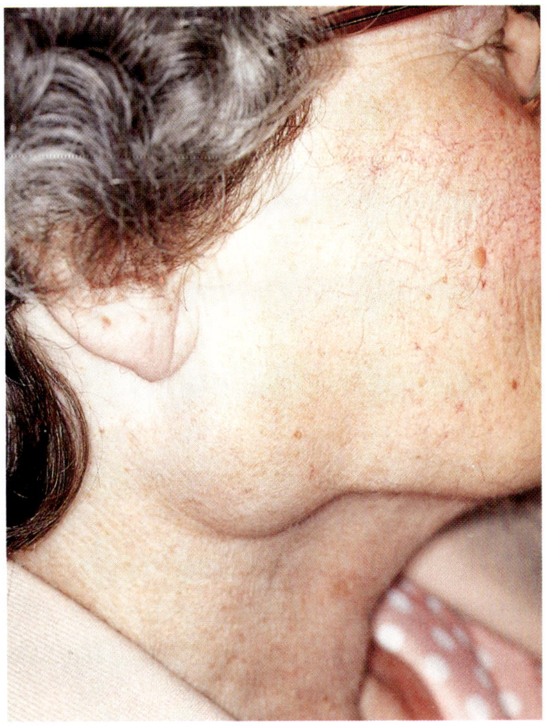

2.23

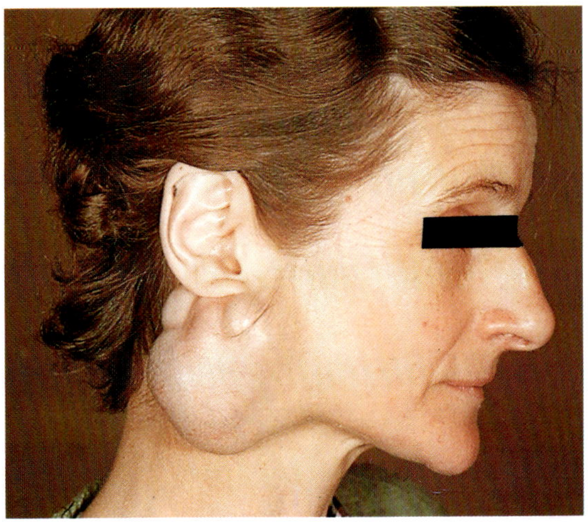

2.24

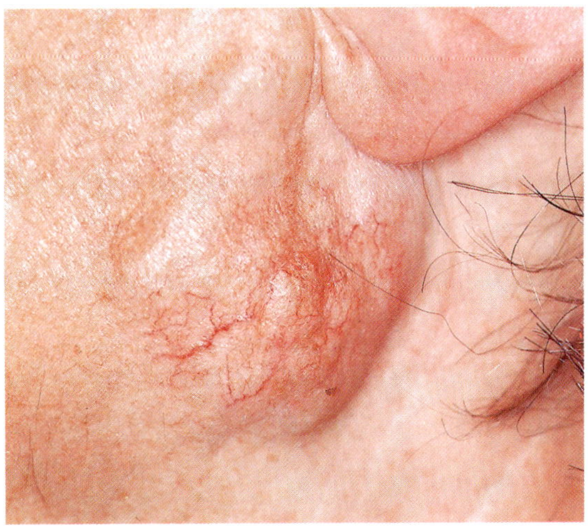

2.25

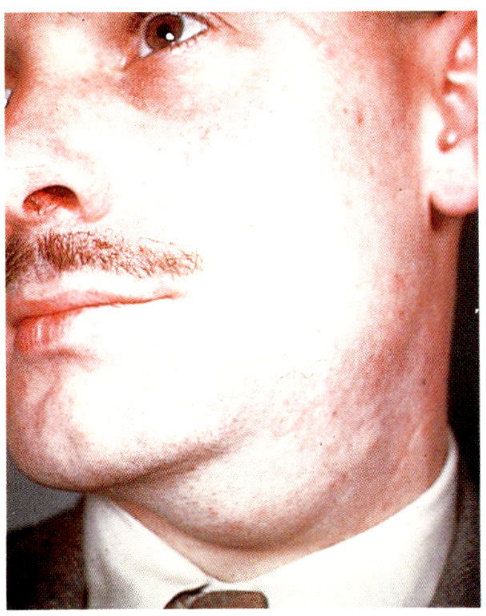

2.26

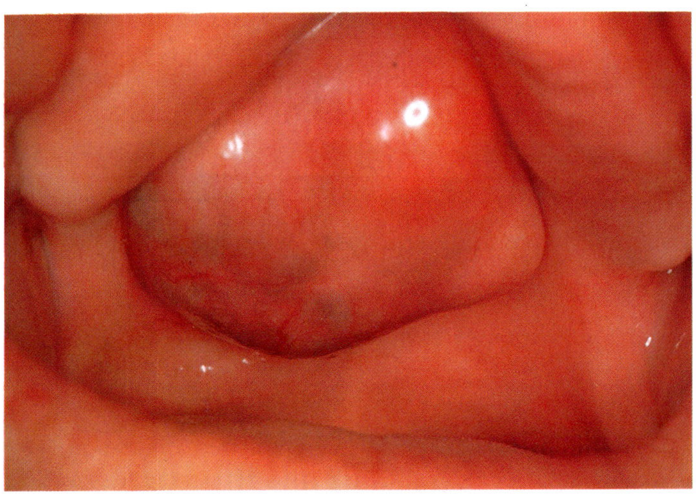

2.27

PLEOMORPHIC SALIVARY ADENOMA (*Mixed salivary tumour*)

Figure 2.22 Salivary gland neoplasms are uncommon and of unknown aetiology, although there is increased incidence in those exposed to atomic or therapeutic irradiation and possibly an association with breast carcinoma. The most common is pleomorphic salivary adenoma (PSA), a benign neoplasm which typically affects middle-aged or elderly persons. There is a slight female predominance and the neoplasm is found mainly in the parotid, as here.

Figure 2.23 The majority of salivary neoplasms are benign; most are PSA; and most affect the parotid. Swellings of the parotid gland typically appear behind and over the angle of mandible and evert the lobe of the ear.

Figure 2.24 PSA is usually painless and has no effect on the facial nerve, despite an often intimate relationship. PSA frequently has a lobulated surface, as here.

Figure 2.25 Malignant change, although uncommon, is suggested by pain, rapid growth, facial palsy, increased vasculature, as shown here, or ulceration.

Figure 2.26 The submandibular gland may be the site of PSA, as here.

Figure 2.27 Intraoral salivary gland neoplasms are most common in the palate, usually in the region of the junction of hard and soft palate. PSA often has a lobulated surface and is slow-growing.

PLEOMORPHIC SALIVARY ADENOMA
(continued)

Figure 2.28 PSA is not only the most common neoplasm of major salivary glands but also of the minor salivary glands of lip, palate and elsewhere. This is a PSA presenting as a small swelling in the upper labial vestibule.

Figure 2.29 A nodule or sometimes a cystic mass, especially in the upper lip, should be considered as a salivary neoplasm until histologically proved otherwise (showing same patient as Figure 2.28).

Figure 2.30 Ulceration is uncommon in PSA, even where the lesion has impinged on a denture, as here.

ADENOID CYSTIC CARCINOMA

Figure 2.31 Adenoid cystic carcinoma is the most common malignant neoplasm of minor salivary glands and is usually seen in the palate as a fairly slow-growing lump which eventually ulcerates. Nevertheless, it is invasive, especially perineurally, and has a poor prognosis.

MUCOEPIDERMOID TUMOUR

Figure 2.32 Neoplasms are rare in the sublingual gland but are typically malignant, such as acinic cell tumour, mucoepidermoid tumour, adenoid cystic tumour, malignant PSA, or adenocarcinoma.

Mucoepidermoid tumour appears to be the most common malignant tumour of salivary glands induced by previous irradiation.

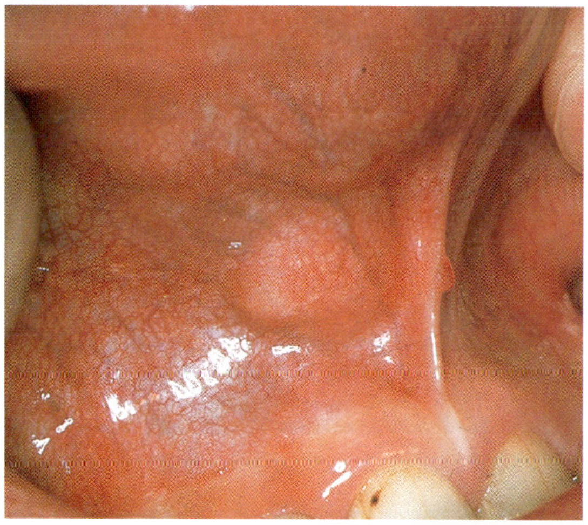
2.28

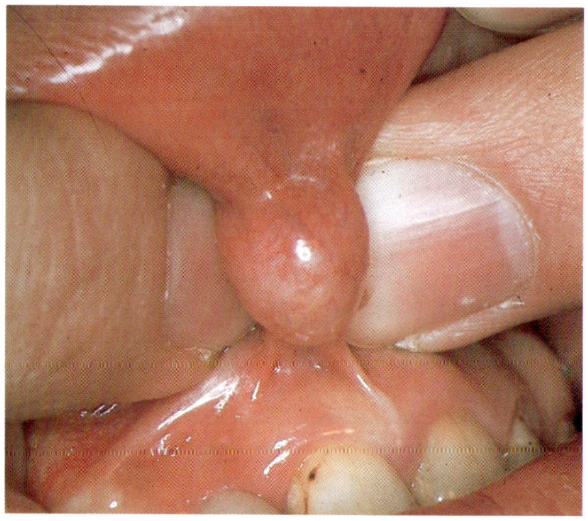
2.29

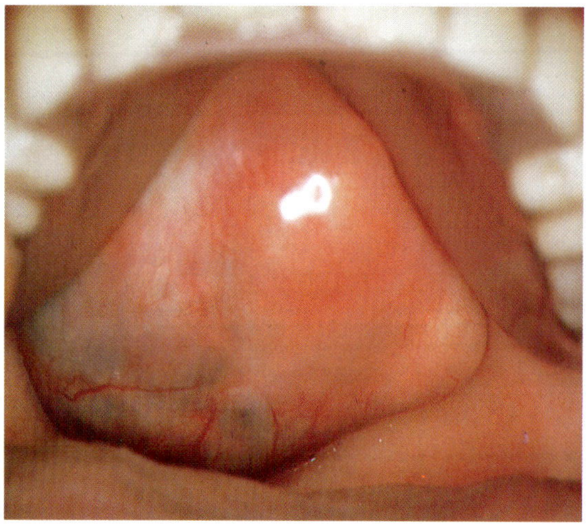
2.30

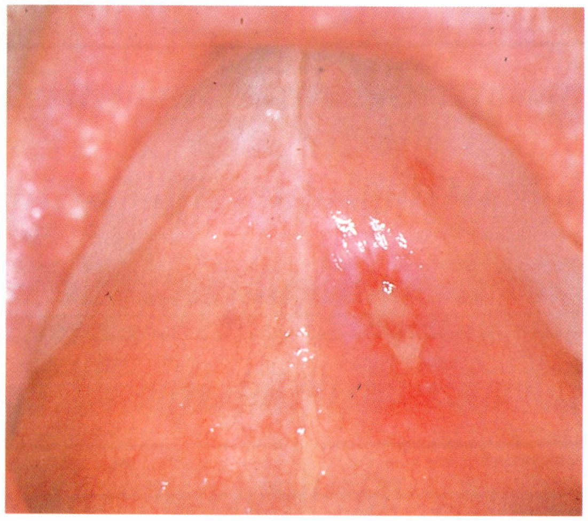
2.31

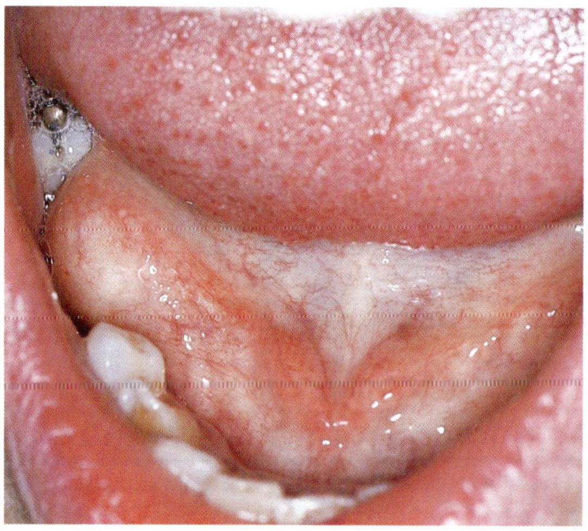
2.32

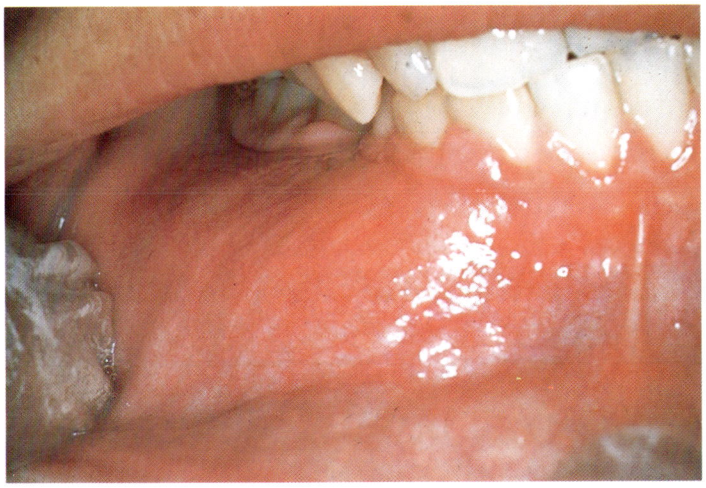

2.33

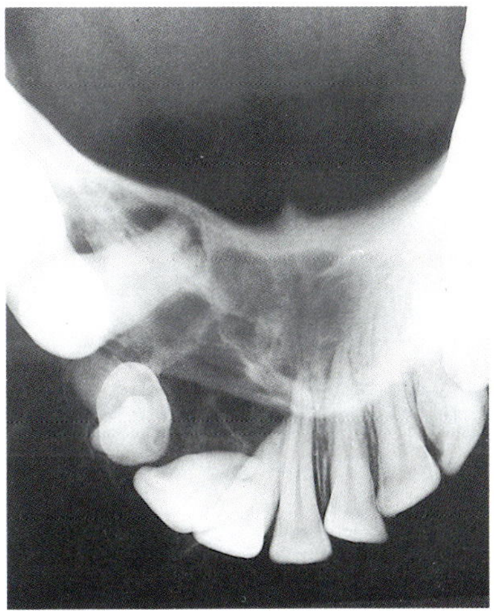

2.34

MYXOMA

Figure 2.33 Myxomas may have an odontogenic origin (odontogenic myxoma), usually affect the mandible, and are most commonly seen in young people. They are slow growing, but pain may be a feature.

Figure 2.34 Bony expansion with cortical destruction, displacement of teeth without root resorption, and a multilocular, or honeycomb appearance, are typical radiographic features.

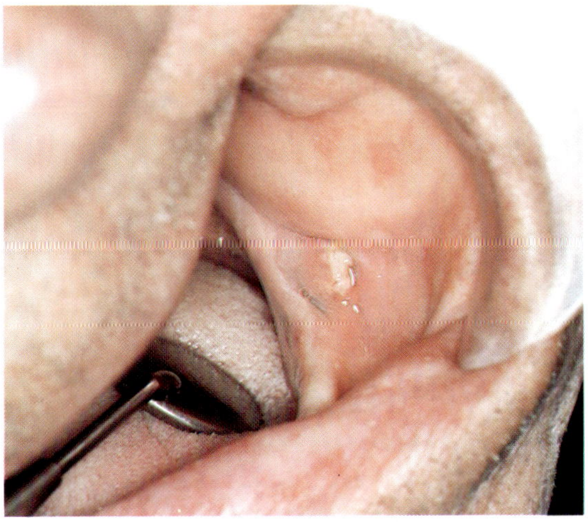

2.35

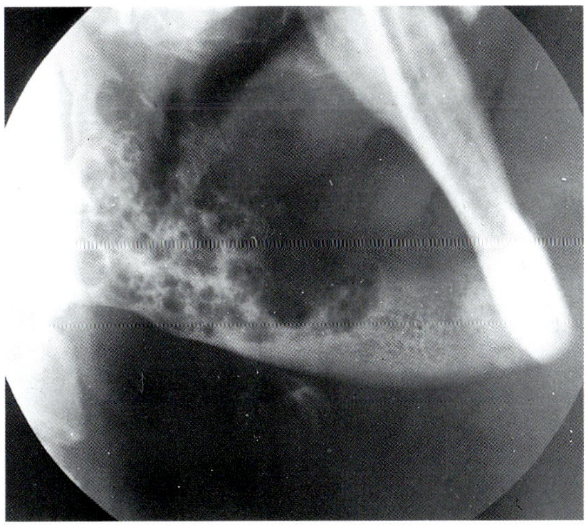

2.36

AMELOBLASTOMA (*Adamantinoma*)

Figure 2.35 This locally invasive odontogenic tumour affects the mandible four times more frequently than the maxilla, and 75 per cent of mandibular lesions are at the angle. Although the lesion may appear at any age, it usually presents in middle age. It grows insidiously, and rarely causes neuropathy or mucosal breakdown. The ulceration in this case was caused by trauma from a denture.

Figure 2.36 The radiographic appearance is generally of a cystic multilocular radiolucency. Bony expansion may be seen. A unilocular appearance is not uncommon, however.

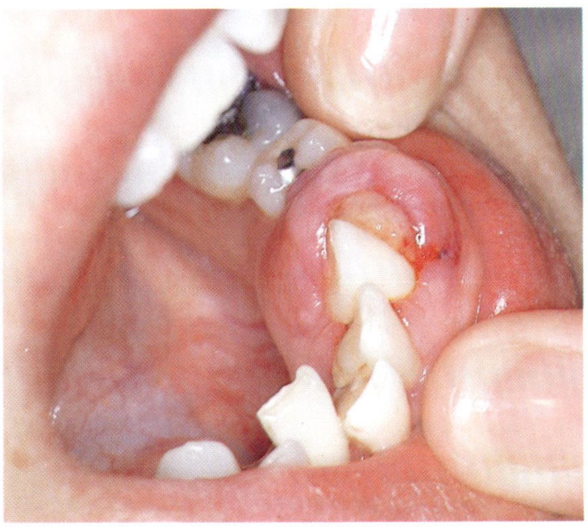

2.37

ADENOMATOID ODONTOGENIC TUMOUR (*Adeno-ameloblastoma*)

Figure 2.37 Although this figure shows a lesion in the mandible, this benign odontogenic tumour is more common in the maxillary canine region.

MALIGNANT MELANOMA

Figure 2.38 Primary oral melanoma is rare. It affects both sexes equally, is more common in coloured patients, and usually appears in or after middle age. Most arise in the palate and many are preceded by melanosis. Some vegetate profusely, as here (a rather extreme example), others remain flattish and spread more deeply. Not all are pigmented. The prognosis is very poor.

METASTATIC NEOPLASM

Figure 2.39 Blood-borne metastases are rare in the oral soft tissues and most are seen in the mandible, especially the angle and body. They virtually all present with pain or anaesthesia, expansion of the jaw, or loosening of the teeth. This was a metastatic carcinoma of the bronchus. Metastases to the jaws are usually from carcinomas of the breast or bronchus, thyroid, kidney, colo-rectum, stomach, prostate or uterus.

Figure 2.40 Metastatic lymphatic spread is a particular feature of carcinomas of the oral and perioral regions, and is a poor prognostic finding. This patient had a carcinoma of the tongue, and the cervical lymph node swelling was the presenting feature.

Figure 2.41 Rarely, metastases in cervical lymph nodes ulcerate the skin.

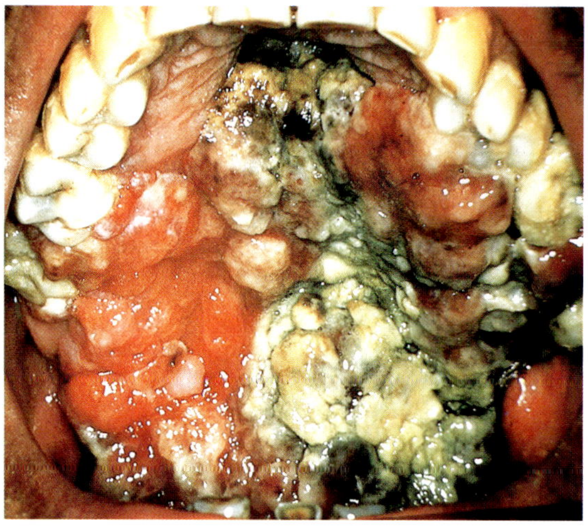

2.38

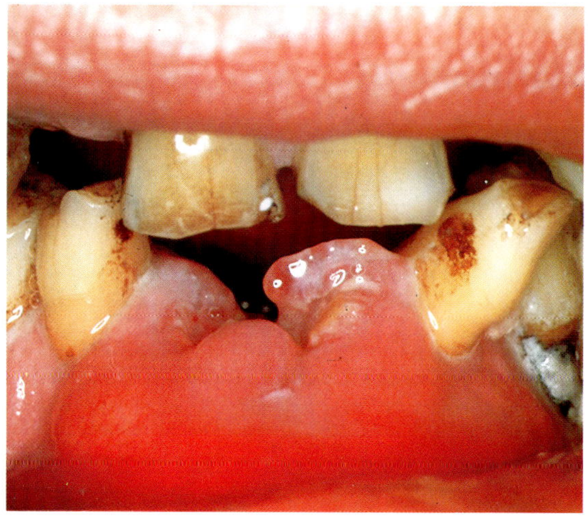

2.39

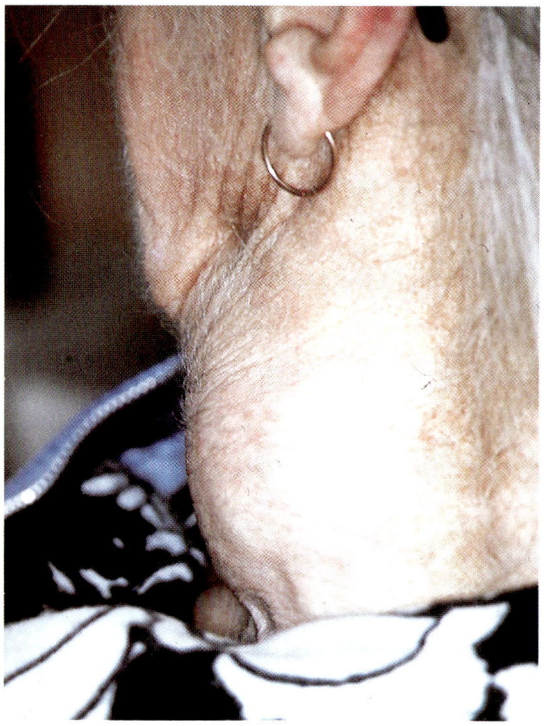

2.40

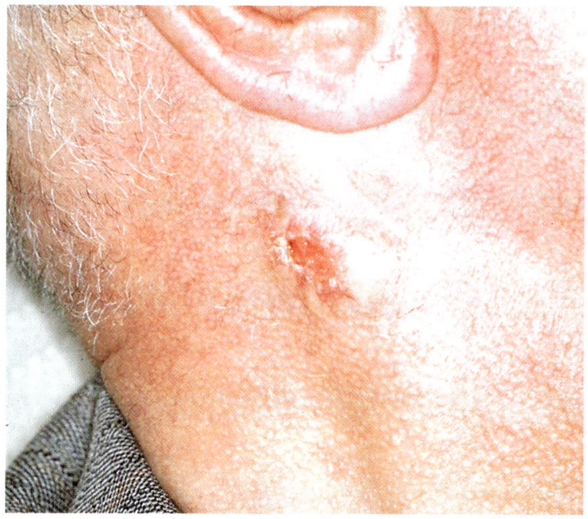

2.41

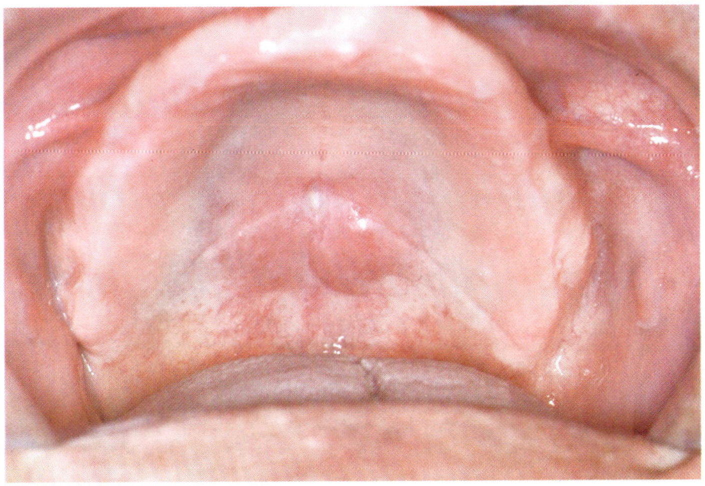

2.42

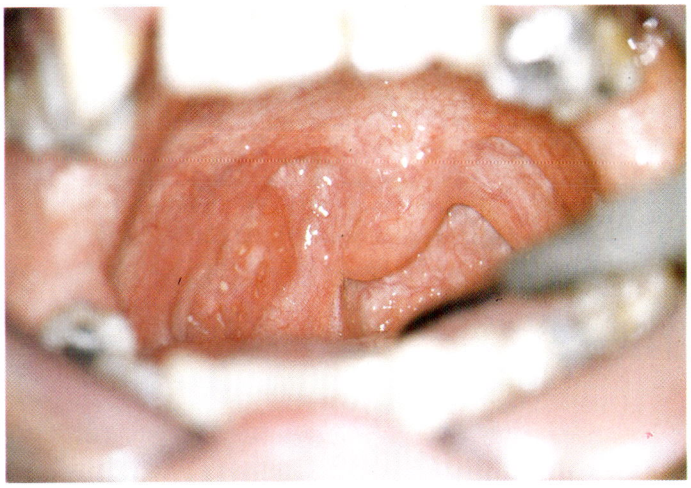

2.43

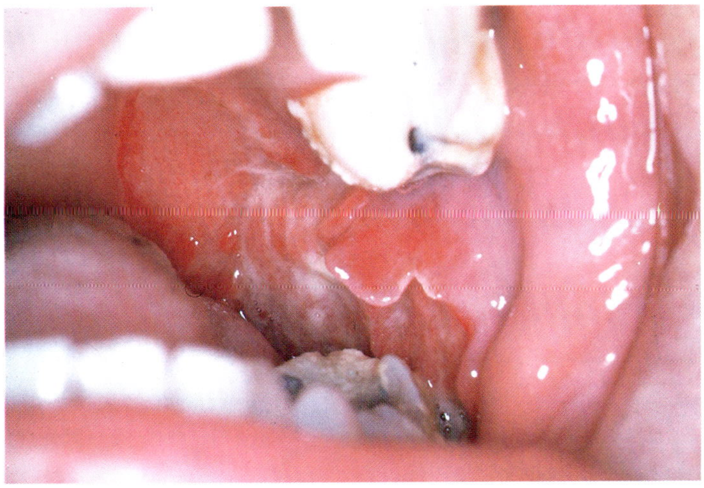

2.44

LYMPHOMA

Figure 2.42 Lymphomas are rare in the mouth, although cervical lymph node involvement is common. Usually lymphomas present as ulcers or swellings – this patient has a swelling over the palate from Hodgkin's lymphoma.

Figure 2.43 Non-Hodgkin's lymphoma in the right tonsil.

Figure 2.44 Non-Hodgkin's lymphoma commonly affects the oropharynx, particularly the tonsillar region, and usually presents as a diffuse painless swelling that eventually ulcerates. There is an increased prevalence in HIV infection (see also Sjögren's syndrome, page 184).

LYMPHOMA (*continued*)

Figure 2.45 African Burkitt's lymphoma is associated with Epstein-Barr virus and typically affects children before the age of 12–13 years. The jaws, particularly the mandible, are common sites of presentation. Massive swelling, which ulcerates in the mouth, may be seen. Radiographically, the teeth may appear to be 'floating in air'.

Figure 2.46 The association of non-African Burkitt's lymphoma with Epstein-Barr virus is tenuous and the disease is less common. Here there is an ulcerated lump arising from the mandible, but the disease may cause oral pain, paraesthesia or increasing tooth mobility.

The jaws are less frequently involved in this type of Burkitt's lymphoma. Discrete radiolucencies in the lower third molar region, destruction of lamina dura and widening of the periodontal space may be seen on radiography.

LYMPHOSARCOMA

Figure 2.47 The initial sign of a lymphosarcoma is often diffuse progressive local swelling, seen here over the mandibular angle. Growth can be very rapid and blood-borne metastasis widespread.

Patients with lymphocytic lymphomas are also predisposed to develop squamous carcinomas of the head and neck, possibly owing at least partly to the chemotherapy.

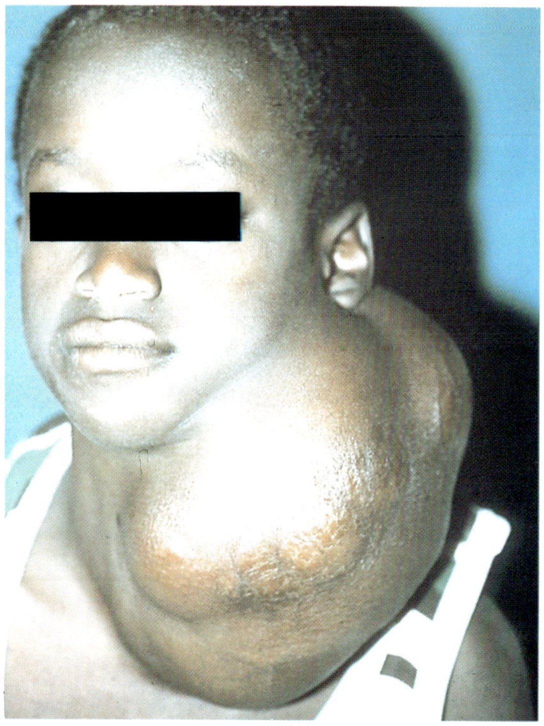

2.45

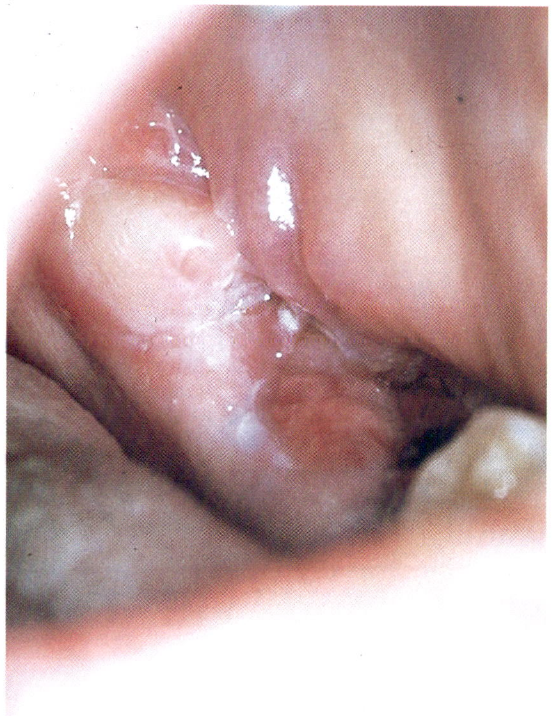

2.46

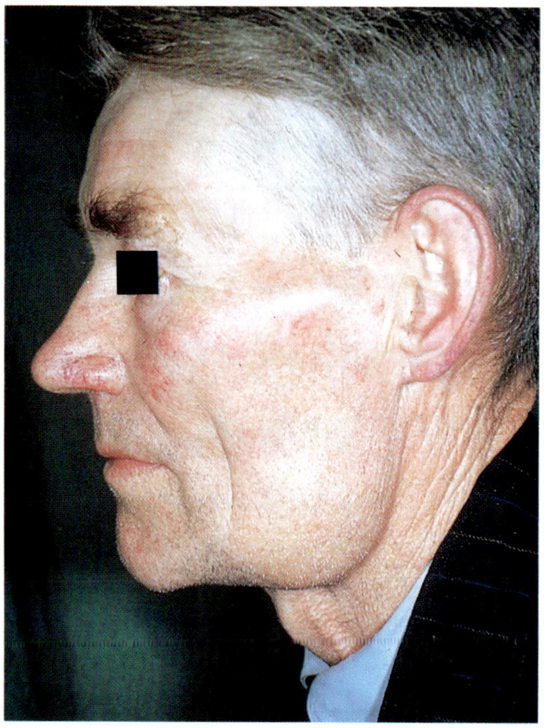

2.47

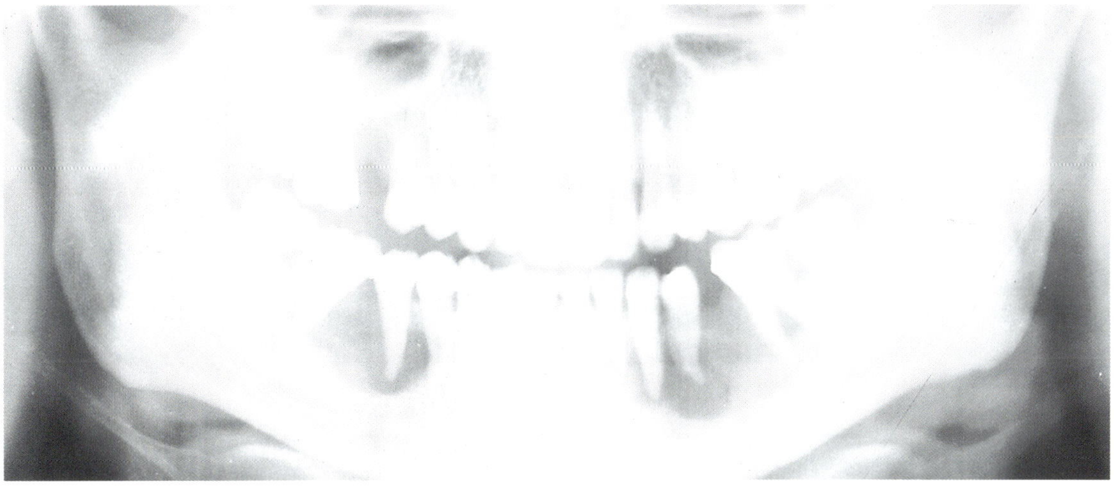

2.48

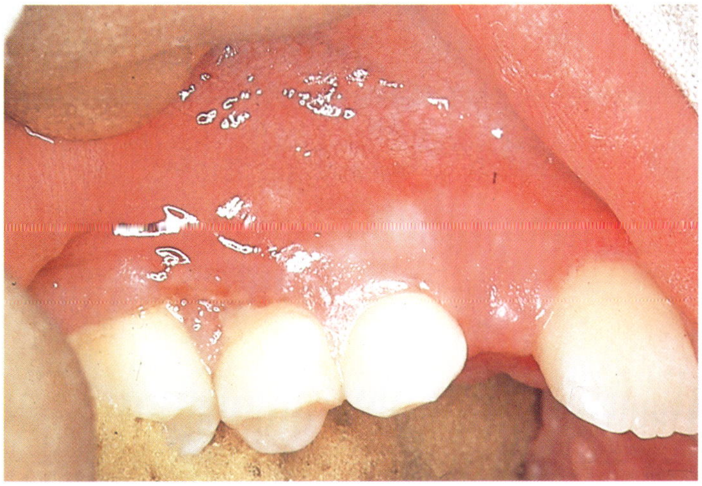

2.49

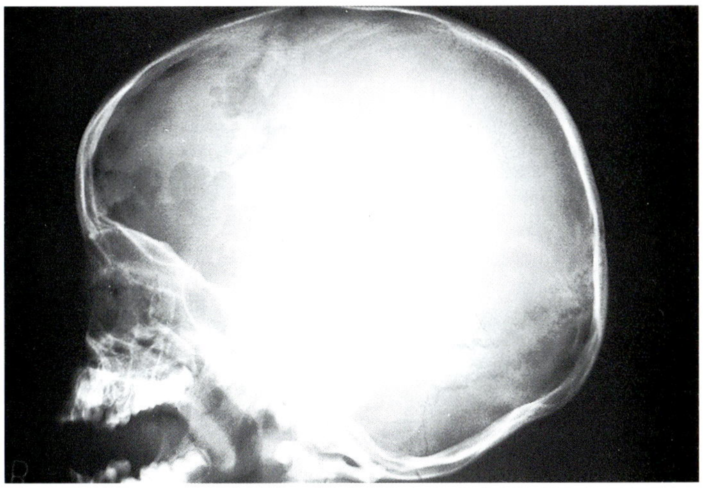

2.50

LANGERHAN'S CELL HISTIOCYTOSES

Figure 2.48 Langerhan's cell histiocytoses are a group of disorders, formerly termed histiocytosis X, arising from Langerhan's cells. Hand-Schüller-Christian disease, as here, appears at 3–6 years of age with osteolytic jaw lesions and loosening of teeth (floating teeth), diabetes insipidus and exophthalmos.

Figure 2.49 Eosinophilic granuloma is a localized benign form of histiocytosis where there are painless osteolytic bone lesions and, sometimes, mouth ulcers. The affected teeth may loosen.

Figure 2.50 Letterer-Siwe disease is an acute disseminated and usually lethal form of histiocytosis in children under the age of 3 years. There are bone lesions, skin lesions, fever, lymphadenopathy and hepatosplenomegaly.

MYCOSIS FUNGOIDES

Figure 2.51 Mycosis fungoides is a predominantly cutaneous T cell neoplasm that may produce oral plaques, infiltrates or ulcers, especially on the tongue. Incidentally, this patient also has erythema migrans.

MULTIPLE MYELOMA (*Myelomatosis*)

Figure 2.52 Myelomatosis is a malignant disorder of plasma cells, affecting predominantly the bone marrow. Most commonly found in males over 50 years of age, it particularly affects the skull and axial skeleton. The jaws may be involved but soft tissue lesions are rare.

Figure 2.53 The symptomatic stage is preceded by the presence in plasma of an M-type (monoclonal) plasma protein, raised ESR, and proteinuria. Renal dysfunction may eventually arise.

Clinically there may be anaemia, bone pain, swelling, paraesthesia or, occasionally, pathological fractures. Radiography shows multiple punched-out radiolucencies.

Ultimately, there may be circulatory impairment, Raynaud-type phenomena or bleeding tendency caused by the paraproteins. Amyloidosis may be seen. There is a predisposition to recurrence of varicella zoster virus infection.

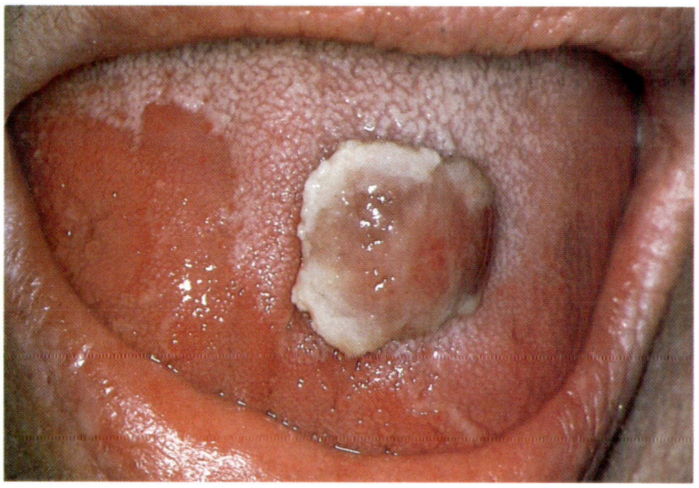

2.51

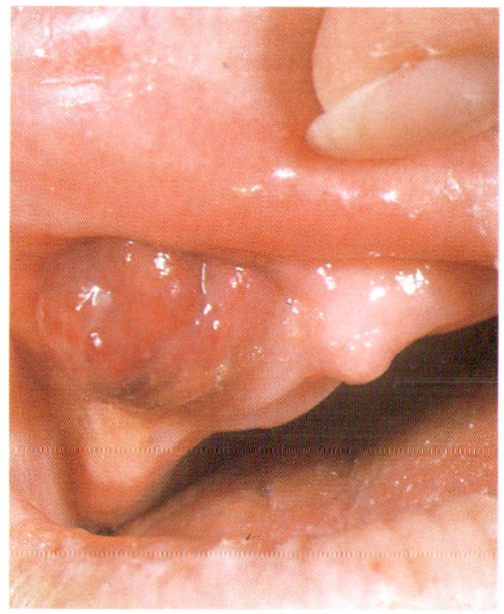

2.52

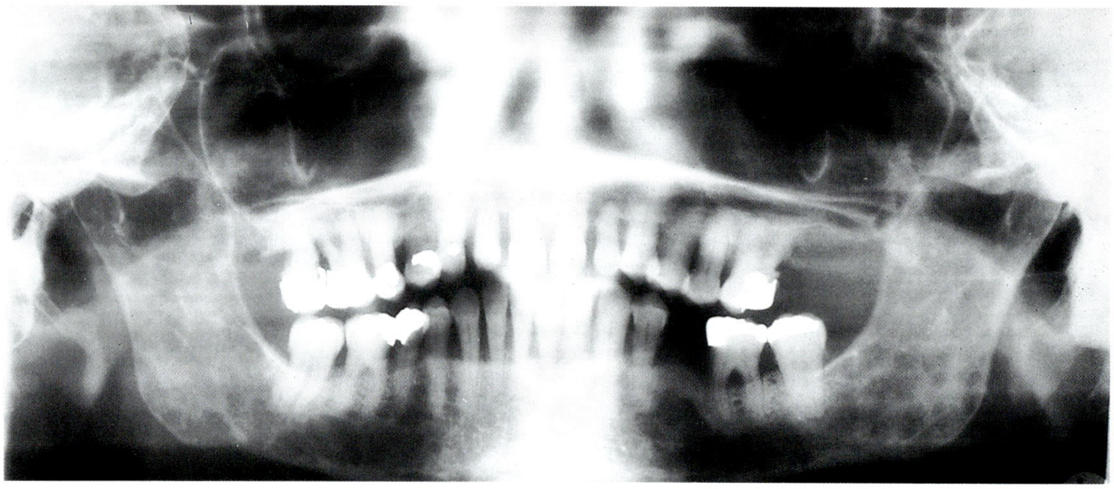

2.53

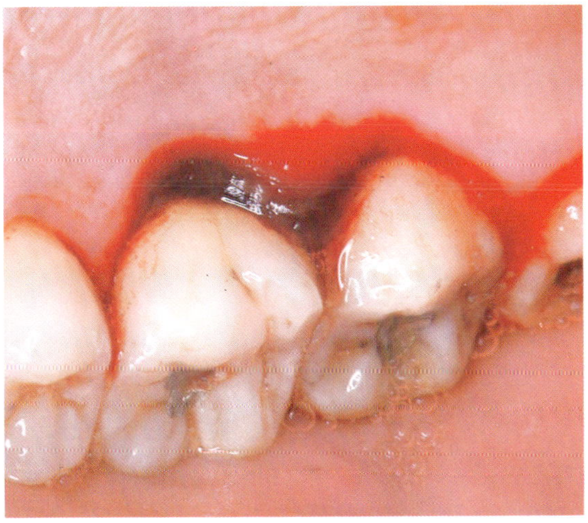

2.54

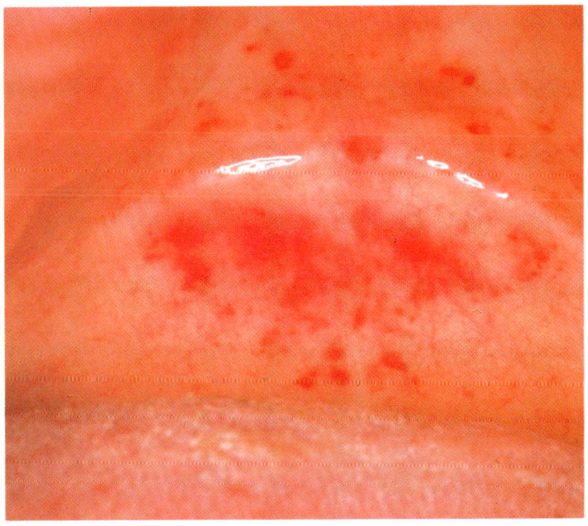

2.55

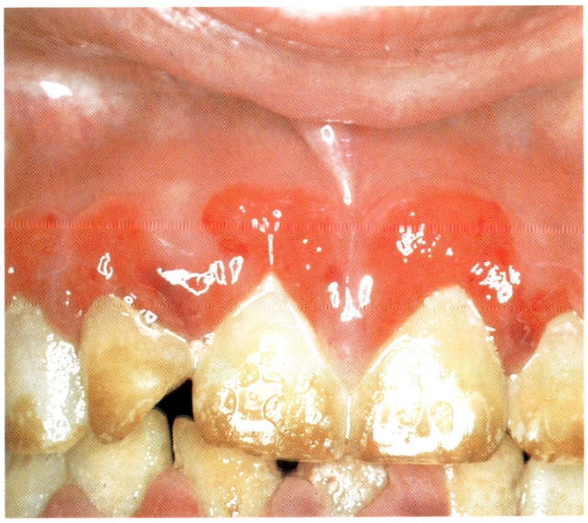

2.56

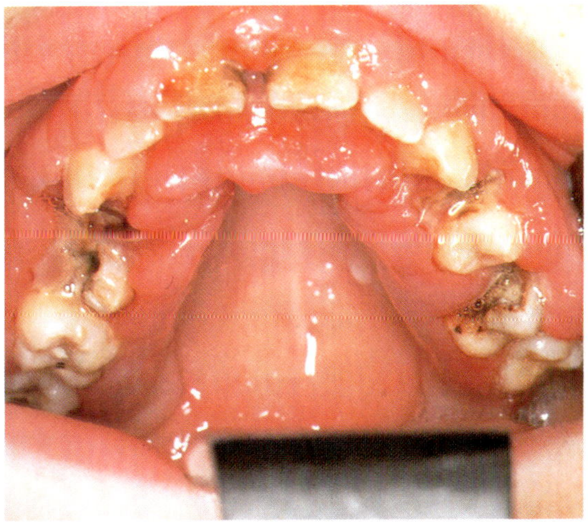

2.57

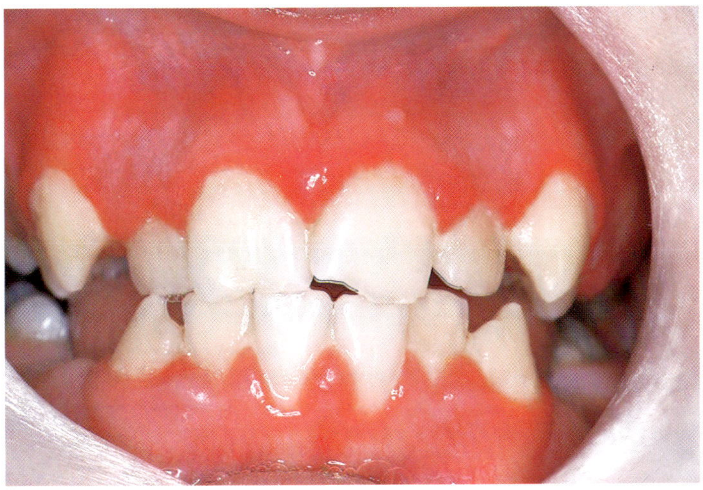

2.58

LEUKAEMIA

Figure 2.54 Replacement of bone marrow by leukaemic tissue leads to crowding out of other cellular elements and consequent anaemia and thrombocytopenia. Spontaneous gingival haemorrhage is common. There are no oral features that distinguish reliably between the different leukaemias.

Figure 2.55 Oral purpura is common, particularly where there is trauma, such as the suction exerted by an upper denture. Chemotherapy may aggravate the bleeding tendency.

Figure 2.56 Gingival haemorrhage can be so profuse as to dissuade the patient from oral hygiene, but this simply aggravates the problem as the gingivae then become inflamed, more hyperaemic and bleed more profusely.

Figure 2.57 Leukaemic deposits in the gingiva occasionally cause gingival swelling. This is a feature especially of myelomonocytic leukaemia.

Figure 2.58 Profuse swelling of the gingiva in myelomonocytic leukaemia.

LEUKAEMIA *(continued)*

Figure 2.59 Simple odontogenic infections can spread widely and be difficult to control, as in this periapical infection in a leukaemic patient.

Non-odontogenic oral infections are common in leukaemic patients and involve a range of organisms including *Staphylococcus aureus*, *Pseudomonas aeruginosa*, *Klebsiella pneumoniae*, *Staphylococcus epidermidis*, *Escherichia coli*, enterococci, herpes simplex or varicella-zoster viruses, Candida species, Aspergillus, Mucor and, occasionally, other opportunists.

Figure 2.60 Mouth ulcers are common in leukaemia. Some are associated with cytotoxic therapy, some with viral or bacterial infection, and some are non-specific.

Figure 2.61 Erythroleukaemia or Di Guglielmo's disease is a rare disorder, characterized by proliferation of erythropoietic cells, with anaemia and hepatosplenomegaly but no lymphadenopathy. Oral ulceration and pallor, as shown here, and purpura are the main features.

Figure 2.62 Microbial infections are common in the mouth and can be a significant problem to the leukaemic patient. Candidosis is extremely common, as shown here. Of the viral infections, recurrent intraoral herpes simplex is also common. This patient has a dendritic ulcer, caused by herpes simplex virus.

Figure 2.63 Recurrent herpes labialis is common in leukaemic patients. The lesions can be extensive and, because of the thrombocytopenia, there is often bleeding into the lesion, as here.

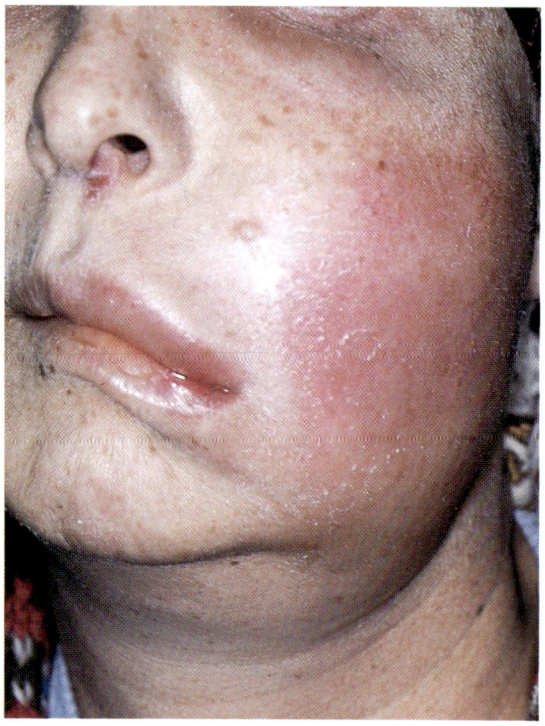

2.59

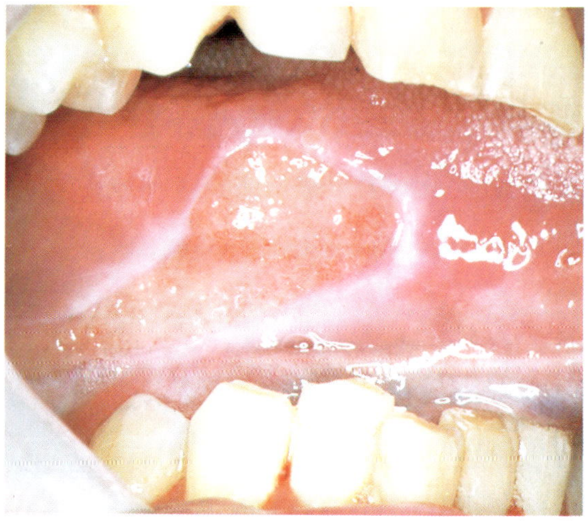

2.60

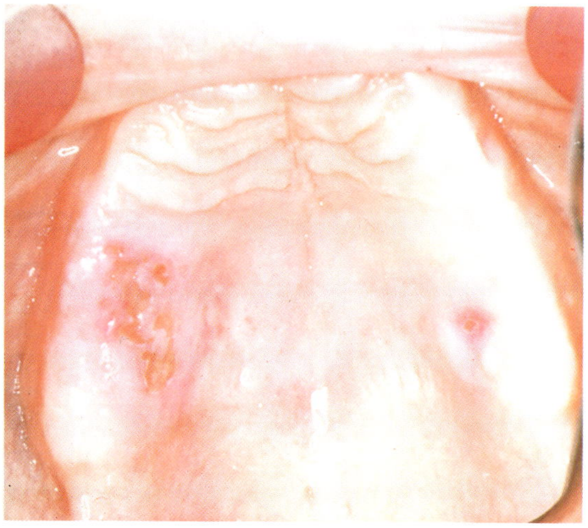

2.61

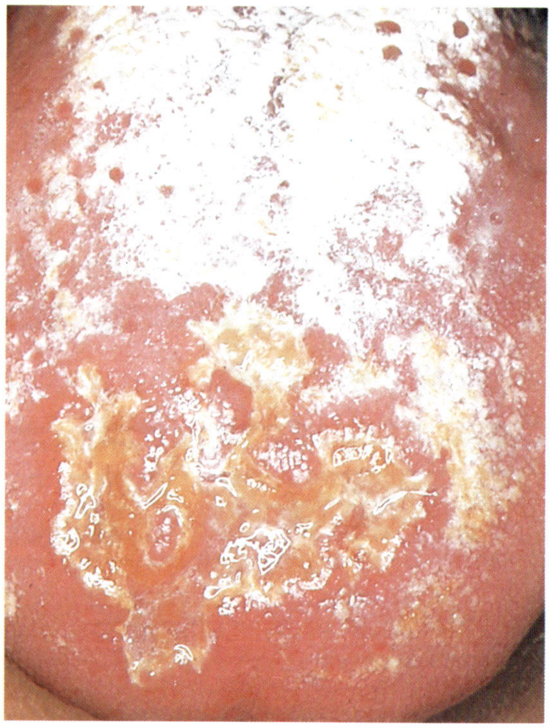

2.62

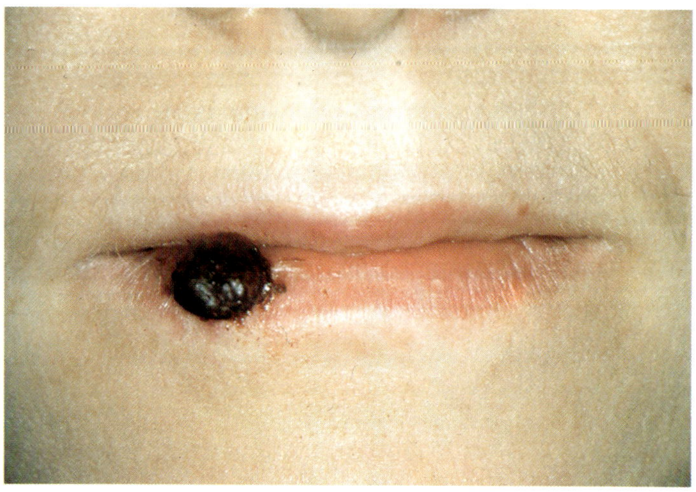

2.63

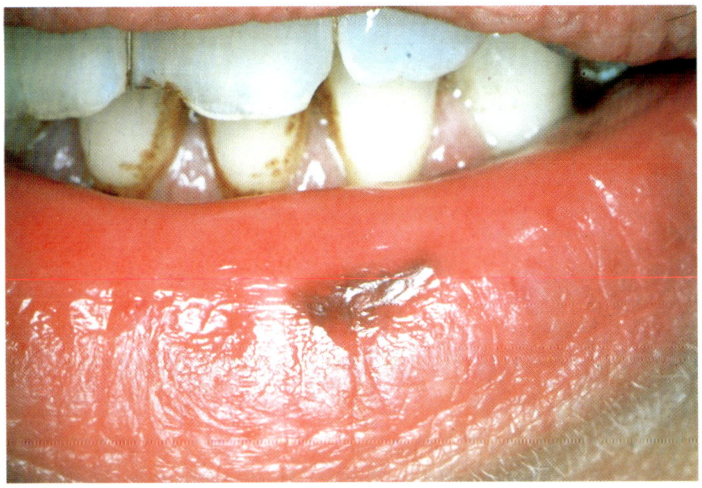
2.72

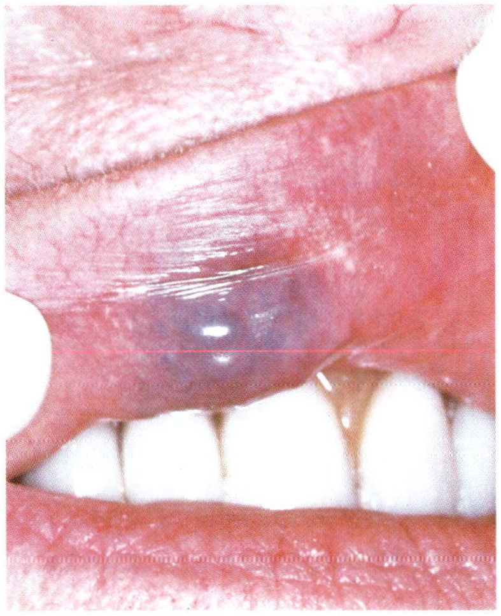
2.73

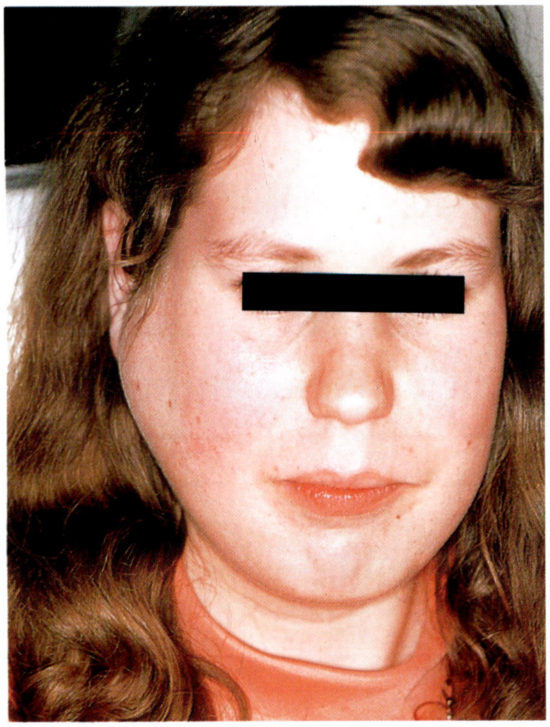
2.74

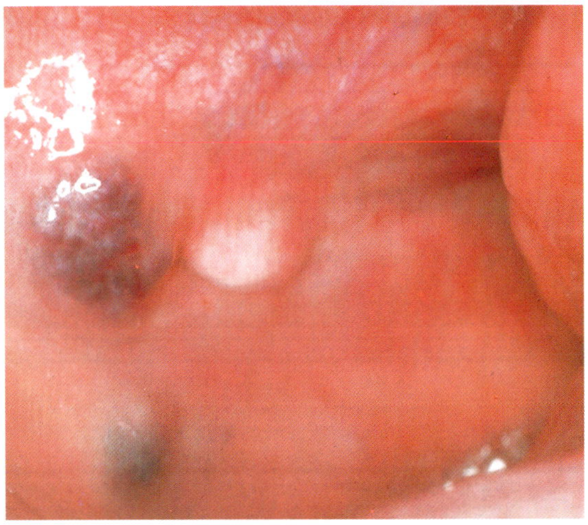
2.75

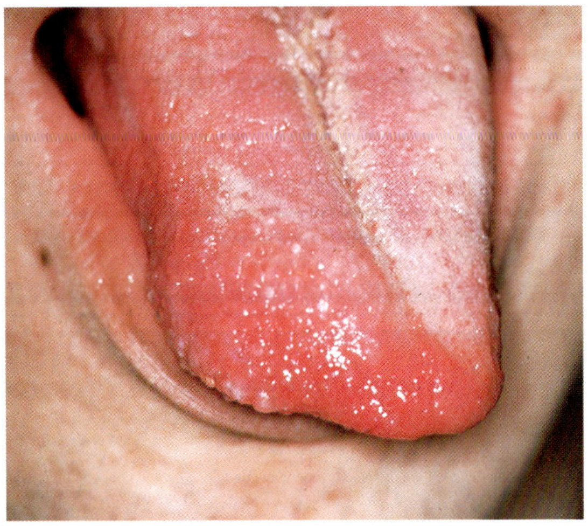
2.76

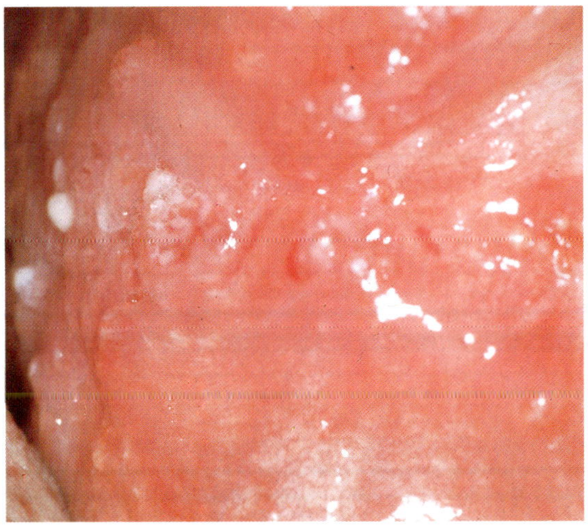
2.77

EPHELIS (*Freckle*)

Figure 2.72 These circumscribed melanotic macules, typically smaller than 0·5 cm, appear on sun-exposed areas in childhood, owing to a local increase in melanin production, in a normal number of melanocytes. Although usually affecting the skin, ephelides may occasionally involve mucous membranes, as here.

HAEMANGIOMA

Figure 2.73 Haemangiomas are fairly common hamartomas in the mouth, especially on the lip.

Figure 2.74 Facial disfiguration here was caused by an haemangioma, although the appearance simulates a parotid swelling.

MAFFUCCI'S SYNDROME

Figure 2.75 Cavernous haemangiomas in the buccal mucosa, adjacent to the parotid papilla. Haemangiomas are typically in the tongue in Maffucci's syndrome, when they are associated with multiple enchondromas elsewhere.

LYMPHANGIOMA

Figure 2.76 Lymphangioma is an hamartoma most common in the anterior tongue or lip.

Figure 2.77 The typical 'frogspawn' appearance of the surface is seen in this lymphangioma of the buccal mucosa.

3

Endocrine, nutritional and metabolic diseases and immunity disorders

CONGENITAL HYPOTHYROIDISM (*Cretinism*)

Figure 3.1 Short stature, mental handicap, and coarse facies are the most obvious features of cretinism. Oral changes include macroglossia, delayed eruption and hypoplasia of the teeth.

DIABETES MELLITUS

Figure 3.2 The oral changes in diabetes are non-specific and seen mainly in severe insulin-dependent diabetics. Parodontal abscesses, infections, and rapid peridontal breakdown are the most obvious features. This figure shows gingivitis in the lower anterior region and an abscess above the right lateral incisor which proved to be a periapical abscess related to the non-vital and discoloured central incisor.

Figure 3.3 Severe periodontal breakdown in a diabetic (there is a healing lesion of herpes labialis on the upper lip).

Other oral lesions in diabetes may include sialosis, median rhomboid glossitis, glossodynia, and lichenoid lesions induced by hypoglycaemic drugs. Dry mouth may be caused by dehydration in diabetes. Mucormycosis is a rare complication.

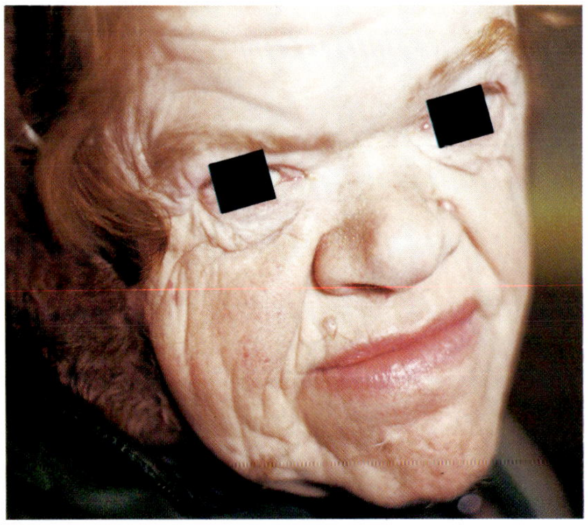

3.1

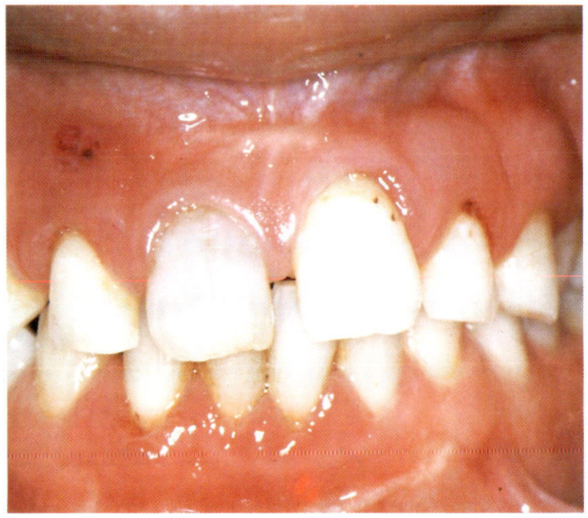

3.2

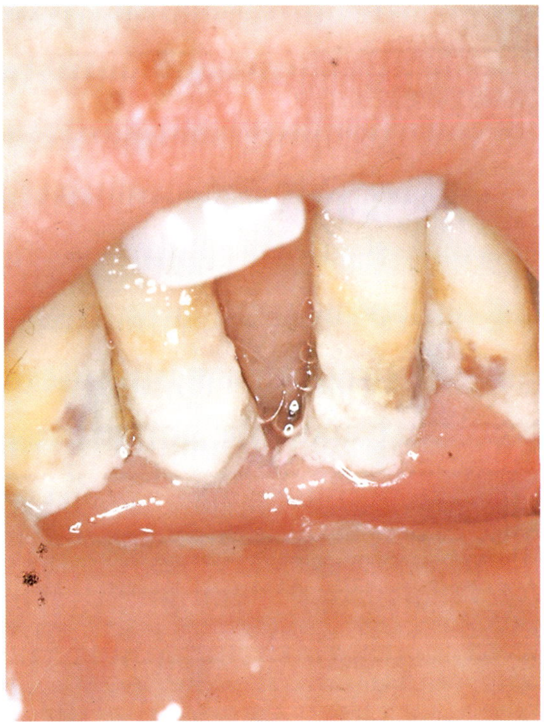

3.3

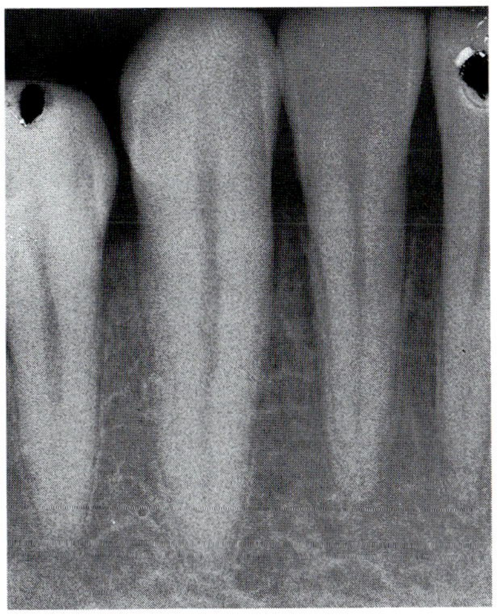

3.4

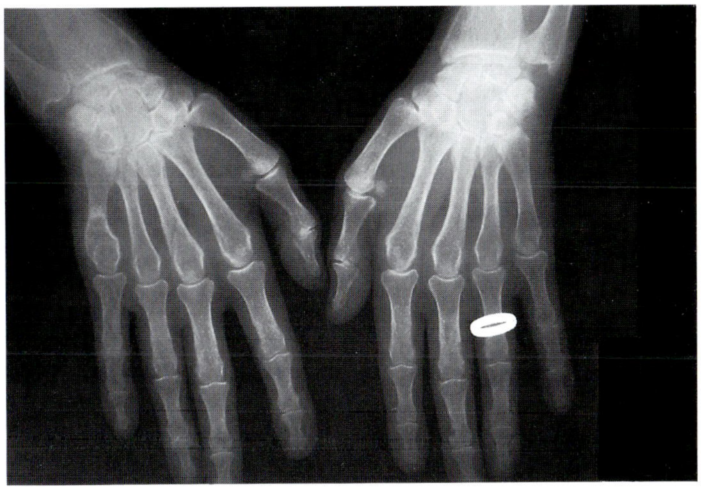

3.5

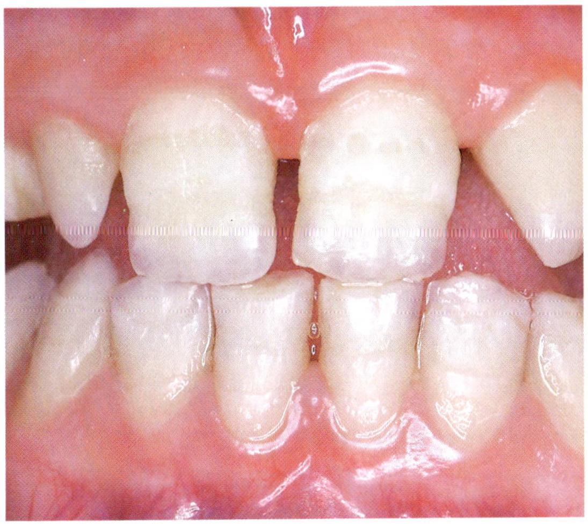

3.6

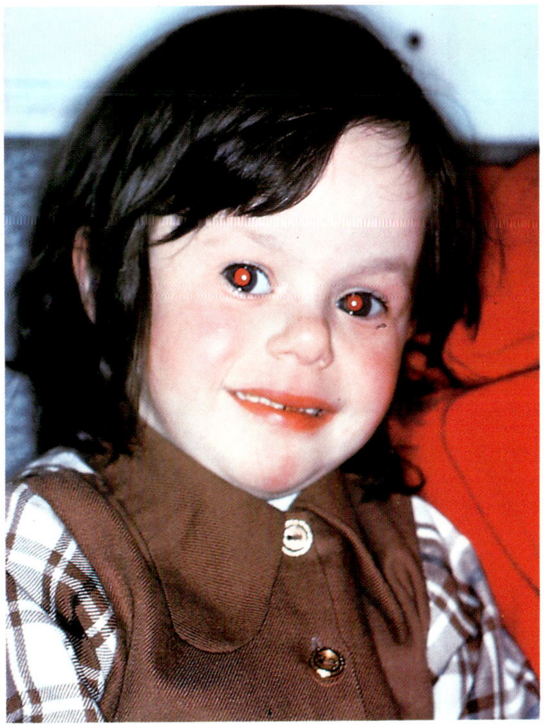

3.7

HYPERPARATHYROIDISM

Figure 3.4 Skeletal changes in primary hyperparathyroidism typically include generalized rarefaction, and sometimes lytic lesions (osteitis fibrosa cystica) but an almost pathognomonic oral change is the loss of the lamina dura, shown here. Almost all patients with primary hyperparathyroidism have skeletal lesions microscopically indistinguishable from the central giant cell granuloma of bone (brown tumours). Skull and jaw involvement is a late complication.

Figure 3.5 The characteristic radiographic sign is subperiosteal bone resorption, and 'tufting' of terminal phalanges, as shown here.

CONGENITAL HYPOPARATHYROIDISM

Figure 3.6 In congenital hypoparathyroidism, there may be severe hypoplasia of the teeth, as shown here, shortened roots and retarded eruption.

Rare patients with candida-endocrinopathy syndrome and with Di George syndrome also have chronic mucocutaneous candidosis (see page 30), as well as hypoparathyroidism.

Acquired hypoparathyroidism produces facial tetany but no oral manifestations.

Figure 3.7 Pseudohypoparathyroidism: elfin facies, short stature, short metatarsals and metacarpals, calcified basal ganglia and enamel hypoplasia are features of this rare, complex, dominant disorder, possibly sex-linked. Parathyroid hormone is secreted, but the end organs are unresponsive. There is also an association with other endocrine disorders, particularly hypothyroidism.

ACROMEGALY

Figure 3.8 Acromegaly results from increased growth hormone secretion by a pituitary adenoma.

Mandibular prognathism, generalized thickening of soft tissues, including the tongue, and spacing of the teeth are typical of acromegaly.

Figure 3.9 Spaced teeth.

Figure 3.10 Large hands.

Figure 3.11 Enlarged pituitary fossa, as a result of the causal pituitary adenoma, and enlarged supraorbital ridges and mandible are obvious on this radiograph. Headache and tunnel vision (bitemporal hemianopia) may result eventually as the pituitary neoplasm enlarges.

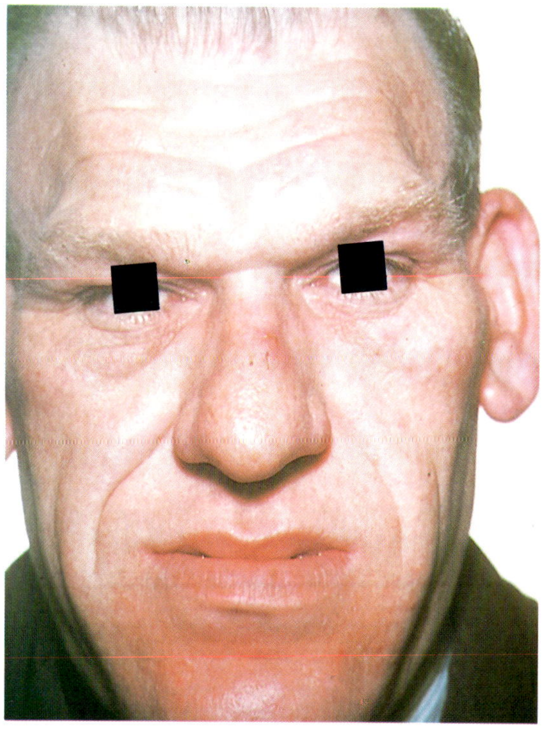

3.8

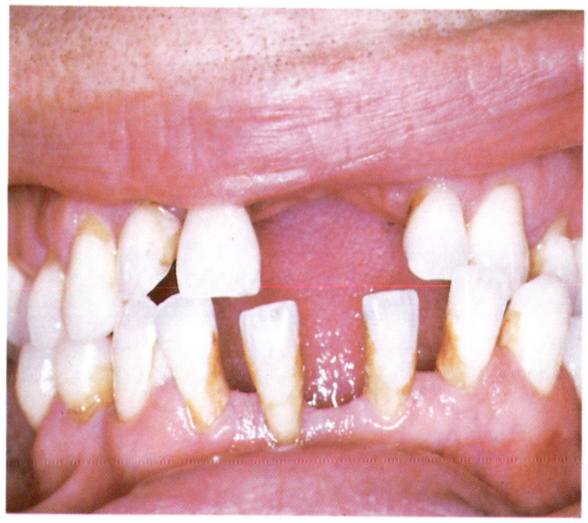

3.9

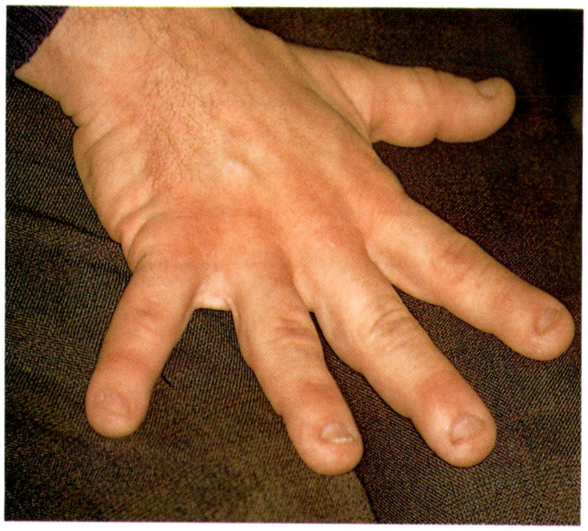

3.10

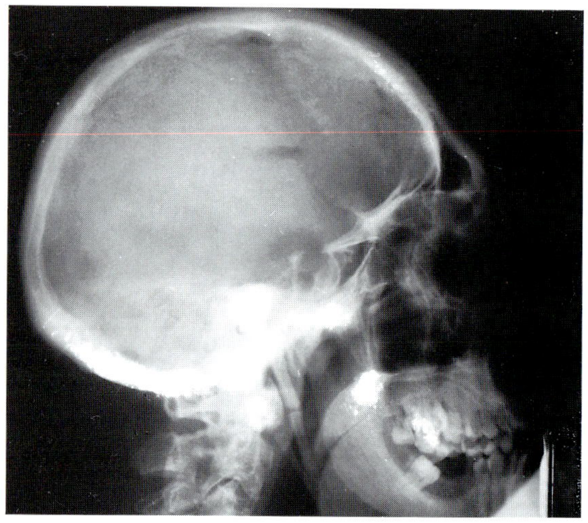

3.11

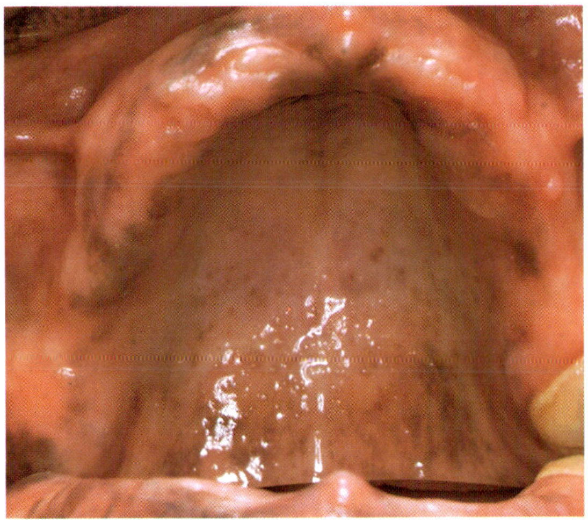

3.12

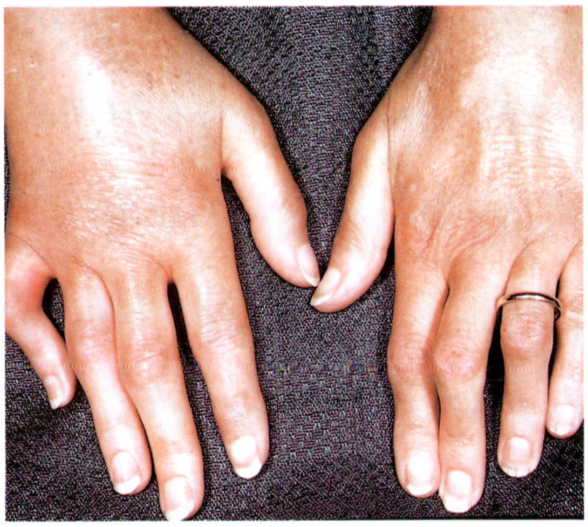

3.13

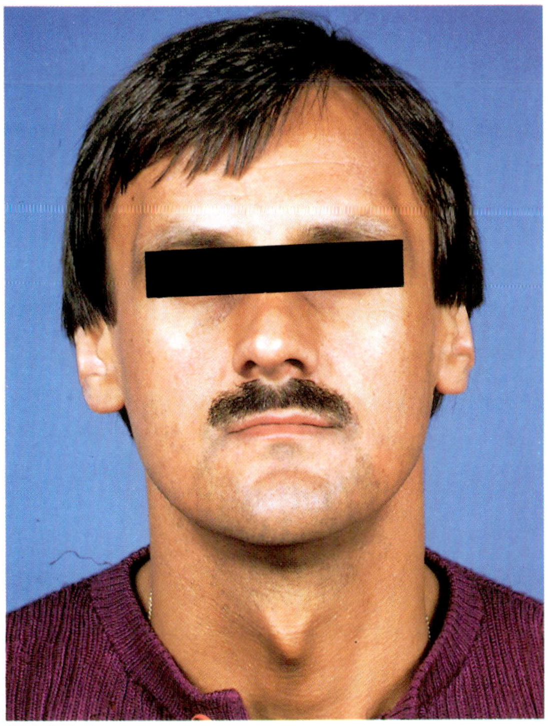

3.14

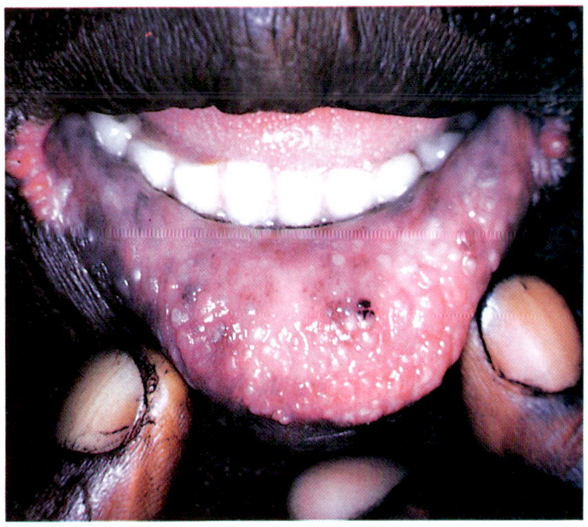

3.15

ADDISON'S DISEASE (*Hypo-adrenocorticism*)

Figure 3.12 Addison's disease is hypo-adrenocorticism, often of autoimmune aetiology, but may be caused by tumour, tuberculosis or, rarely, histoplasmosis. Lower plasma cortisol levels result in increased pituitary secretion of ACTH and precursor hormones with MSH like activity.

Oral hyperpigmentation of a brown, grey or black colour is typical of Addison's disease, although most patients with oral hyperpigmentation prove to have other causes.

Figure 3.13 Generalized Addisonian skin hyperpigmentation.

There are occasional associations of Addison's disease with other diseases, particularly autoimmune diseases, such as the probable TASS syndrome of thyroiditis, Addison's disease, Sjögren's syndrome and sarcoidosis. This patient also has incidental Dupuytren's contractures.

Figure 3.14 Facial hyperpigmentation in Addison's disease. Similar hyperpigmentation is also seen in Nelson's syndrome (increased ACTH production after bilateral adrenalectomy).

MULTIPLE ENDOCRINE ADENOMA SYNDROME TYPE III

Figure 3.15 Oral mucosal neuromas are associated with medullary cell carcinoma of the thyroid, phaeochromocytoma and, occasionally, hyperparathyroidism in the type III multiple endocrine adenoma syndrome. Patients may have a Marfanoid habitus.

VITAMIN B DEFICIENCY

Figure 3.16 Atrophic glossitis in a child with malabsorption syndrome. The tongue is completely depapillated and smooth. Oral ulcers and angular stomatitis are also common features. This particular child had coeliac disease, associated with selective IgA deficiency (see page 64).

Figure 3.17 Angular stomatitis is seen particularly in vitamin B_{12} and in riboflavin deficiency, and is also seen in iron or folate deficiency. The most common cause of angular stomatitis, however, is candidosis (see page 29).

VITAMIN B_{12} DEFICIENCY

Figure 3.18 Atrophic glossitis. In Western countries, vitamin B_{12} deficiency is rarely dietary in origin. Usually it is due to pernicious anaemia, gastric or small intestinal disease. Gastric bypass surgery for morbid obesity is a cause recently described.

Figure 3.19 Red lines or red patches, as shown here on the ventrum of the tongue (Moeller's glossitis), are fairly typical of early vitamin B_{12} deficiency.

Figure 3.20 Pernicious anaemia is characterized often by premature greying of the hair and blue eyes, and may progress to neurological damage, especially subacute combined degeneration of the spinal cord.

DEFICIENCY OF HAEMATINICS

Figure 3.21 Deficiency of haematinics (iron, vitamin B_{12}, or folic acid) can manifest with glossitis, angular stomatitis and mouth ulcers, shown here. A significant proportion of patients with classical clinical aphthae prove to be deficient in an haematinic.

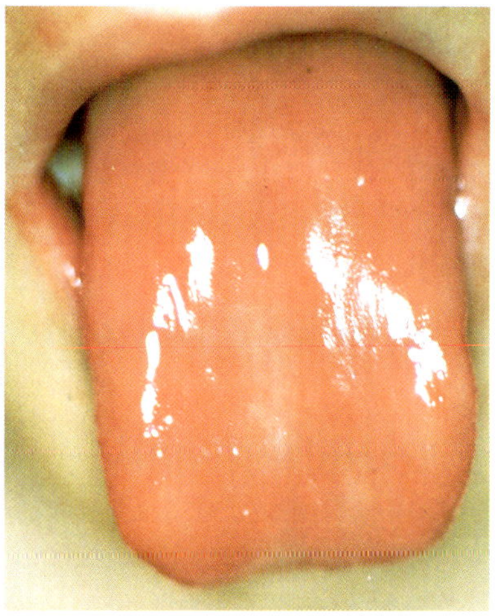

3.16

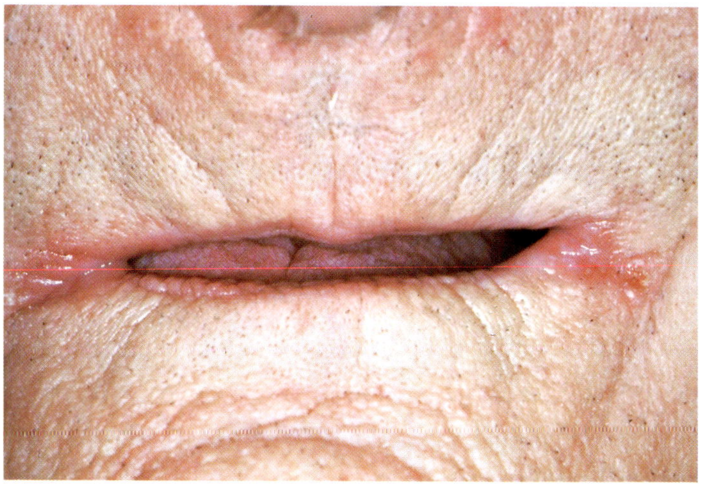

3.17

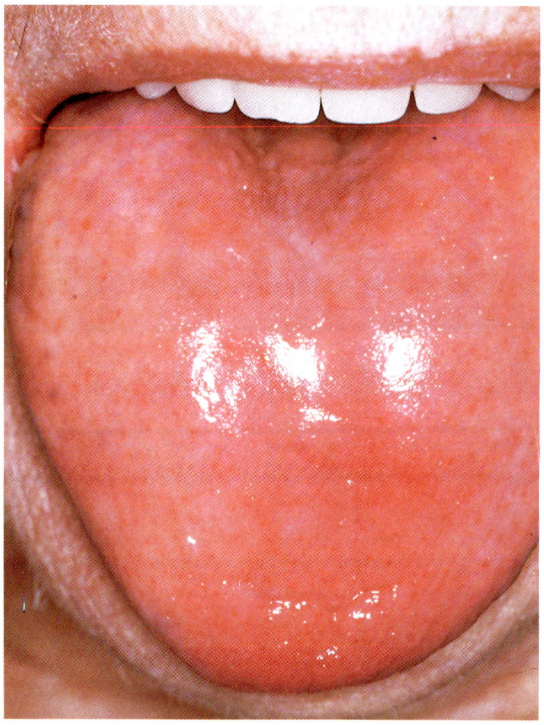

3.18

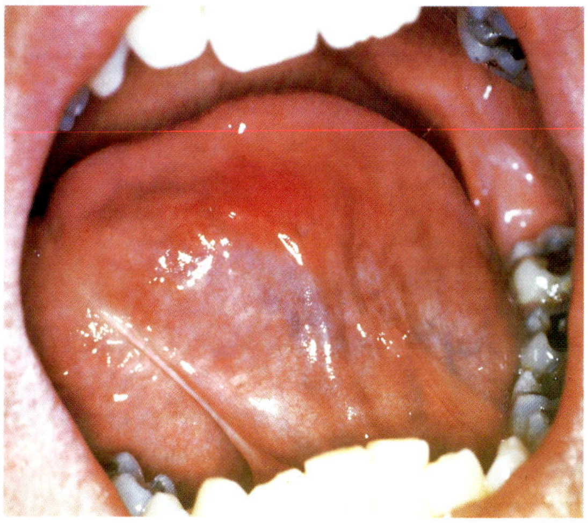

3.19

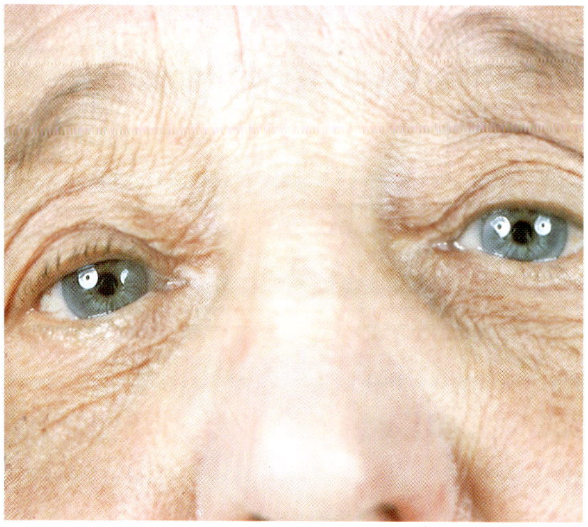

3.20

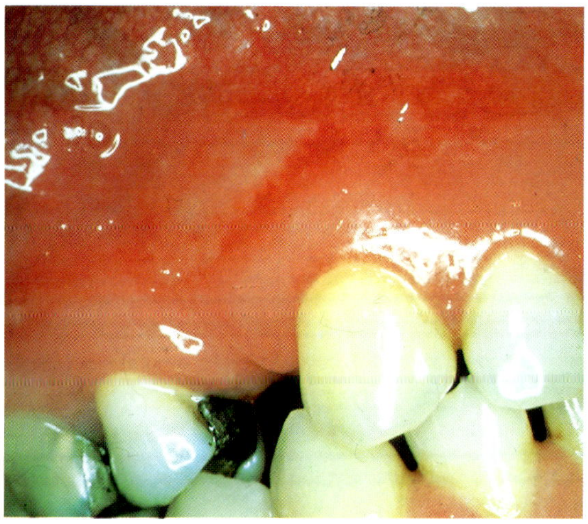

3.21

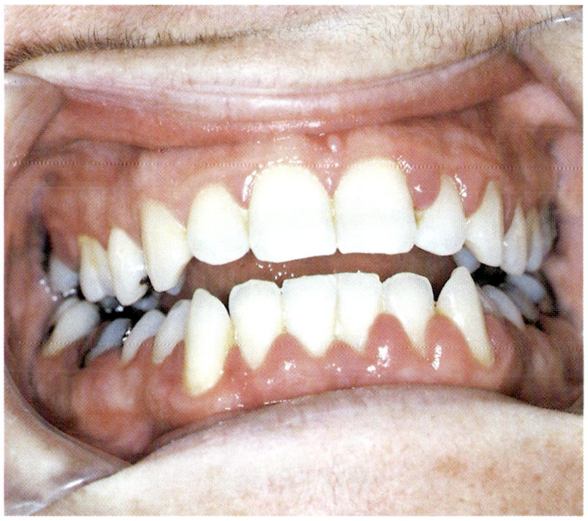
3.22

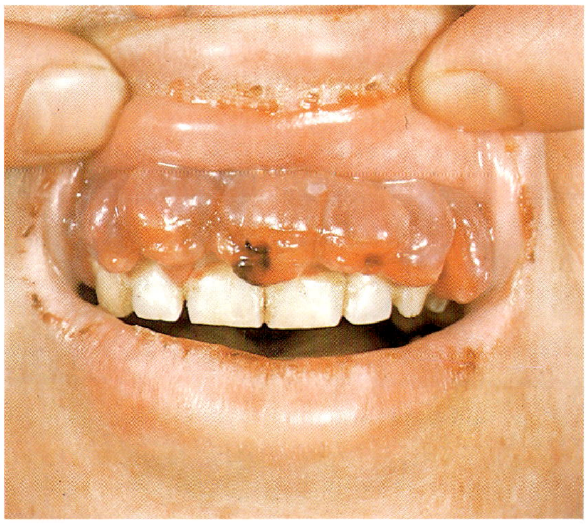
3.23

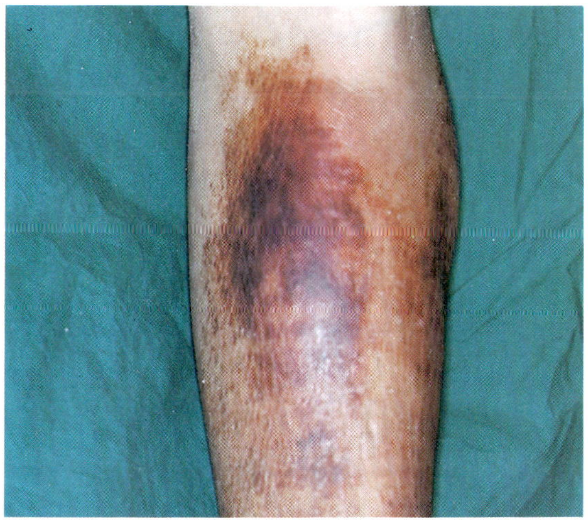
3.24

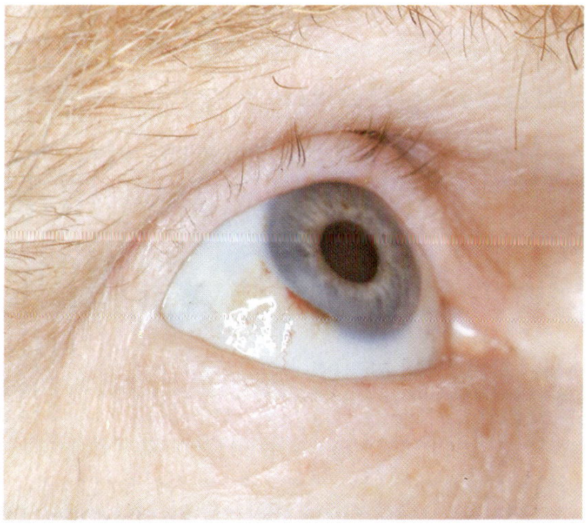
3.25

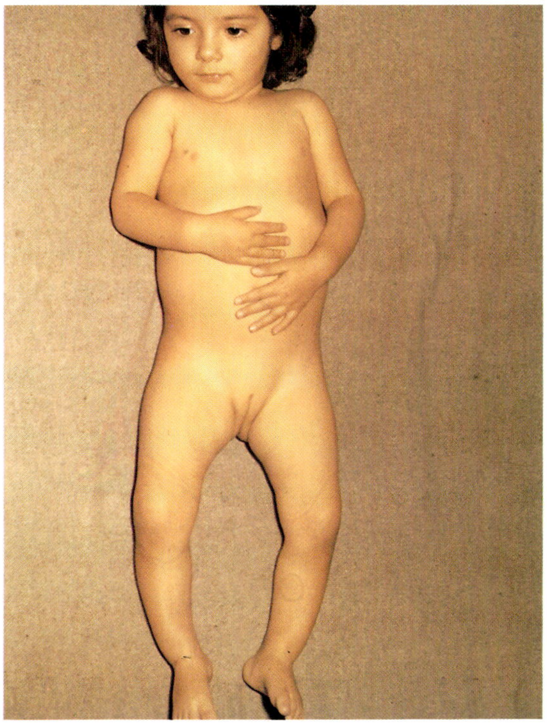
3.26

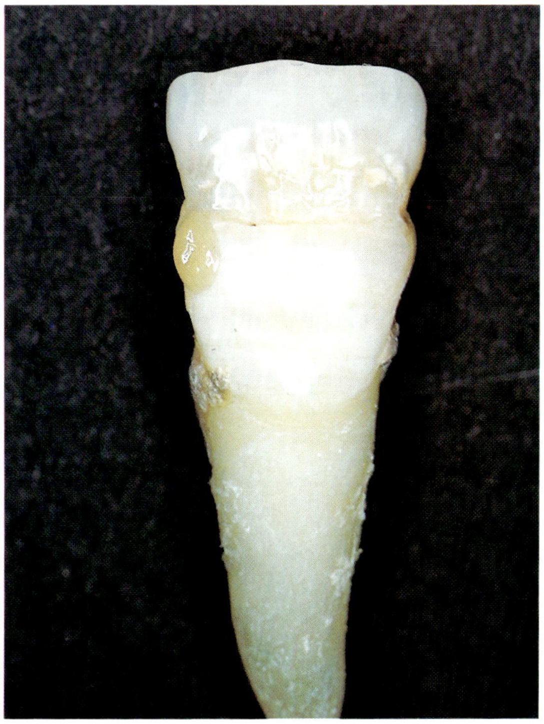
3.27

SCURVY
(*Vitamin C deficiency*)

Figure 3.22 Although rare in Western countries, scurvy is an occasional cause of gingival hyperplasia, as here. Most patients develop scurvy because they have an abnormal diet, lacking in fresh vegetables.

Figure 3.23 Gingival hyperplasia with purpura in severe scurvy is reminiscent of leukaemia.

Figure 3.24 Perifollicular haemorrhages are typical of scurvy but occasionally there may be more severe purpura, as here. Cutaneous bleeding is most obvious on the legs and buttocks.

Figure 3.25 Small subconjunctival haemorrhage in scurvy.

RICKETS
(*Vitamin D deficiency*)

Figure 3.26 Rickets is uncommon in Western countries, but has been recorded recently in Asian patients living in environments where they are exposed to relatively little sunlight and with a diet rich in phytate (found in chuppatti flour), which chelates dietary calcium.

Figure 3.27 Enamel hypoplasia has been seen only in extremely severe rickets where tooth eruption may also be retarded (see also renal rickets, page 160).

AMYLOIDOSIS

Figure 3.28 Amyloidosis is a group of diseases in which one of a range of materials is deposited in tissues. Deposits are sufficiently large in size to give a characteristically fibrillar structure on electron microscopy, and green birefringence on polarization microscopy after Congo Red staining. Amyloid L arises from immunoglobulin light chains, amyloid A, from amyloid A protein, and others are from prealbumin, gamma-trace protein, or beta-2-microglobulin.

Primary amyloidosis (that associated with plasma cell dyscrasias) particularly affects males over the age of 50 years and is the type of amyloid most commonly associated with deposits in the oral mucosa and sub-endocardium. Macroglossia is typical. The tongue is large, firm and indurated and may show red nodules and/or petechiae, especially at the lateral margins.

The tongue may also be involved in beta-2-microglobulin amyloidosis in patients on long-term haemodialysis and the palate may be red and swollen in Franklin's gamma heavy-chain disease.

Figure 3.29 Petechiae, ecchymoses or blood-filled blisters may be seen, as there is an acquired deficiency of blood coagulation factor X in patients with the light chain type of amyloid found in plasma cell dyscrasias.

Figure 3.30 Subconjunctival haemorrhage in the patient shown in Figure 3.29, who subsequently died from amyloid nephropathy, detected through his heavy proteinuria and glycosuria.

Secondary types of amyloidosis – most of those associated with deposits other than of light chains – rarely affect the mouth.

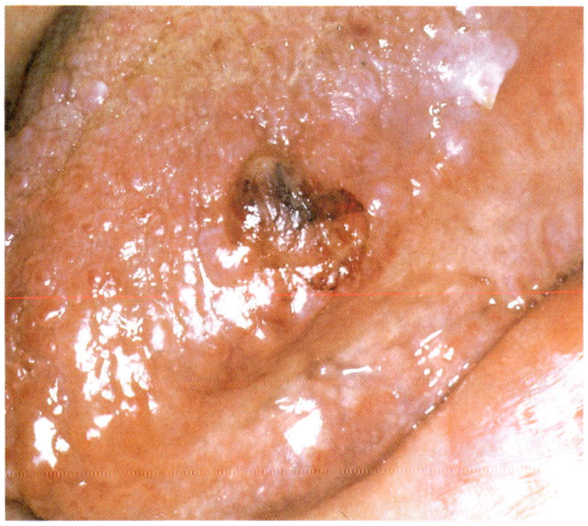

3.28

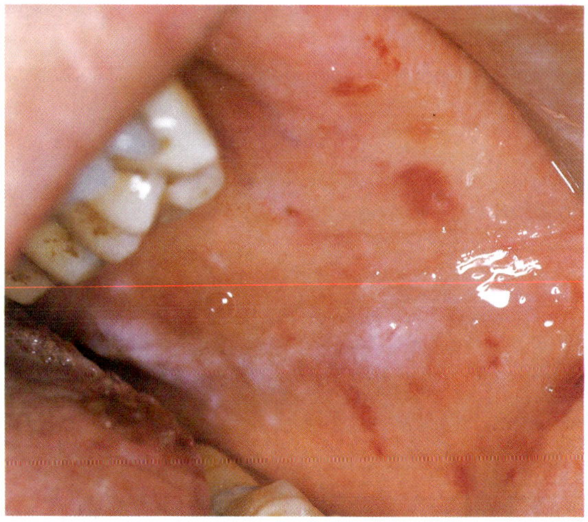

3.29

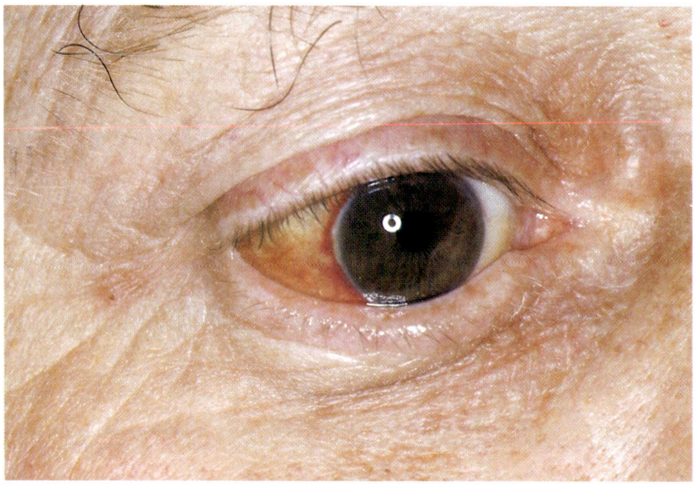

3.30

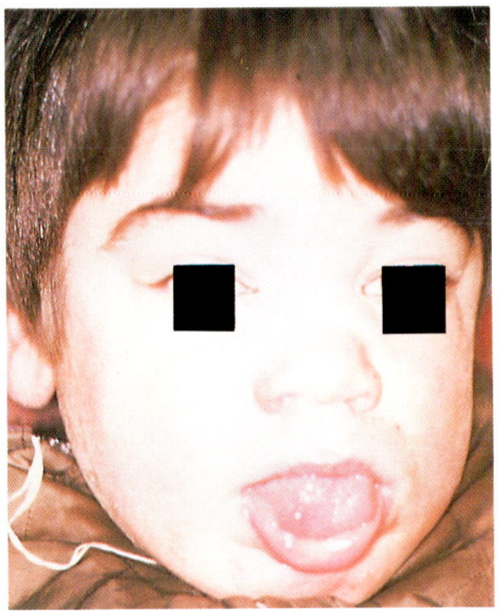

3.31

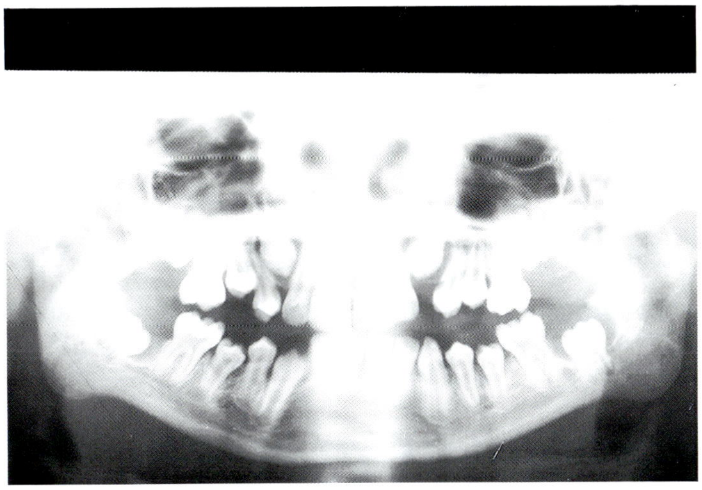

3.32

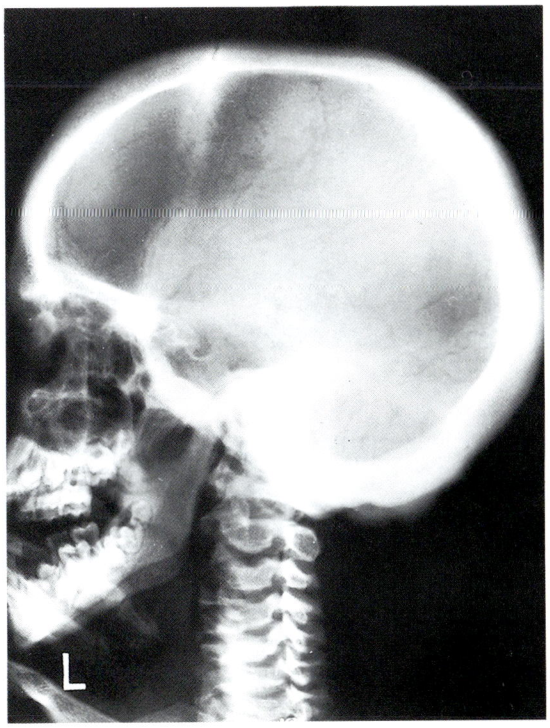

3.33

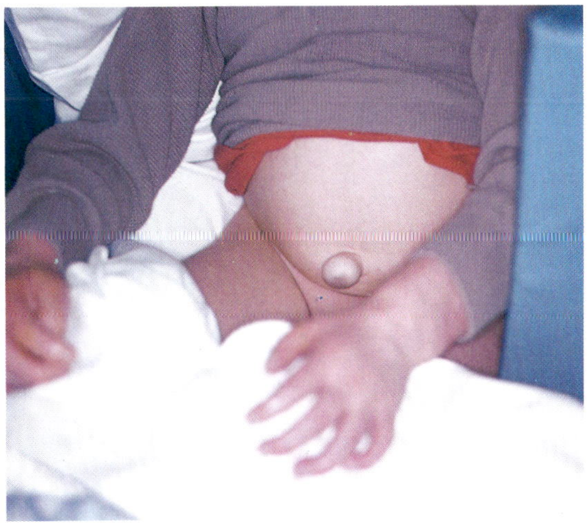

3.34

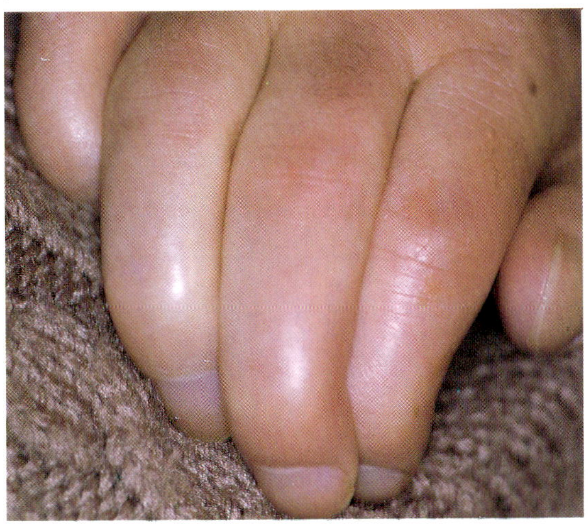

3.35

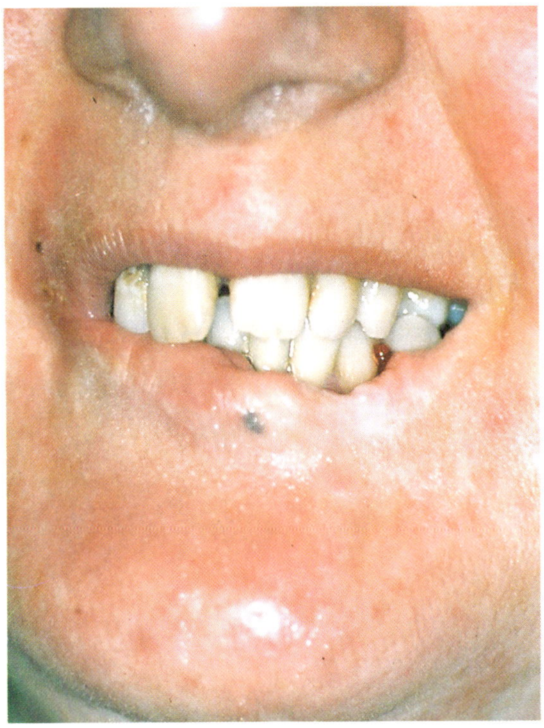

3.36

MUCOPOLY-SACCHARIDOSIS (*Hurler's syndrome or gargoylism*)

Figure 3.31 Deficiency of mucopolysaccharidases leads to the accumulation of mucopolysaccharides (glycosaminoglycans) and one of a number of syndromes, characterized by dwarfism, hirsutism, coarse features, and macroglossia, often with mental handicap, deafness, cardiac failure and corneal clouding. Hurler's syndrome is the most common of these disorders.

Figure 3.32 Hurler's syndrome manifests in early childhood with deteriorating mental and physical development. There are frequent upper respiratory infections, cardiomegaly and murmurs. Delayed or incomplete eruption of teeth, as here, and radiolucent lesions around the crowns of the lower second molars may be seen, as well as temporo-mandibular joint anomalies.

Figure 3.33 The head is large with premature closure of sagittal and metopic sutures. The pituitary fossa is boot- or slipper-shaped.

Figure 3.34 Hepatosplenomegaly causes abdominal swelling, and umbilical hernia is common.

Figure 3.35 Characteristic 'claw hand' occurs because the joints cannot be fully extended. There are also flexion contractures in many other joints. Talipes is common.

LESCH-NYHAN SYNDROME

Figure 3.36 Sex-linked hyperuricaemia, owing to deficiency of the enzyme hypoxanthine guanine phosphoribosyl transferase, is associated with mental handicap, choreoathetosis, and self-mutilation especially of the tongue and lip.

SELECTIVE IgA DEFICIENCY

Figure 3.37 Selective IgA deficiency is the most common primary (genetically determined) immune defect. Some patients are healthy but those who also lack IgG_2 suffer recurrent respiratory infection, autoimmune disorders and atopy. Many have mouth ulcers, and there may be a reduced protection against dental caries.

AGAMMA-GLOBULINAEMIA (*Bruton's syndrome*)

Figure 3.38 Panhypoimmunoglobulinaemia affects males almost exclusively, and presents mainly with recurrent pyogenic respiratory infections. Several patients with mouth ulcers have been recorded.

Figure 3.39 Severe infections in the neonate can disturb odontogenesis, causing enamel hypoplasia. In the past, tetracycline treatment caused tooth discoloration, as here.

CELL-MEDIATED IMMUNODEFICIENCY

Figure 3.40 Chronic oral candidosis, which may present, as here, with angular stomatitis, is an early and prominent feature in any cell-mediated immune defect, and there is a predisposition to recurrent lesions of herpes simplex and varicella-zoster virus.

Figure 3.41 Oral thrush is an early feature of many T lymphocyte defects.

Figure 3.42 Herpes labialis is often reactivated during immunosuppression of the cellular response, as in this patient on systemic corticosteroids.

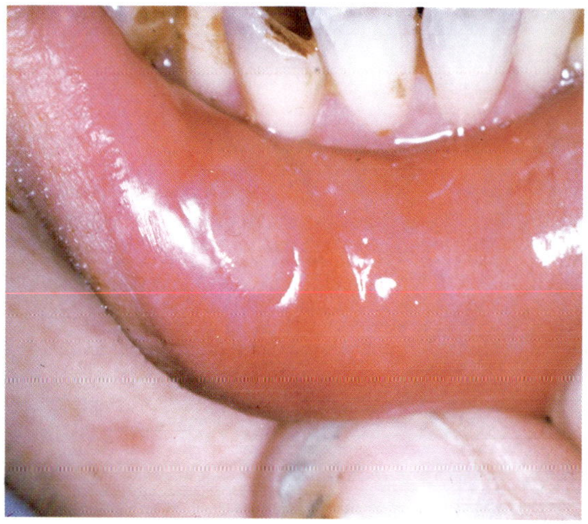

3.37

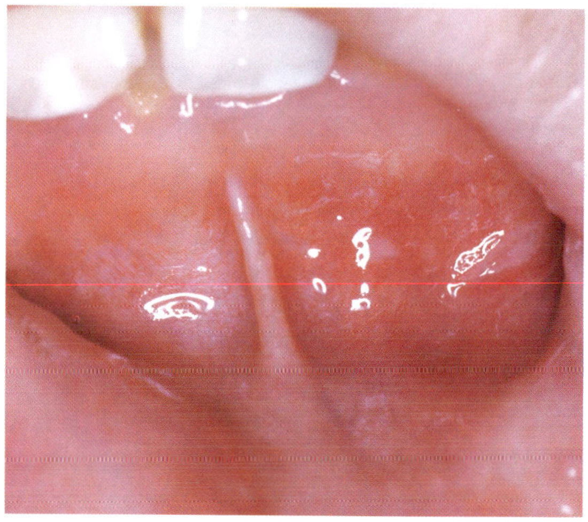

3.38

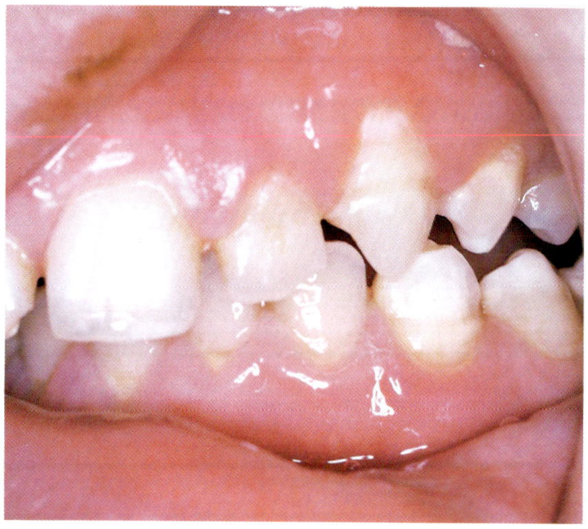

3.39

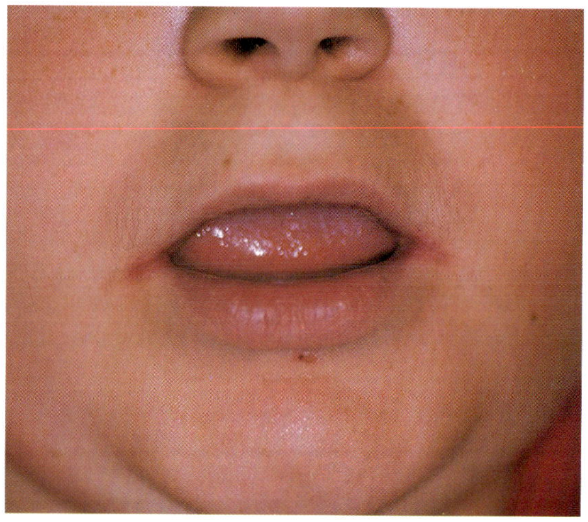

3.40

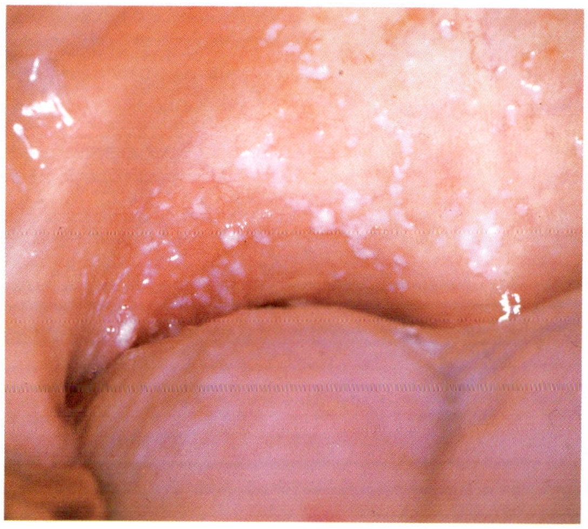

3.41

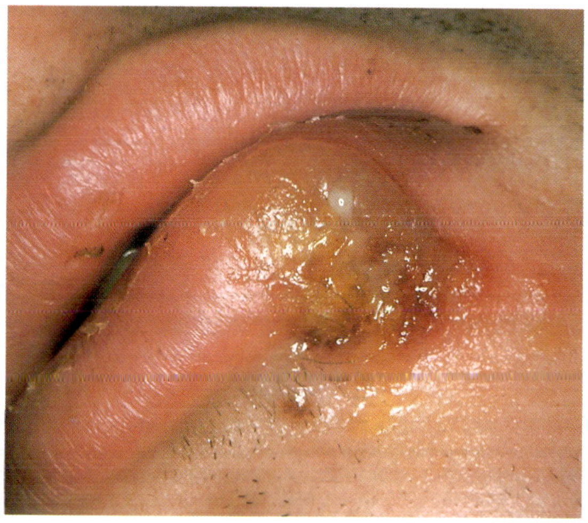

3.42

4

Diseases of the blood and blood-forming organs

IRON DEFICIENCY

Figure 4.1 The most common cause of iron deficiency in Western countries is chronic haemorrhage. When bone marrow iron stores are depleted, there is a stage of iron deficiency without anaemia (sideropenia) before red cell changes are evident. Angular stomatitis is one oral manifestation which may be seen in the pre-anaemic stage as well as in anaemia.

Figure 4.2 Angular stomatitis is soreness and sometimes fissuring at the commissure. Usually of local aetiology, related to candidosis beneath an upper denture, it is occasionally precipitated by a deficiency of iron, folate or vitamin B (see also page 29).

Figure 4.3 Besides angular stomatitis, this patient also has a sore red depapillated tongue (glossitis). Although deficiency of iron or other haematinics can cause sore tongue with atrophic glossitis, many haematinic deficient patients with a sore tongue have no obvious organic lesion. Oral ulceration is sometimes a manifestation of iron deficiency.

Figure 4.4 Spoon-shaped nails (koilonychia) which tend to split are typical of iron deficiency anaemia.

Other deficiency anaemias are discussed in Chapter 3. Haemoglobinopathies such as sickle cell anaemia and thalassaemias may present with maxillary hyperplasia owing to marrow overgrowth.

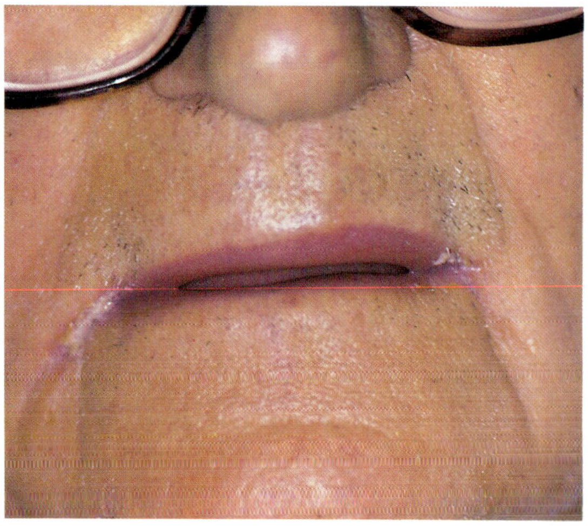

4.1

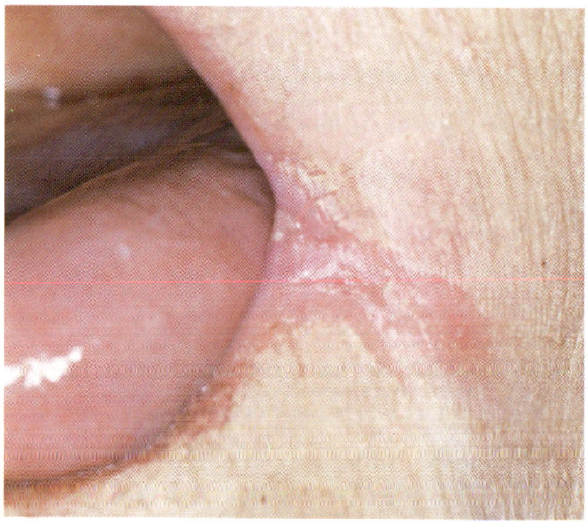

4.2

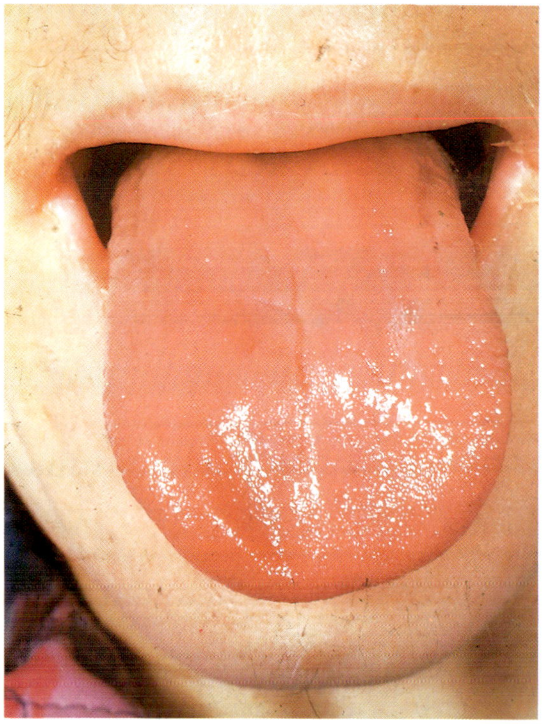

4.3

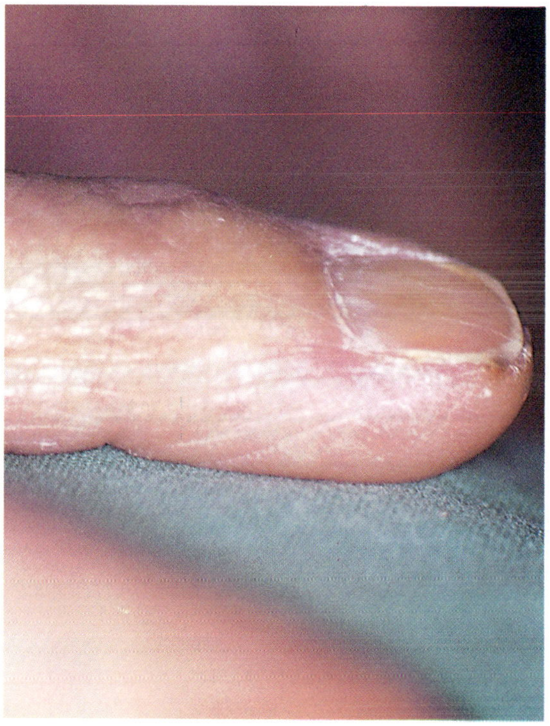

4.4

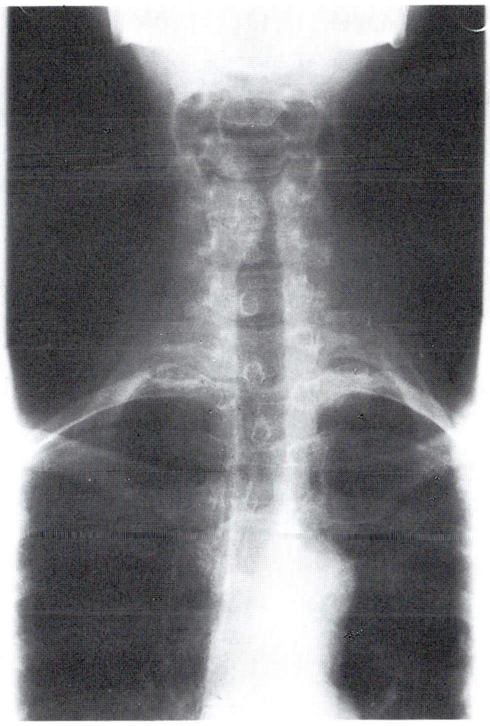

4.5

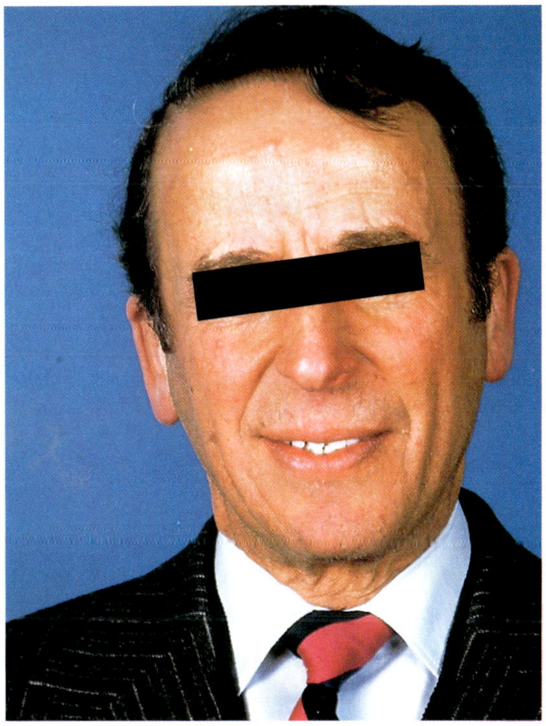

4.6

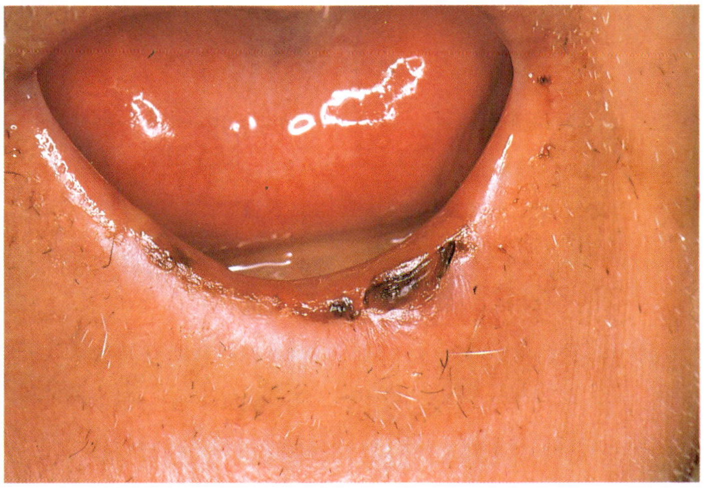

4.7

PLUMMER-VINSON SYNDROME (*Patterson-Kelly syndrome*)

Figure 4.5 In this syndrome (sideropenic dysphagia), patients typically are middle-aged with dysphagia, caused by an oesophageal web, often with candidosis, hypochromic microcytic anaemia, koilonychia and a depapillated tongue. There is a predisposition to post-cricoid carcinoma, illustrated here, and to oral carcinoma.

POLYCYTHAEMIA RUBRA VERA

Figure 4.6 Polycythaemia rubra vera is a primary myeloproliferative disorder characterized by increased numbers of red cells (giving a plethoric appearance, as here), increased granulocytes, and increased but dysfunctional platelets.

Figure 4.7 Cytotoxic therapy of the disease may lead to neutropenic oral ulceration and an increased bleeding tendency, as here. Secondary polycythaemia is associated with compensatory or inappropriate erythropoietin release in cardiorespiratory disease, heavy smoking, or in association with a variety of tumours, such as renal carcinoma or cerebellar haemangioblastoma, and recently has been associated with malignant fibrous histiocytoma of the parotid gland.

MYELODYSPLASTIC SYNDROME

Figure 4.8 In this syndrome, there is a functional neutropenia as a result of disordered granulopoiesis. The lingual ulcer in this myelodysplastic patient notably lacks an inflammatory halo.

APLASTIC ANAEMIA

Figure 4.9 Clinical features of aplastic anaemia depend on the predominant cell type affected and aplastic anaemia may therefore present as signs and symptoms of thrombocytopenia, leukopenia, anaemia or a combination of all three (pancytopenia). In this case, thrombocytopenia is most profound and spontaneous purpuric or ecchymotic haemorrhages of the skin and mucous membrane are the presenting features.

Figure 4.10 Leucopenia (particularly neutropenia) leads to decreased resistance to infection, manifest as severe ulceration, often associated with opportunistic organisms. Typically there is, as in agranulocytosis, only a minimal red inflammatory halo around the ulcers.

Bone marrow transplantation is often the treatment for aplastic anaemia. Oral complications include mucositis, candidosis, parotitis, graft-versus-host disease with lichenoid or sclerodermatous reactions, and infections with herpes viruses or fungi, such as aspergillus (see page 33). Xerostomia predisposes to caries.

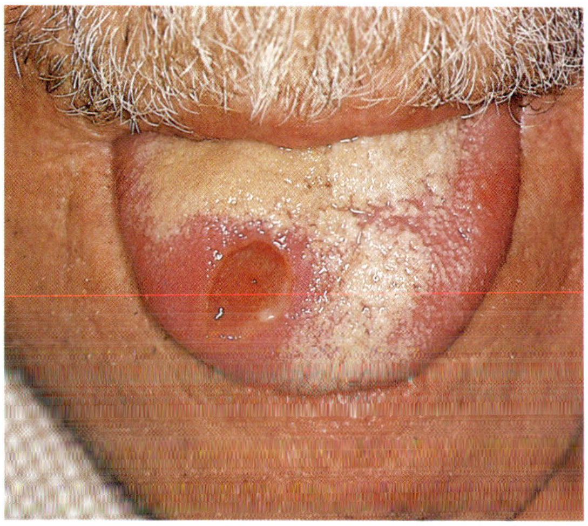

4.8

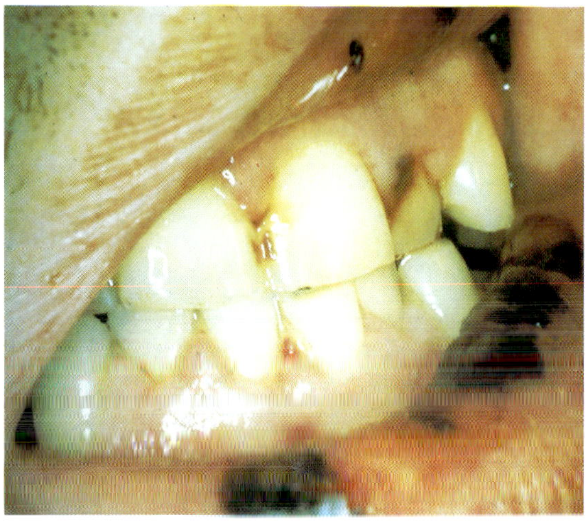

4.9

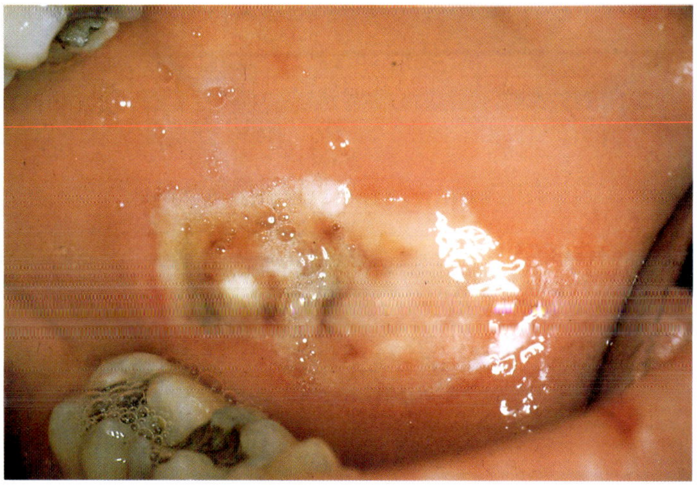

4.10

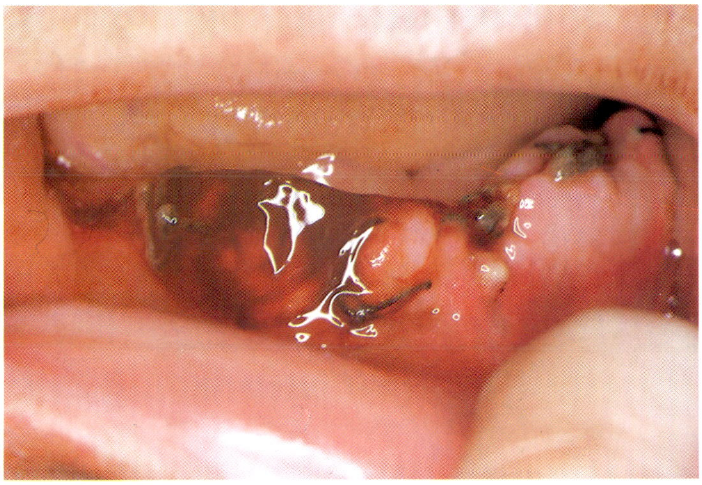

4.11

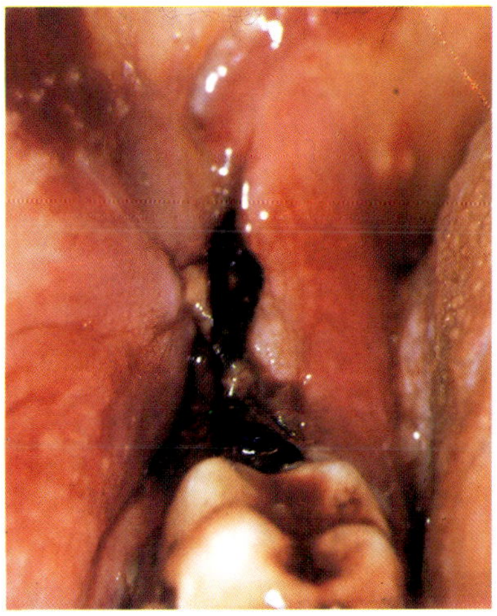

4.12

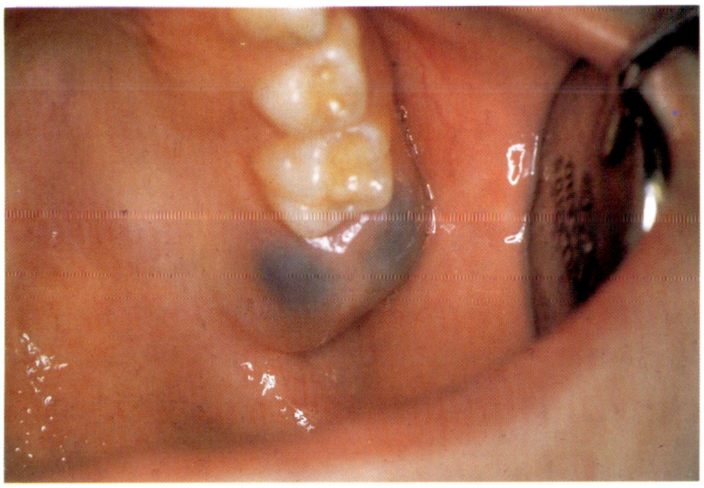

4.13

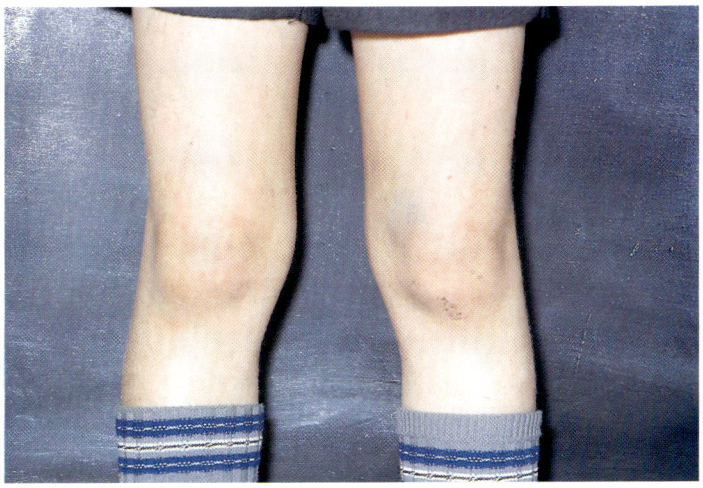

4.14

HAEMOPHILIAS

Figure 4.11 Defects of blood coagulation factors, unlike thrombocytopenia, do not predispose to spontaneous gingival haemorrhage, oral petechiae or ecchymoses. Any breach of the mucosa, however, especially tooth extraction, can lead to persistent bleeding that is occasionally fatal. Haemorrhage after extraction here was controlled with factor VIII replacement. Surgery must only be carried out with factor VIII replacement.

Figure 4.12 One danger is that haemorrhage into the fascial spaces, especially from surgery in the lower molar region, can track into the neck and embarrass the airway. This patient had von Willebrand's disease. The combined factor VIII defect and platelet abnormality in von Willebrand's disease can sometimes be more serious than classic haemophilia A.

Figure 4.13 Tooth eruption and exfoliation are usually uneventful but, occasionally, as here, there can be a small bleed into the follicle (of the upper left first molar) in this patient.

Figure 4.14 Haemophilia A (classic haemophilia) is ten times as common as haemophilia B (Christmas disease). Deep haemorrhage is a serious complication of both. Trauma predisposes to bleeding, though it can be spontaneous. Haemarthrosis, as here, can be crippling.

HIV infection may manifest orally in patients given blood transfusions, or factor replacement before heat-treated factors were available.

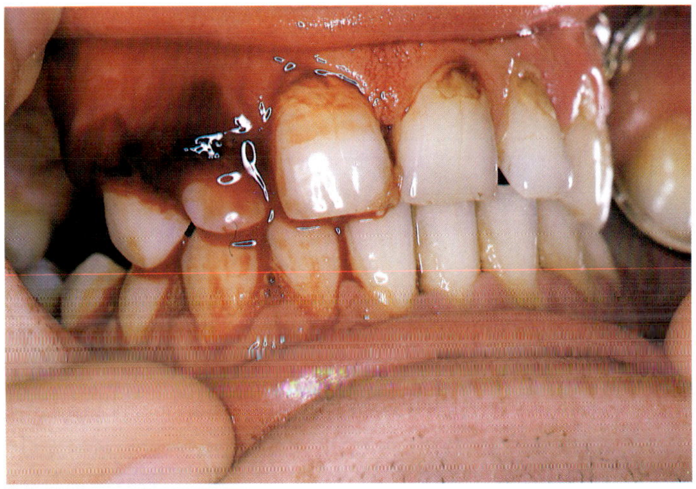

4.15

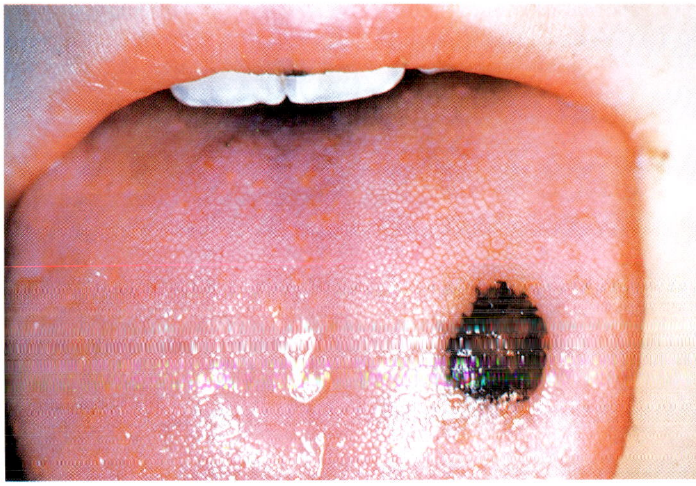

4.16

THROMBOCYTOPENIA

Figure 4.15 Spontaneous gingival bleeding is often an early feature in platelet deficiencies or defects.

Figure 4.16 Oral petechiae and ecchymoses appear mainly at sites of trauma but can be spontaneous. Post-extraction bleeding may be a problem.

Figure 4.17 Petechiae appear mainly in the buccal mucosa, on the lateral margin of the tongue, and at the junction of hard and soft palates – sites readily traumatized.

Figure 4.18 Petechiae and ecchymoses appear readily on the skin, especially if there is trauma. Even the pressure from a sphygmomanometer can cause petechiae during the measurement of blood pressure.

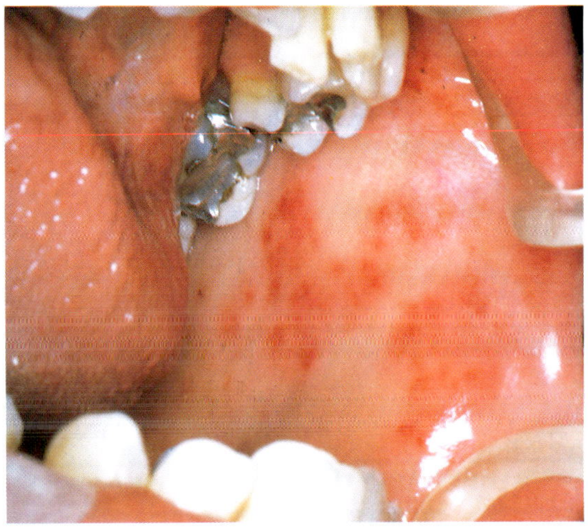

4.17

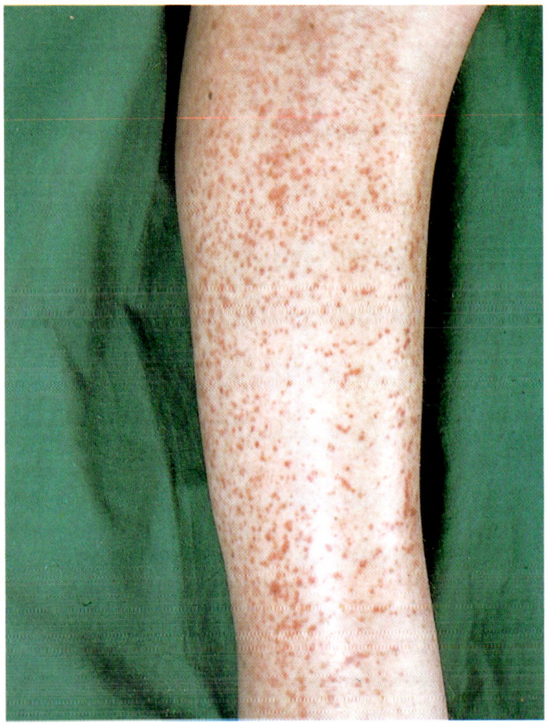

4.18

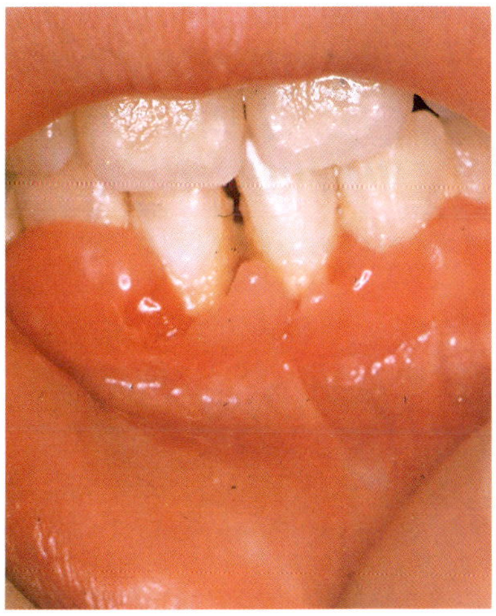

4.19

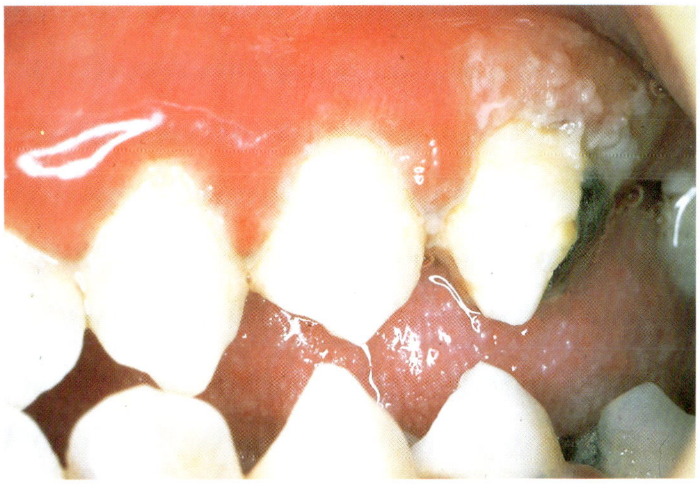

4.20

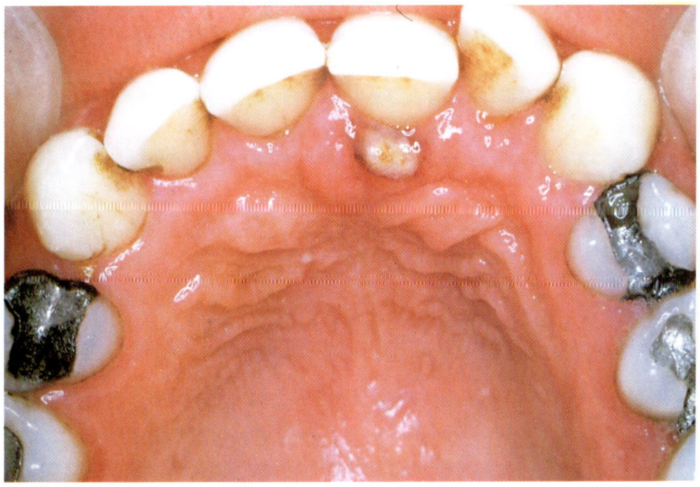

4.21

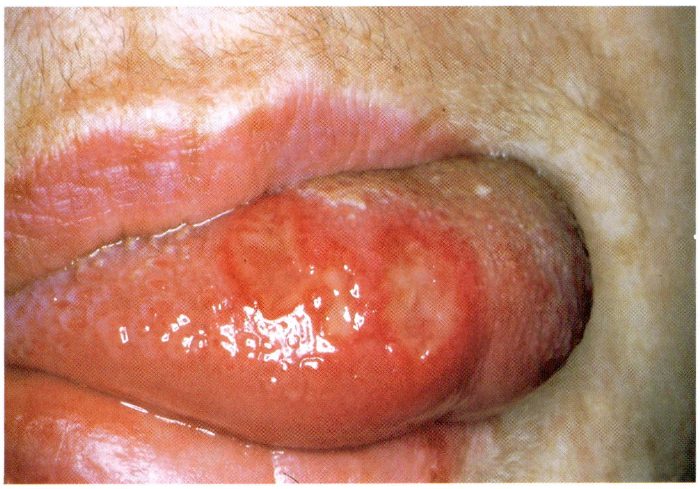

4.22

CHRONIC NEUTROPENIA

Figure 4.19 Neutropenias predispose to rapidly destructive periodontal disease and to oral ulceration.

CYCLIC NEUTROPENIA

Figure 4.20 Early onset: neutropenia may be cyclical with a drop in polymorphonuclear neutrophil count, and sometimes other leukocytes, every 21 days. Destructive periodontal disease, recurrent ulcerative gingivitis and recurrent mouth ulcers are frequent manifestations, as in this 14-year-old boy who had a history, dating from early childhood, of recurrent pyogenic infections.

Figure 4.21 Late onset: recurrent mouth ulcers are a common presentation of cyclic neutropenia. Palatal ulceration in this site is rare in aphthae and suggested an immune defect which proved to be neutropenia.

Figure 4.22 Late onset: recurrent mouth ulcers in neutropenias, leukaemias, and some cell-mediated immune defects are sometimes intraoral herpes simplex recurrences.

Gangrene may be seen in patients with neutropenia or rare neutrophil defects such as acatalasia (seen mainly in Japan, Korea, Israel and Switzerland).

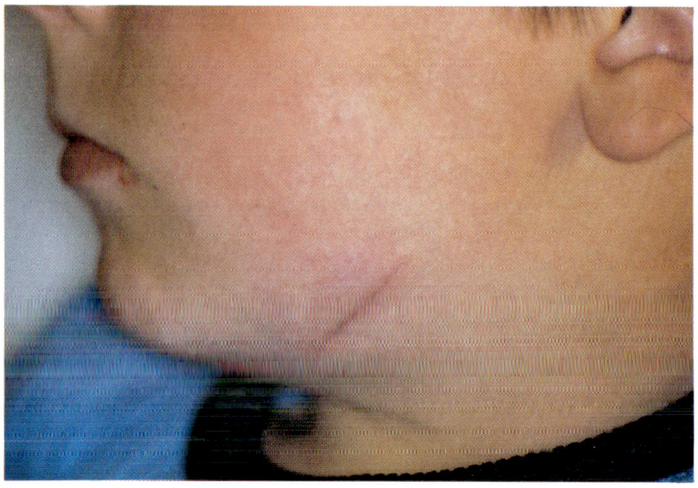

4.23

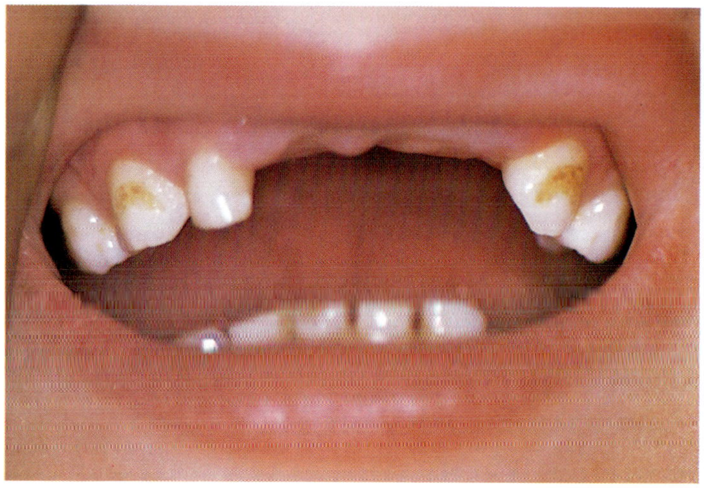

4.24

CHRONIC GRANULOMATOUS DISEASE (*CGD*)

Figure 4.23 This predominantly sex-linked leukocyte defect in which neutrophils and monocytes are defective at killing catalase-positive micro-organisms presents typically with cervical lymph node enlargement and suppuration (a submandibular node abscess has been drained here).

Figure 4.24 Recurrent infections in early childhood may result in enamel hypoplasia. The tooth loss here, however, was from a road traffic accident. CGD also predisposes to oral ulceration and periodontal destruction. Other types of neutrophil defect also predispose to ulcers and accelerated periodontitis (see page 115).

5

Mental disorders

ORAL DYSAESTHESIA
(*Burning mouth syndrome, glossopyrosis, glossodynia*)

Figure 5.1 A burning sensation in the mouth, especially the tongue, may be caused by infection such as candidosis, vitamin deficiency, diabetes or lesions such as erythema migrans. In some patients, no organic cause can be established, the tongue appears normal, and there may be a psychogenic basis. Affected patients are often females of middle age or older and the burning sensation *may* be relieved by eating. Anxiety about cancer is found in many.

ATYPICAL FACIAL PAIN

Figure 5.2 Persistent, dull, boring pain, especially in the maxilla, in the absence of identifiable organic disease, is seen in some psychiatric disorders, such as depression. Most patients affected with this atypical facial pain are females of middle age or older. This is an extreme example of a patient who is wearing a large bandage to help 'relieve' the pain, perhaps an attention-seeking device.

Patients with psychogenically-related orofacial symptoms not infrequently bring in diaries, graphs or notes outlining their complaints, which are often of pain, bad taste in the mouth, non-existent slime, lumps, dry or wet mouth, and are often multiple. A 'syndrome of oral complaints' has even been described.

PSYCHOGENIC ORAL DISEASE

Figure 5.3 A feature sometimes seen in these patients is a remarkable degree of tongue protrusion to the extent that the epiglottis can be seen, as here.

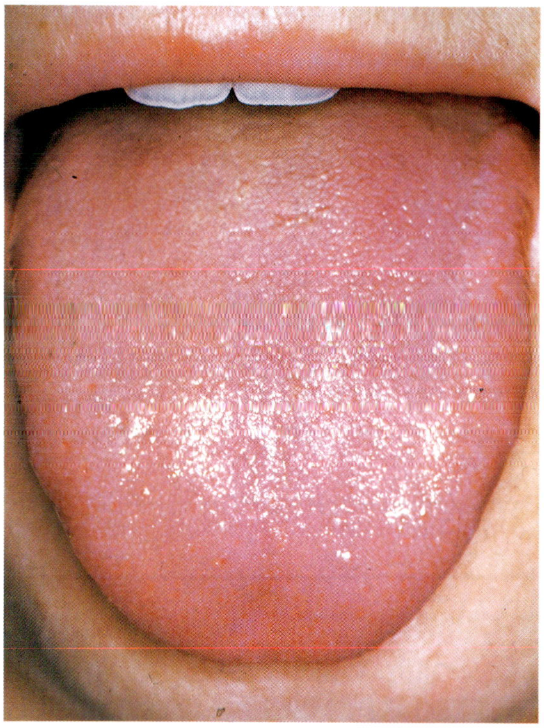

5.1

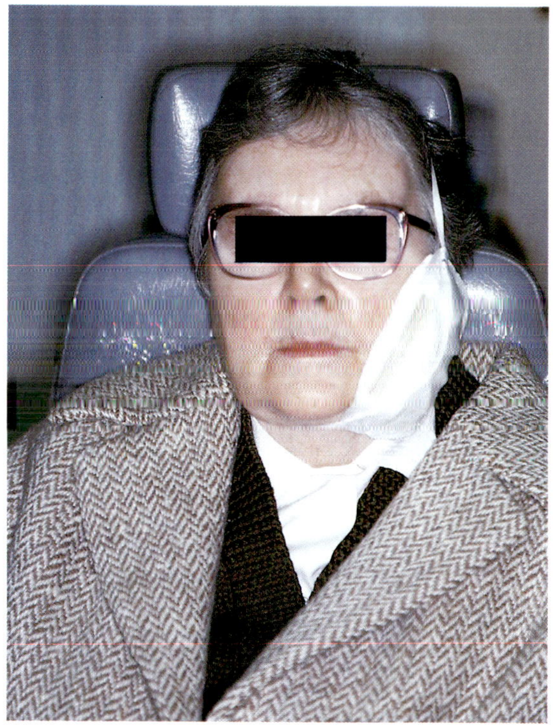

5.2

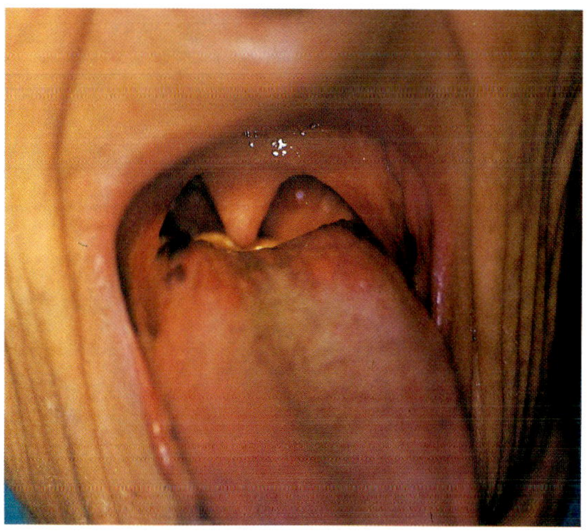

5.3

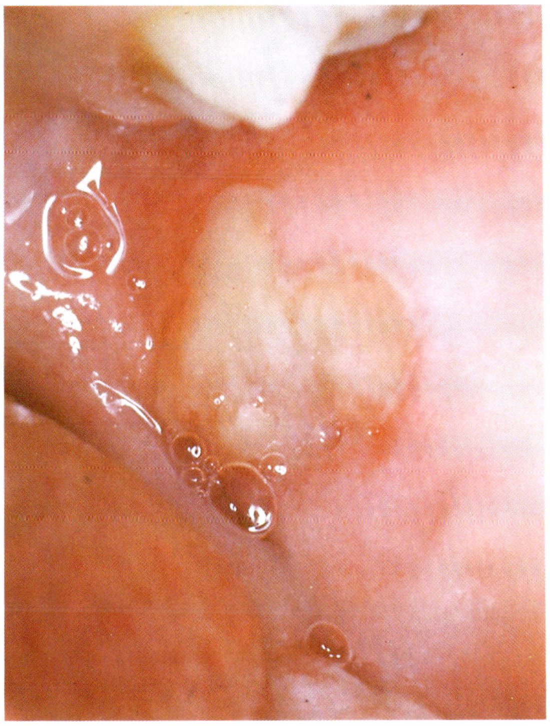

5.4

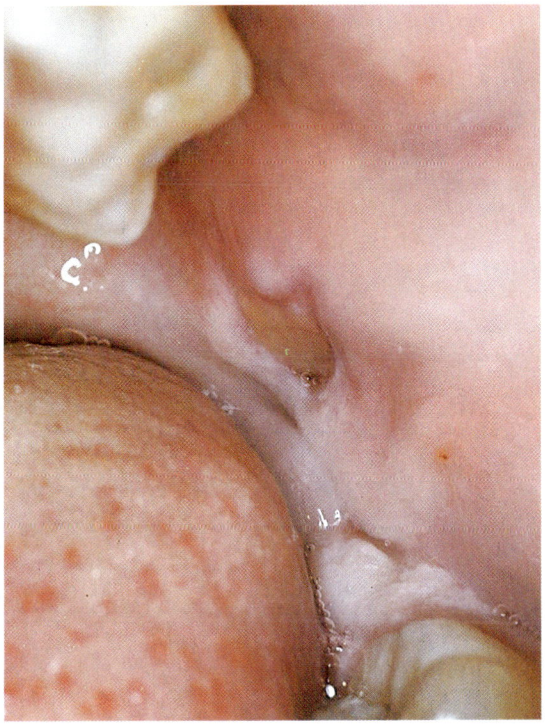

5.5

SELF-MUTILATION

Figure 5.4 Factitious or artefactual lesions are seen in some disturbed or mentally handicapped patients; in patients with Lesch-Nyhan syndrome (page 63); in Gilles de la Tourette syndrome (tic, coprolalia and copropraxia); where there is sensory loss in the area (see page 78) and where there is congenital indifference to pain as in familial dysautonomia (Riley-Day syndrome). This oral ulcer appeared in a child whose father had just left home to be away for some weeks (see Figure 5.5).

Figure 5.5 The ulcer shown in Figure 5.4 began to heal just after the father returned home.

6

Diseases of the nervous system

TRIGEMINAL NEURALGIA (*Paroxysmal trigeminal neuralgia*)

Figure 6.1 Neuralgia in the trigeminal region can have many causes. If organic causes such as multiple sclerosis or tumour cannot be demonstrated it is termed benign paroxysmal trigeminal neuralgia. This affects mainly the middle-aged or elderly and causes intermittent lancinating pain, usually in one division or branch in the sensory distribution of the trigeminal nerve. There are no organic manifestations but, if there is a trigger zone on the face, patients are understandably reluctant to touch the area – as in this patient who was reluctant to shave his right upper lip.

Figure 6.2 Treatment is usually medical (typically carbamazepine) but surgery such as cryoanalgesia may be required. Neurosurgery is rarely required and then may leave a sensory defect. This patient was left with a numb left cheek and nose after neurosurgery and constantly traumatizes the area.

SENSORY LOSS IN THE TRIGEMINAL AREA

Figures 6.3 The trigeminal nerve arises from the pons and runs through the posterior and middle cranial fossa. The most common causes of sensory loss are iatrogenic – here, local anaesthesia, after which the patient accidentally traumatized the lip. Removal of lower third molars, and mandibular osteotomies are other common iatrogenic causes.

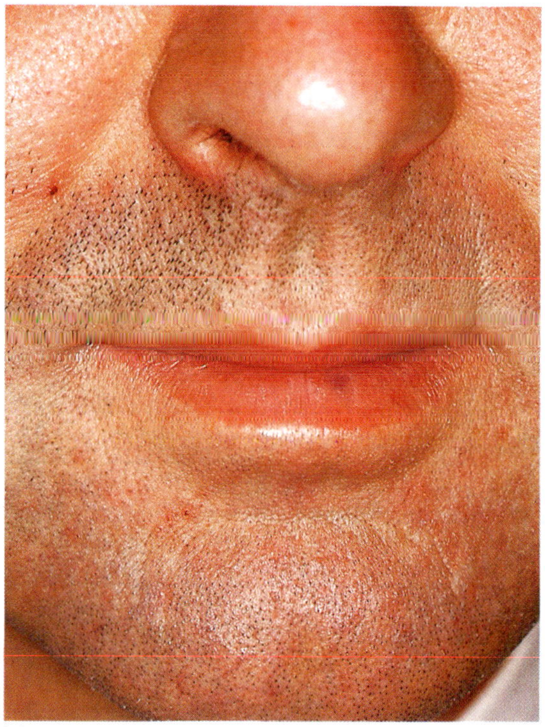

6.1

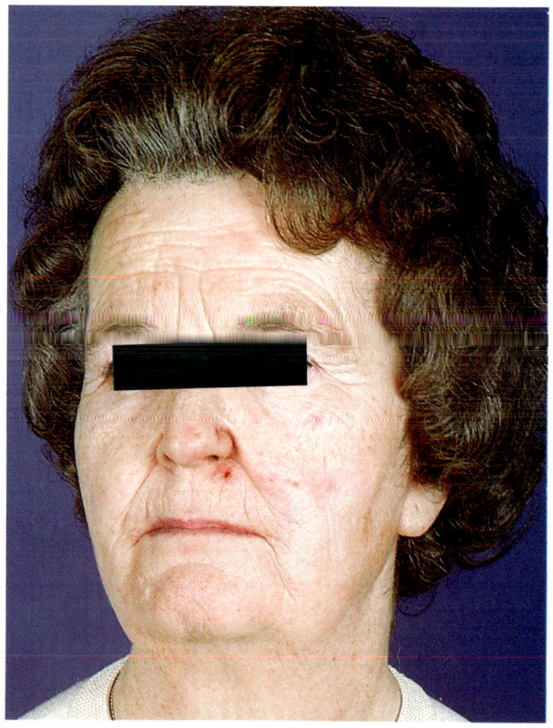

6.2

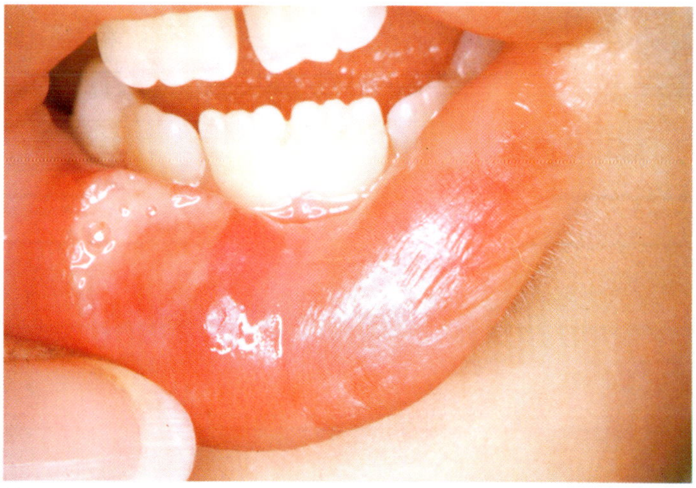

6.3

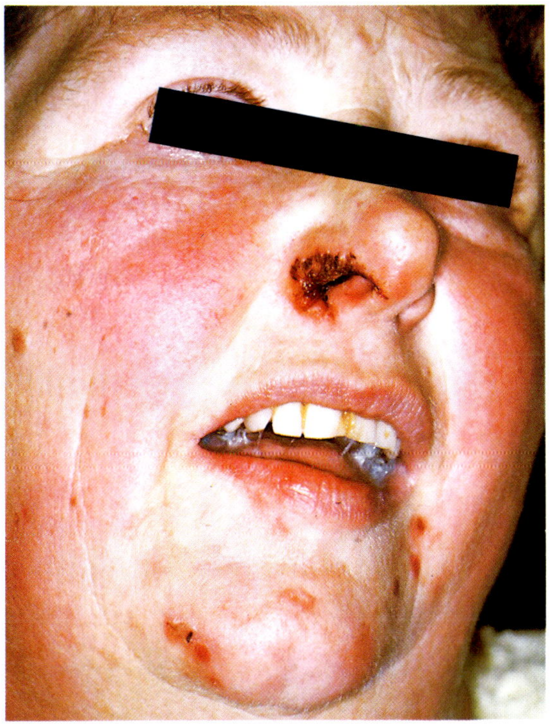

6.4

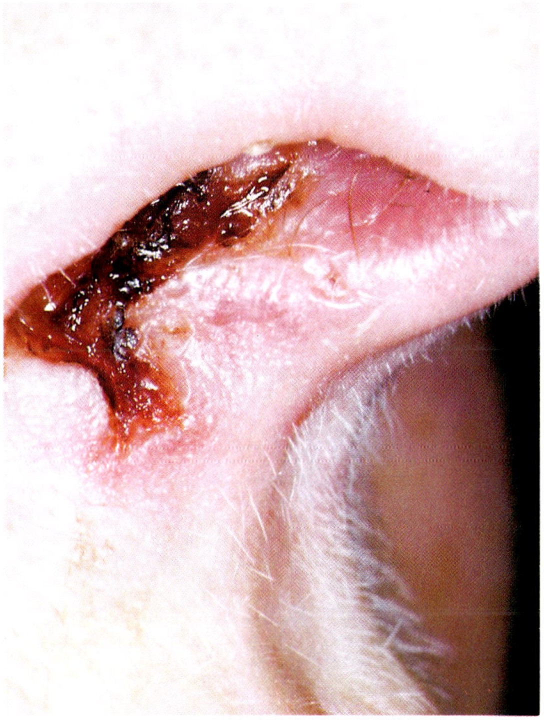

6.5

Figures 6.4 and 6.5 Sensory loss may be central in origin (cerebrovascular disease and anomalies, syringobulbia, cerebral neoplasm, or trauma) or peripheral (trauma, neoplasm or infection). This patient had a cerebral neoplasm resulting in lesions of cranial nerves V and VI. Subsequently she repeatedly traumatized her nose and mouth on the right side. Trophic ulceration has also been reported.

Other causes include bone disease; drugs; neuropathy, a premonitory feature in the occasional patient with trigeminal neuralgia; an acute spontaneously resolving idiopathic neuropathy; and neuropathy associated with systemic sclerosis, mixed connective tissue disease or other autoimmune states.

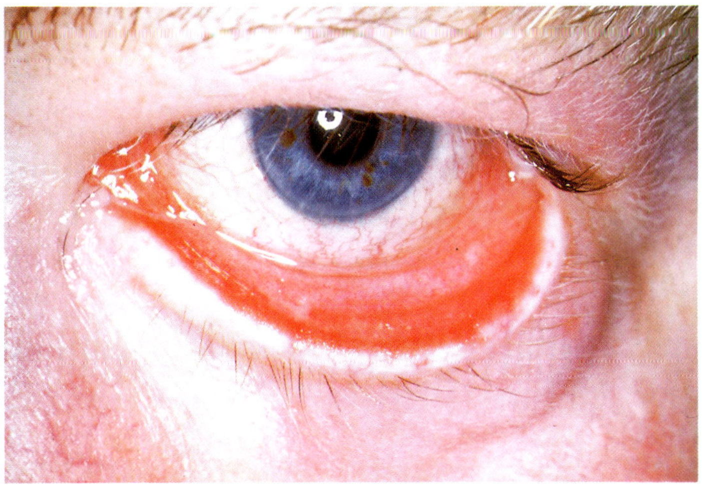

6.6

CEREBROVASCULAR ACCIDENT

Figure 6.6 One of the most common causes of facial palsy is stroke, when there is often unilateral facial palsy with ipsilateral hemiplegia. This patient had a stroke affecting his left side. An upper motor neurone lesion as in a stroke, causes paralysis mainly of the contralateral lower face, but involuntary movement is preserved: for instance, laughing can still produce facial movement. Perhaps the greatest danger from facial palsy is to the eye on the affected side, since poor eyelid closure and defective corneal reflex exposes the cornea to damage.

BELL'S PALSY

Figure 6.7 Bell's palsy is an acute lower motor neurone facial palsy of unknown aetiology, possibly viral. Figures 6.7–6.9 show a patient during and after an attack of right-sided palsy.

Typically, Bell's palsy affects young or middle-aged patients and is acute and unilateral, often preceded by mild pain around the ear region and sometimes a degree of hypo-aesthesia. The mouth droops on the side affected – the patient's right in this instance.

Although usually a mononeuropathy, Bell's palsy may be part of a more widespread cranial or even peripheral polyneuropathy. There are occasional associations with diabetes and with lymphoma.

Figure 6.8 One complete side of the face is paralysed. Attempts to smile or to whistle reveal the motionless affected side. The eyelids cannot be closed tightly on that side. Absence of the efferent arc of the corneal reflex presents a hazard to the eye.

Figure 6.9 Most cases resolve spontaneously in a few weeks but it may be prudent to give a short course of systemic corticosteroids to try and avoid permanent nerve damage, as was done here.

Lower motor neurone facial palsy is a rare disorder which may be congenital (Moebius' syndrome); or caused by varicella-zoster virus (Ramsay-Hunt syndrome, see page 8) or by HIV, or seen in association with sarcoidosis (Heerfordt's syndrome, see page 33), Melkersson-Rosenthal syndrome, (see page 157), Guillain-Barre syndrome, leprosy (see page 3), Kawasaki disease (mucocutaneous lymph node syndrome) or Lyme disease (tick-borne infection with *Borrelia burgdorferi*).

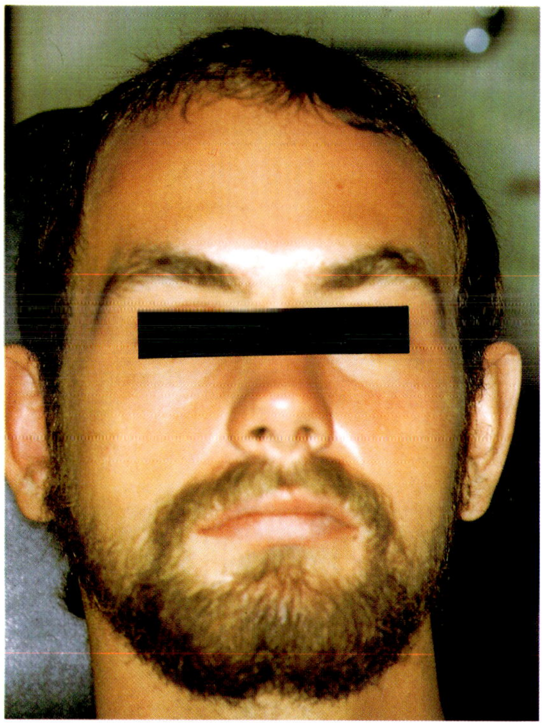

6.7

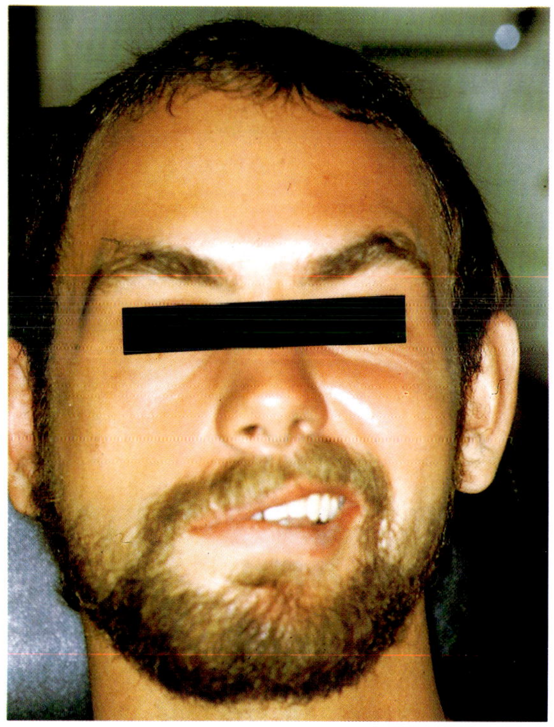

6.8

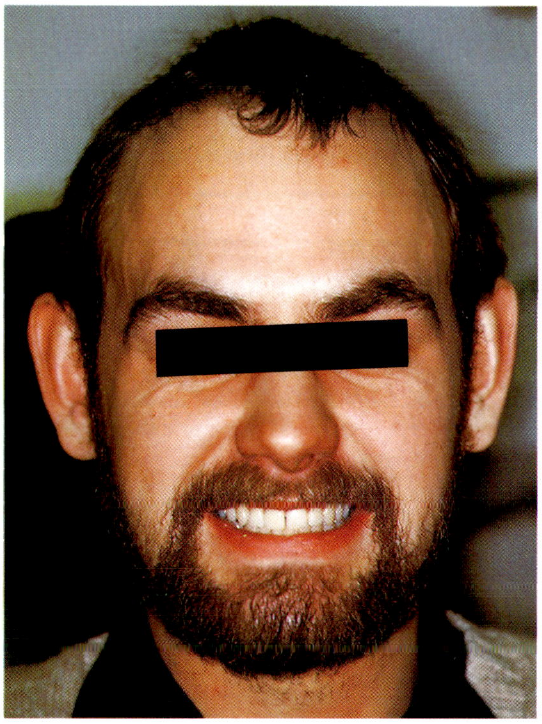

6.9

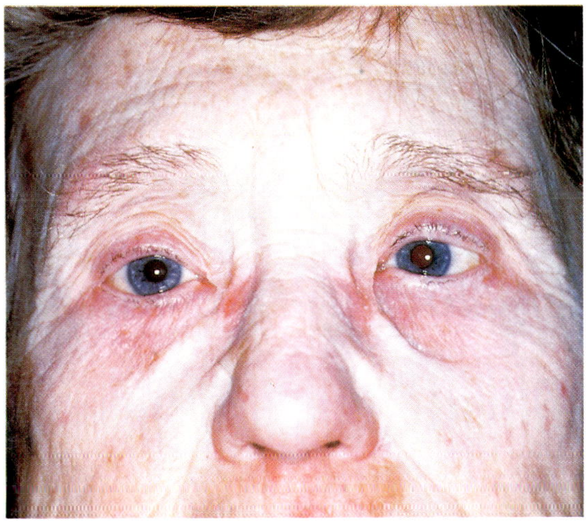

6.10

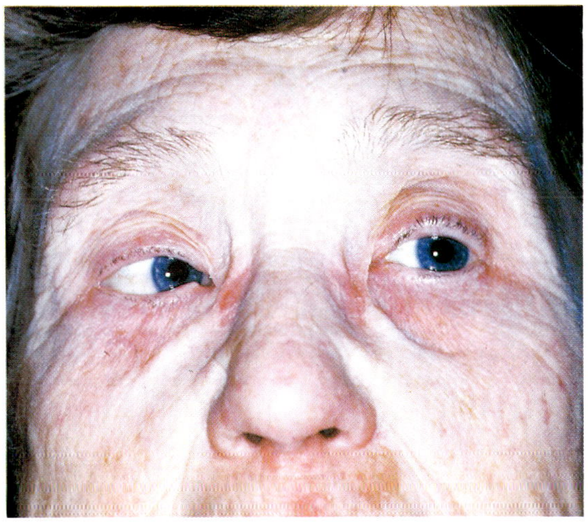

6.11

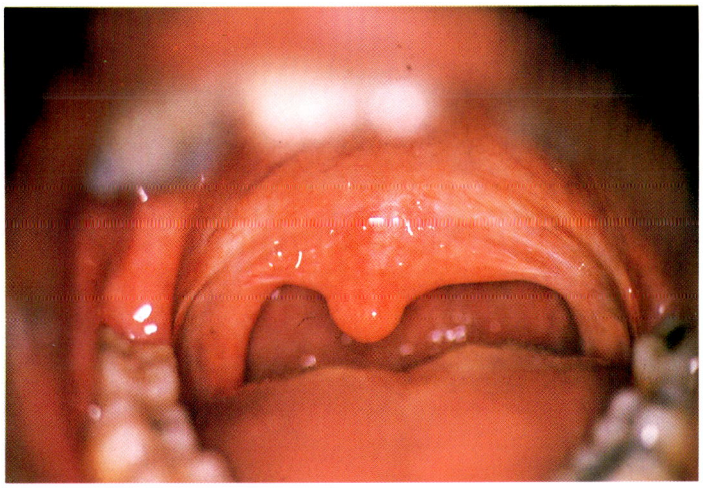

6.12

ABDUCENT NERVE LESION

Figures 6.10 and 6.11 The abducent (cranial nerve VI) arises from the pons, has the longest intracranial course of any cranial nerve, and can be damaged by lesions in the posterior or middle cranial fossae, or the orbit. It supplies the lateral rectus muscle which abducts the eye. This shows a patient with a left abducent nerve palsy.

GLOSSOPHARYNGEAL AND VAGUS NERVE PALSY

Figure 6.12 The palatal sensation and, therefore, the gag reflex are impaired. The uvula deviated to the right – away from the affected side. This patient had deficits of cranial nerves IX to XII inclusive (bulbar palsy) from a posterior cranial fossa neoplasm.

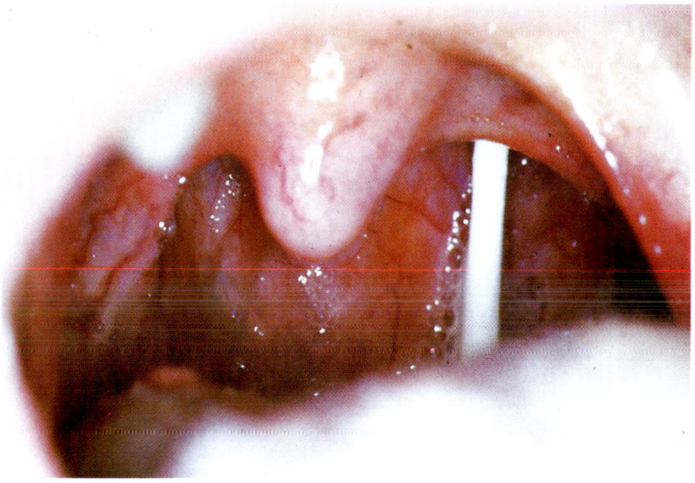

6.13

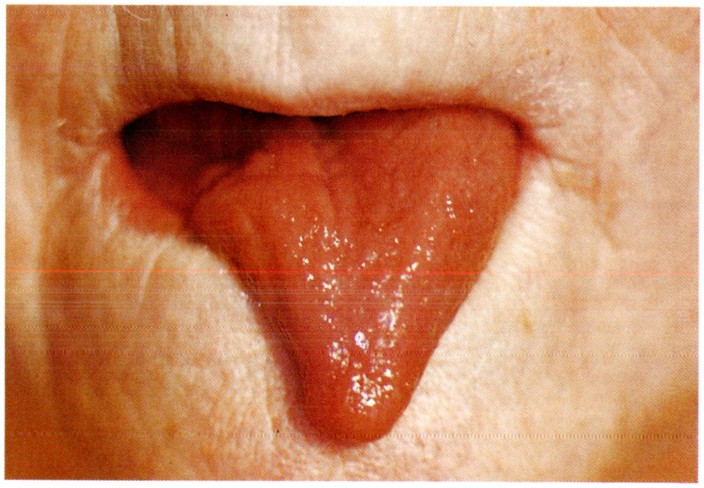

6.14

LATERAL MEDULLARY SYNDROME

Figure 6.13 Occlusion of the inferior artery of the lateral medulla oblongata, or occasionally of the posterior inferior cerebellar artery or vertebral artery, produces a syndrome of contralateral impairment of pain and thermal sense (damage to the spinothalamic tract); ipsilateral Horner's syndrome (damage to the sympathetic tract); hoarseness, dysphagia, and ipsilateral palatal palsy, as shown here (IX and X cranial nerve palsies); sensory loss over the ipsilateral face (damage to V nerve nuclei); vestibular signs; and loss of taste (damage to tractus solitarius).

Asymmetry of the soft palate is demonstrated here by the naso-gastric tube which marks the midline.

HYPOGLOSSAL NERVE LESION

Figure 6.14 The hypoglossal nerve arises from the medulla and supplies motor fibres to most tongue muscles. Lower motor neurone lesions are rare but cause paralysis and wasting of the ipsilateral half of the tongue, as in this patient. On protrusion, the tongue often deviates to the affected side.

7

Diseases of the circulatory system

PERIARTERITIS NODOSA (*Polyarteritis nodosa, PAN*)

Figure 7.1 Periarteritis nodosa is a necrotizing vasculitis of small- and medium-sized arteries, affecting mainly males and often related to previous infection with hepatitis B virus. Arthralgia, angina, hypertension and renal disease are the main features. Oral nodules, bleeding or ulcers may be seen.

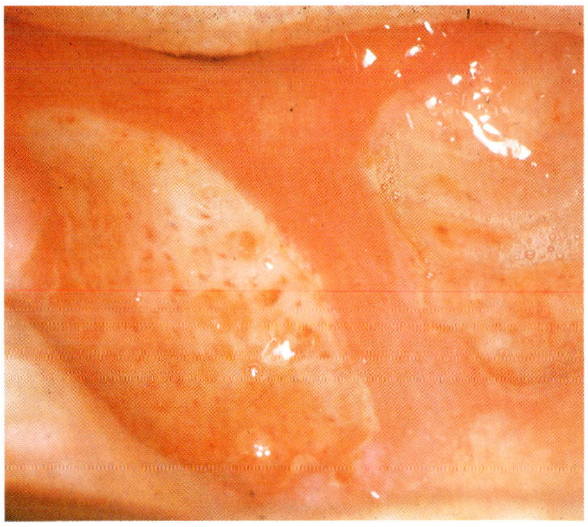

7.1

WEGENER'S GRANULOMATOSIS

Figure 7.2 This is a rare disorder with granulomatous lesions in the respiratory tract, almost pathognomonic gingival lesions (resembling strawberries) and, later, necrotizing glomerulonephritis. Gingival swelling, mucosal ulcers or delayed wound healing are the oral features.

Occasionally, a limited form of the disease, involving only one or two organ systems, is seen.

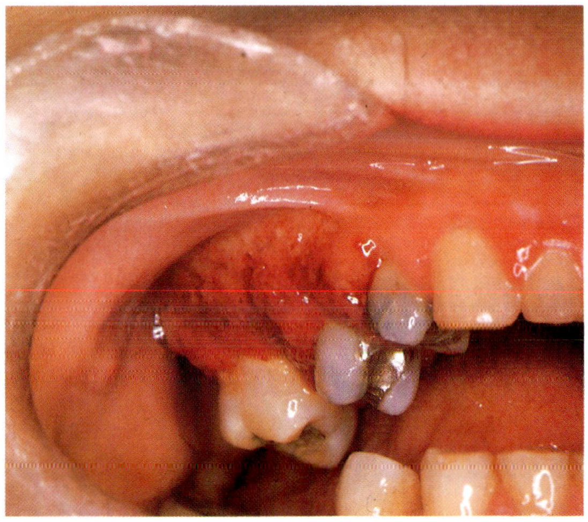

7.2

MIDLINE GRANULOMA (*Idiopathic midfacial granuloma syndrome*)

Figure 7.3 This is a group of rare disorders starting in the nasal or paranasal tissues, causing destruction of the facial bones, and sometimes progressing to a reticulosis. This clinical syndrome can result from Stewart's granuloma, lymphomatoid granulomatosis or polymorphic reticulosis.

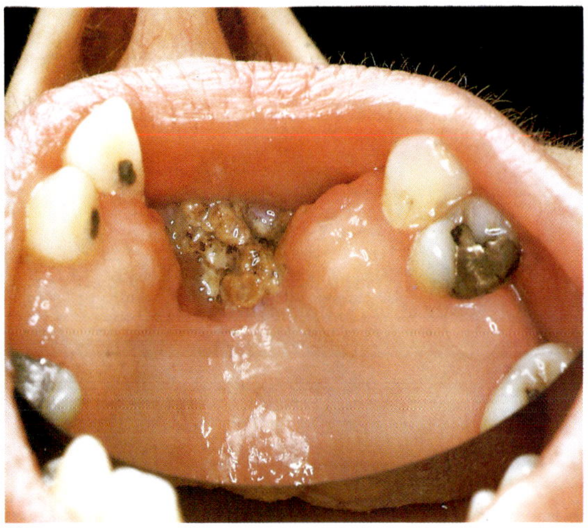

7.3

SUBLINGUAL VARICES

Figure 7.4 Dilated lingual veins give rise to varices, common in the elderly, and are of no special significance. There are occasional associations with varices elsewhere in the body, including the jejunum and scrotum.

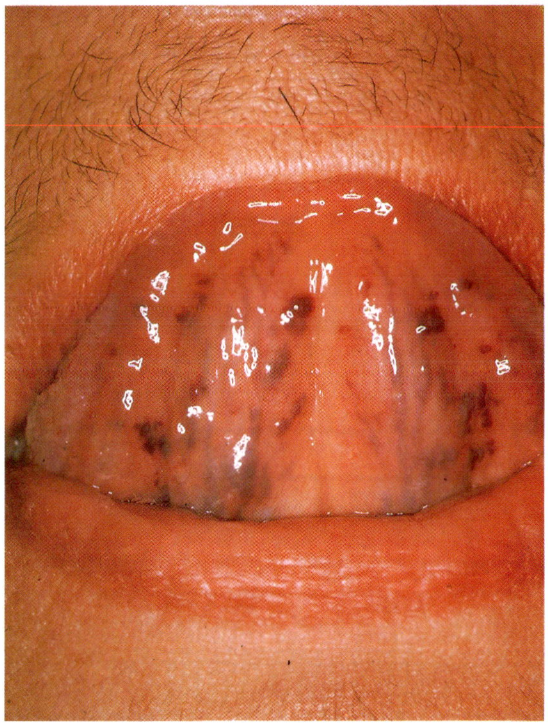

7.4

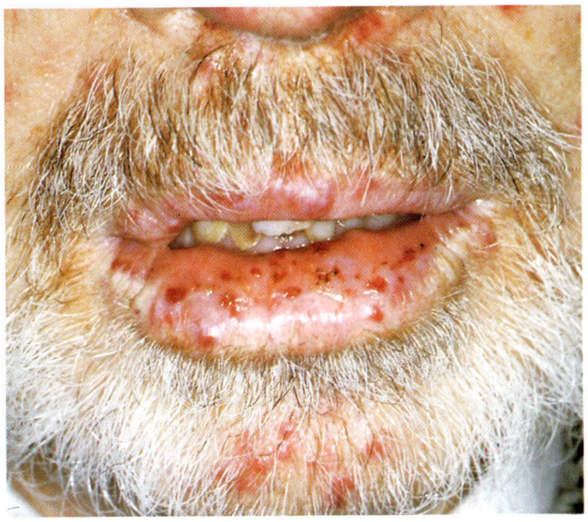

7.5

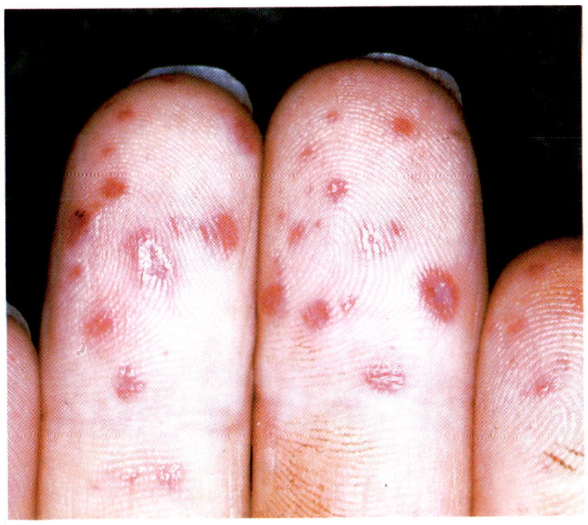

7.6

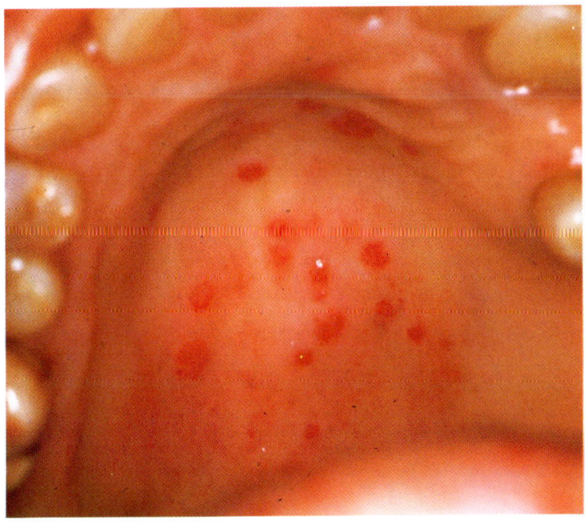

7.7

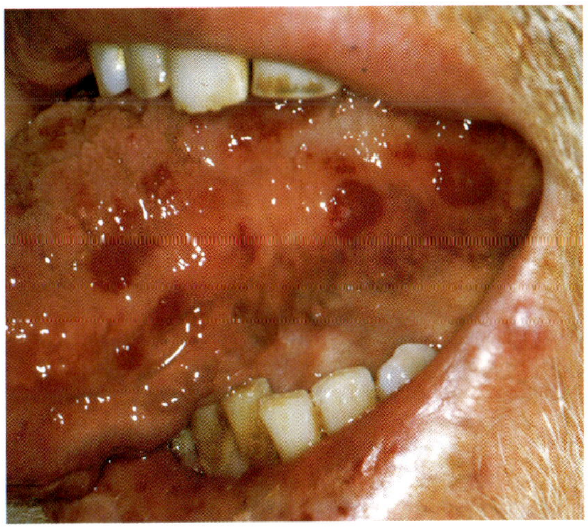

7.8

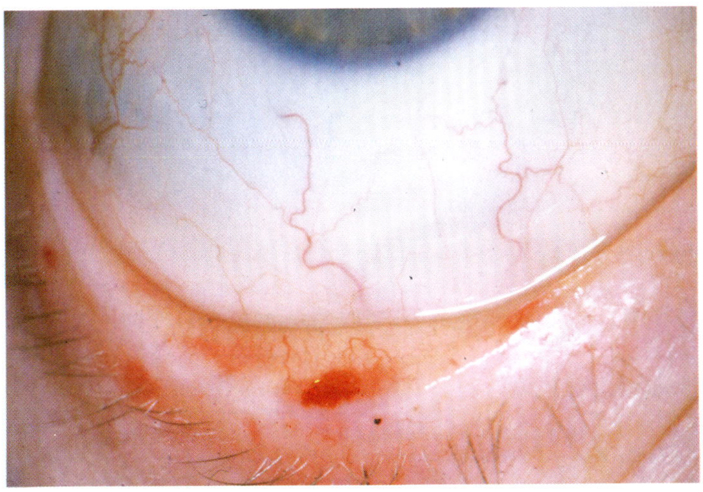

7.9

HEREDITARY HAEMORRHAGIC TELANGIECTASIA (*Osler-Rendu-Weber syndrome*)

Figure 7.5 Hereditary haemorrhagic telangiectasia (HHT) is an autosomal dominant condition characterized by mucosal and cutaneous telangiectases which appear on the lips and perioral, often well after birth.

Figure 7.6 Occasional telangiectases appear on the extremities, particularly on the palmar surfaces of the digits.

Figure 7.7 Mucosal telangiectases are found in the mouth, nasal, and alimentary mucosa. Chronic haemorrhage almost invariably produces anaemia.

Figure 7.8 Pronounced telangiectases on the tongue in this patient caused repeated haemorrhage, leading eventually to severe anaemia and then cardiac failure.

Figure 7.9 Occasional telangiectases affect other mucosae, such as the conjunctiva. Retinal telangiectases predispose to intraocular bleeding. Pulmonary arteriovenous fistulae, central nervous system and hepatic vascular anomalies predispose to complications. HHT has occasional associations with von Willebrand's disease, and with IgA deficiency.

8

Diseases of the respiratory system

STREPTOCOCCAL TONSILLITIS

Figure 8.1 Caused by *Streptococcus pyogenes* (Lancefield Group A, beta haemolytic streptococcus), the incubation period of 2–4 days is followed by sore throat, dysphagia and fever. Usually children are affected. The uvula, tonsils and pharynx are diffusely red, with punctate white or yellow tonsillar exudates. Complications are rare but can include otitis media, quinsy, sinusitis, rheumatic fever or glomerulonephritis.

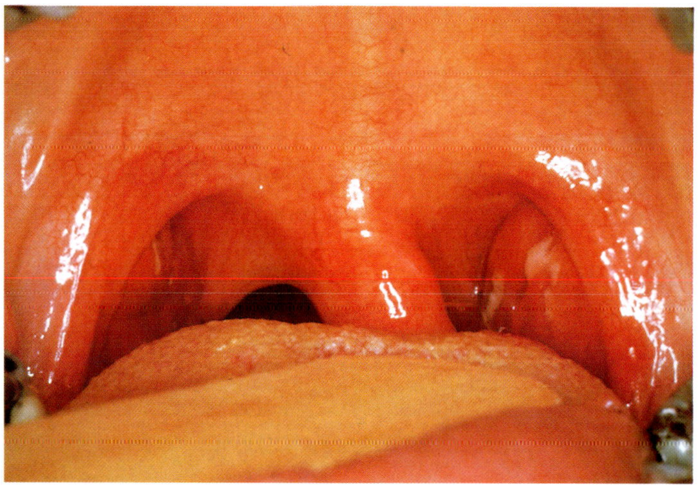

8.1

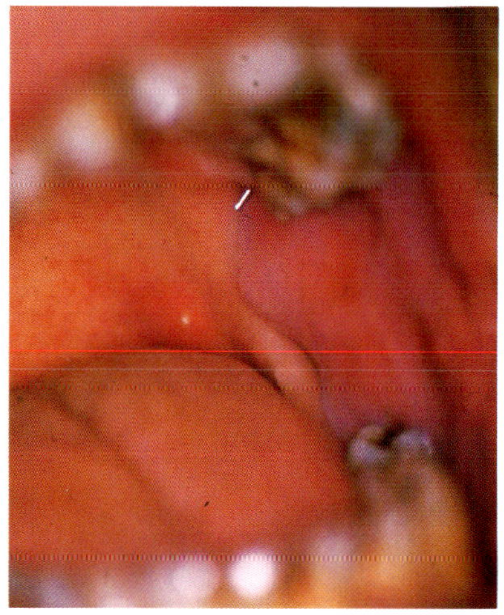

8.2

QUINSY (*Peritonsillar abscess*)

Figure 8.2 Peritonsillar abscess, although usually following *Streptococcus pyogenes* infection, typically contains a variety of oropharyngeal micro-organisms. The abscess causes severe pain, dysphagia and trismus before pointing, as shown here, and discharging.

INFLUENZA

Figure 8.3 Oral lesions have not often been reported in influenza but ulcers, pericoronitis, gingivitis and soft palate hyperaemia have been described. This teenager developed mouth ulcers and mild gingivitis after an episode of influenza.

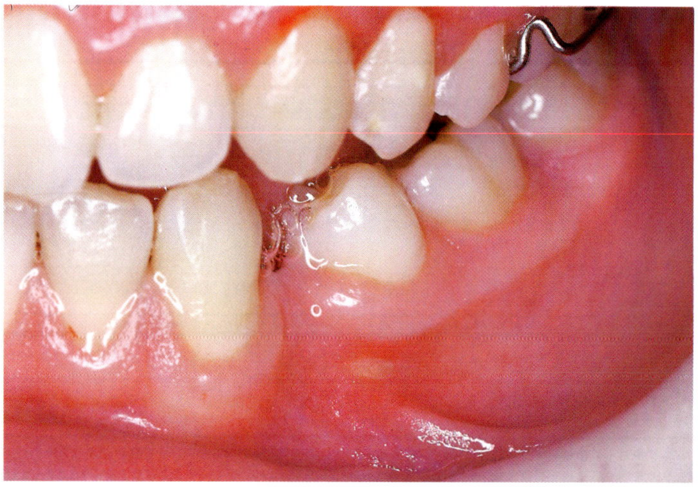

8.3

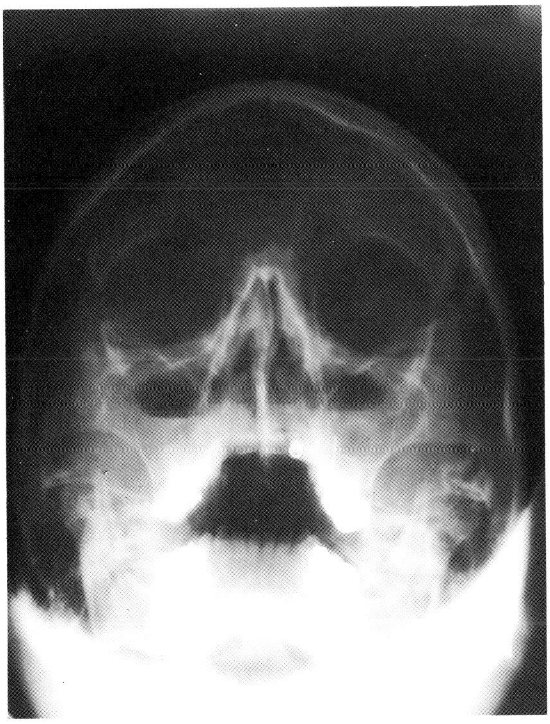

8.4

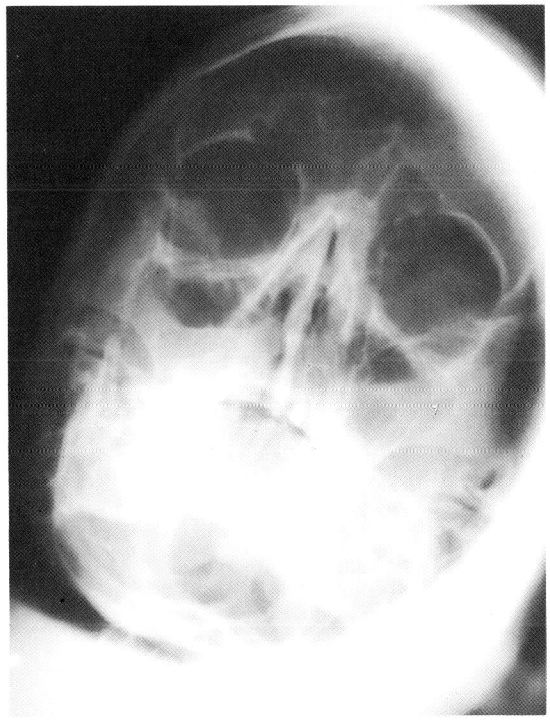

8.5

MAXILLARY SINUSITIS

Figure 8.4 Acute sinusitis is usually preceded by an upper respiratory tract viral infection but occasionally follows an oroantral fistula or displacement of a tooth or root into the sinus. Pain is felt over the antrum, especially on moving the head, and the ipsilateral premolars and molars may be tender to percussion. Transillumination or occipitomental radiography show opacities in the lower half of each antrum in this patient.

Figure 8.5 Tilting the head shows that the bilateral antral opacities are fluid.

Sinusitis is also a complication of cystic fibrosis, Kartagener's syndrome (immobile cilia and dextrocardia) and various immunodeficiencies. Such patients may also have enamel hypoplasia.

9

Diseases of the digestive system

HYPODONTIA

Figure 9.1 Isolated hypodontia is fairly common, may have a genetic basis, and affects mainly the permanent dentition, particularly third molars, second premolars or, as here, upper lateral incisors. The right upper deciduous lateral incisor is retained, a common occurrence when the permanent successor is missing.

Teeth may be apparently missing in many cases because they are impacted and thus fail to erupt. Rarely, eruption is delayed because of systemic disease, such as cretinism or Down's syndrome.

Figure 9.2 Congenital absence of several teeth: the retained lower deciduous central incisors are discoloured because they are non-vital, having been worn down by attrition which has caused pulpal exposure, as shown, and pulp necrosis. The permanent central incisors are congenitally absent.

Figure 9.3 Occasionally several teeth are congenitally absent, as here.

Figure 9.4 Radiograph showing several missing teeth in an otherwise healthy person (same patient as in Figure 9.1).

Figure 9.5 Hypodontia associated with systemic disorders: hypodontia is a feature of local disorders such as cleft palate, and of many systemic disorders. In some, the teeth are present but fail to erupt; in others, such as ectodermal dysplasia, shown here, or incontinentia pigmenti, they are truly missing (see page 208). Rarely, all teeth are absent (anodontia).

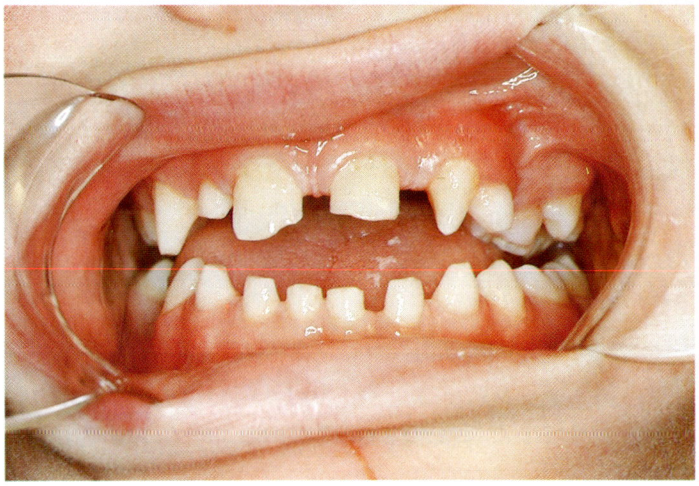

9.1

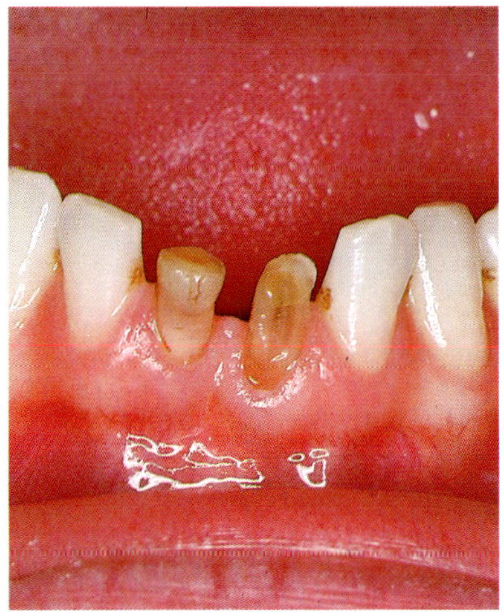

9.2

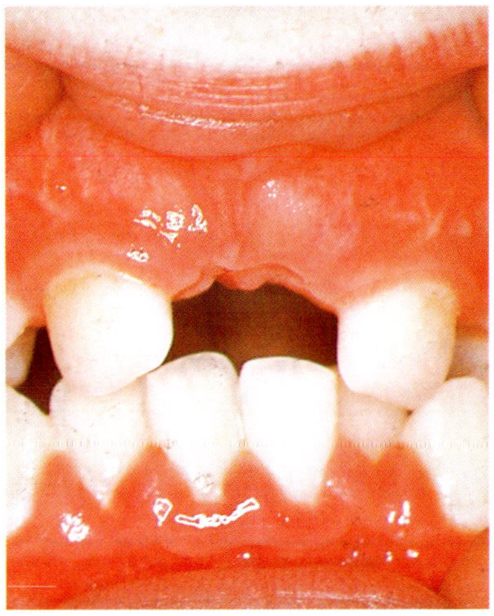

9.3

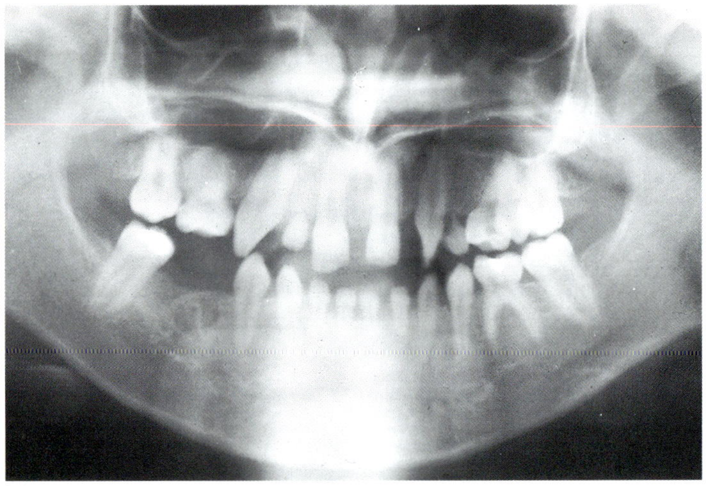

9.4

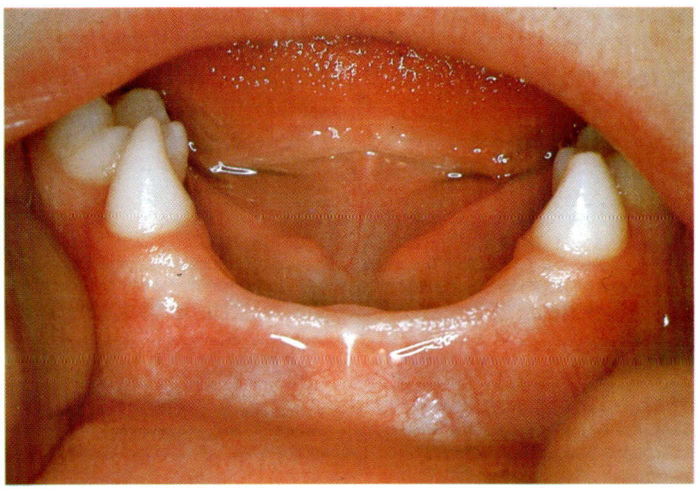

9.5

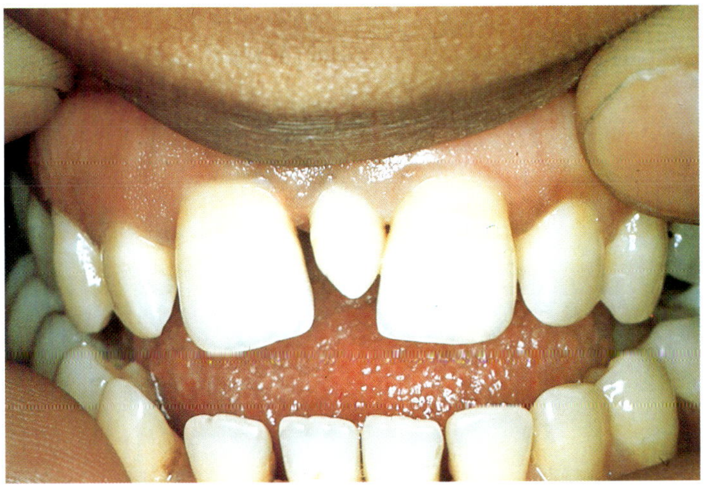

9.6

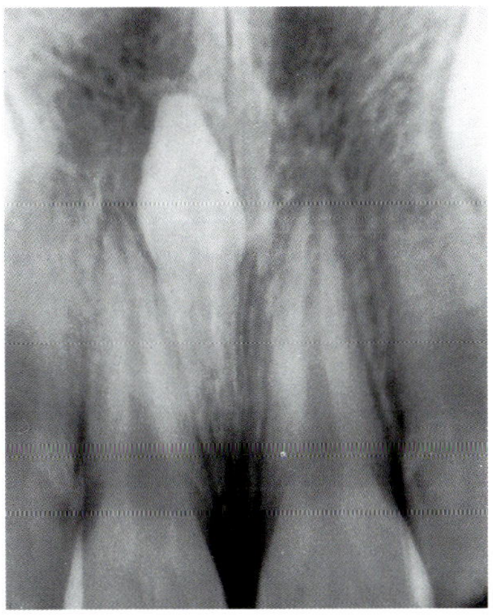

9.7

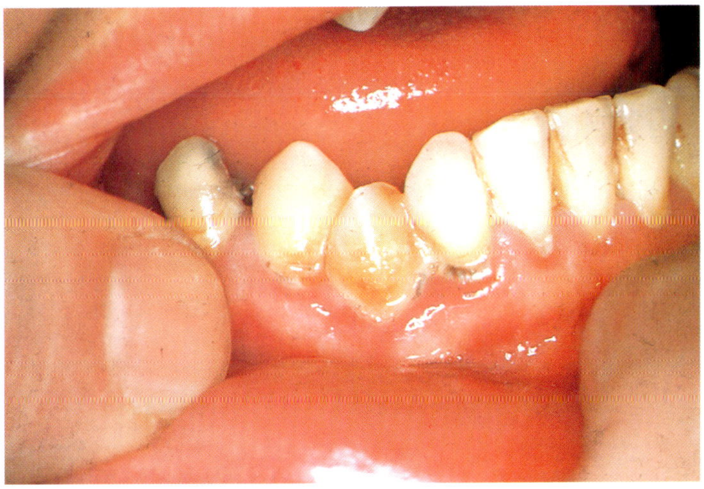

9.8

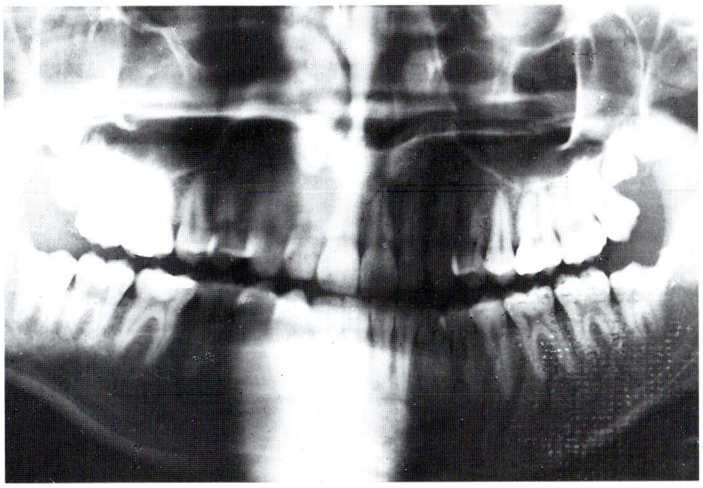

9.9

HYPERDONTIA

Figure 9.6 Additional teeth are usually of simple conical shape (supernumerary) and are most common in the upper incisor region. If midline, as here, the tooth is termed a mesiodens (see also Figure 9.7). Supernumerary teeth may cause malocclusion, occasionally impede tooth eruption, or, rarely, are the site of cyst formation.

Figure 9.7 Although a mesiodens may erupt, sometimes it is, as here, inverted.

Figure 9.8 Additional teeth often erupt in an abnormal position, as has this supernumerary canine or premolar. This may predispose to caries or periodontal disease.

Figure 9.9 Four maxillary molars can be seen on each side. They resemble normal teeth and are thus termed supplemental (or sometimes distodens).

Supernumerary teeth are usually seen in otherwise healthy patients but occasionally are a manifestation of a systemic disorder such as cleidocranial dysplasia (see page 198) or Gardner's syndrome (see page 130).

FUSION

Figure 9.10 Fusion (union of two normally separate, adjacent tooth germs) gives rise to a large tooth with one tooth obviously missing from the series, unless the fusion is with a supernumerary tooth.

Figure 9.11 Fusion may be complete along the length of the teeth or may involve roots alone.

Figure 9.12 Fused or geminated teeth may give rise to poor aesthetics and sometimes malocclusions.

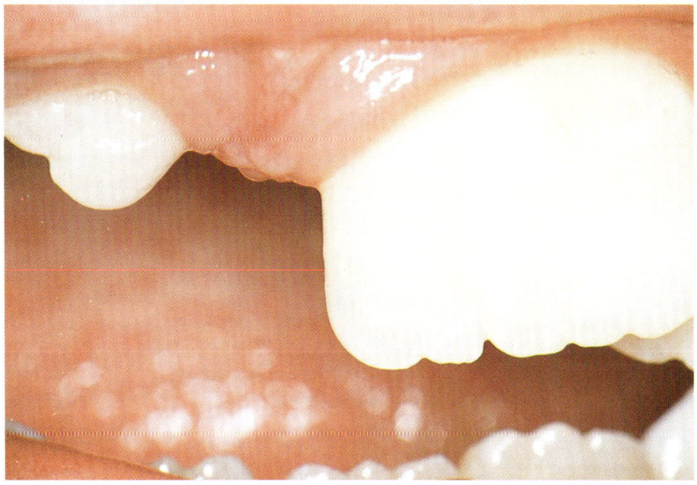

9.10

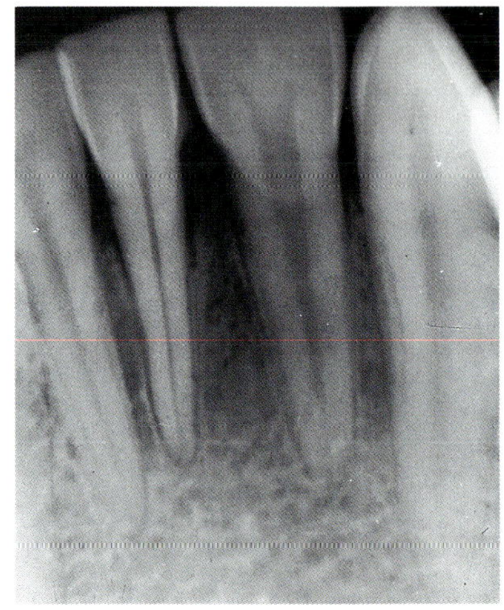

9.11

GEMINATION (*Geminated odontome*)

Figure 9.13 An odontome is a developmental malformation of dental tissues. Gemination is a result of incomplete attempted division of a tooth germ. Usually seen in the incisor region, the crowns may be separate or divided by a shallow groove as in the right upper central incisor. However, the root is shared.

Figure 9.14 It is often difficult to differentiate gemination from fusion: the terms 'double tooth' or 'twinning' are therefore sometimes used.

Figure 9.15 Double teeth are seen most commonly, but not invariably, in the incisor and canine regions and may be seen in the deciduous and permanent dentitions.

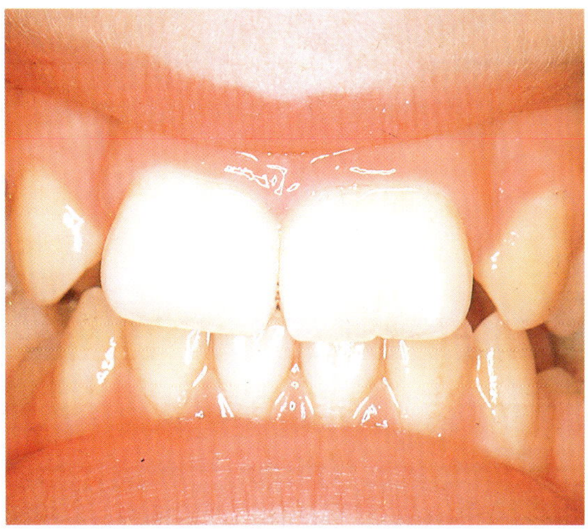

9.12

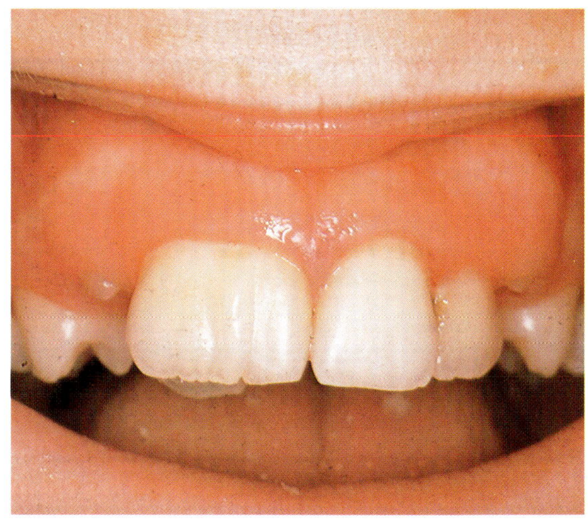

9.13

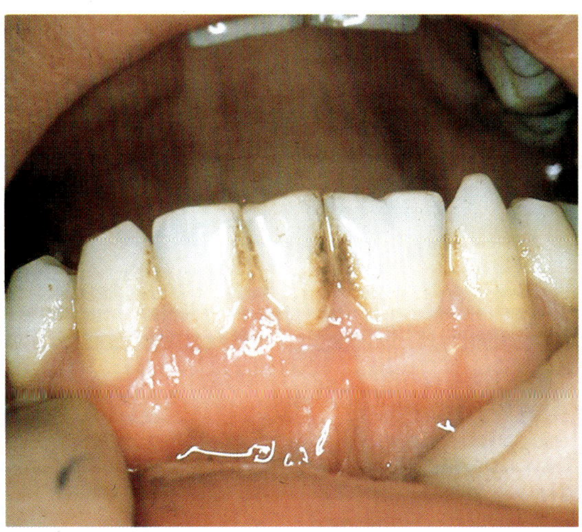

9.14

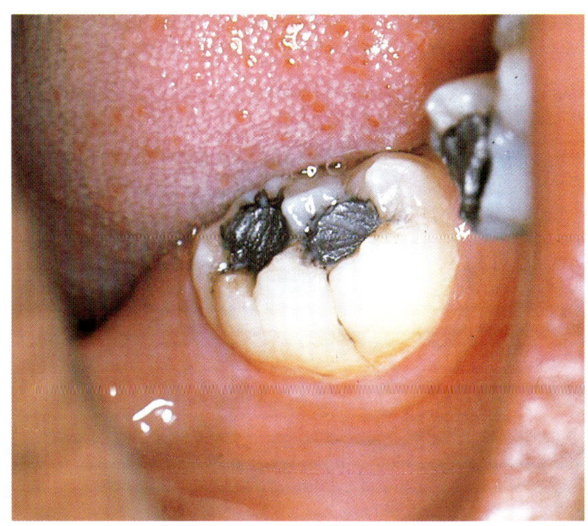

9.15

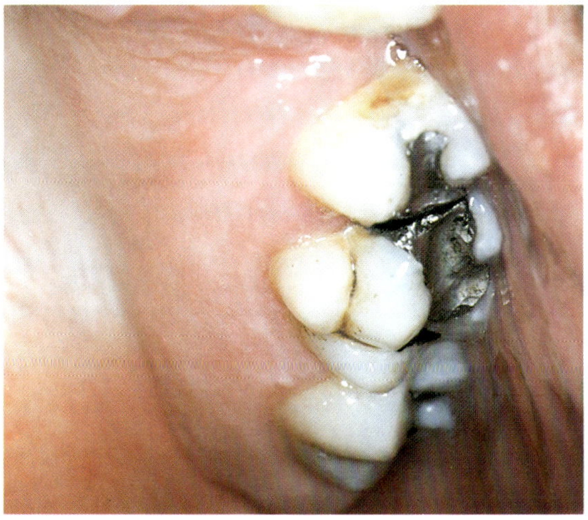

9.16

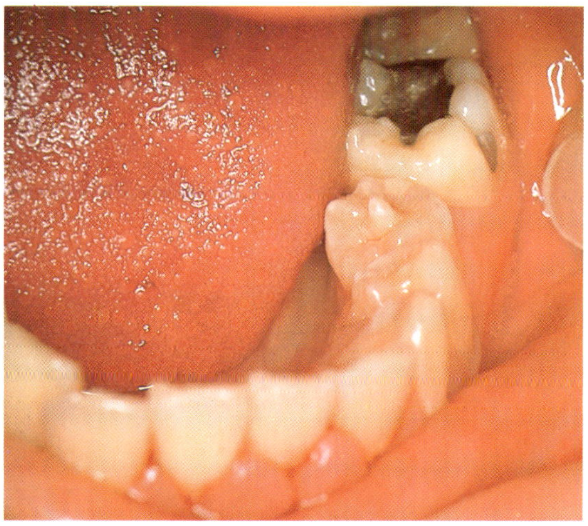

9.17

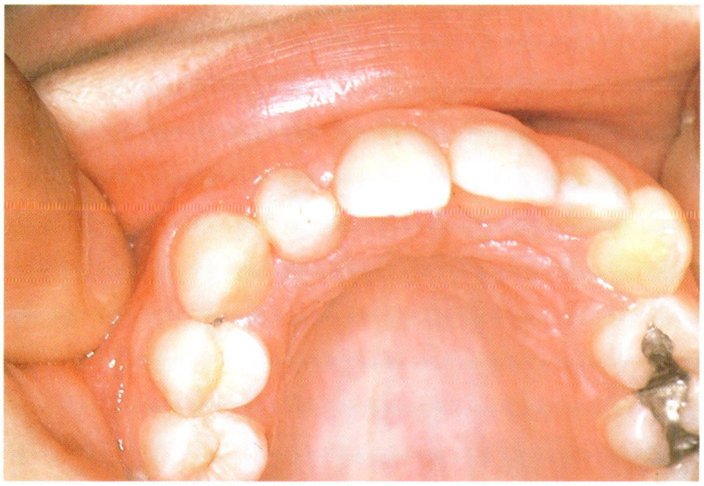

9.18

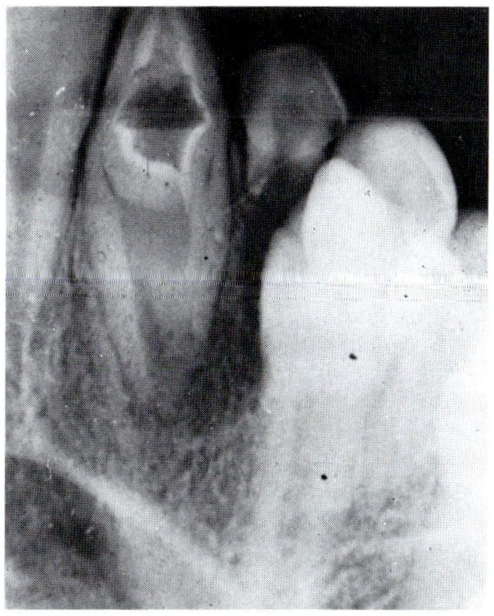

9.19

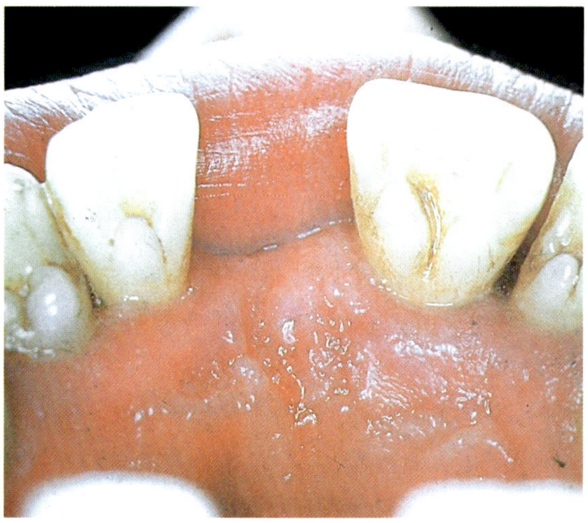

9.20

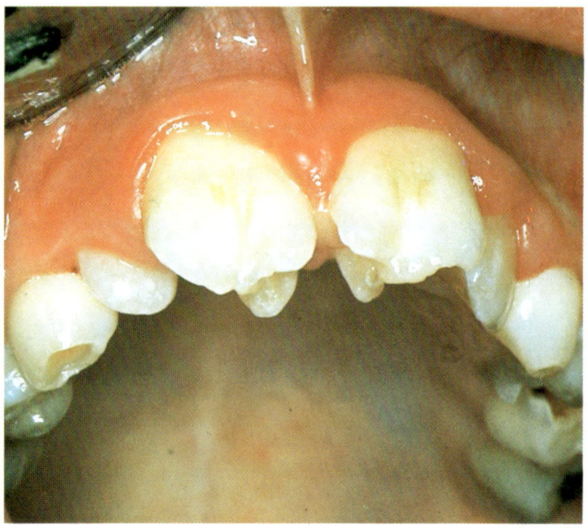

9.21

CUSP OF CARABELLI

Figure 9.16 This is an anatomical variant – a palatal cusp on the upper first molar.

EVAGINATED ODONTOME (*Dens evaginatus*)

Figure 9.17 A small occlusal nodule is seen, especially in mongoloid races. Since the nodule contains a pulp horn, pulpitis is not uncommon when there is attrition.

INVAGINATED ODONTOME (*Dilated odontome, dens in dente*)

Figure 9.18 Invagination of enamel and dentine in the *dens in dente* may also dilate the affected tooth.

Figure 9.19 Ameloblasts invaginate during development to form a pouch of enamel such that a radiograph shows what resembles a tooth within a tooth. This odontome is prone to caries development in the abnormal pouch.

PROMINENT TUBERCULES OR CUSPS

Figure 9.20 Prominent tubercles.

Figure 9.21 Teeth are occasionally malformed with a large palatal cusp, to the extent that they have a talon cusp configuration.

PEG-SHAPED LATERAL INCISOR

Figure 9.22 This is the most common anomaly of tooth shape and produces a cosmetic problem.

ENAMEL NODULE (*Enameloma, enamel pearl*)

Figure 9.23 A small circular mass of enamel is seen on the tooth surface near the cemento-enamel junction.

Figure 9.24 Sometimes the enamel nodule contains dentine and pulp. Nodules are most common on maxillary teeth.

TAURODONTISM

Figure 9.25 Taurodontism is the term applied to teeth that clinically look normal but on radiograph resemble those of ungulates (hence the Latin origin, *taurus,* a bull). The crown is long, the roots short. Taurodontism is usually a simple racial trait but may rarely be associated with some chromosome anomalies such as Klinefelter's syndrome; tricho-dento-osseous syndrome; orofacial-digital syndrome; ectodermal dysplasia; or amelogenesis imperfecta.

Figure 9.26 Taurodont teeth lack a pronounced constriction at the neck of the tooth and are parallel-sided. The floor of the pulp chamber is lower than normal and the pulp appears extremely large. Taurodontism usually affects permanent molars, especially the lower second molar, sometimes only one in the arch, but may affect teeth in the deciduous dentition.

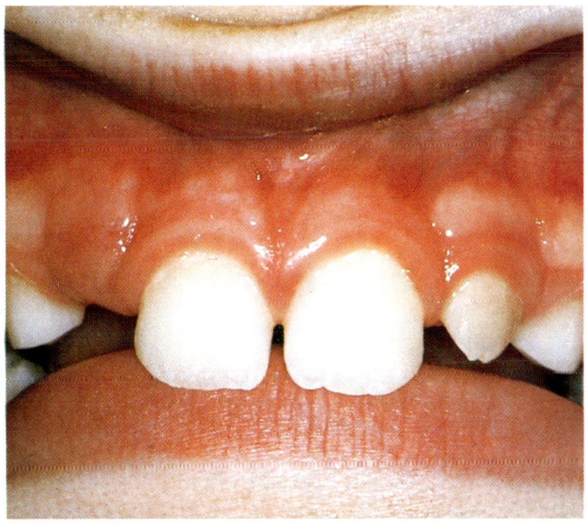

9.22

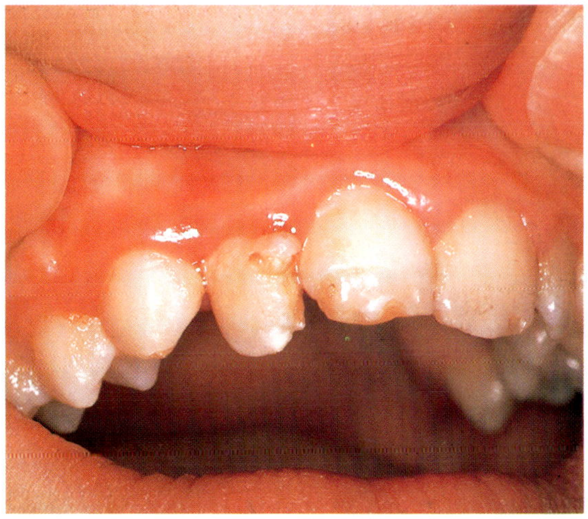

9.23

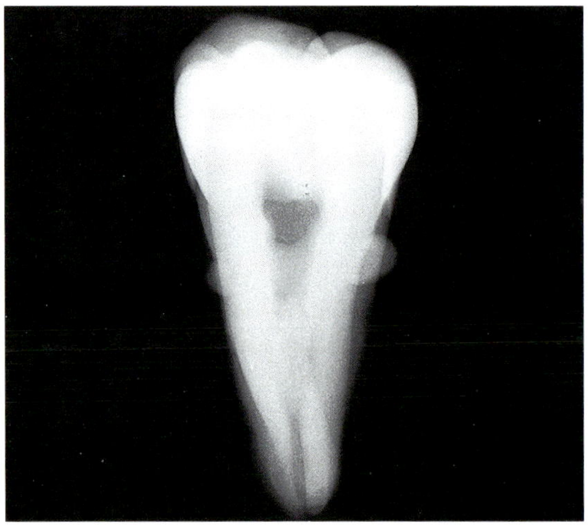

9.24

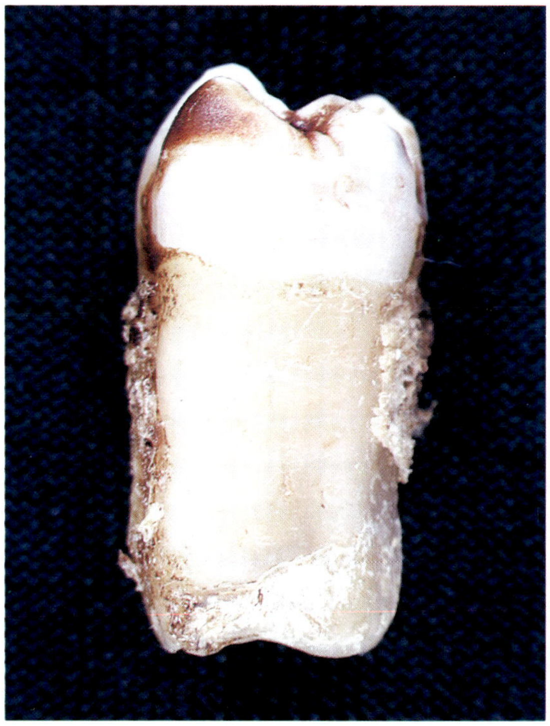

9.25

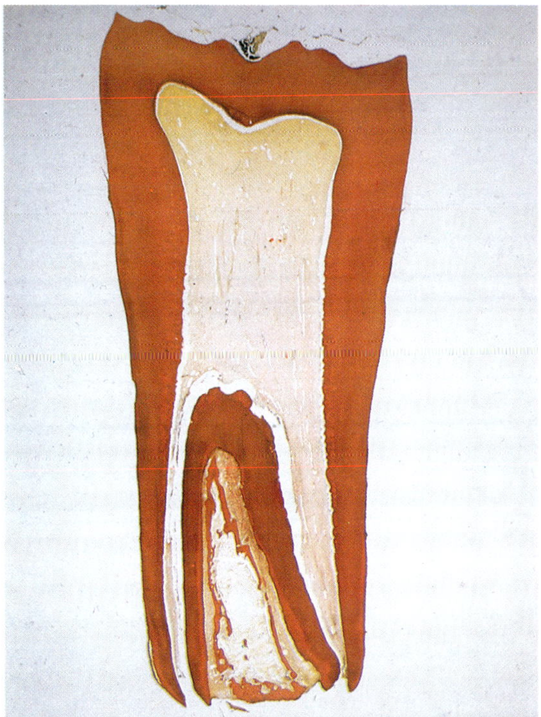

9.26

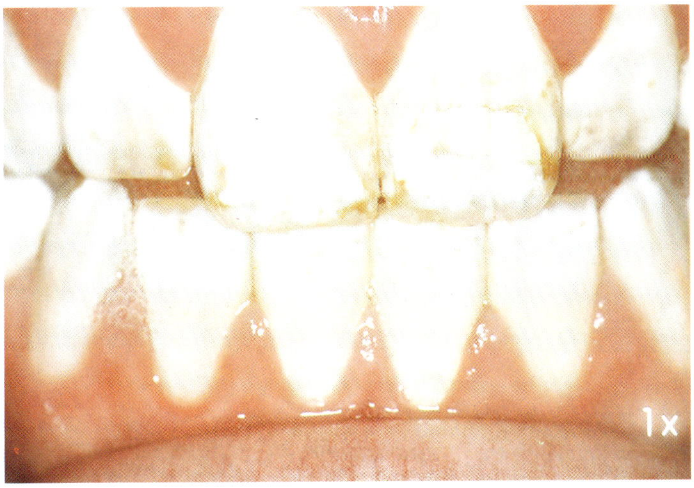
9.27

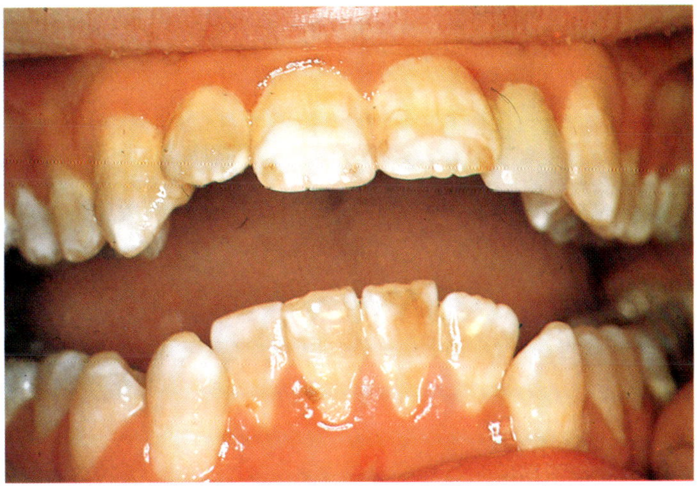
9.28

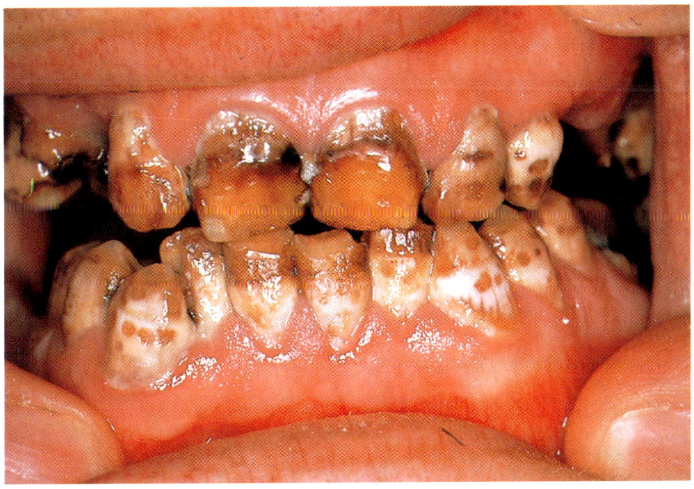
9.29

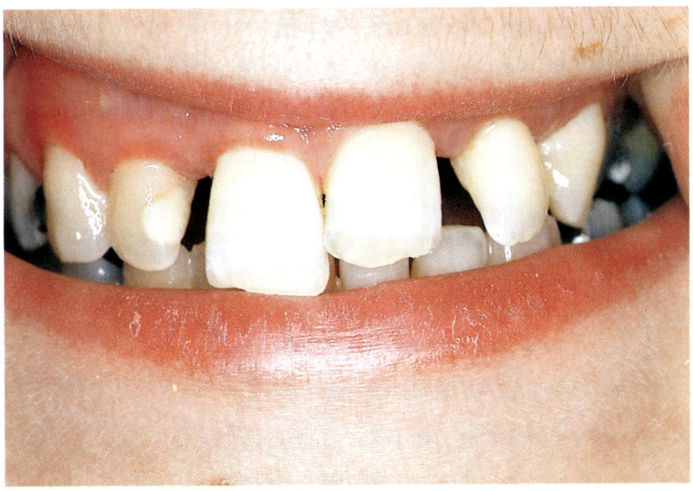
9.30

FLUOROSIS

Figure 9.27 Mottling of the enamel may be seen where the fluoride in drinking water exceeds about 2 ppm or excess fluoride is taken via other sources, although in the mildest form it may not produce a cosmetic defect. Mottling in mild fluorosis is usually seen as white flecks or patches. Brown staining and pitting is seen in more severe fluorosis. The mottling here is enough to require the cosmetic crowning of the upper anterior teeth.

Figure 9.28 Mottling more severe than in Figure 9.27.

Figure 9.29 Severe fluorosis causes opacity and brown and white staining and pitting of the entire enamel. This can be difficult clinically to differentiate from amelogenesis imperfecta (page 99).

NON-FLUORIDE ENAMEL OPACITIES

Figure 9.30 Whitish flecks are not uncommon and are often idiopathic.

ENAMEL HYPOPLASIA

Figure 9.31 Tooth development can be disturbed by constitutional disturbances such as childhood fevers, cystic fibrosis and gastroenteritis, producing a linear pattern of defects corresponding to the site of amelogenesis at the time ('chronological' hypoplasia). Horizontal pits or grooves are usually seen in the incisal third of the crowns of permanent teeth. Intrauterine infections such as rubella, or metabolic disturbances, may cause hypoplasia of the deciduous dentition.

Figure 9.32 In this case, mottling and hypoplasia of the deciduous dentition was caused by intrauterine disease – here by pseudohypoparathyroidism (see page 57). Enamel hypoplasia may also appear in the absence of any identifiable cause.

DILACERATION

Figure 9.33 Trauma to a developing tooth may produce distortion and dilaceration – a bend.

ISOLATED HYPOPLASIA (*Turner tooth*)

Figure 9.34 Infection of, or trauma to, a deciduous tooth, may cause hypoplasia of the underlying permanent successor.

Figure 9.35 This lower second premolar was deformed after an abscess on the predecessor deciduous molar. The malformed Turner tooth has subsequently become carious.

Figure 9.36 Comparison of a normal premolar (on the reader's left) with a Turner tooth shows the degree of deformity that can result.

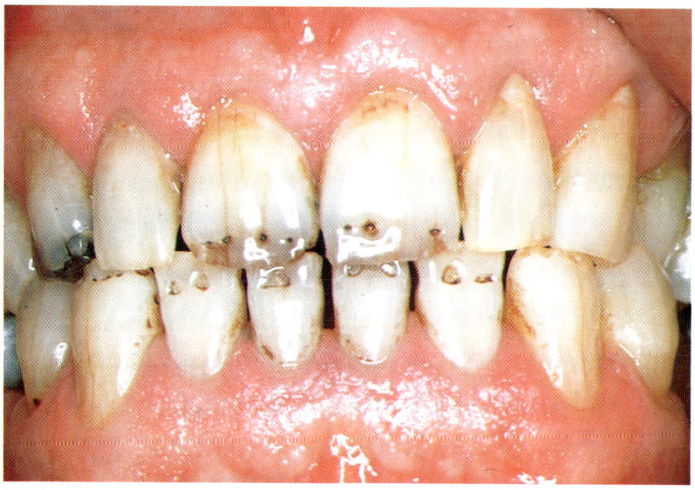

9.31

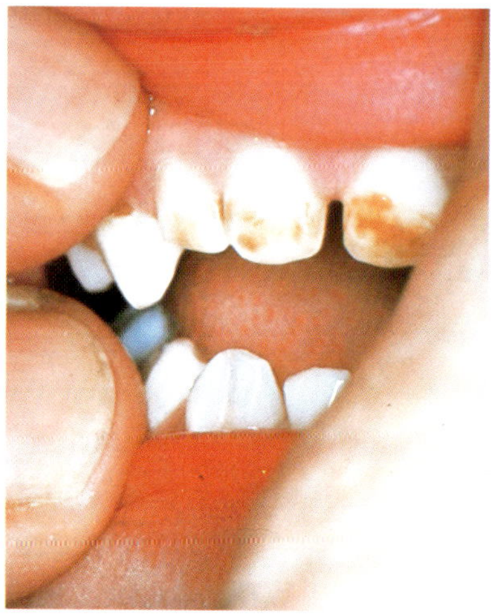

9.32

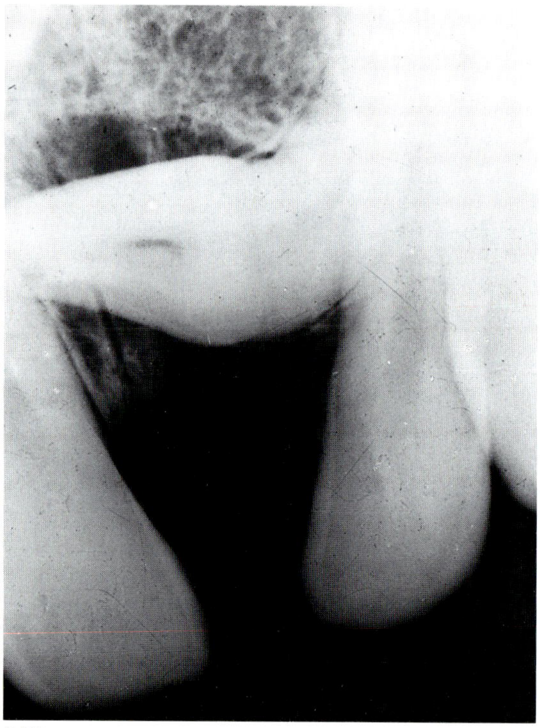

9.33

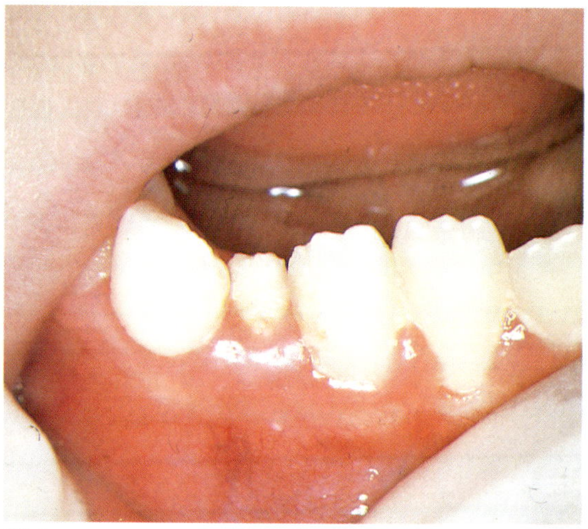

9.34

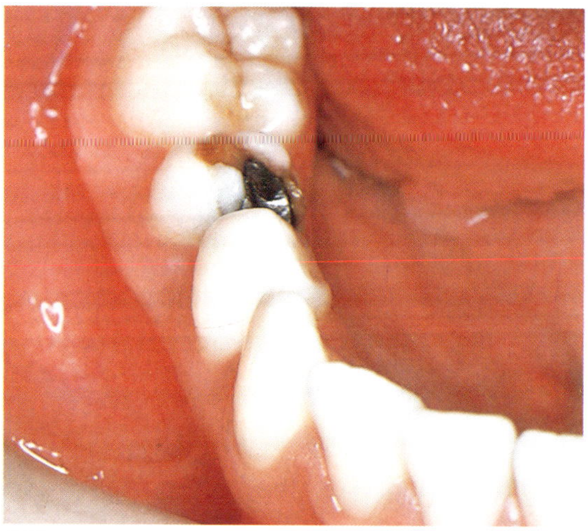

9.35

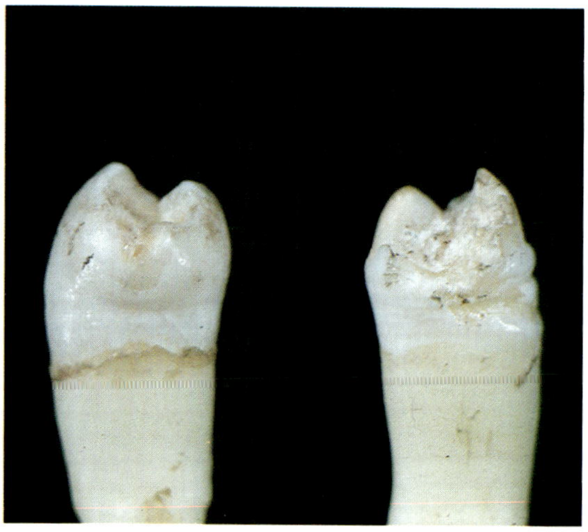

9.36

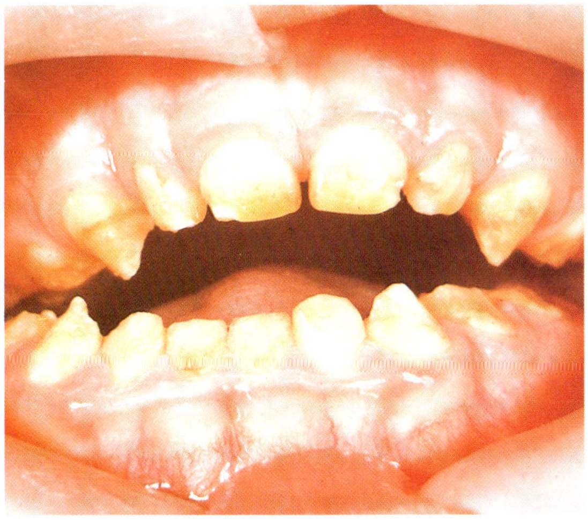

9.37

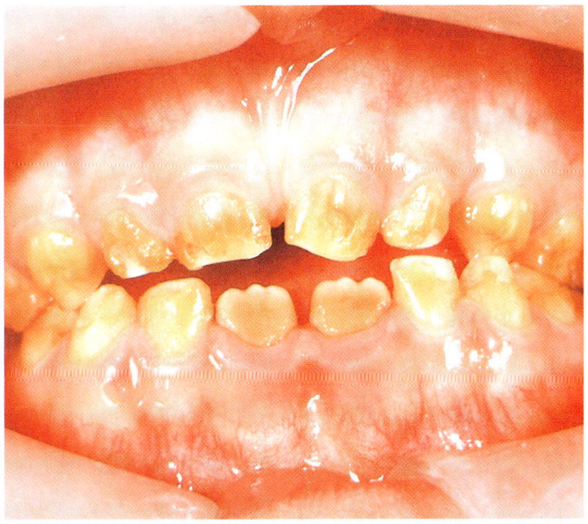

9.38

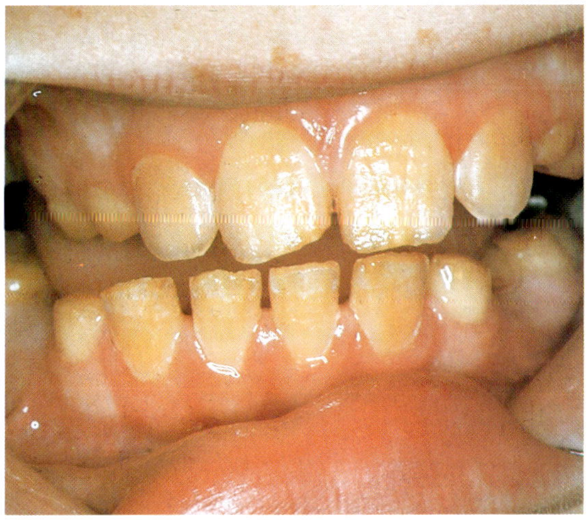

9.39

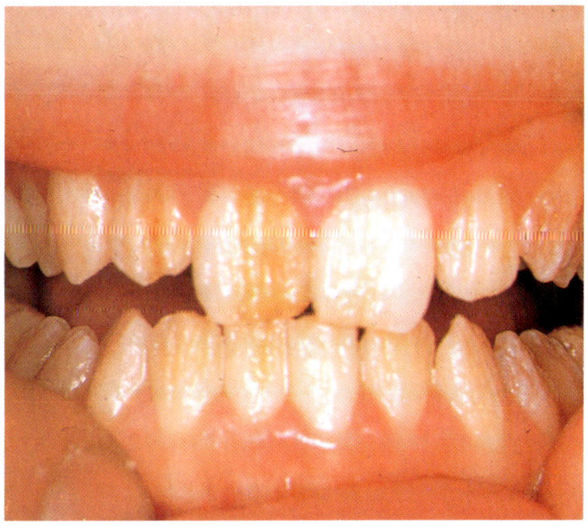

9.40

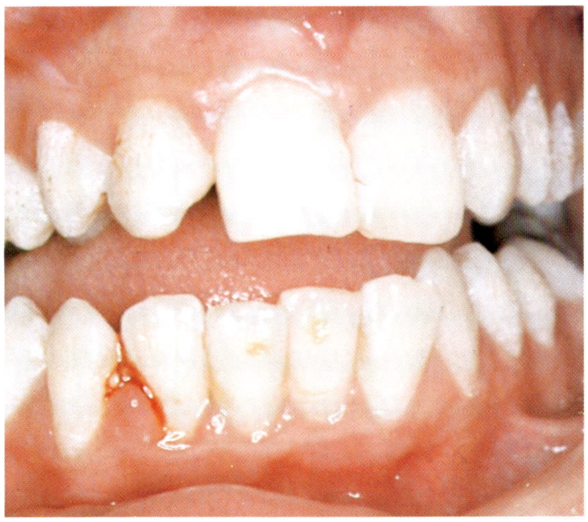

9.41

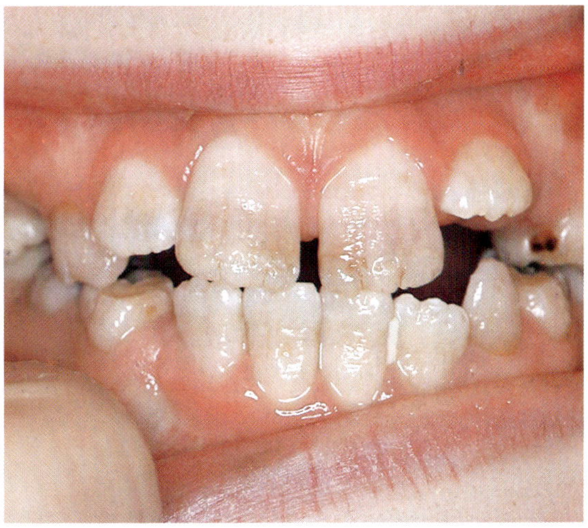

9.42

AMELOGENESIS IMPERFECTA

Figure 9.37 Amelogenesis imperfecta is the term applied to a number of rare genetically-determined disorders of enamel formation. This figure shows an affected primary dentition.

There are three main types of amelogenesis imperfecta: in hypoplastic types the enamel is thin; in hypocalcified types it is of normal thickness but weak and soft; and in hypomaturation types it can be pierced with a probe.

Figure 9.38 This illustration is of a sibling of the patient in Figure 9.37, and shows the genetic basis and the fact that the primary and secondary dentitions (the permanent central incisors are erupting) are both affected.

Figure 9.39 Hereditary enamel hypoplasia: an autosomal dominant type – the enamel matrix is defective, although calcification is normal (note the vertical ridging).

Figure 9.40 A more extreme example of hereditary enamel hypoplasia: a sex-linked dominant type.

Figure 9.41 Pitting and grooving is seen in some types of hereditary enamel hypoplasia.

Figure 9.42 A more extreme example of the type of hereditary enamel hypoplasia shown in Figure 9.41.

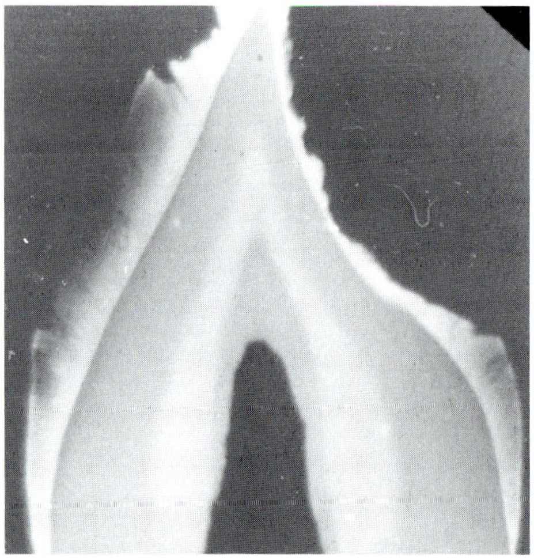

9.43

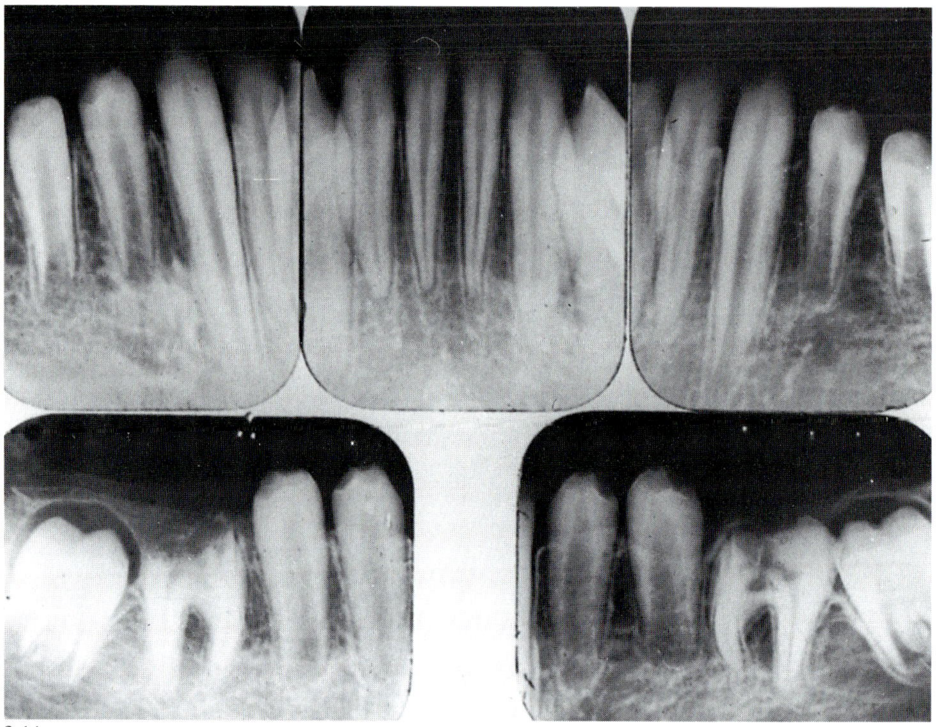

9.44

AMELOGENESIS IMPERFECTA (*continued*)

Figures 9.43 and 9.44 Radiographs show enamel deficiencies.

Figure 9.45 Hereditary enamel hypocalcification is the second main type of amelogenesis imperfecta – the matrix is normal but calcification defective. The soft enamel may wear away rapidly, as in this example, to leave only the dentine core.

Figure 9.46 In this example, there is almost complete breakdown of the dentition, and incidental calculus deposition.

Figure 9.47 Hereditary enamel hypomaturation: opaque white flecks or patches in an autosomal dominant variety of hypomaturation, the third type of amelogenesis imperfecta ('snow capped' teeth).

Figure 9.48 A variant affecting permanent first molars only.

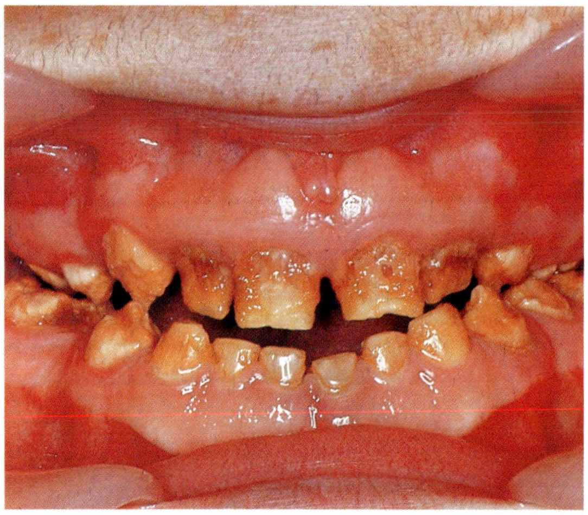

9.45

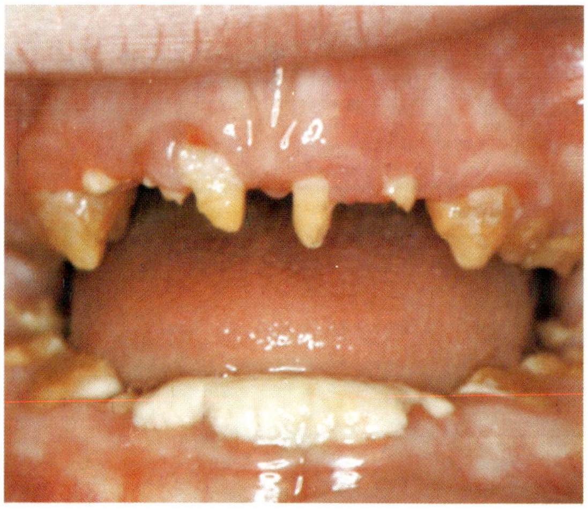

9.46

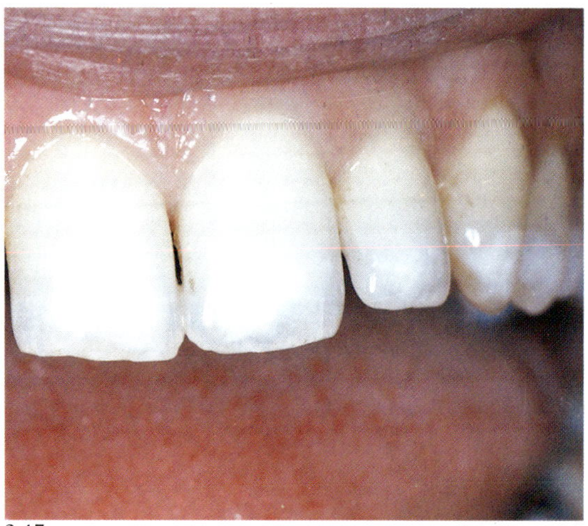

9.47

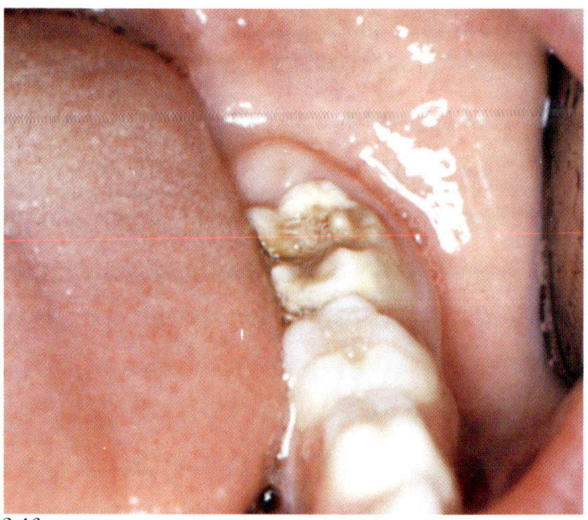

9.48

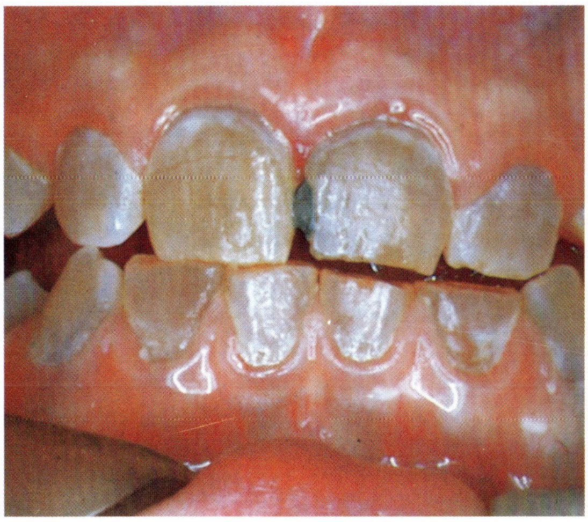

9.49

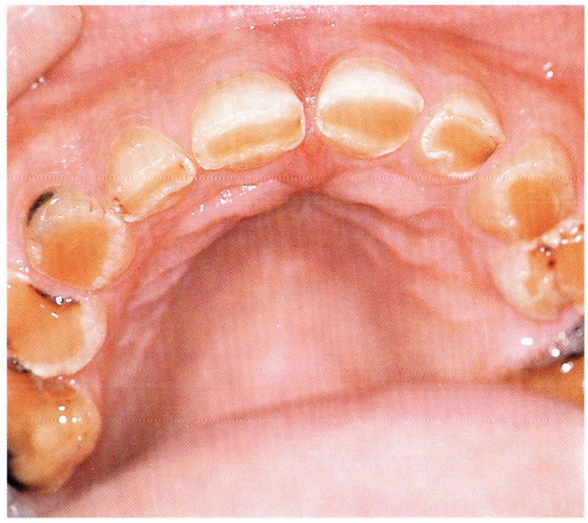

9.50

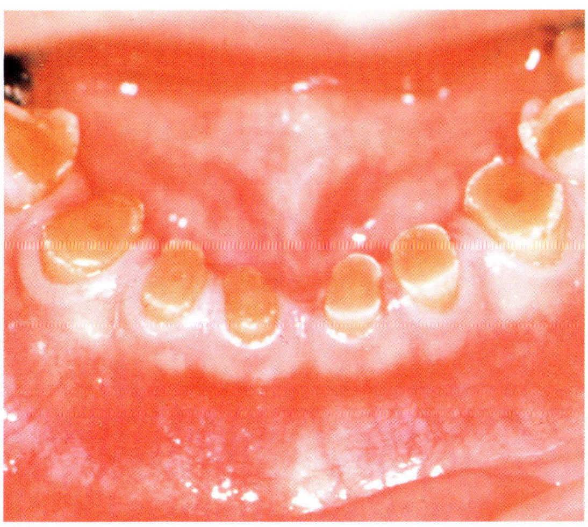

9.51

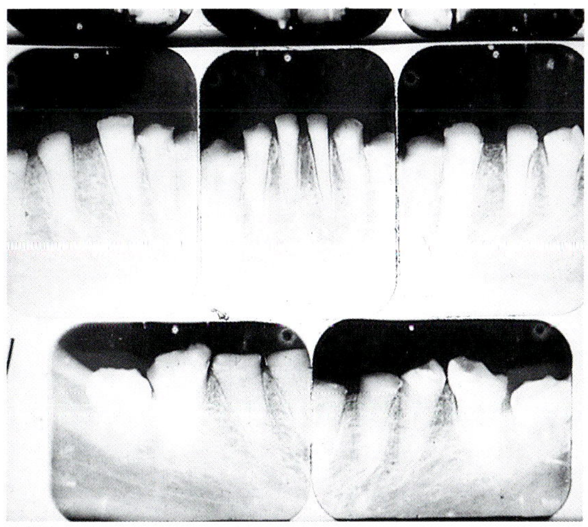

9.52

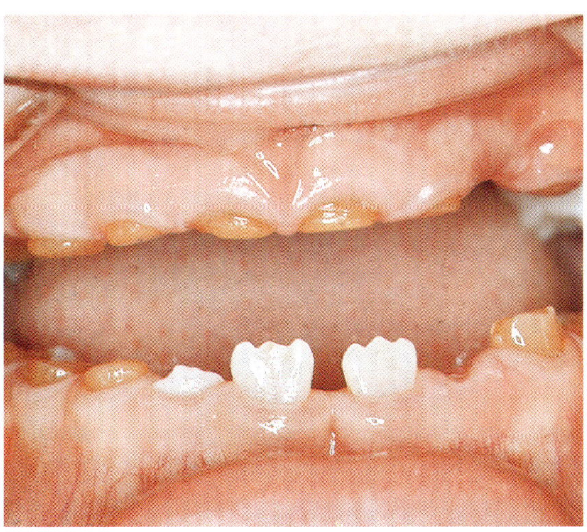

9.53

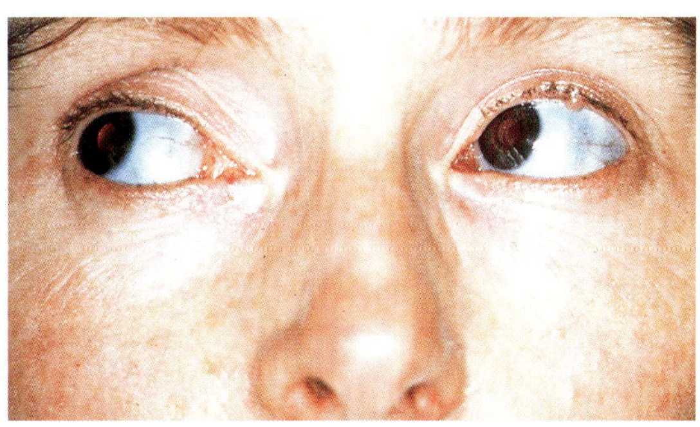

9.54

DENTINOGENESIS IMPERFECTA

Figure 9.49 Dentinogenesis imperfecta is an autosomal dominant condition in which the dentine is abnormal in structure and is translucent. This illustration shows Type I dentinogenesis imperfecta, with translucent brown teeth, but teeth may vary in colour from grey to blue or brown.

Figure 9.50 The tooth crowns are bulbous and the roots short. The enamel, though normal, is poorly adherent to the abnormal dentine and chips and wears.

Figure 9.51 Ultimately the teeth are worn flat by attrition but, fortunately, the pulp chambers are obliterated by secondary dentine and, therefore, are not exposed. The roots, however, fracture easily.

Figure 9.52 Pulp obliteration can be seen on radiography.

Figure 9.53 The deciduous dentition is often more severely affected than the permanent, especially in this variant – coronal dentine dysplasia or Type II dentine dysplasia. Radiographs show flame-shaped pulp chambers and narrow pulp canals. There may be several pulp stones in most teeth. Hereditary opalescent dentine is an alternative term for Type II dentinogenesis imperfecta.

Figure 9.54 Type III dentinogenesis imperfecta is associated with osteogenesis imperfecta. The deciduous dentition is more severely affected than the permanent teeth. Dentinogenesis imperfecta appears frequently in those patients with osteogenesis imperfecta who have normal, rather than blue, sclerae (illustrated here).

DENTINOGENESIS IMPERFECTA (*continued*)

Figure 9.55 In Type IV dentinogenesis imperfecta, dentine formation ceases after the initial mantle layer, leaving teeth that are shell-like.

NATAL TEETH

Figure 9.56 Rarely, teeth are present at, or soon after, birth, and have been described even at 26 weeks' gestation. They may cause no trouble but may ulcerate the tongue, as here, or the breast if suckling. Usually the teeth involved are lower incisors of the normal primary dentition: occasionally they are supernumeraries. Rarely, there are associations with Ellis-van Creveld syndrome; pachyonychia congenita; Hallermann-Streiff syndrome, or steatocystoma multiplex.

Figure 9.57 If there are problems from natal teeth, radiographs should be taken before extractions are contemplated. Extractions are best restricted to those teeth that are supernumeraries or are very loose and in danger of being inhaled.

TERATOMA

Figure 9.58 Cystic ovarian teratomas (dermoid) may, as here, contain well-formed teeth.

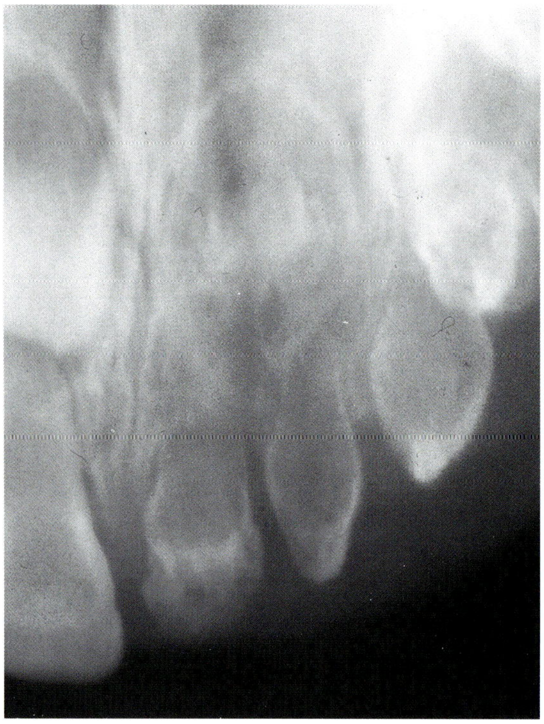

9.55

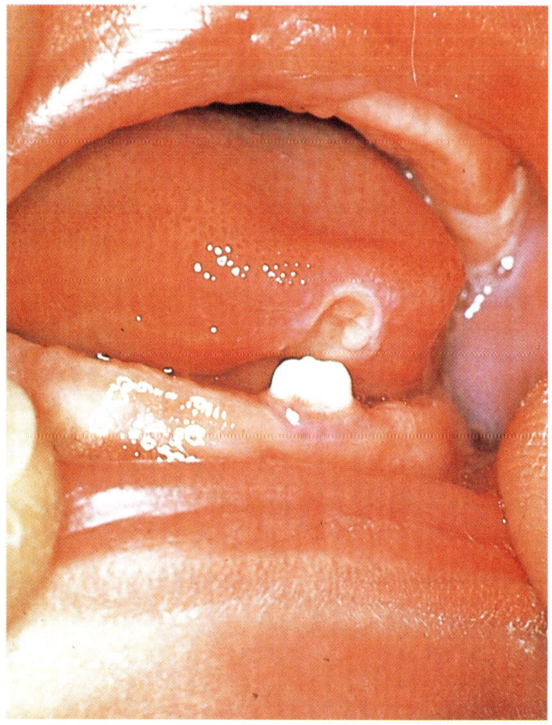

9.56

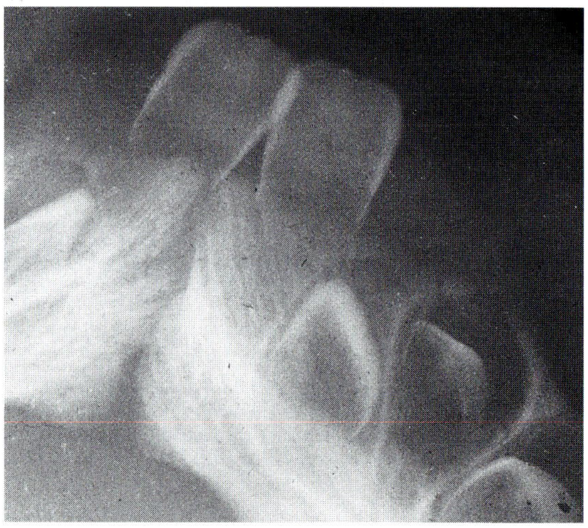

9.57

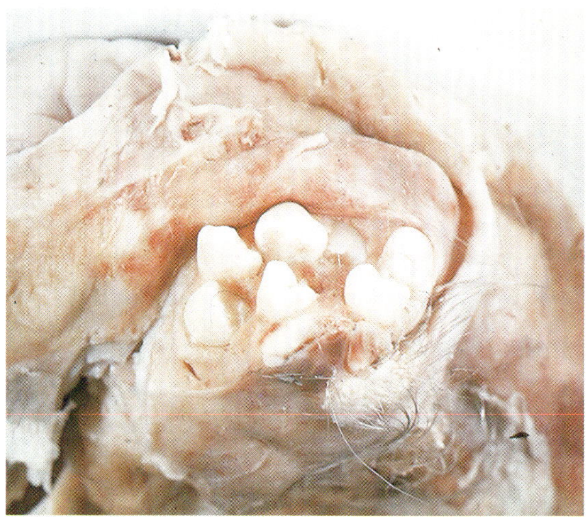

9.58

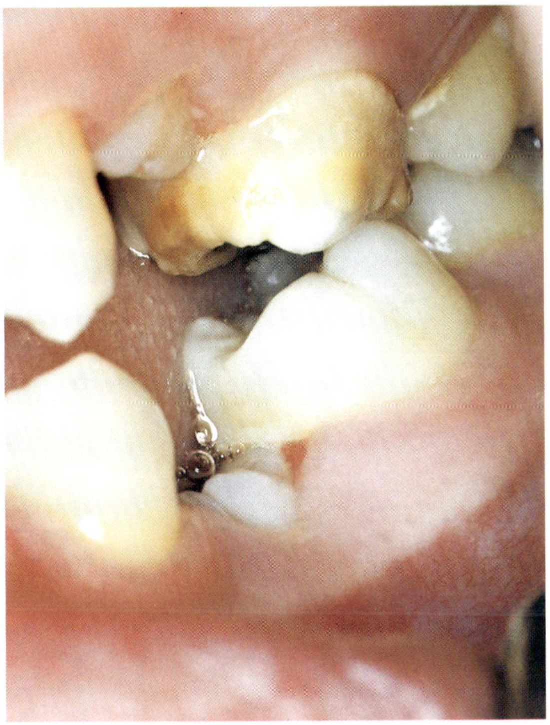

9.59

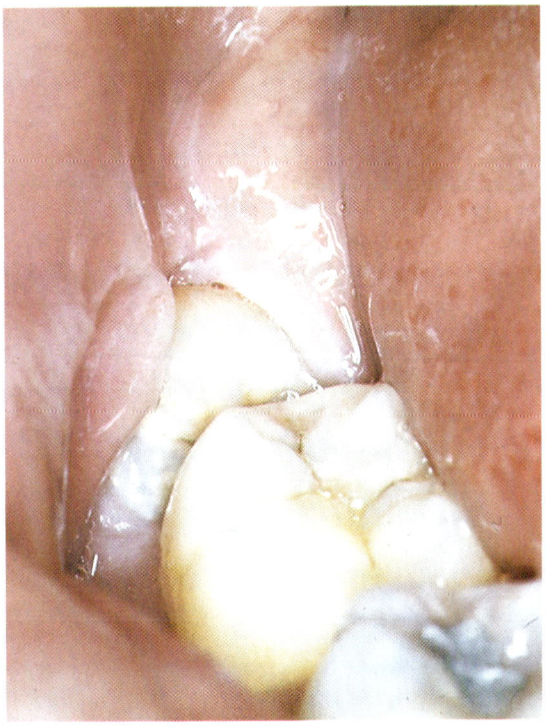

9.60

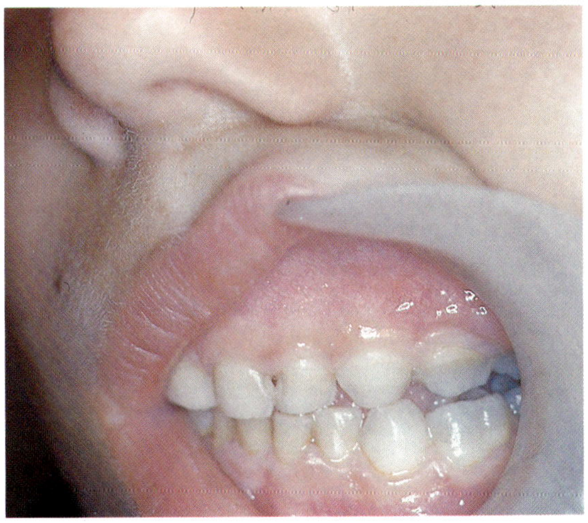

9.61

RETAINED PRIMARY TOOTH

Figure 9.59 Primary teeth are commonly retained if the successor is missing (see page 92). Usually this is of little consequence but occasionally, as here, particularly in the case of lower deciduous molars, the tooth fails to maintain its occlusal relationship (infraocclusion or submergence).

IMPACTED TEETH

Figure 9.60 Lower third molars (as here) are the most common teeth to impact, that is, fail to erupt fully because of insufficient space. Canines and second premolars as well as other teeth also impact commonly. Impacted teeth may well be asymptomatic but occasionally cause pain, usually from caries or pericoronitis, or are the site of dentigerous cyst formation.

BILE PIGMENT STAINING

Figure 9.61 Haemolytic disease of the newborn (icterus gravis neonatorum) is now rare but more infants survive with hyperbilirubinaemia of other cause. Jaundice in either case may cause enamel hypoplasia in the deciduous dentition, which may have a greenish colour, as in this case.

Congenital erythropoietic porphyria may cause yellow to brown-red tooth discoloration.

TETRACYCLINE STAINING

Figure 9.62 Tetracycline is taken up by developing teeth and by bone. If given to pregnant or nursing mothers or to children under the age of 8 years, the tooth crowns become discoloured, initially being yellow but darkening with time. This shows very clearly here, since the permanent teeth that formed after the drug was given in pregnancy have a normal appearance.

Figure 9.63 Staining of the permanent dentition – yellow and brown bands of staining – is most obvious at the necks of the teeth where the thinner enamel allows the colour of the stained dentine to show through. Staining is greater the larger the dose of tetracycline, and is worse with tetracycline than with oxytetracycline.

Figure 9.64 More severe staining of the permanent dentition. Staining is most obvious in light-exposed anterior teeth. The tooth of normal colour is a supernumerary tooth that clearly developed at a time after tetracyclines had been given.

Figure 9.65 Even in older children, tetracyclines cause staining but by then most tooth crowns have formed. The staining then affects the roots – as in this lower third molar.

Figure 9.66 Affected teeth may fluoresce bright yellow under ultraviolet light and this helps to distinguish tetracycline staining from dentinogenesis imperfecta. Fluorescence is also seen in undecalcified sections viewed under ultraviolet light.

Nitrofurantoin has also been reported to cause tooth discoloration.

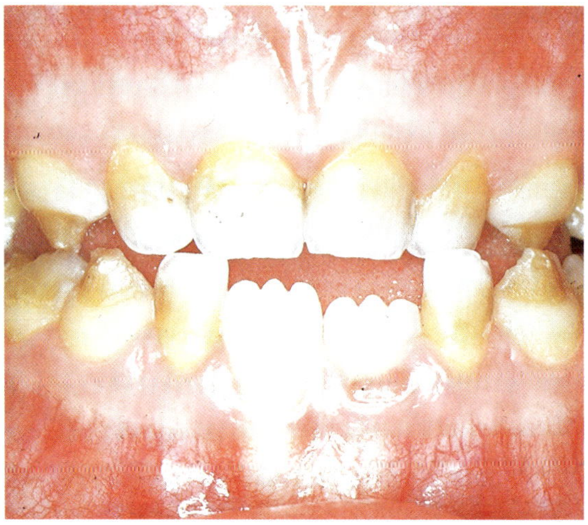

9.62

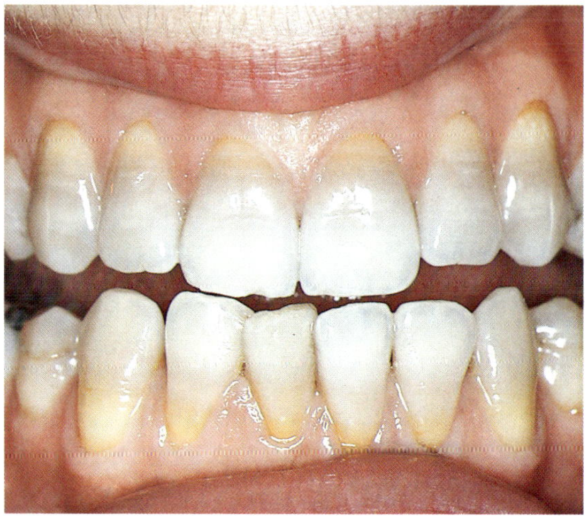

9.63

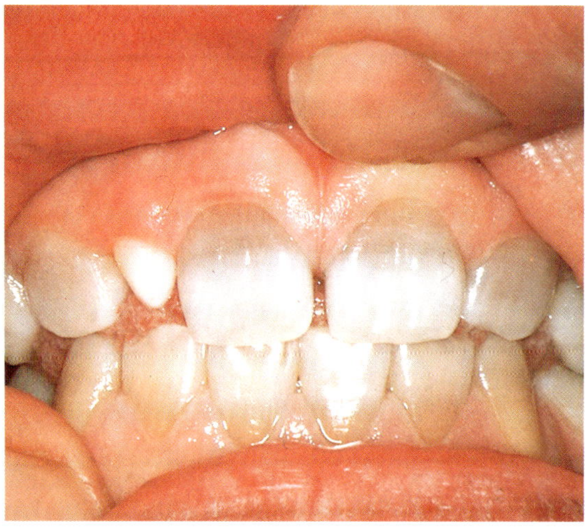

9.64

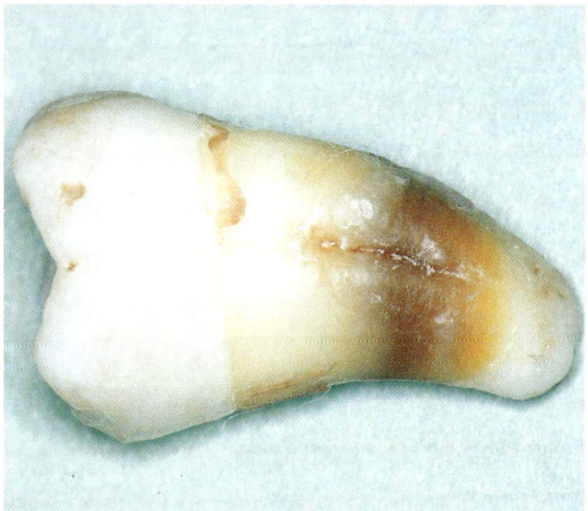

9.65

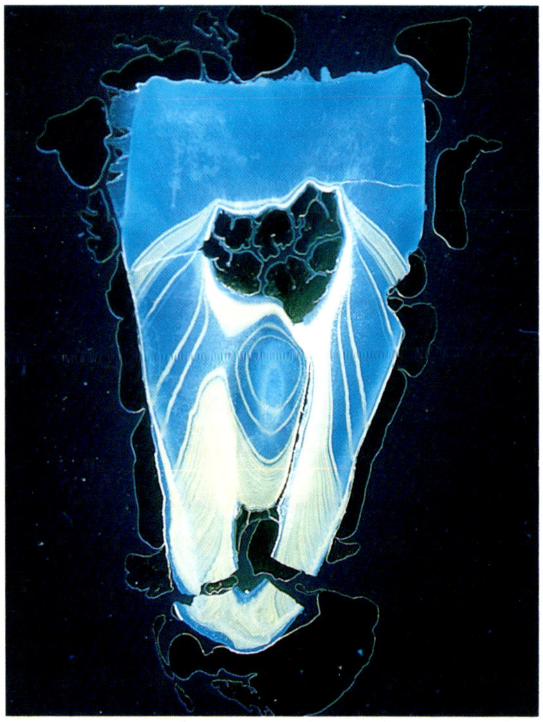

9.66

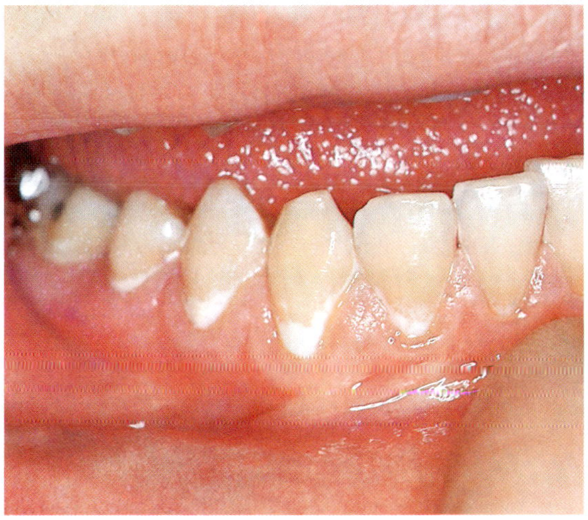

9.67

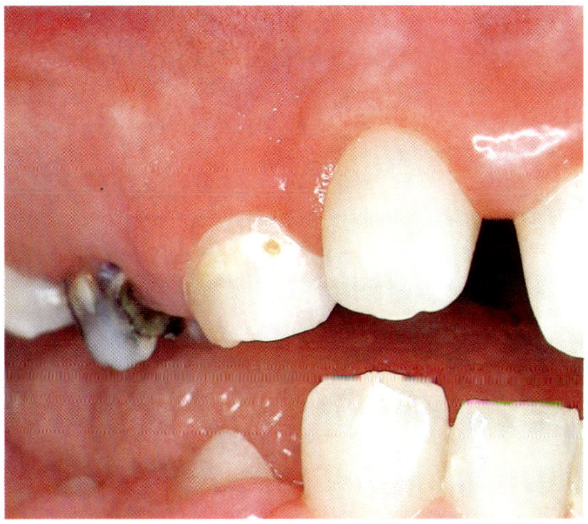

9.68

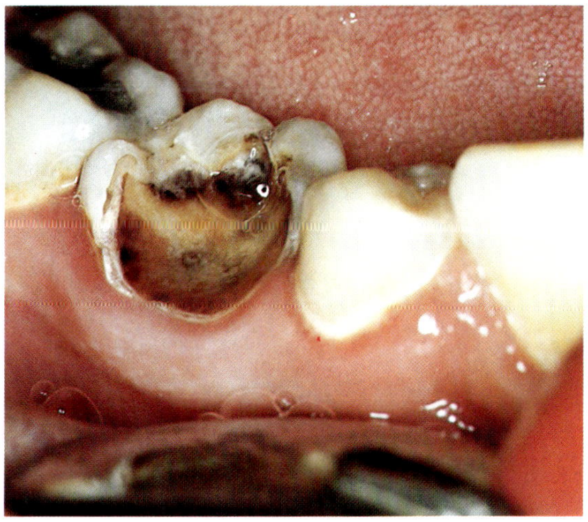

9.69

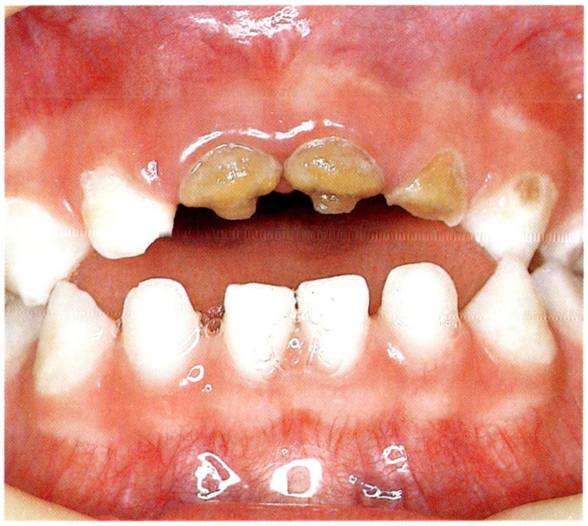

9.70

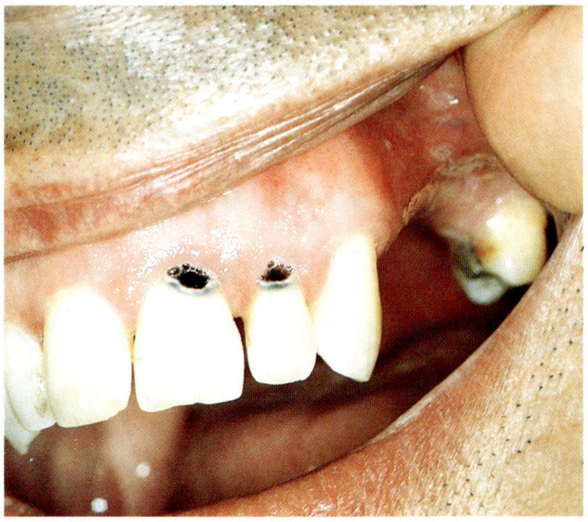

9.71

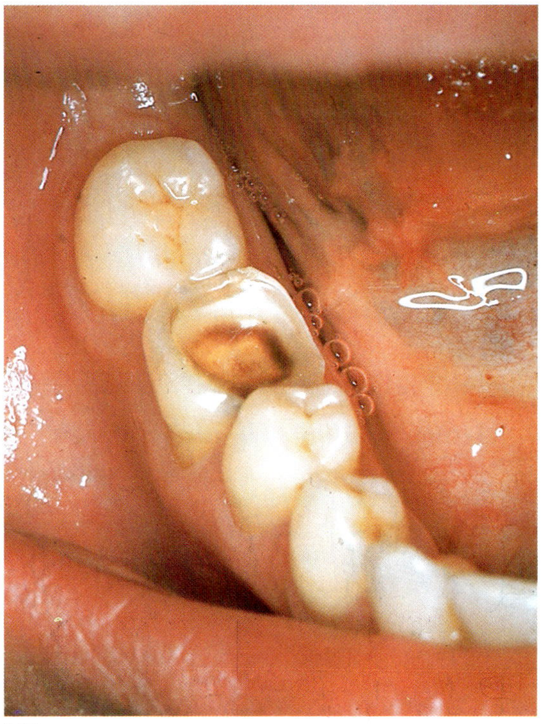

9.72

DENTAL CARIES

Figure 9.67 Decalcification beneath the bacterial plaque that accumulates in stagnation areas, such as close to the gingival margin, produces an opaque whitish band. At this early stage, where there is no cavitation, the lesion is reversible if diet is changed and fermentable carbohydrates reduced or excluded. Fluoride aids remineralization.

Figure 9.68 This is an upper deciduous canine tooth with early caries. The carious enamel breaks down to form a cavity, as shown.

Figure 9.69 The enamel has been undermined and fractured away. The carious dentine is discoloured and this shows through the enamel. Pulpal involvement is inevitable in such carious teeth.

Figure 9.70 Rampant caries, affecting mainly the upper incisors in a child using a sugar/fruit juice mix in a bottle to help her sleep at night.

Figure 9.71 Arrested caries: change in dietary habits (particularly a reduction in frequency of fermentable carbohydrate intake), fluoride treatment, and improved oral hygiene can arrest the progress of caries. Lesions shown here at the cervical margins then darken and become static.

Figure 9.72 Any change in local environment that makes the carious lesions self-cleansing, for example, loss of a tooth adjacent to an interproximal lesion, or fracture of cusps overlying a lesion, may cause arrest of the caries.

In contrast, xerostomia for any reason significantly predisposes to caries.

ATTRITION

Figure 9.73 Attrition is wearing away of tooth substance by mastication. It is most obvious where the diet is coarse or where there is a parafunctional habit such as bruxism. The incisal edges and cusps wear with more loss of dentine than enamel, leading to a flat or hollowed surface.

Figure 9.74 Unless attrition is rapid, the pulp is protected by obliteration with secondary dentine.

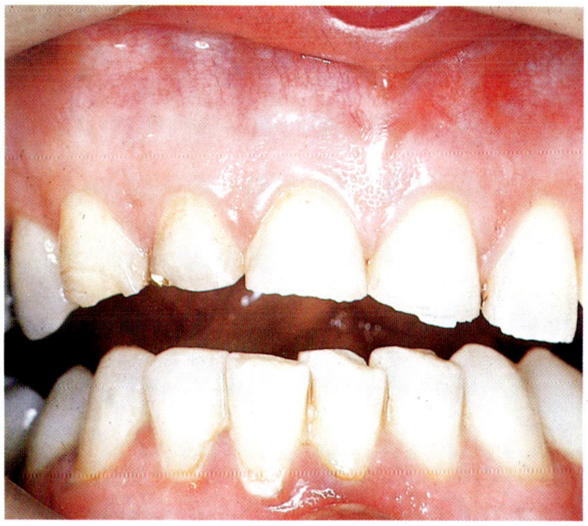

9.73

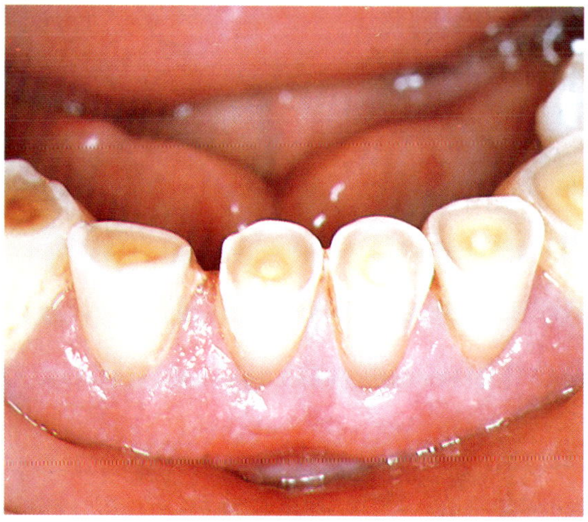

9.74

ABRASION

Figure 9.75 Abrasion is wearing away of tooth substance by a habit such as toothbrushing. Brushing with a hard brush and coarse dentifrice may abrade the neck of the tooth. The gingiva recedes but is otherwise healthy. The cementum and dentine wear but the harder enamel survives, resulting in a notch. Eventually, the tooth may fracture, as shown.

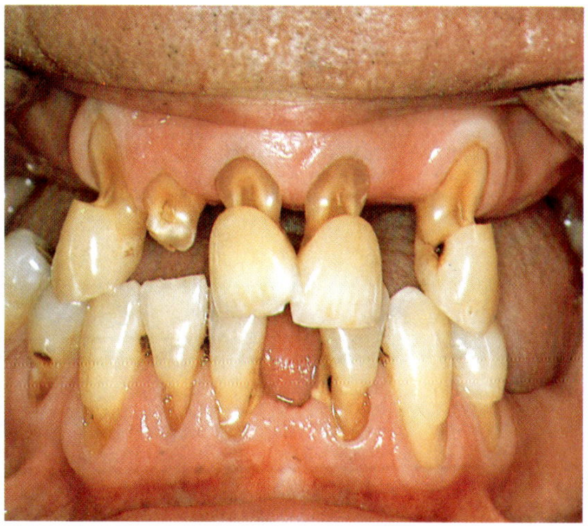

9.75

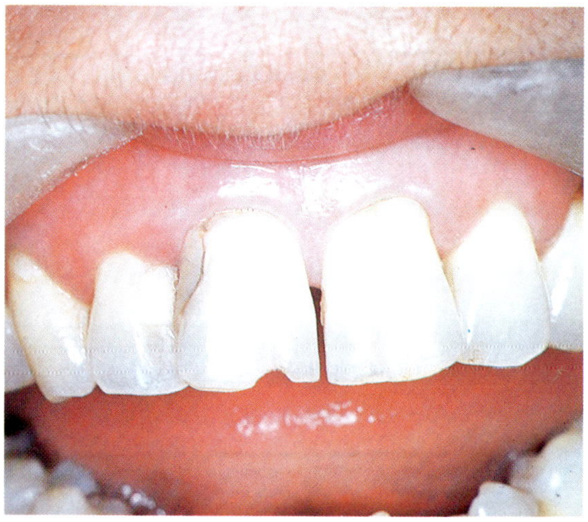

9.76

LOCALIZED DAMAGE

Figure 9.76 Seamstress' notch: holding pins, nails, etc, between the teeth can produce a variety of lesions. This patient held pins in her teeth during her work as a seamstress.

Figure 9.77 Self-mutilation for aesthetic reasons, according to tribal custom: there is also a degree of fluorosis.

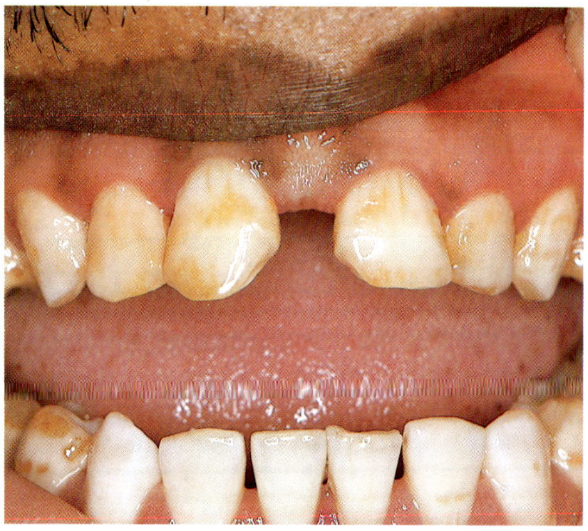

9.77

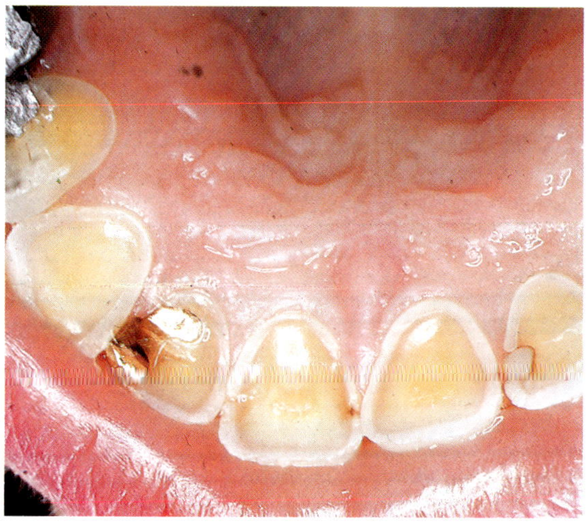

9.78

EROSION

Figure 9.78 Erosion is the loss of tooth substance caused by acids. Citrus fruits or carbonated beverages may produce such lesions. Habitual sucking of oranges has caused erosion of these incisors. Rarely, occupational exposure to acids may produce erosion, and even the low pH of indoor swimming pools may be a cause.

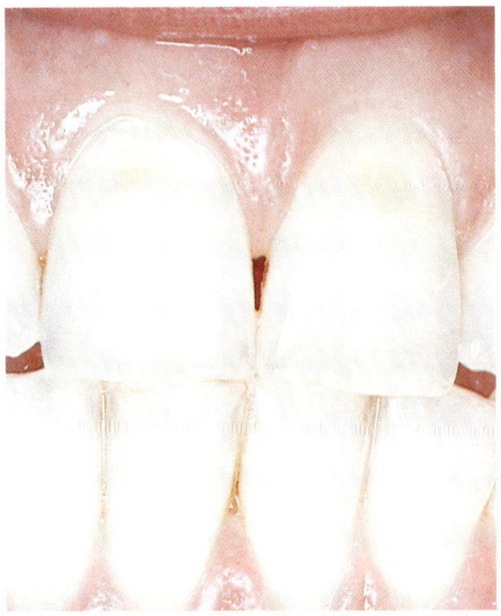

9.79

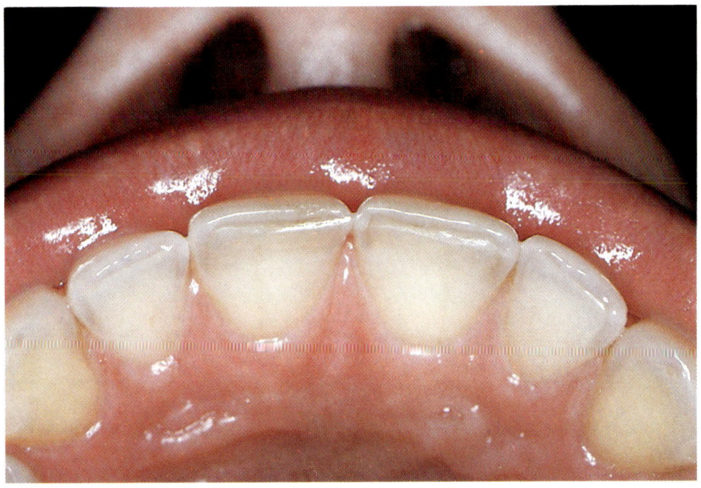

9.80

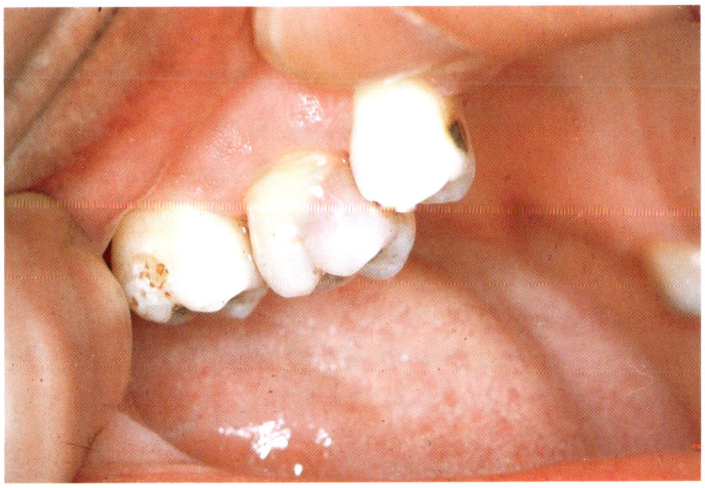

9.81

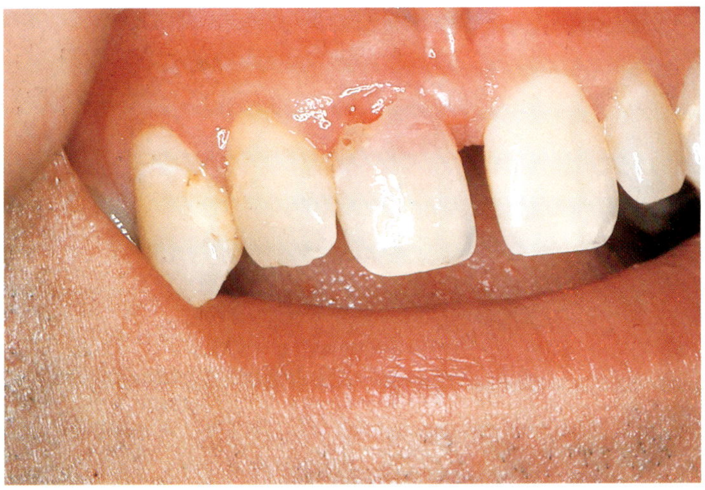

9.82

BULIMIA NERVOSA

Figure 9.79 Repeated gastric regurgitation over a prolonged period may cause erosion, mainly of the palatal surfaces of the upper teeth. This is seen especially in bulimia nervosa. Figure 9.79 and 9.80 show a patient with bulimia nervosa.

Figure 9.80 Other features not shown include enlargement of salivary glands (mainly parotids) which appears to be sialosis; possible conjunctival suffusion and oesophageal tears (caused by retching); and Russell's sign – abrasions on the back of the hand or fingers caused by using the hand to touch the throat to induce vomiting.

INTERNAL RESORPTION (*Pink spot*)

Figure 9.81 The upper first permanent molar shows pink spot. In this, dentine is spontaneously resorbed from within. The pulp is eventually exposed.

Incidentally, the dark brown lesion on the premolar is a result of interproximal caries that has arrested. The lesion on the second molar is a cavity from which the restoration has been lost.

EXTERNAL RESORPTION

Figure 9.82 Resorption may progress from the external surface, eventually to involve the pulp.

The canine has a synthetic restoration. The white semilunar line is decalcification that occurred some years earlier, when the oral hygiene was not so good and the gingiva not so far receded.

HYPERCEMENTOSIS

Figure 9.83 Hypercementosis is usually a consequence of periapical periodontitis, or may affect isolated functionless teeth. Paget's disease of bone may be complicated by hypercementosis (see page 189).

ANKYLOSIS

Figure 9.84 There is bony ankylosis and no evidence of a periodontal ligament in this deciduous molar, which is retained and in infraocclusion because the permanent successor is absent.

POST-ERUPTIVE COLOUR CHANGE OF TEETH

Figure 9.85 Metal-staining: a rare cause of colour change affecting many teeth is occupational, such as in workers with chromium (here) or lead (page 118). Isolated teeth that discolour are usually non-vital or carious.

Figure 9.86 Non-vital tooth: pulp necrosis from caries or trauma is the usual cause of a non-vital (dead) tooth. The tooth progressively darkens, sometimes to a brownish colour as shown here, and also becomes more brittle.

HYPERPLASTIC PULPITIS (*Pulp polyp*)

Figure 9.87 Only when the coronal pulp is widely exposed and there is a very good blood supply does the pulp survive trauma or infection. This situation can occur in young persons, and the pulp becomes hyperplastic and epithelialized.

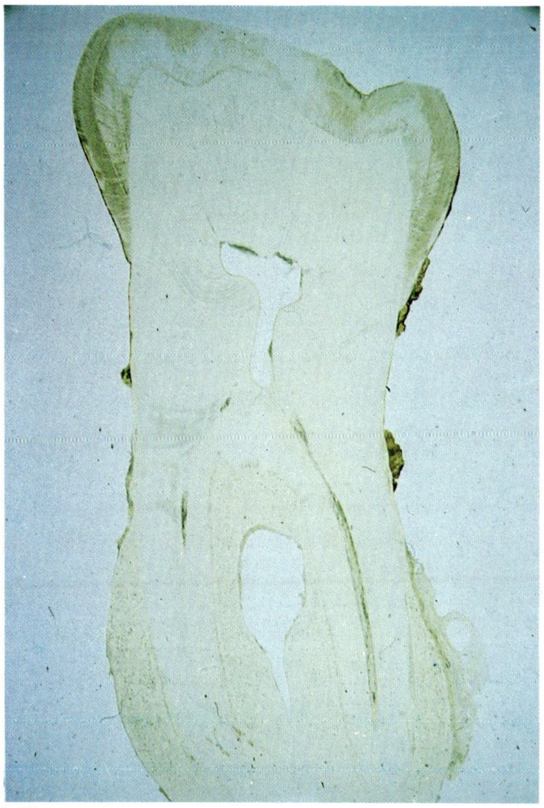

9.83

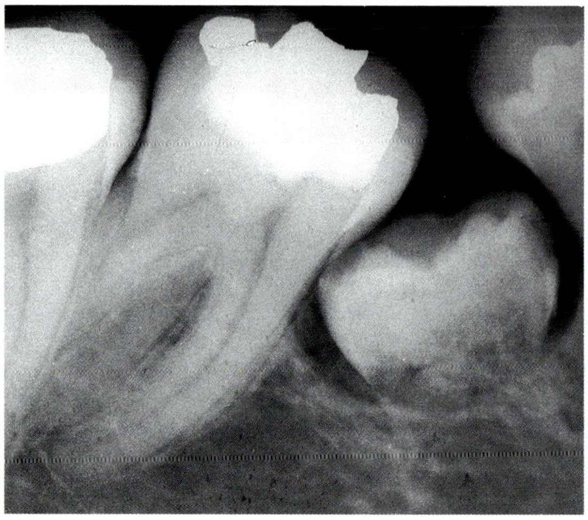

9.84

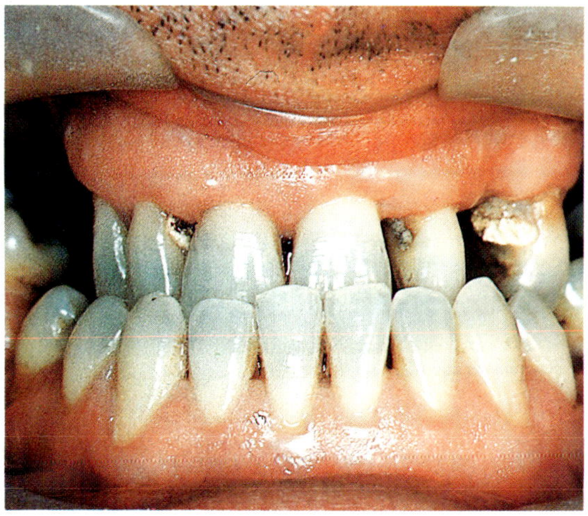

9.85

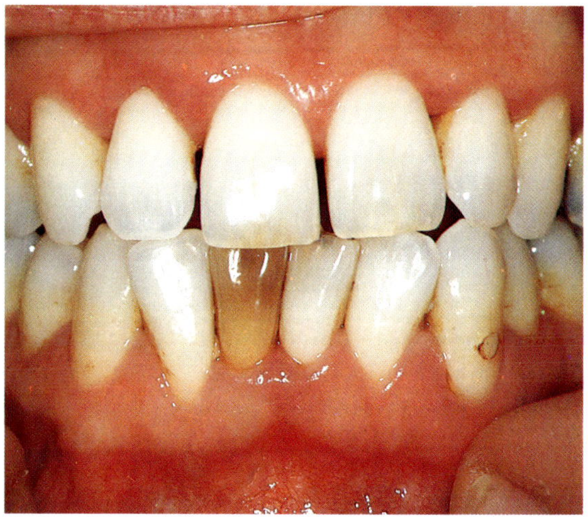

9.86

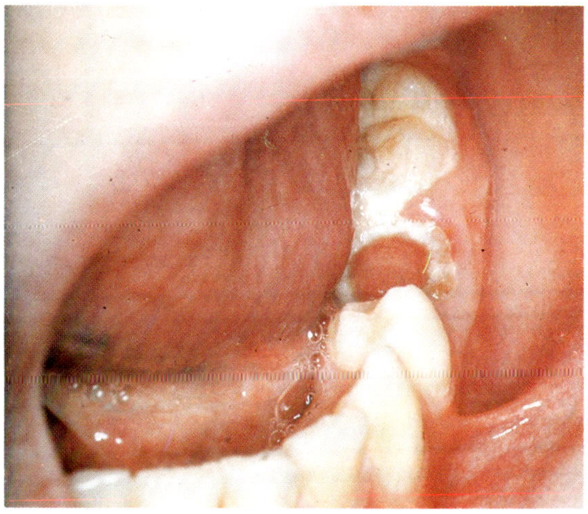

9.87

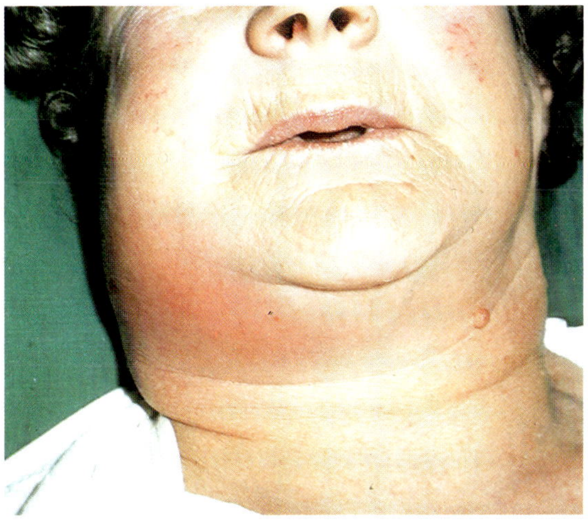

9.88

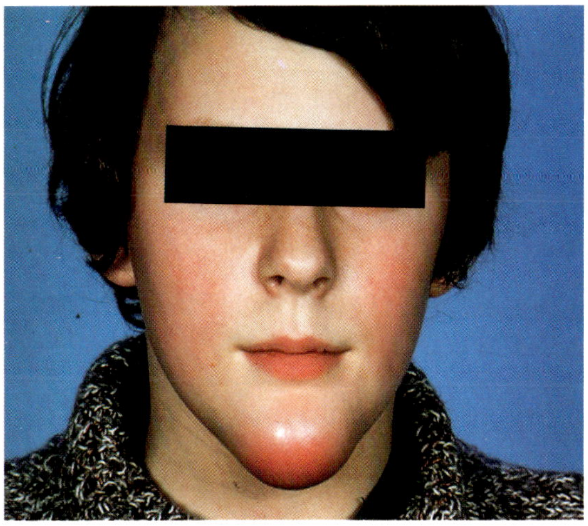

9.89

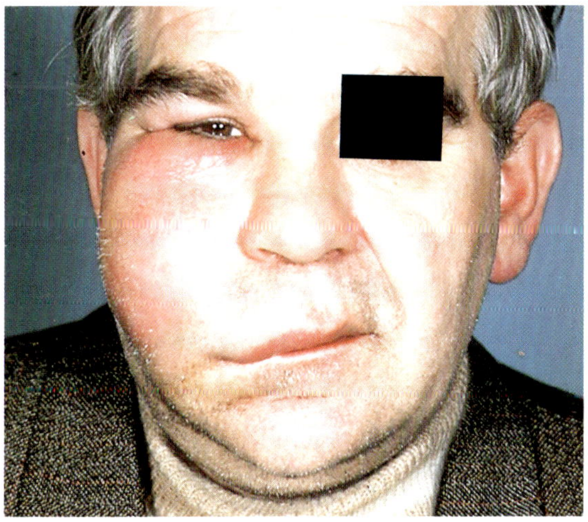

9.90

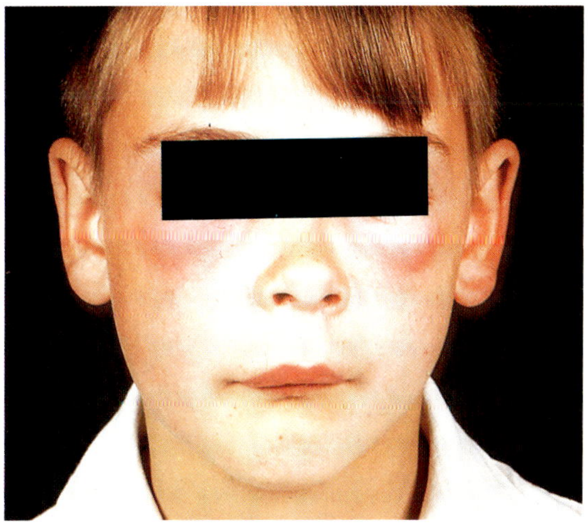

9.91

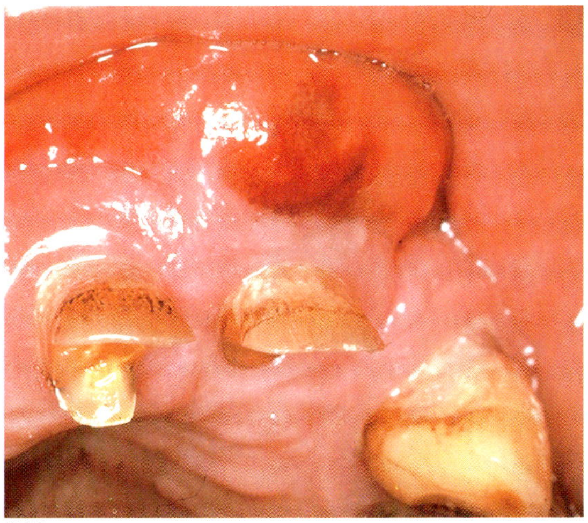

9.92

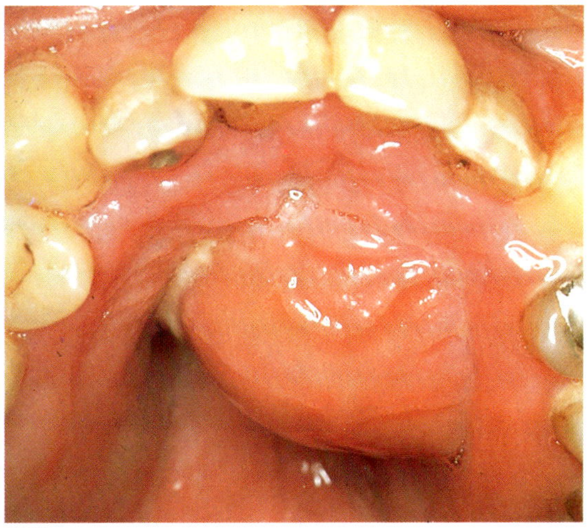

9.93

PERIAPICAL ABSCESS (*Dental abscess, odontogenic abscess*)

Figure 9.88 An abscess is often a sequel of pulpitis caused by dental caries but may arise in relation to any non-vital tooth. A mixed bacterial flora is implicated, although the role of anaerobes such as fusobacteria and bacteroides species is increasingly recognized. Pain and facial swelling, here from an abscess on a lower molar, are characteristic.

Figure 9.89 Inflammatory swelling resulting from a dental abscess on a lower incisor. Not all dental abscesses cause facial swelling, however.

Figure 9.90 Periapical abscess on an upper premolar causing infraorbital swelling.

Figure 9.91 Swelling of the infraorbital region and upper lip from a periapical abscess on an upper incisor.

Figure 9.92 Most dental abscesses produce an intraoral swelling, typically on the labial or buccal gingiva. This large, tender, inflammatory swelling which is about to discharge, is related to pulp exposure from attrition.

Figure 9.93 Although most periapical abscesses cause swelling buccally, abscesses on maxillary lateral incisors and those arising from the first molar tend to present palatally. The lateral incisor involved here has a deep, carious palatal pit which caused pulp necrosis.

PERIAPICAL ABSCESS
(continued)

Figure 9.94 Bone destruction caused by a periapical abscess on the carious lower permanent molar shows well on this radiograph.

Figure 9.95 The periapical abscess here resulted from trauma, rendering the upper deciduous incisor non-vital.

Figure 9.96 Once the abscess discharges, the acute inflammation, pain and swelling resolve and a chronic abscess develops discharging from a sinus – usually buccally, as here.

Figure 9.97 Extraction, or endodontic therapy, of a tooth affected with a periapical abscess removes the source of infection. Here, the pus is discharging through the extraction socket.

Figure 9.98 Occasionally, abscesses – especially those of lower incisors or molars – discharge extraorally. This sinus arose from a dental abscess on the lower canine.

Figure 9.99 This sinus was related to an abscess on the lower first premolar.

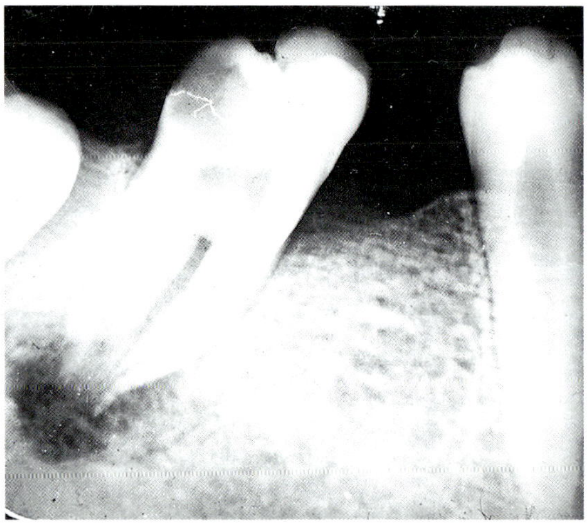
9.94

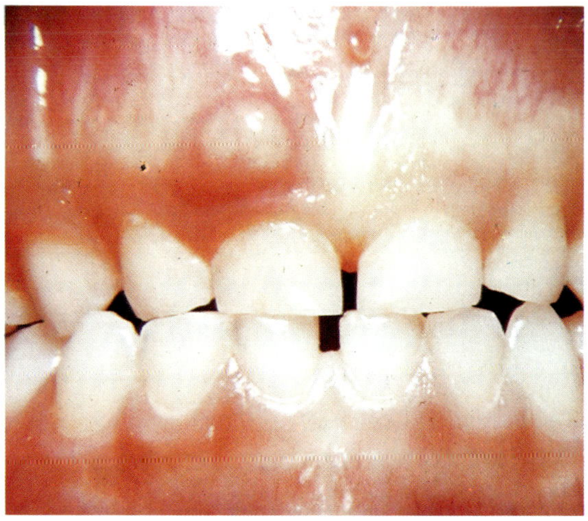
9.95

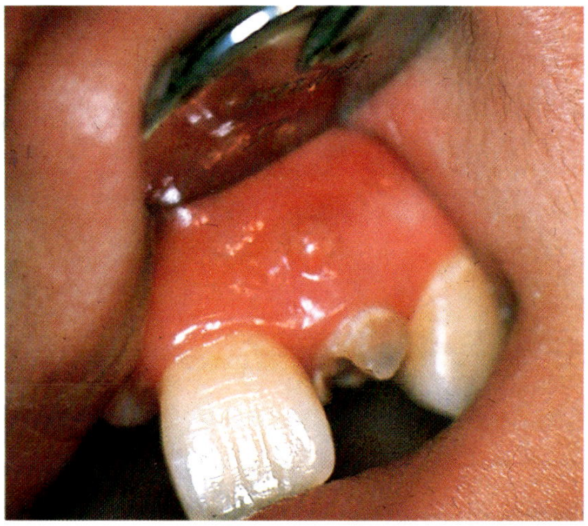
9.96

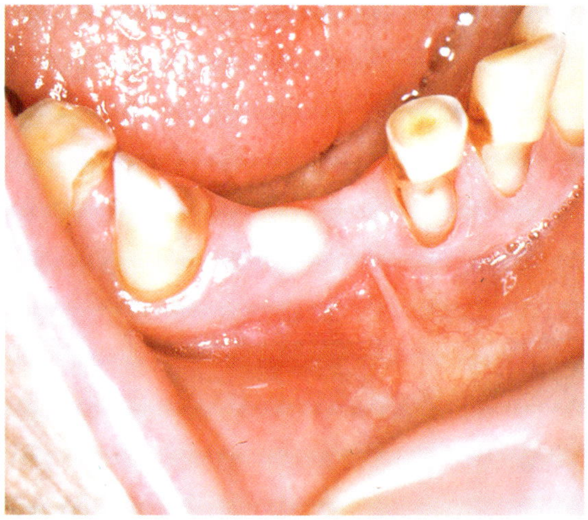
9.97

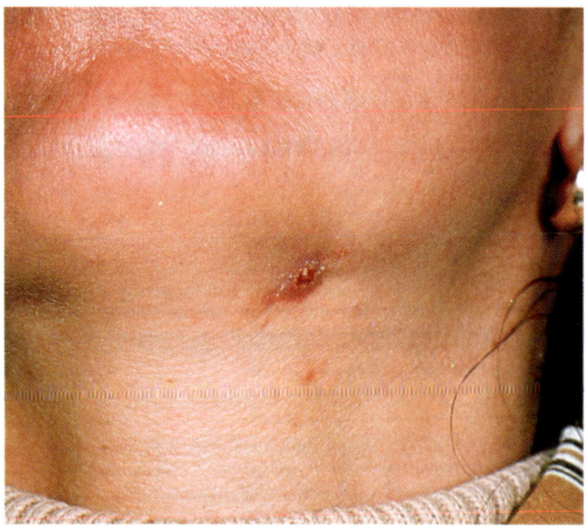
9.98

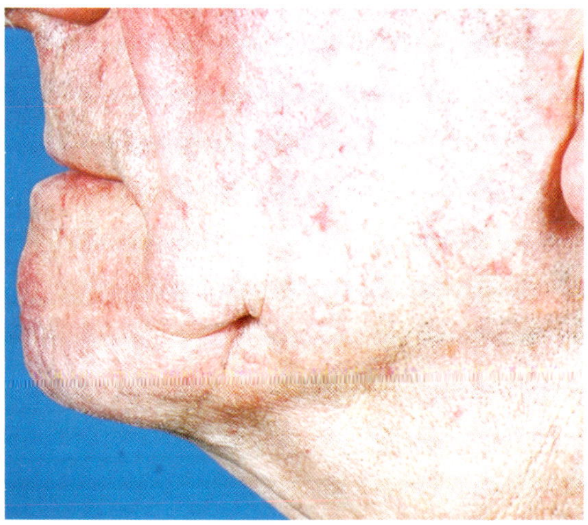
9.99

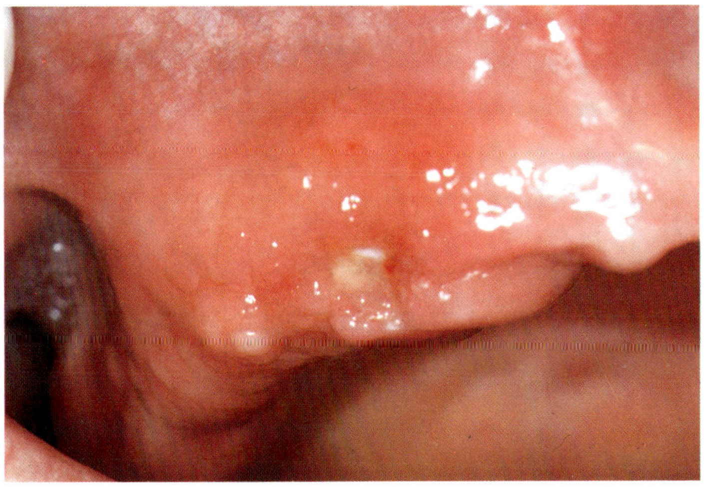

9.100

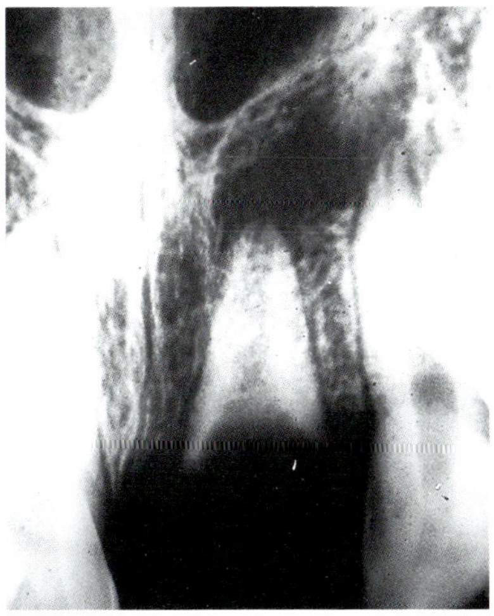

9.101

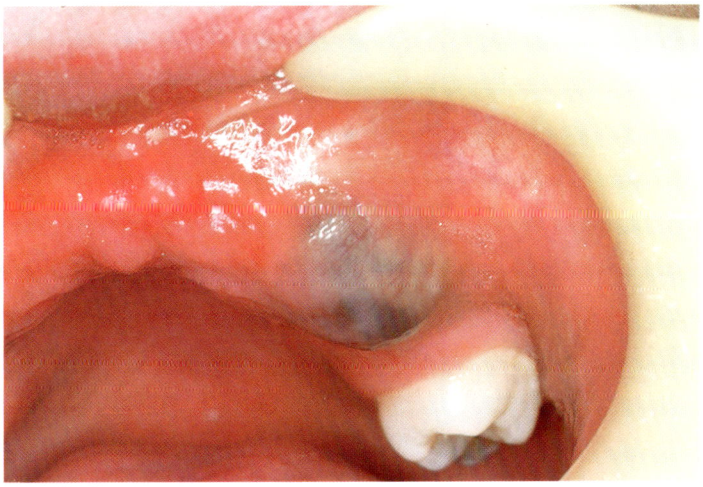

9.102

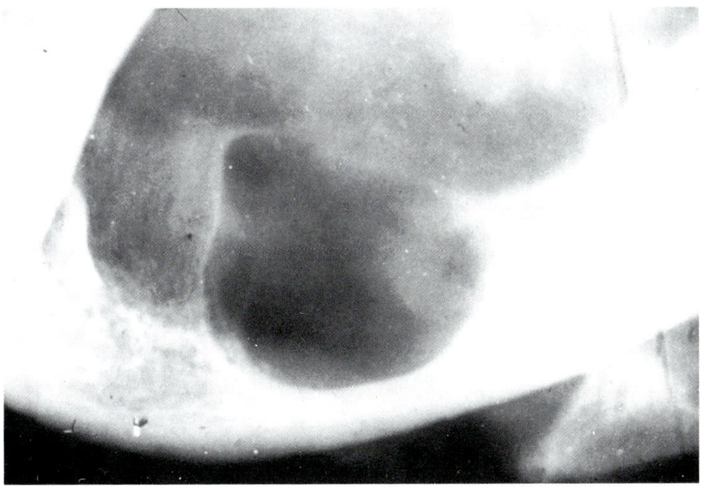

9.103

PERIAPICAL CYST
(*Radicular or dental cyst*)

Figure 9.100 A granuloma may arise at the apex of a non-vital tooth and may occasionally develop into a cyst from proliferation of epithelial rests in the area (cell rests of Malassez). Here, there is a retained root in the maxilla with swelling from a cyst. Many periapical cysts involve upper lateral incisors since these not infrequently become carious and the pulp can be involved relatively rapidly.

Figure 9.101 Most odontogenic cysts are periapical cysts. A periapical cyst may well be asymptomatic and often is a chance radiographic finding. It may present as a swelling (usually in the labial sulcus) or may become infected and present as an abscess. There is a cyst here on the incisor root.

A small periapical cyst may remain attached to, and be extracted with, the causal root or tooth, or resolve with endodontic therapy.

RESIDUAL CYST

Figure 9.102 A periapical cyst left *in situ* after the causal root or tooth is removed, may continue to expand, termed a residual cyst. The bluish swelling of the cyst is shown here.

Figure 9.103 This oblique lateral radiograph is of a residual mandibular cyst. A residual cyst is almost invariably unilocular but may expand to an appreciable size. It may be asymptomatic, may be detected as a swelling, a chance radiographic finding, pathological fracture, or may rarely become infected and present as an abscess.

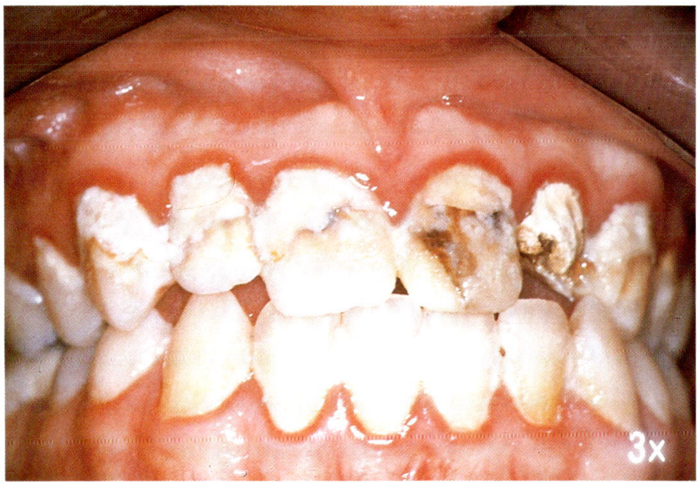

9.104

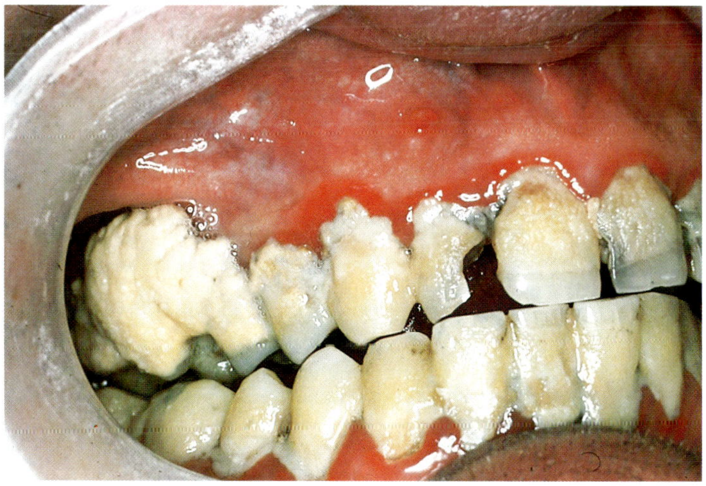

9.105

CHRONIC MARGINAL GINGIVITIS

Figure 9.104 Most of the population have a degree of gingivitis. Chronic marginal gingivitis is caused by the accumulation of dental bacteria plaque on the tooth close to the gingiva. If plaque is not removed it calcifies to become calculus which aggravates the condition by facilitating plaque accumulation.

Figure 9.105 Inflammation of the margins of the gingiva is painless and often the only features are gingival bleeding on eating or brushing, some halitosis, and erythema, swelling, and bleeding on probing. If left uncorrected this may slowly and painlessly progress to periodontitis and tooth loss.

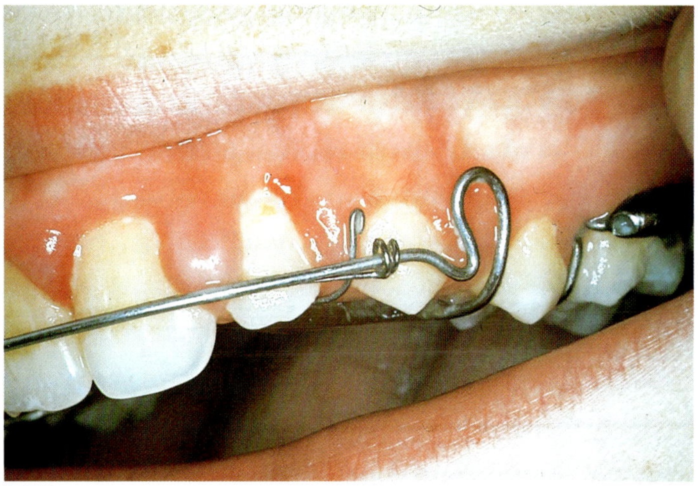

9.106

CHRONIC HYPERPLASTIC GINGIVITIS

Figure 9.106 Gingivitis may be hyperplastic, especially where there is mechanical irritation, or mouth-breathing, or sometimes with the use of the oral contraceptive or other drugs. Here, mouth-breathing and poor oral and appliance hygiene are responsible.

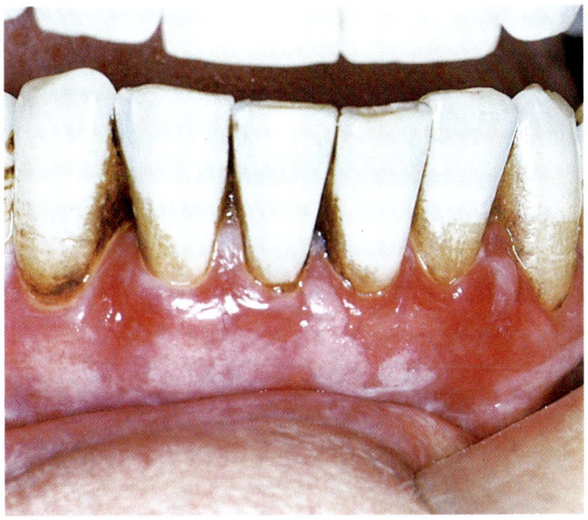

9.107

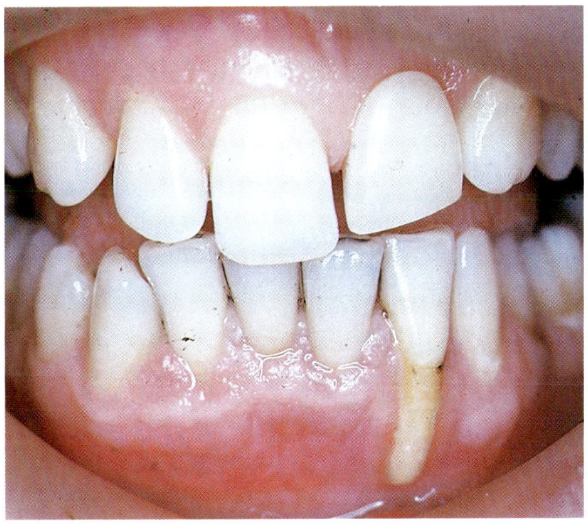

9.108

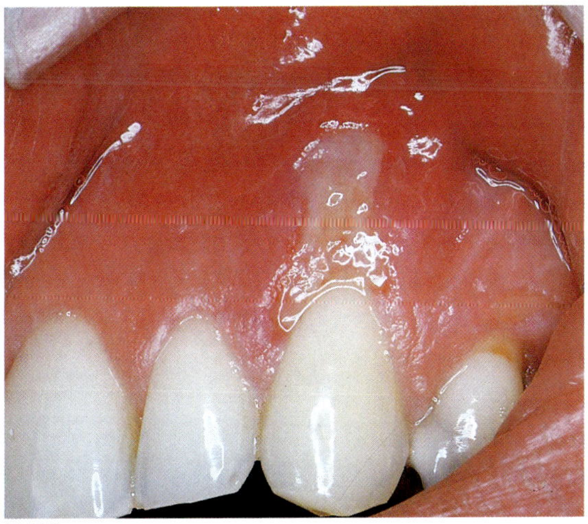

9.109

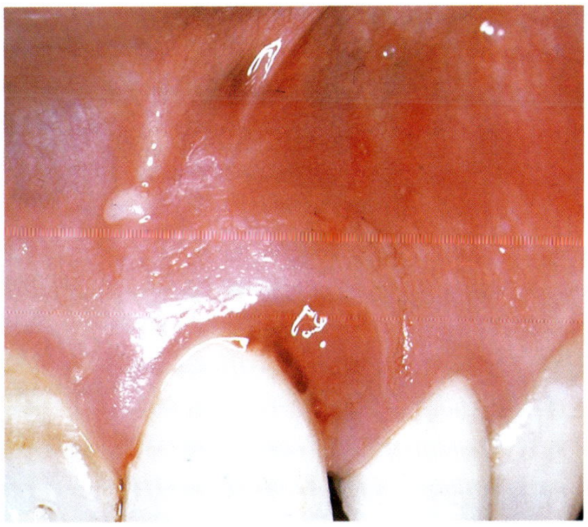

9.110

DESQUAMATIVE GINGIVITIS

Figure 9.107 Desquamative gingivitis differs from marginal gingivitis in that there is erythema over the attached gingiva, extending into the vestibule: indeed, the gingival margins may be spared. Mainly seen in middle-aged or elderly females, desquamative gingivitis is typically caused by lichen planus, pemphigoid, or, occasionally, by pemphigus.

LOCALIZED GINGIVAL RECESSION

Figure 9.108 Isolated recession has exposed the root of this lower lateral incisor. Incidentally the central incisor has an artificial crown.

ARTEFACTUAL GINGIVAL RECESSION

Figure 9.109 Self-induced ulcers of the gingival margin are not rare. The upper canine region seems a common site, and this may be a form of Munchausen's syndrome.

GINGIVAL ABSCESS

Figure 9.110 Gingival infection, or a foreign body, may initiate a gingival abscess. Here it is the result of cement pushed into the tissues during cementing the crown on the central incisor.

LATERAL PERIODONTAL ABSCESS (*Parodontal abscess*)

Figure 9.111 Lateral periodontal abscesses are seen almost exclusively in patients with chronic periodontitis, but may follow impaction of a foreign body, or are related to a lateral root canal on a non-vital tooth. Debris and pus cannot escape easily from the pocket and therefore an abscess, with pain and swelling results.

Figure 9.112 Lateral periodontal abscesses usually discharge either through the pocket or buccally, but more coronal than a periapical abscess.

Figure 9.113 The probe has been gently inserted into a pocket to show continuity with the labial sinus.

ACUTE PERICORONITIS

Figure 9.114 Inflammation of the operculum over an erupting or impacted tooth is common. The lower third molar is the site most commonly affected and patients complain of pain, trismus, swelling and halitosis. There may be fever and regional lymphadenitis, and the operculum is swollen, red and often ulcerated.

Figure 9.115 Migratory abscess of the buccal sulcus: acute pericoronitis appears in relation to the accumulation of plaque and trauma from the opposing tooth. Immune defects may predispose.

A mixed flora is implicated and fusobacteria and bacteroides recognized to be important. Pus usually drains from beneath the operculum but may, in a migratory abscess of the buccal sulcus, track anteriorly as shown.

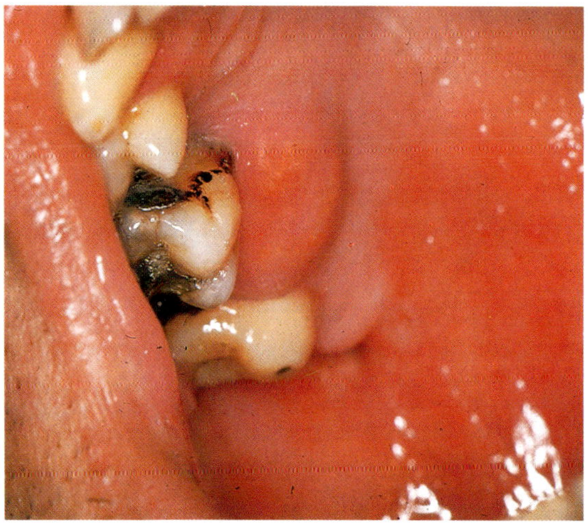

9.111

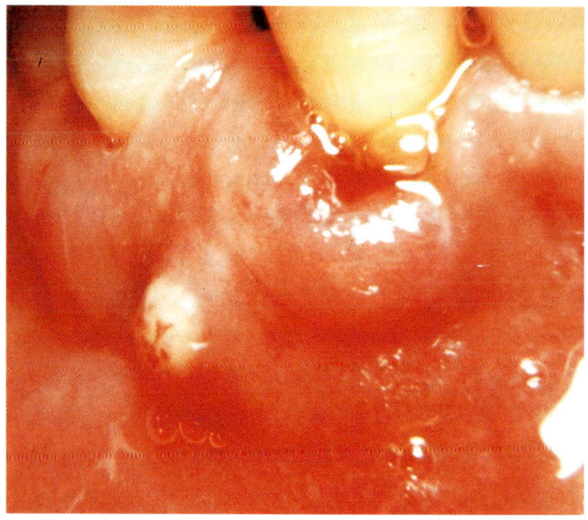

9.112

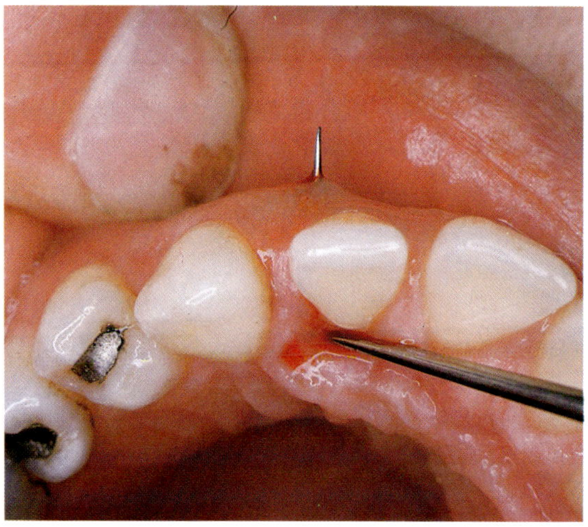

9.113

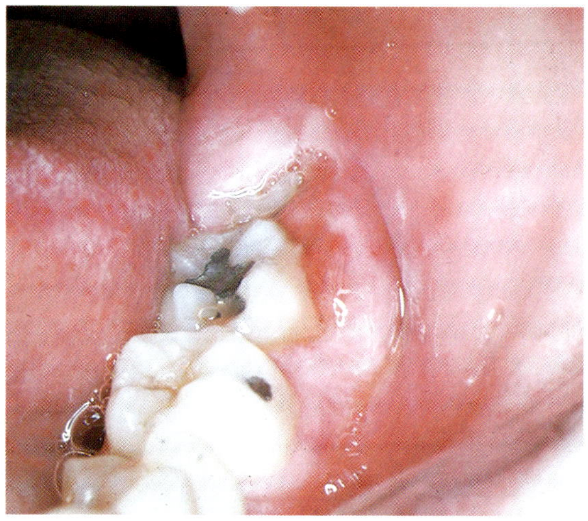

9.114

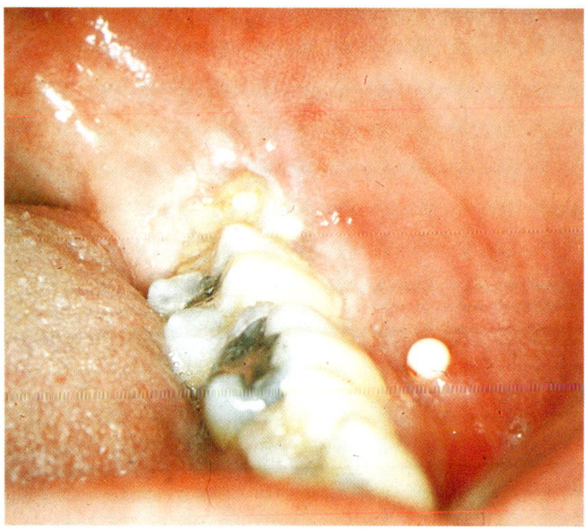

9.115

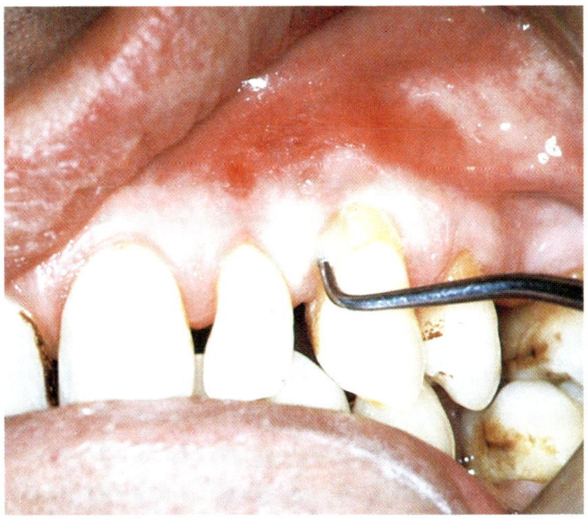

9.116

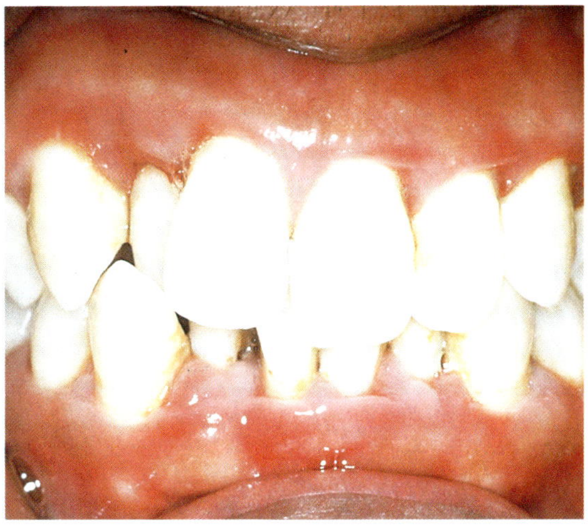

9.117

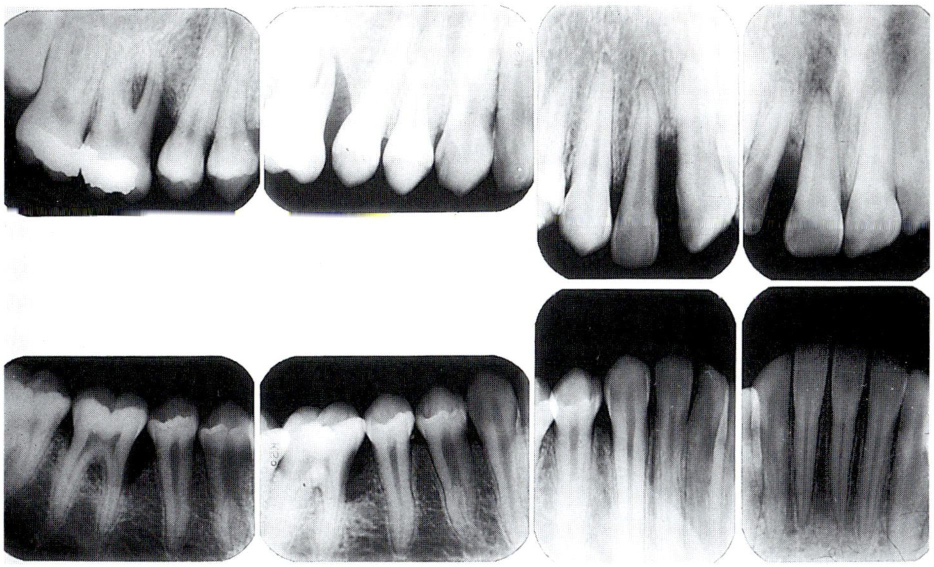

9.118

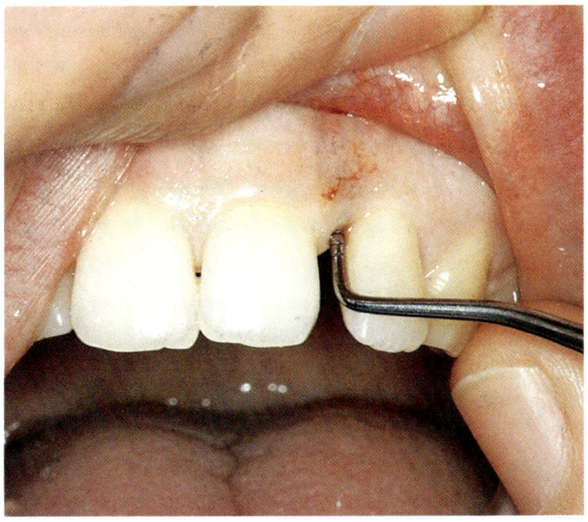

9.119

PERIODONTITIS

Figure 9.116 Chronic periodontitis is common, related to plaque accumulation, and progresses from marginal gingivitis. The features are those of marginal gingivitis but, with destruction of alveolar bone support, there is increasing tooth mobility, teeth may drift, and there is deep pocket formation.

Figure 9.117 Accelerated periodontitis: rare patients still develop periodontitis despite good control of plaque. A range of systemic causes may underlie this accelerated periodontitis, notably diabetes mellitus, white cell dyscrasias including neutrophil defects and neutropenias, and other immune defects including AIDS.

Figure 9.118 Rapidly progressive periodontitis is the term applied to adults – typically females in their early 30s – who, despite good oral hygiene and general health, develop periodontitis. Minor neutrophil defects may be responsible.

Figure 9.119 Localized juvenile periodontitis: localized destruction, classically in the permanent incisor and first molar regions, is seen in some adolescents or young adults in the absence of poor oral hygiene or gross systemic disease. Juvenile periodontitis (periodontosis) is seen especially in females, and in Afro-Asians and may be associated with minor defects of neutrophil function and microorganisms such as *Actinobacillus actinomycetemcomitans* and capnocytophaga. Similar periodontal destruction can be seen in Down's syndrome, type VIII Ehlers-Danlos syndrome, and hypophosphatasia.

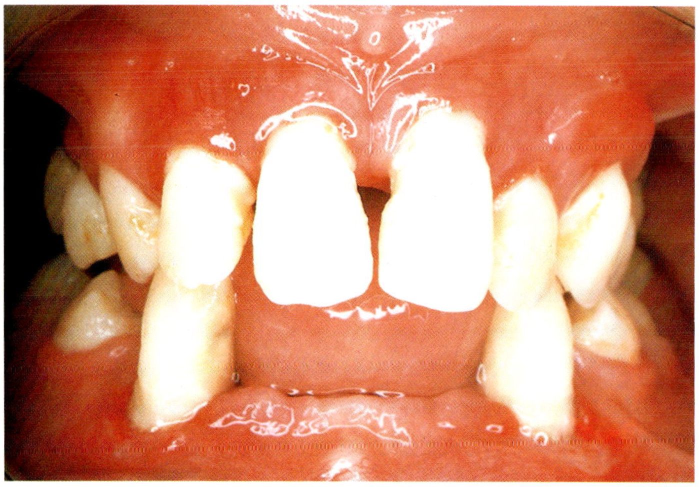

9.120

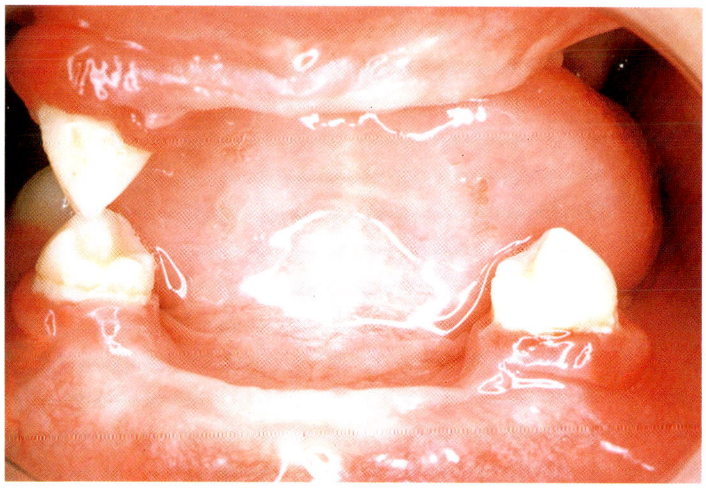

9.121

PAPILLON-LEFÈVRE SYNDROME

Figure 9.120 The Papillon-Lefèvre syndrome is a rare, genetically–linked disorder of pre-pubertal periodontitis, in association with palmar-plantar hyperkeratosis. Virtually all deciduous teeth are involved and the permanent dentition is usually also affected.

Figure 9.121 Most of the deciduous teeth are lost by the age of 4 years, and the permanent teeth by age 16.

Figure 9.122 The soles are usually affected more severely than the palms. The dura mater may be calcified as may the tentorium or choroid.

Figure 9.123 Hyperkeratosis of the palms.

A rare variant of the Papillon-Lefèvre syndrome, not illustrated here, includes arachnodactyly and tapered phalanges as well as the above features.

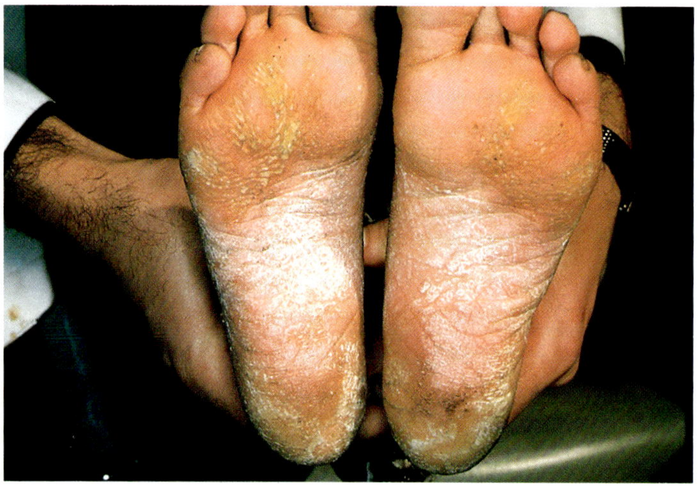

9.122

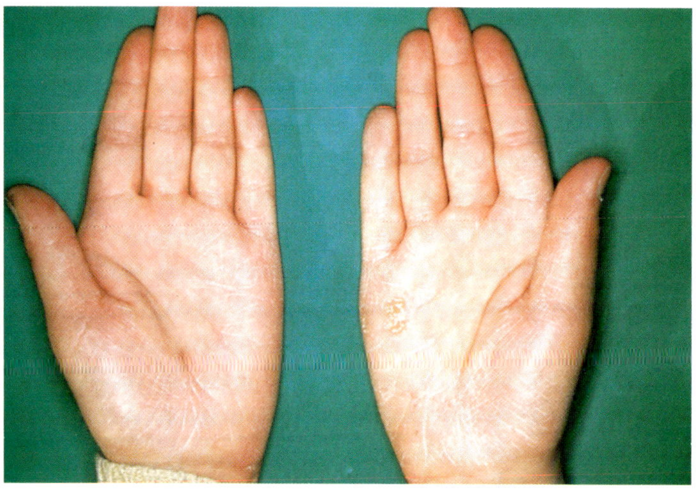

9.123

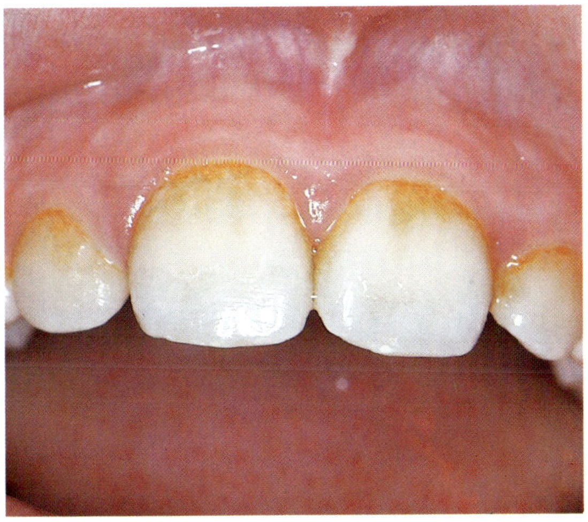
9.124

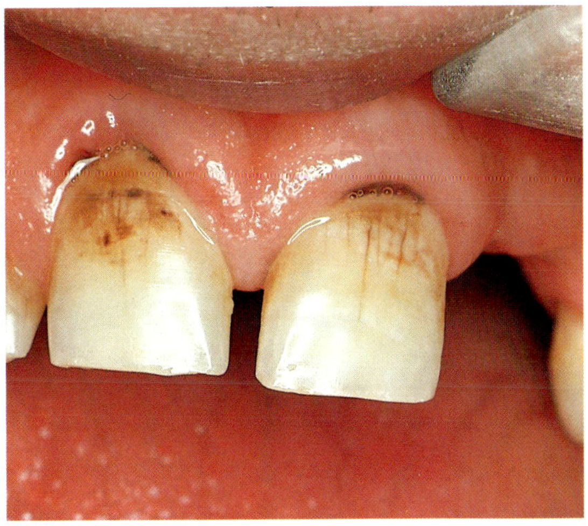
9.125

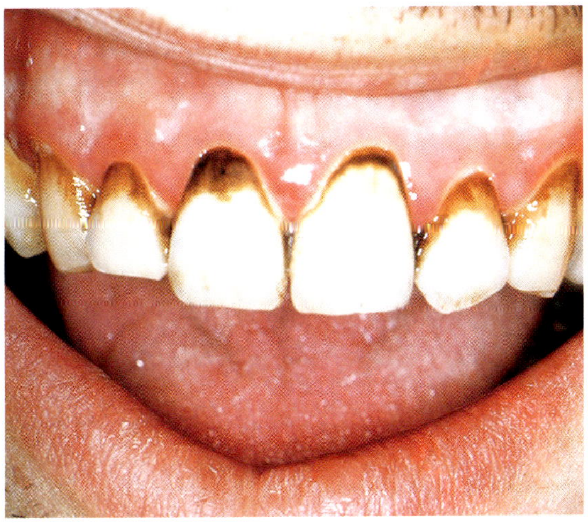
9.126

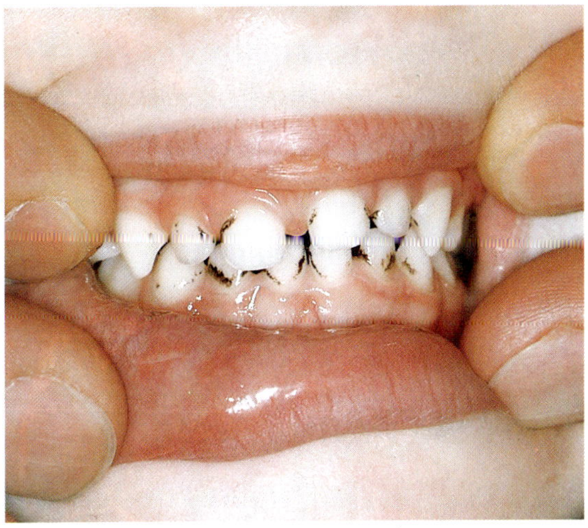
9.127

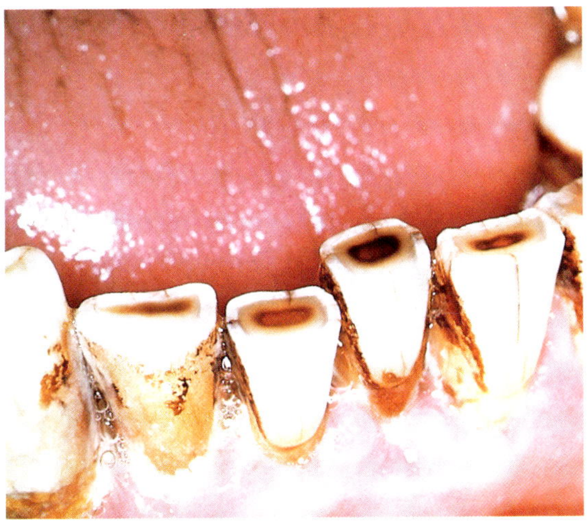
9.128

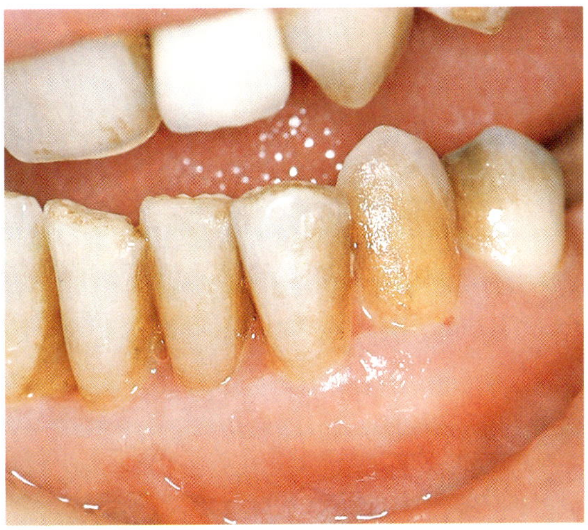
9.129

STAINING

Figure 9.124 Orange stain is believed to be caused by chromogenic bacteria. Extrinsic staining of the teeth can be of various colours and is more likely to appear where oral hygiene is poor or where coloured foods/drinks are taken. Betel chewing, for example, can stain the teeth brown.

Figure 9.125 Brown stain: extrinsic staining is concentrated mainly where plaque accumulates, such as between the teeth and close to gingival margins, and in pits and fissures.

Figure 9.126 Brown stain can be caused by stannous fluoride tooth pastes, as here, and other substances.

Figure 9.127 Black stain is of unknown aetiology and is unusual in that it seems to be associated, by an unknown mechanism, with caries-resistance. It is seen in clean mouths.

Black-staining of teeth is carried out deliberately for cosmetic reasons in some communities.

Green stain is more common, especially in children with poor oral hygiene, and may result from breakdown of blood pigment after gingival haemorrhage, or from chromogenic bacteria.

Figure 9.128 'Nicotine' stain: cigarette smoking, or tobacco chewing, especially in a person with poor oral hygiene, can cause staining. Dentine exposed here by attrition also stains dark brown. Staining can also be produced by chewing habits such as use of betel or khat.

Figure 9.129 Chlorhexidine stain: chlorhexidine is an effective oral antiseptic and binds to dental plaque where it can produce discoloration, especially in drinkers of tea or coffee.

STAINING *(continued)*

Figure 9.130 Iron stain: iron preparations taken orally may produce extrinsic staining of teeth.

Figure 9.131 Lead stain: lead-induced pigmentation is rare and usually follows accidental or occupational exposure. Deposits of lead sulphide in the gingival margin may produce a black 'lead line', especially where oral hygiene is poor.

MATERIA ALBA

Figure 9.132 This is an extreme example of poor oral hygiene – a mentally handicapped patient whose teeth were virtually never cleaned. The teeth are covered with calculus, plaque and debris from food.

DENTAL CALCULUS

Figure 9.133 Supragingival calculus: if plaque is not removed it readily calcifies to produce calculus (tartar), especially in sites close to salivary duct orifices, lingual to the lower incisors and buccal to upper molars.

Figure 9.134 Before oral cleansing: calculus is covered with plaque, cannot be removed by toothbrushing, and is associated with periodontal disease.

Figure 9.135 After cleansing: the teeth pictured in Figure 9.134 professionally cleaned. The extent of periodontal destruction and consequent recession is clearly seen.

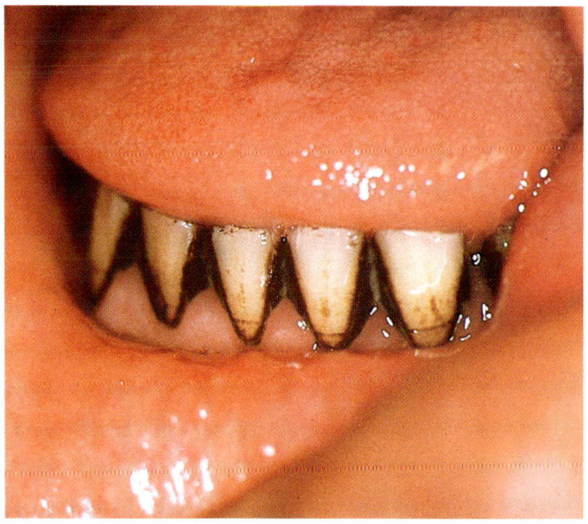

9.130

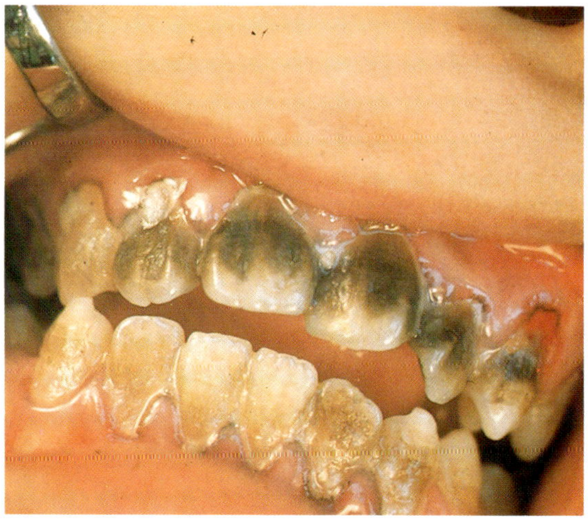

9.131

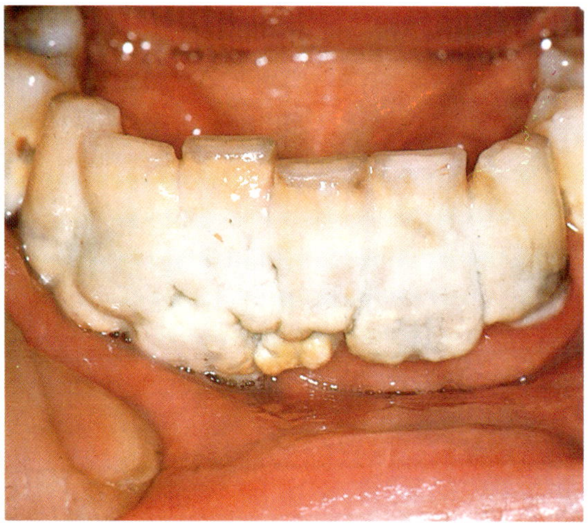

9.132

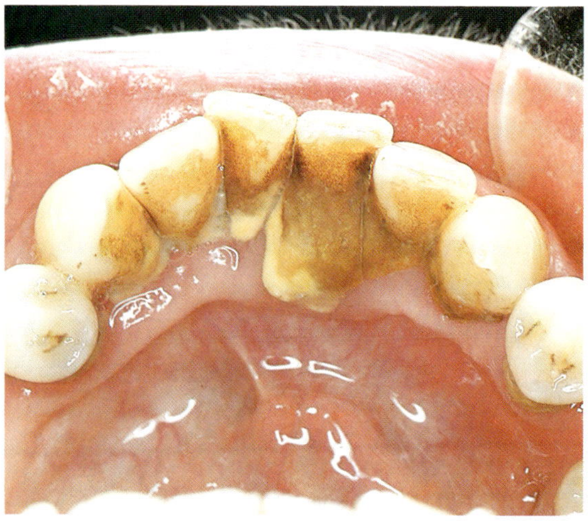

9.133

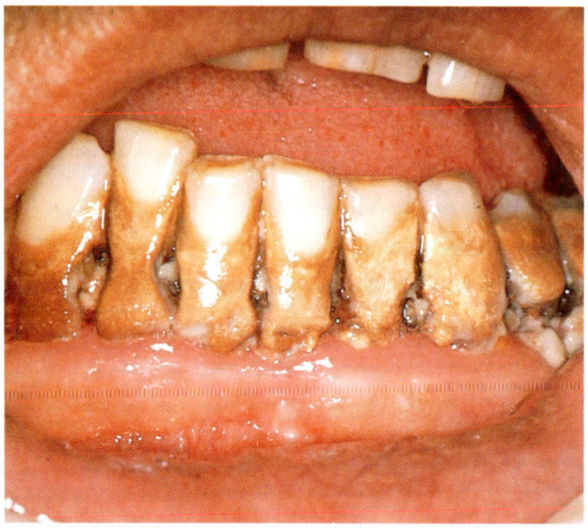

9.134

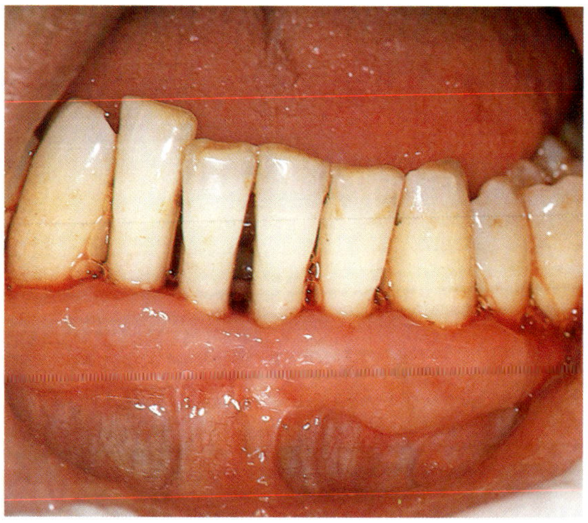

9.135

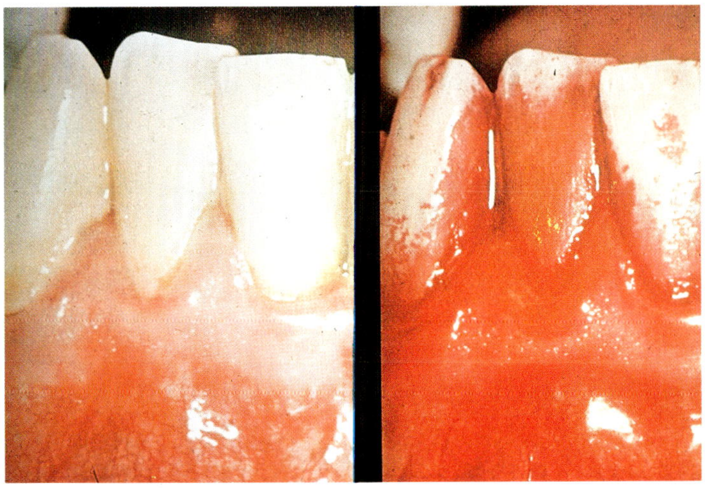

9.136

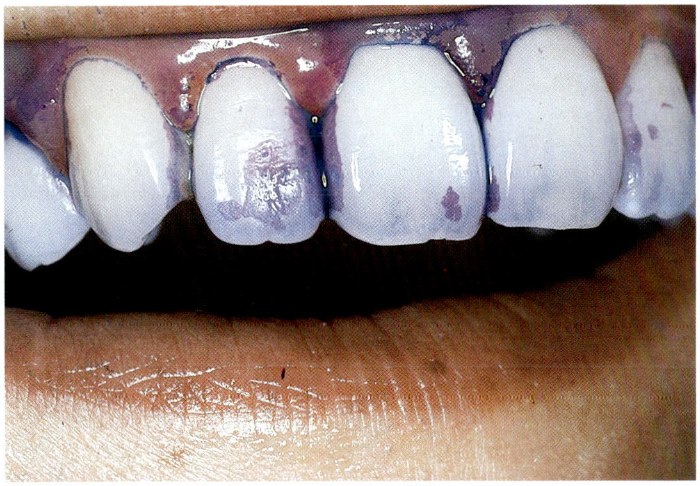

9.137

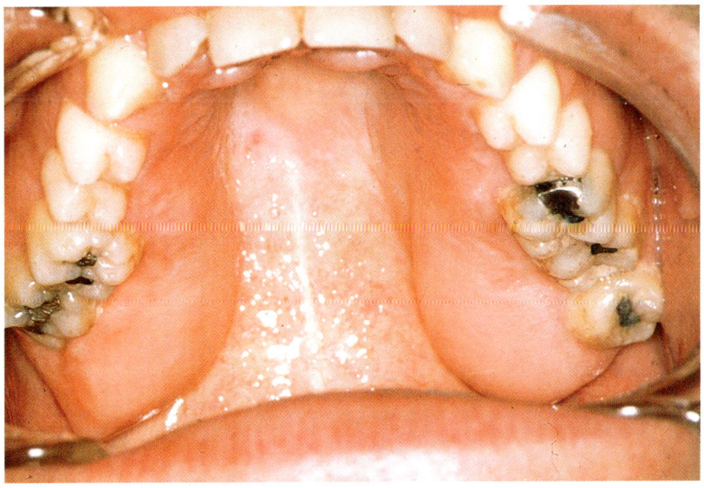

9.138

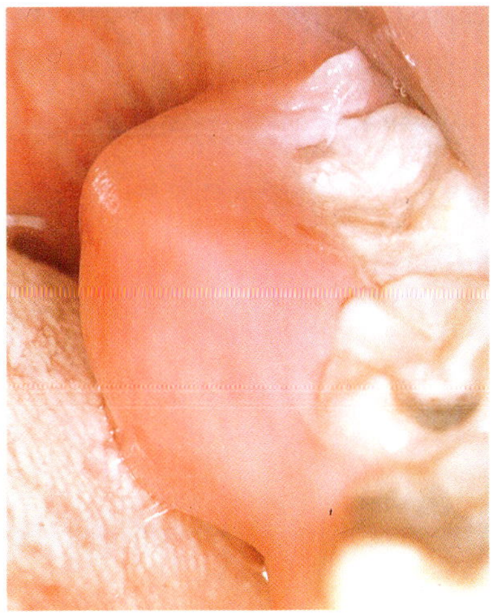

9.139

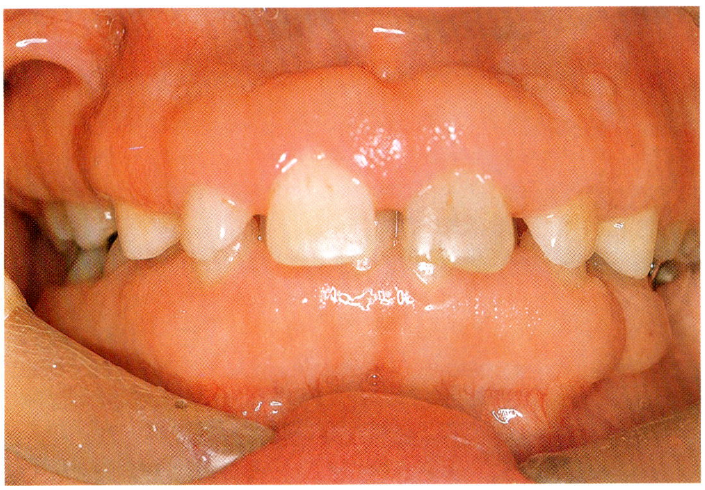

9.140

DENTAL BACTERIAL PLAQUE

Figure 9.136 Plaque is not especially obvious clinically, although teeth covered with plaque lack the lustre of clean teeth. Various solutions can be used to disclose the plaque.

Figure 9.137 Even after thorough toothbrushing, plaque often remains between the teeth unless they are flossed.

GINGIVAL FIBROMATOSIS

Figure 9.138 Enlarged maxillary tuberosities in a localized form of gingival fibromatosis.

Figure 9.139 Occasionally fibromatosis is found in the posterior mandibular region.

Figure 9.140 Hereditary gingival fibromatosis: a familial condition, in which generalized gingival fibromatosis is often associated with hirsutism. Hereditary gingival fibromatosis usually becomes most apparent at the time teeth are erupting.

TRAUMATIC OCCLUSION

Figure 9.141 Trauma can damage the periodontium, often through excessive occlusal stresses and sometimes through direct damage. Here both upper and lower incisors are retroclined and the upper incisors are traumatizing the lower labial gingiva (class II division 2 malocclusion).

Figure 9.142 Periodontal damage from traumatic occlusion: the same patient as Figure 9.141, showing stripping of the periodontium labial to the lower incisors. The upper incisor periodontium may also be traumatized palatally by the lower incisors.

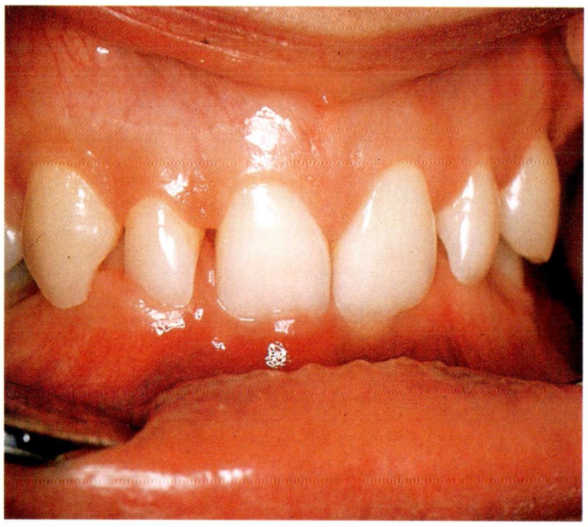

9.141

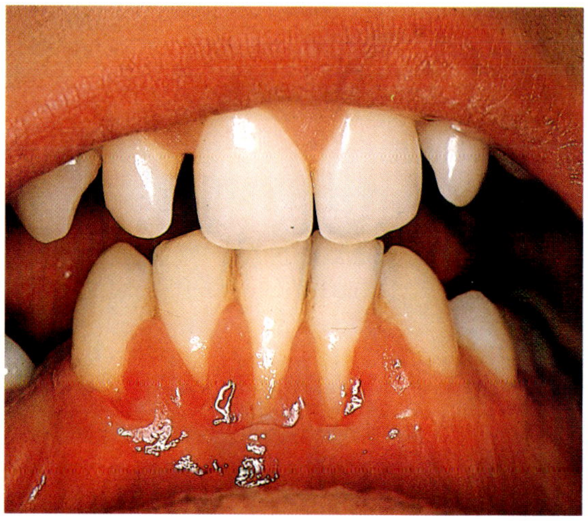

9.142

GINGIVAL CYST

Figure 9.143 Shown here, gingival cysts are rare in adults. They are often solitary and found typically in the mandibular canine or premolar region as a small, painless swelling of the attached or free gingiva, especially near the interdental papilla.

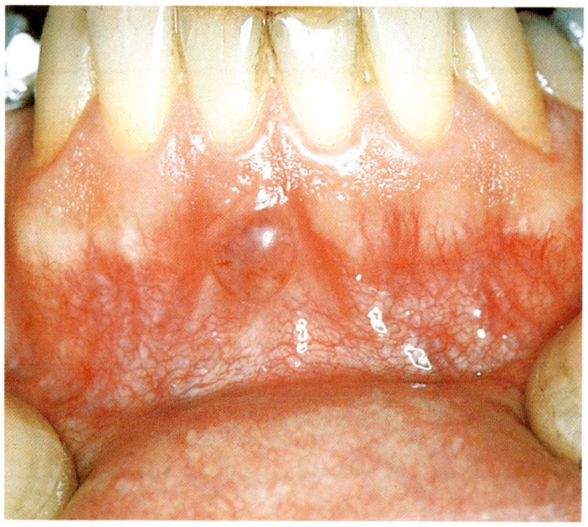

9.143

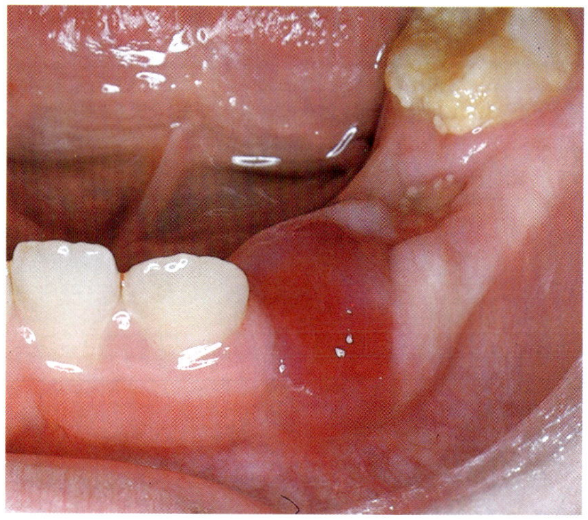

9.144

GIANT CELL GRANULOMA (*Giant cell epulis*)

Figure 9.144 This is a non-neoplastic swelling of proliferating fibroblasts in a highly vascular stroma containing many multinucleate giant cells. It is most common in children, in this region, and after tooth extraction.

Figure 9.145 Giant cell epulides are usually deep red or purple in colour.

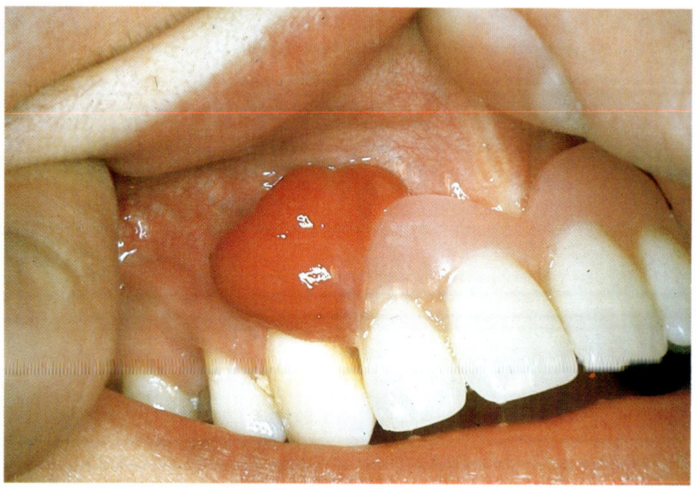

9.145

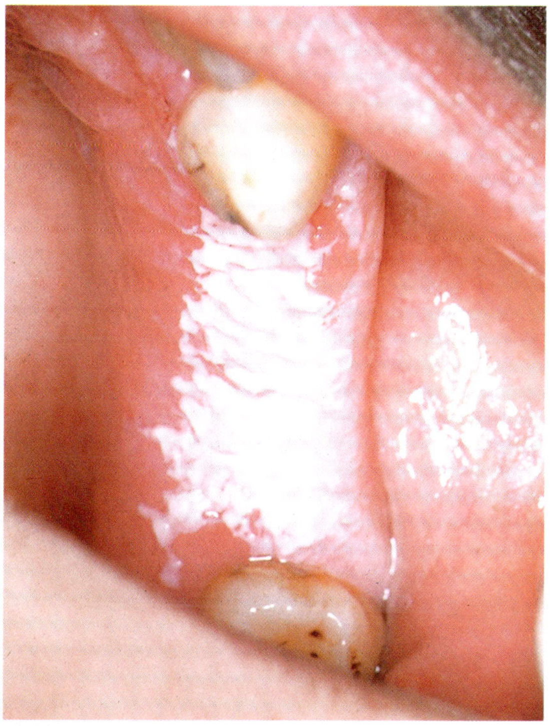

9.146

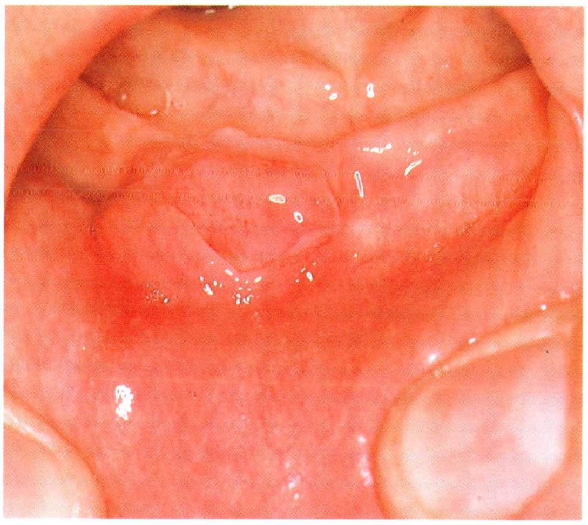

9.147

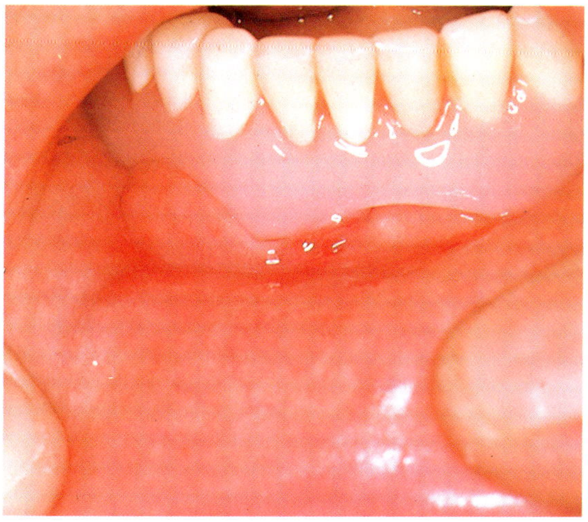

9.148

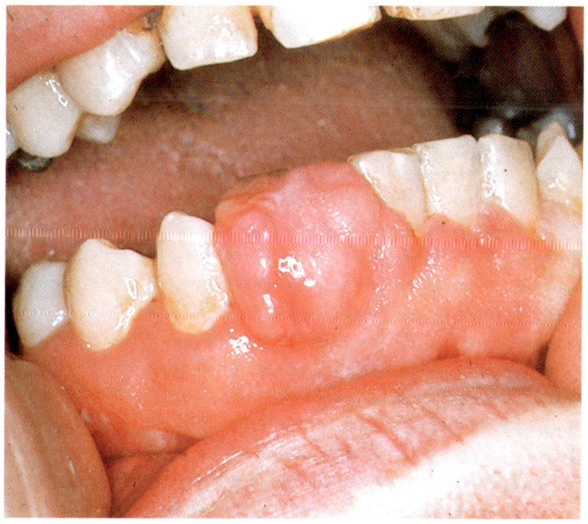

9.149

KERATOSIS (*Leukoplakia*)

Figure 9.146 Keratosis (hyperkeratinization) is fairly common on edentulous ridges and often produced by friction from chewing on the ridge, by smoking or by tobacco-chewing, but some cases are idiopathic, as here.

DENTURE-INDUCED HYPERPLASIA (*Epulis fissuratum*)

Figure 9.147 A denture margin (flange) may cause ulceration of the vestibule, and chronic irritation may produce hyperplasia.

Figure 9.148 The denture fits neatly into the groove between the hyperplastic leaves of tissue (same patient as Figure 9.147). This condition is quite benign but, very occasionally, hyperplasia results from a lesion proliferating beneath and impinging on a denture flange.

FIBROUS EPULIS

Figure 9.149 An epulis is a discrete gingival swelling. Low grade gingival irritation can produce a fibrous epulis – a benign process.

Most epulides are seen in the anterior part of the mouth and most are fibrous epulides.

MALOCCLUSION

Figure 9.150 Typical 'bird face' of mandibular retrusion.

Figure 9.151 Maxillary protrusion: this type of malocclusion is class II division I – compare with that in Figures 9.141 and 9.142.

Figure 9.152 Mandibular protrusion (class III malocclusion): the Hapsburg chin of a prognathic mandible.

Figure 9.153 In mandibular protrusion, the teeth often show reverse overjet with the upper incisors occluding lingual to the lowers.

Figure 9.154 Anterior open bite: the posterior teeth are in occlusion but the incisors fail to meet. Anterior open bites may be caused by increased height of the lower face; tongue posture; dentoalveolar factors; trauma, or thumb-sucking. The upper lateral incisors are also congenitally absent in this patient.

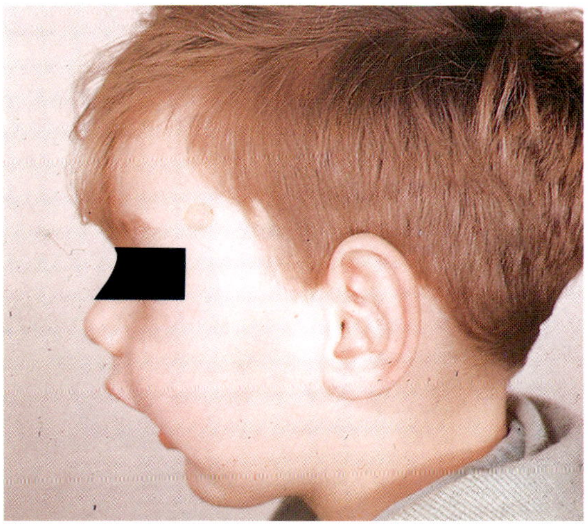

9.150

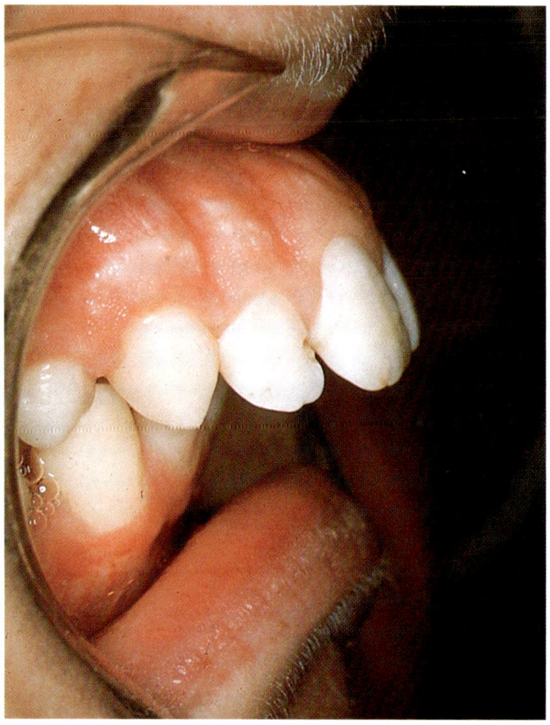

9.151

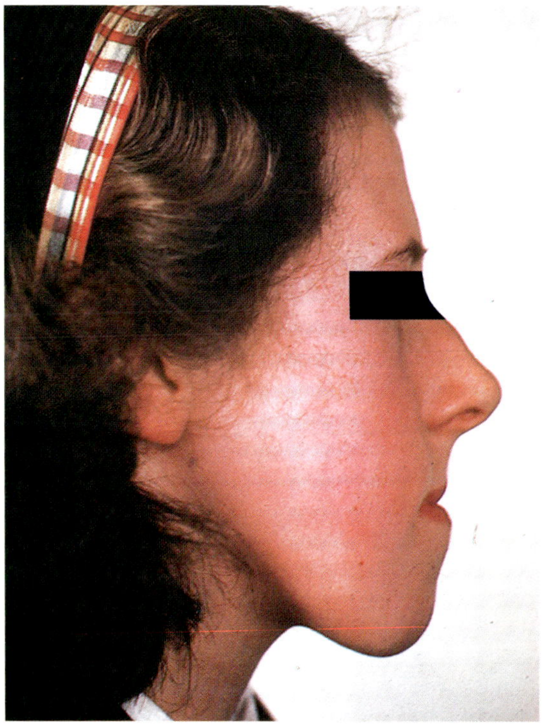

9.152

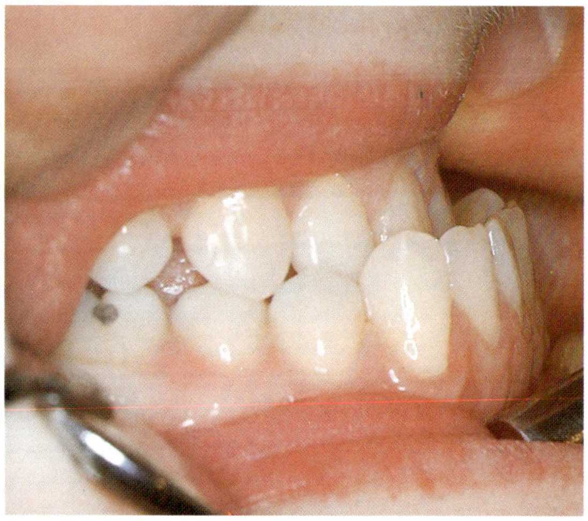

9.153

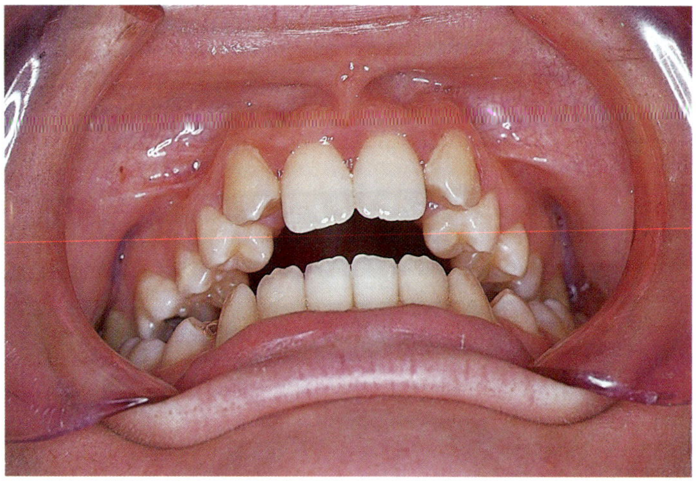

9.154

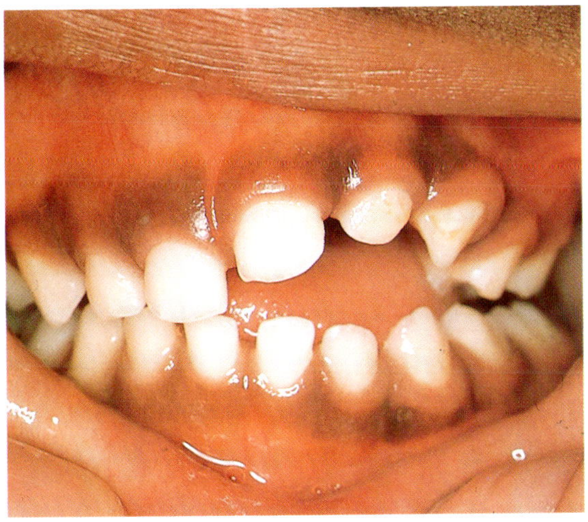

9.155

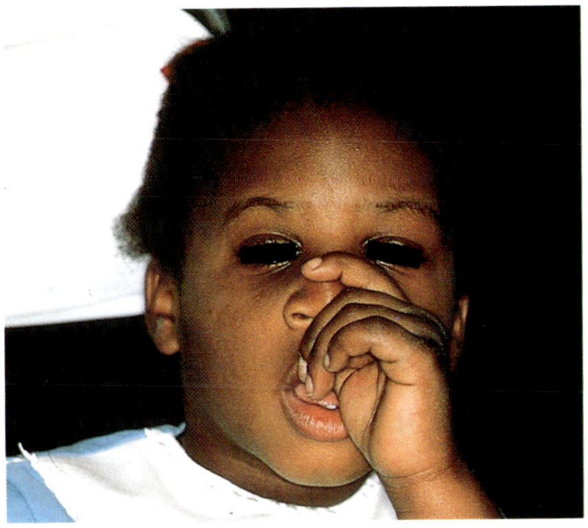

9.156

Figures 9.155 and 9.156 An obvious malocclusion and anterior open bite caused by thumb-sucking.

Figure 9.157 Crowding: the permanent canine normally erupts slightly later than the premolar and lateral incisor and, if there is lack of space in the dental arch (dentoalveolar disproportion), it is crowded out. Second premolars and third molars are the other teeth that may suffer this fate. Any of these teeth, especially lower third molars, may impact.

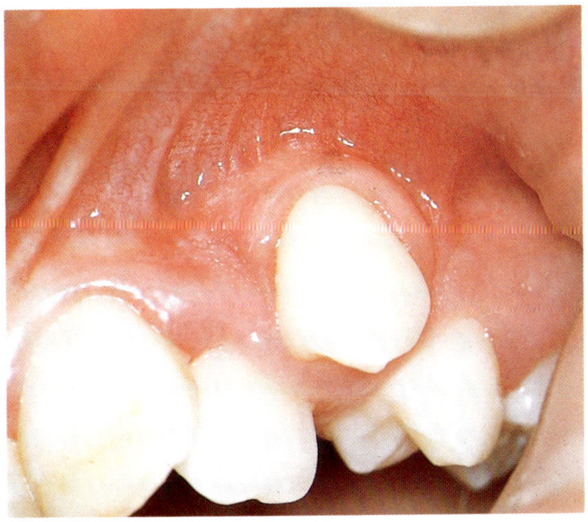

9.157

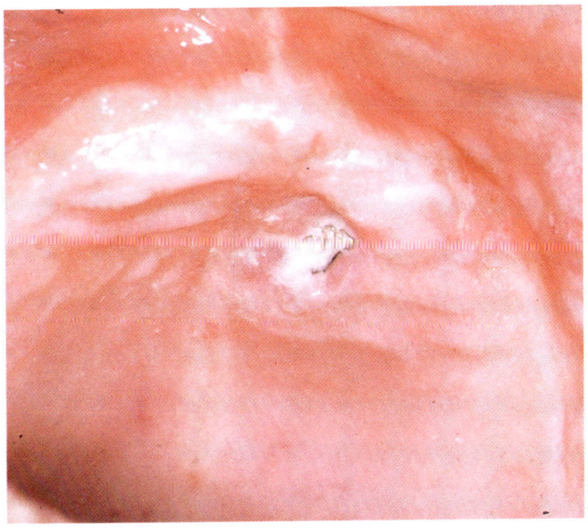

9.158

RETAINED ROOT

Figure 9.158 Retained roots are often asymptomatic but may 'erupt' under a denture, or may give rise to a periapical abscess, or cyst.

ALVEOLAR ATROPHY

Figure 9.159 The alveolar bone of the jaw normally bears the teeth. When teeth are removed, or exfoliate in periodontitis, the alveolar bone atrophies and the jaw occasionally becomes so thin that denture retention is difficult and, in extreme cases, the mandible fractures under relatively little stress.

Osteoporosis may affect the jaws as other bones and is seen particularly in post menopausal women and patients taking systemic corticosteroids.

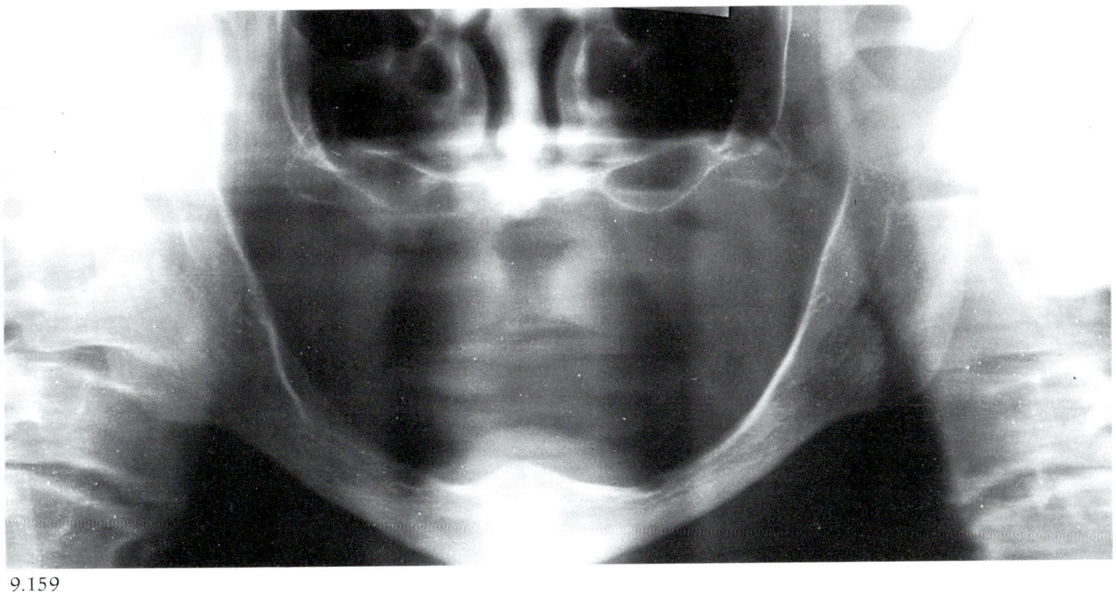

9.159

ERUPTION CYST

Figure 9.160 A cyst often presents clinically as a smooth, rounded swelling with a bluish appearance if there is no overlying bone. Eruption cysts most often involve the deciduous teeth and permanent molars (teeth with no predecessors).

Figure 9.161 Eruption cysts often break down spontaneously as the tooth erupts. The eruption cyst is a type of dentigerous cyst, that is, it surrounds the crown of the tooth.

Figure 9.162 Removal of the operculum (and incidental papilloma) from the cyst reveals an erupting upper first molar.

ODONTOGENIC KERATOCYST (*Primordial cyst*)

Figure 9.163 Odontogenic cysts are often asymptomatic but may produce an intraoral swelling and occasionally an extraoral swelling as here. Odontogenic keratocysts are typically seen in young persons and especially in the mandibular molar region.

Figure 9.164 The odontogenic keratocyst has a tendency to recur after removal. Usually seen in isolation, multiple cysts are a feature of Gorlin's syndrome (see page 214).

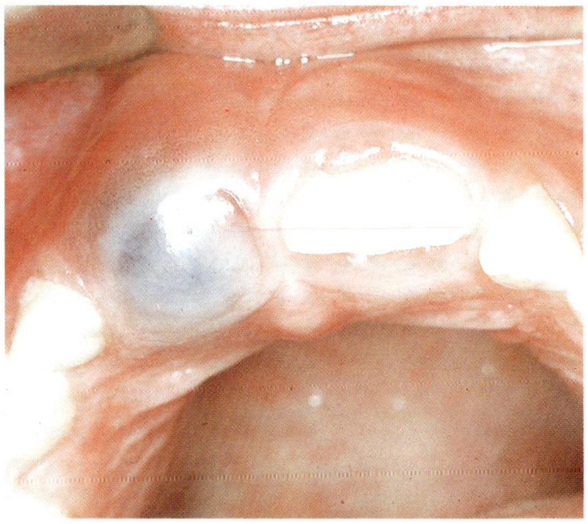

9.160

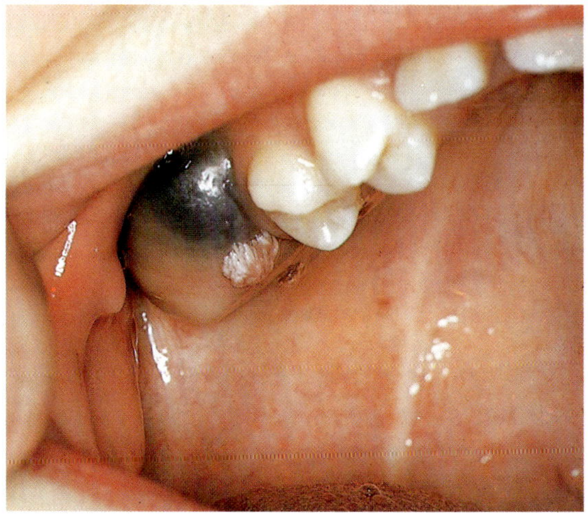

9.161

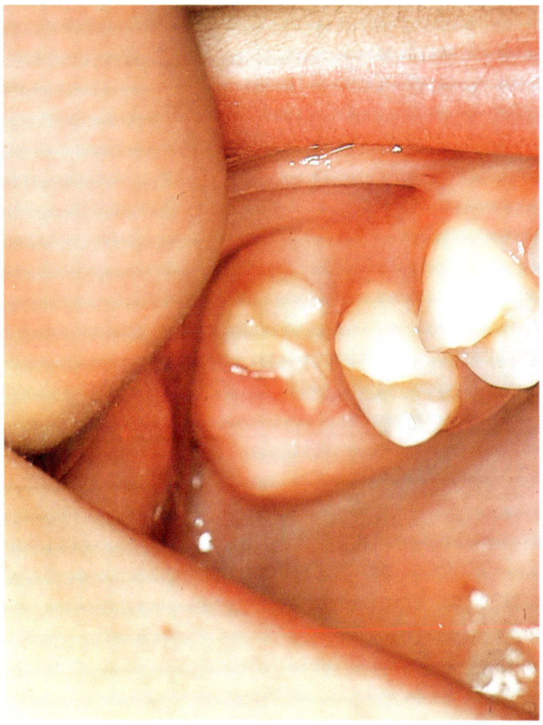

9.162

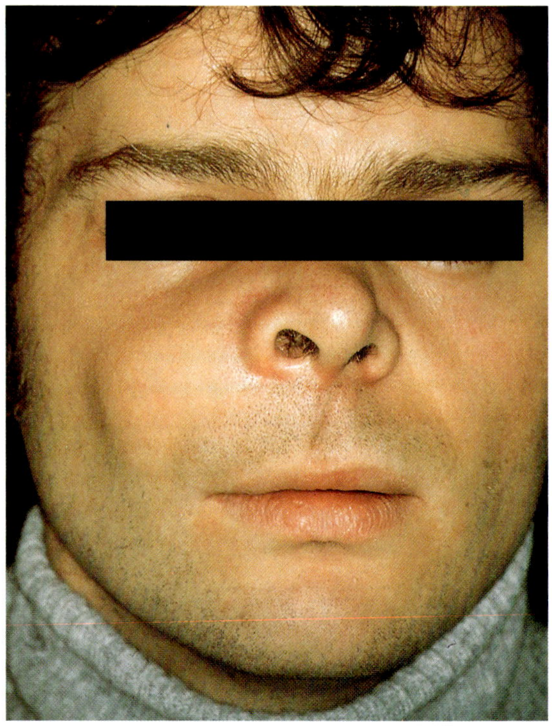

9.163

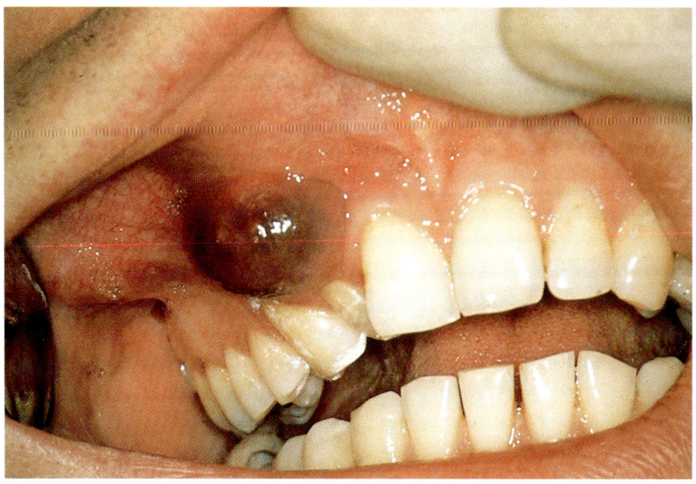

9.164

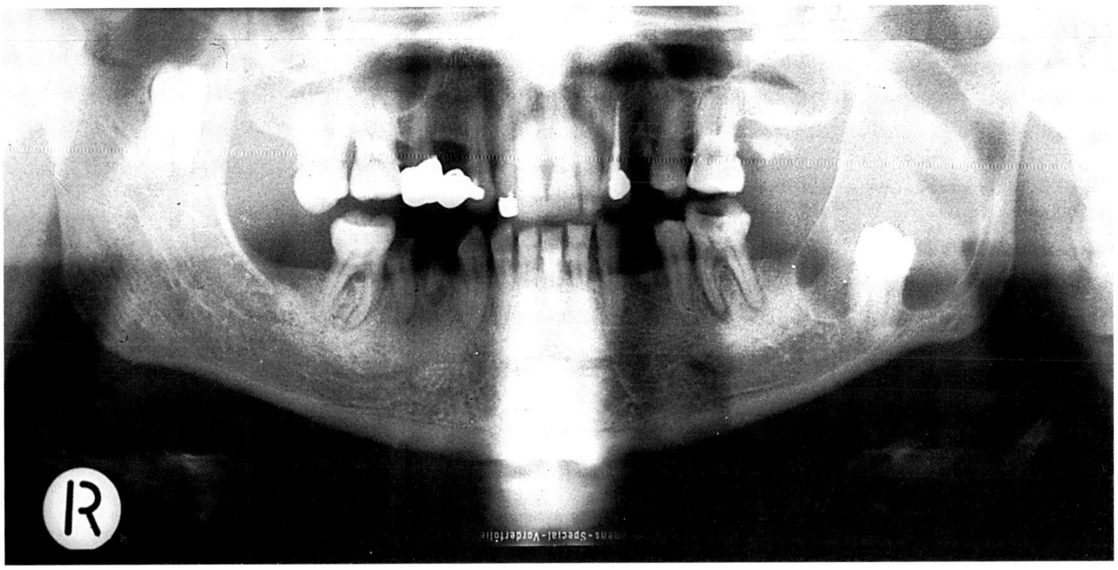

9.165

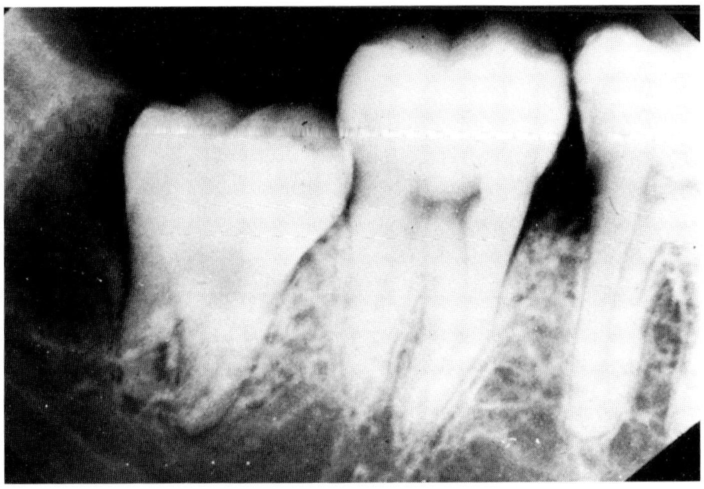

9.166

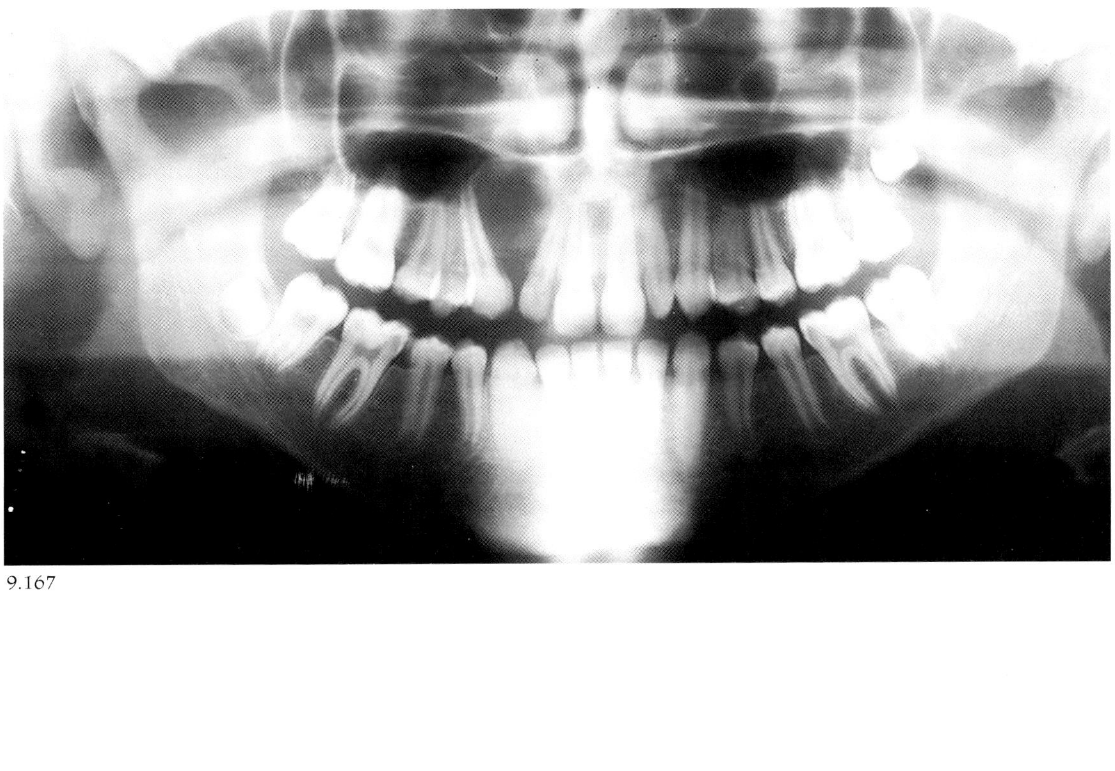

9.167

DENTIGEROUS CYST (*Follicular cyst*)

Figure 9.165 A dentigerous cyst envelops the crown of a tooth and is attached to its neck. Most involve third molars or canine teeth. Here, the left ramus of mandible is occupied by a dentigerous cyst related to a molar, probably the third molar. The other lower third molar is ectopic.

Multiple dentigerous cysts can be a feature of cleidocranial dysplasia (see page 198).

LATERAL PERIODONTAL CYST

Figure 9.166 A lateral periodontal cyst may be follicular in origin; may arise from remnants of the dental lamina; or may be associated with a lateral pulp canal in a non-vital tooth. The cyst here closely resembles a dentigerous cyst.

GLOBULOMAXILLARY CYST

Figure 9.167 A probable misnomer, most cysts in the upper lateral incisor/canine region prove to be odontogenic rather than developmental (non-odontogenic, fissural) cysts. This cyst has displaced the maxillary right canine and lateral incisor teeth.

NASOPALATINE DUCT CYST
(*Incisive canal cyst*)

Figure 9.168 Epithelial remnants related to the nasopalatine canal may give rise to a cyst. If large, the cyst may produce a swelling beneath the upper lip and anterior nares.

Figure 9.169 The swelling may extend to the nasal floor and palatal vault as here, and may discharge a salty fluid. Most nasopalatine cysts are seen in adult males from the age of 40.

Figure 9.170 Dental cysts related to non-vital incisors can be confused with the nasopalatine cyst. Furthermore, the normal incisive canal can be difficult to distinguish radiographically from a cyst, although it is generally accepted that a radiolucency greater than 6 mm in diameter is probably a cyst – as here.

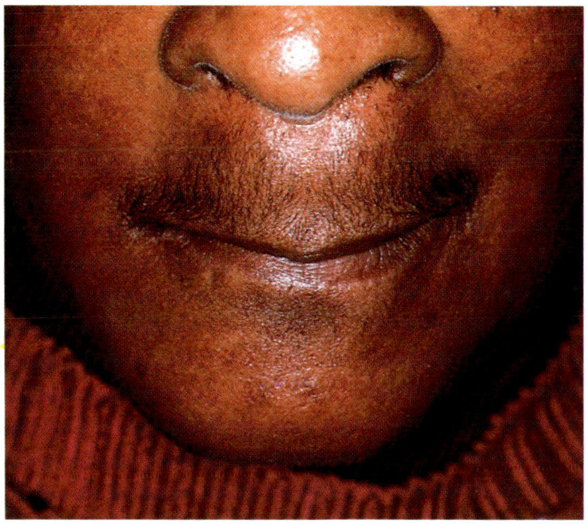

9.168

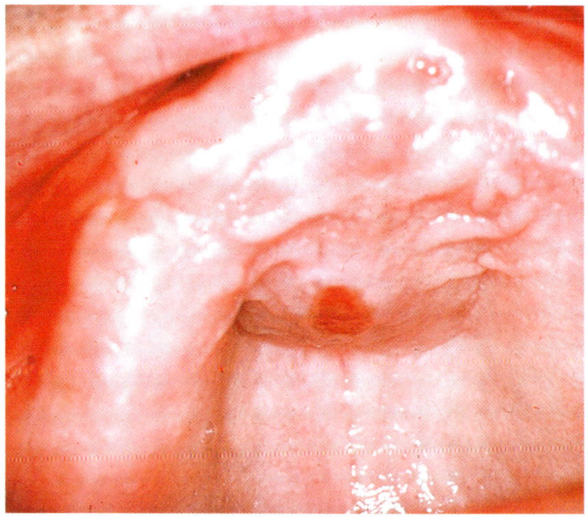

9.169

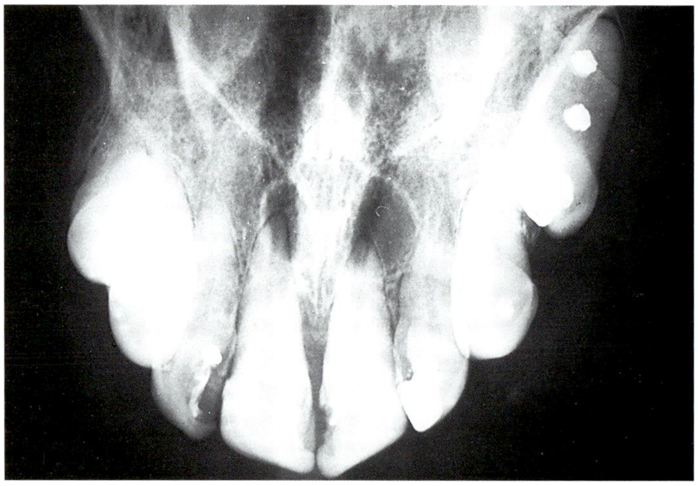

9.170

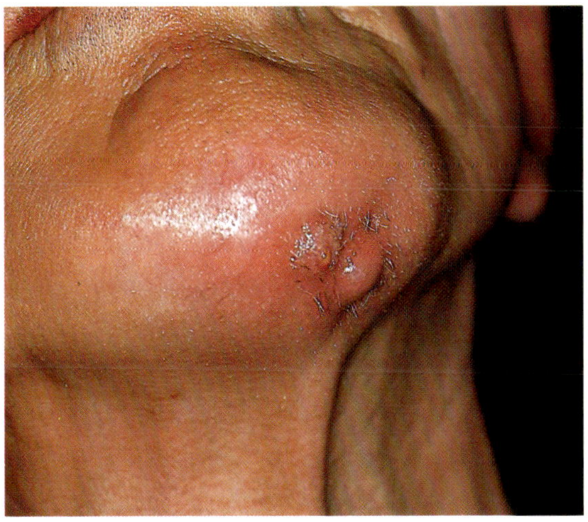

9.171

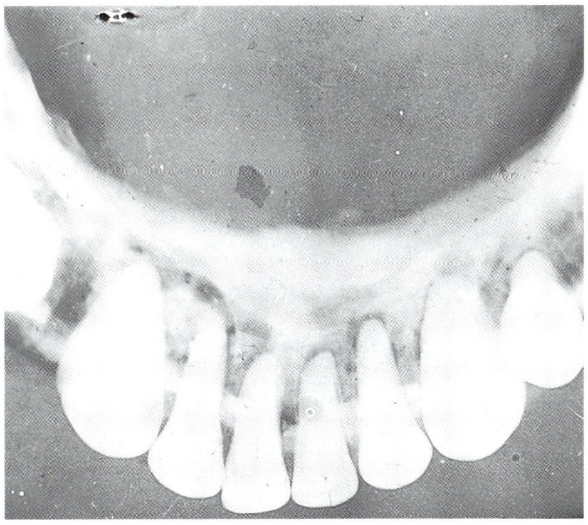

9.172

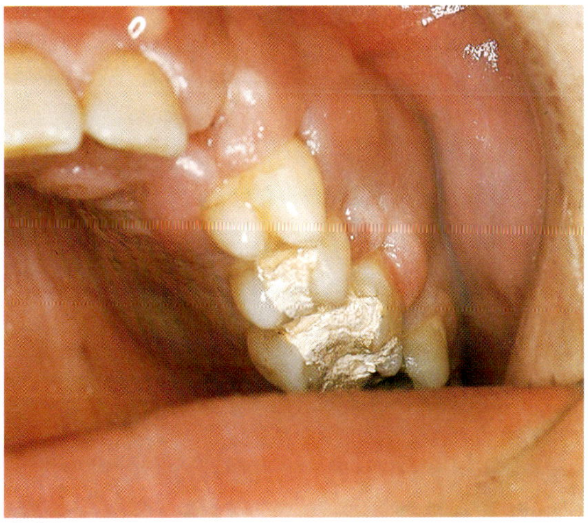

9.173

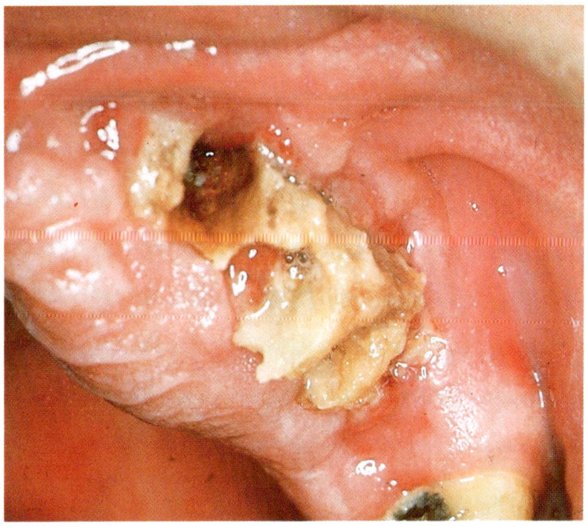

9.174

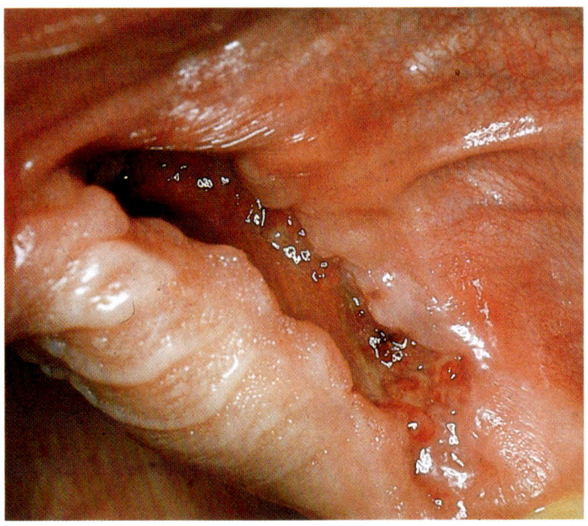

9.175

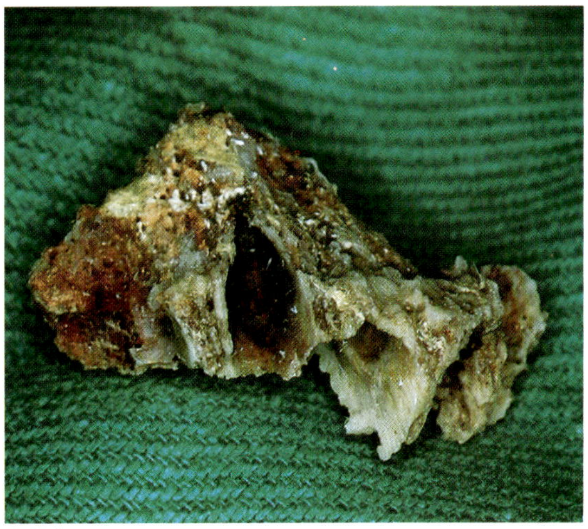

9.176

ACUTE OSTEOMYELITIS

Figure 9.171 Osteomyelitis is an infection of the bone, rare in the jaws. Acute osteomyelitis is seen mainly in the mandible, the infection usually originating from odontogenic infection or trauma. Extreme pain, swelling, labial anaesthesia, tenderness on biting and eventual discharge of pus are the main features.

Figure 9.172 Radiological signs take some weeks to develop but the bone eventually becomes 'moth-eaten', as here.

Figure 9.173 This series, Figures 9.173–9.176, shows a sequence from a patient with rare maxillary osteomyelitis. At this early stage there is pain and swelling by the upper second premolar and first molar which were then extracted.

Figure 9.174 Two months later, a sequestrum has appeared.

Figure 9.175 After a further 2 weeks the necrotic bone sequestrates.

Figure 9.176 The sequestrum.

Osteomyelitis is predisposed by various immune defects, diabetes mellitus, Paget's disease, osteopetrosis, irradiation or local factors, such as foreign bodies.

ACUTE OSTEOMYELITIS
(continued)

Figure 9.177 Acute osteomyelitis is very rare in the maxilla and, when seen, is usually in neonates. It is possible that *Staphylococcus aureus* infects the maxilla, either haematogenously or entering via an oral wound.

CHRONIC OSTEOMYELITIS

Figure 9.178 Proliferative periostitis is an uncommon chronic low grade infection, seen usually in the lower molar region. There are several clinical patterns of chronic osteomyelitis. Periosteal new bone may be seen on this radiograph.

OSTEORADIONECROSIS

Figure 9.179 Endarteritis obliterans, following irradiation of the jaws, predisposes to infection after tooth extraction. This was a not uncommon problem in the past but, with the advent of plesiotherapy and other improved radiotherapeutic techniques and a better understanding by dental surgeons, it is now less common. Here there is a chronic submandibular sinus.

Figure 9.180 A sequestrum is forming slowly. Radiation-scarring with telangiectasia is also evident in the floor of the mouth.

Figure 9.181 Radiography shows the 'moth-eaten' appearance of the mandible and a pathological fracture.

Jaw necrosis was also caused in the past by occupational exposure to red phosphorus, or exposure to heavy metals, and occasionally follows the use of toxic endodontic materials, severe herpes zoster or other infections.

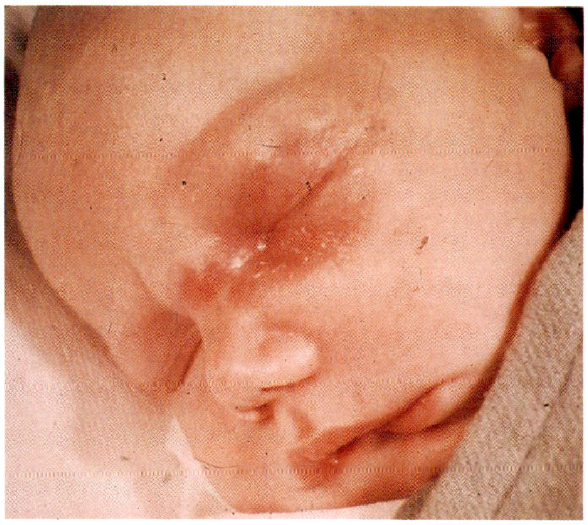

9.177

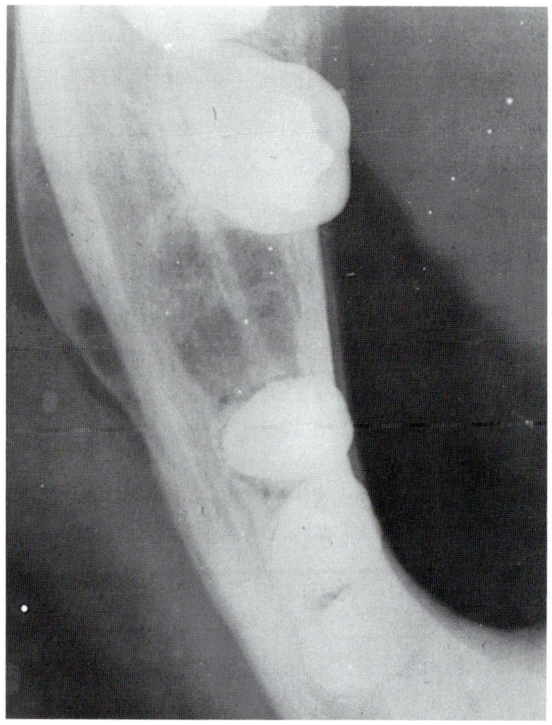

9.178

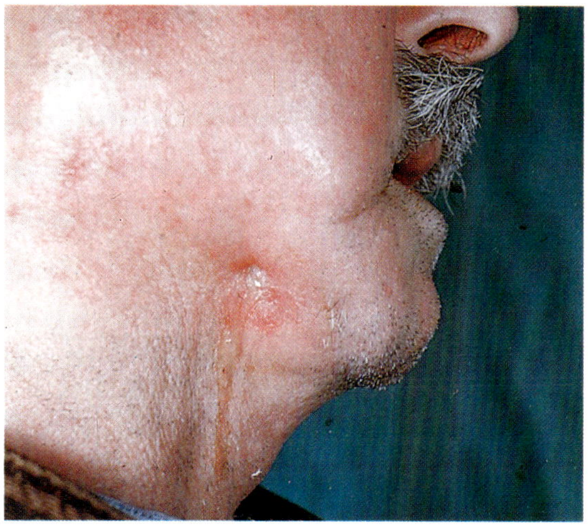

9.179

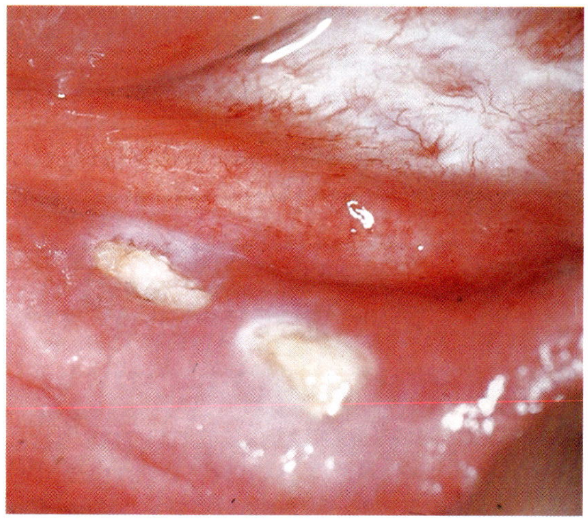

9.180

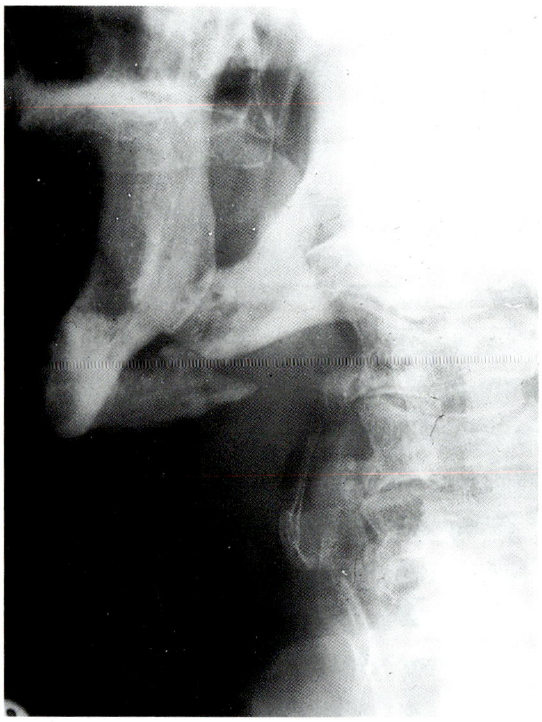

9.181

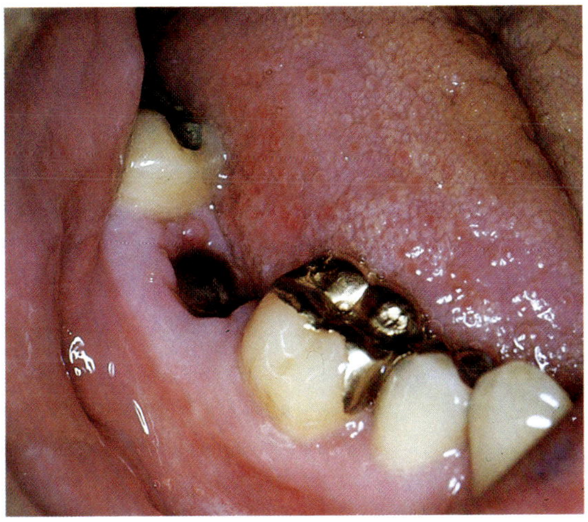

9.182

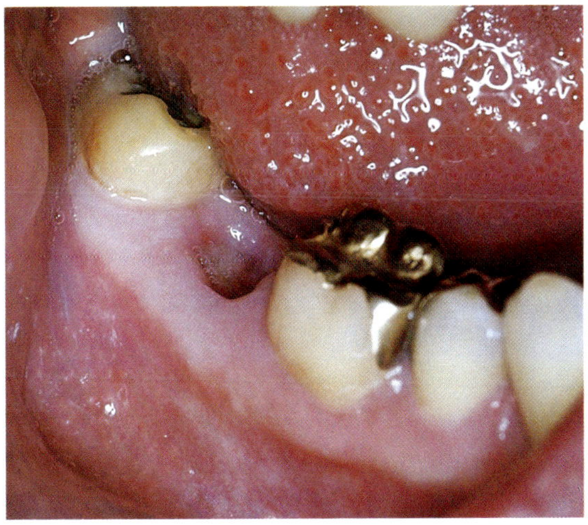

9.183

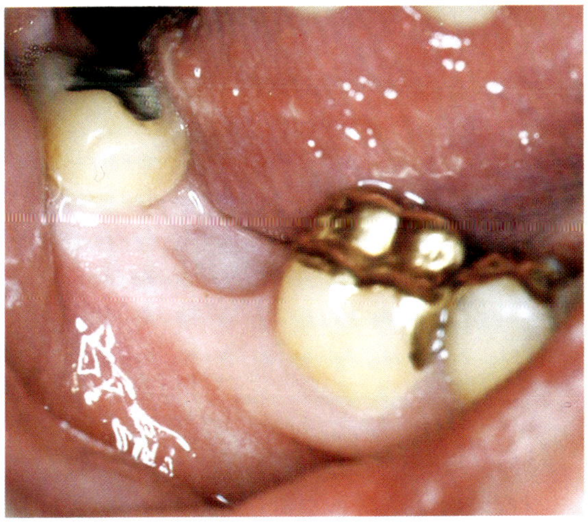

9.184

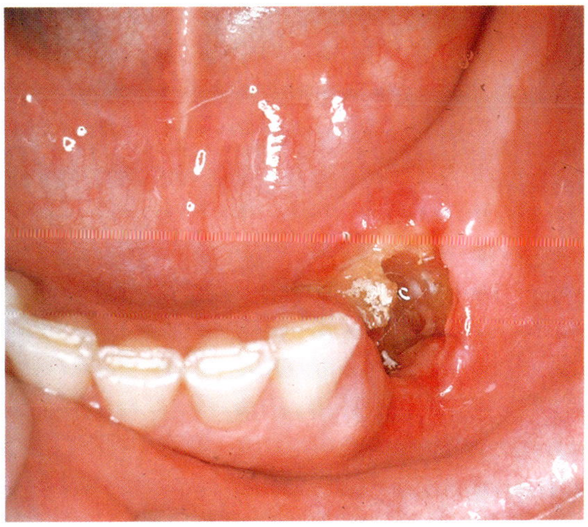

9.185

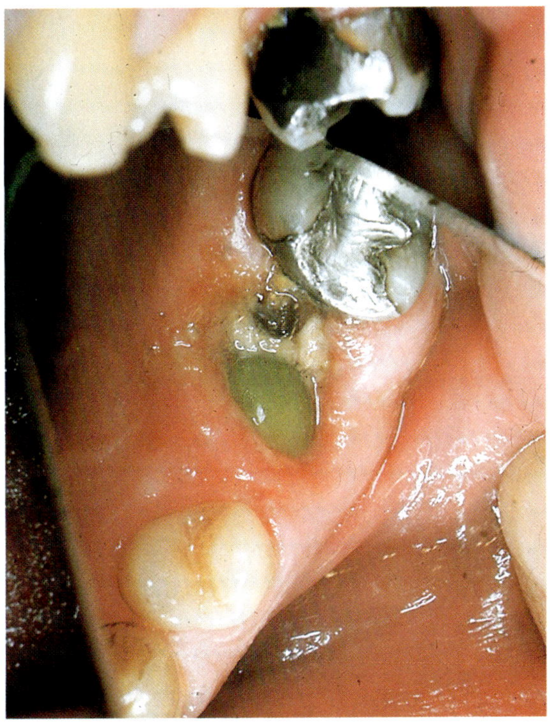

9.186

HEALING EXTRACTION SOCKET

Figure 9.182 Day 1: an extraction socket rapidly fills with blood which normally clots and remains *in situ*. Later post-extraction haemorrhage is usually from mucosal rather than bony vessels.

Figure 9.183 Day 5: the wound contracts. The clot begins to organize.

Figure 9.184 Day 30: the socket is epithelializing and the area will soon appear healed clinically, although radiographically it will still be evident several months later. There will be some remodelling of the alveolar bone.

DRY SOCKET (*Alveolar osteitis*)

Figure 9.185 If the blood clot in an extraction socket breaks down, presumably from the action of fibrinolysins, then the socket is 'dry'. Dry socket manifests with the onset of fairly severe pain 2–4 days after extraction, bad taste in the mouth, and halitosis. The socket has no clot and the surrounding mucosa is inflamed.

Figure 9.186 Dry socket is typically seen after extractions in young persons; in the mandible; in the molar region; after extractions under local anaesthesia; and after traumatic extractions. Oral contraceptive use predisposes to dry socket. Healing is aided if debris (such as the pea here) is irrigated away and the socket dressed.

TORUS MANDIBULARIS

Figure 9.187 Mandibular tori are uni- or bi-lateral bony lumps lingual to the lower premolars. They are of developmental origin and benign.

Figure 9.188 Tori are common but are especially seen in Mongoloid races.

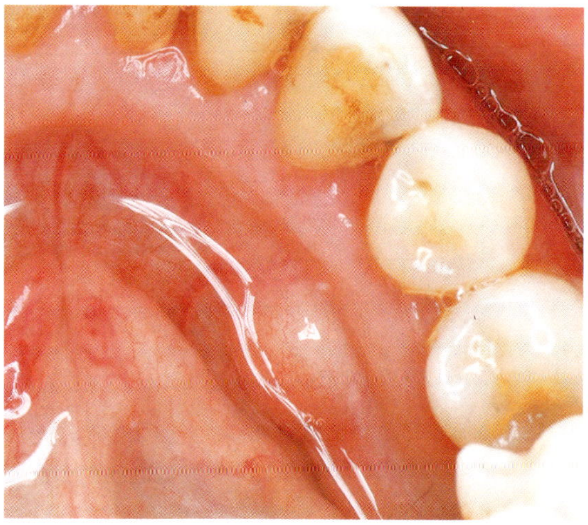

9.187

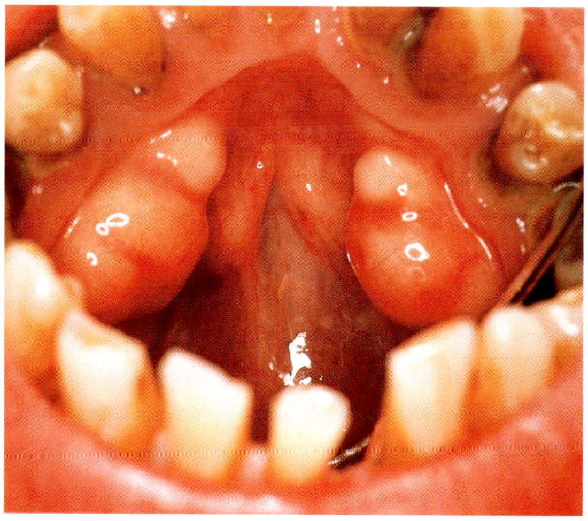

9.188

TORUS PALATINUS

Figure 9.189 Palatal tori are common bony lumps, typically in the midline vault of palate.

Figure 9.190 Palatal tori are most common in Mongoloid races and can sometimes be quite protrusive. Again, they are benign.

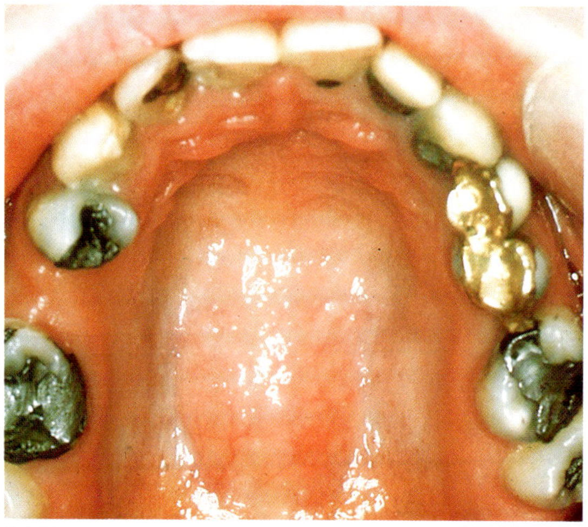

9.189

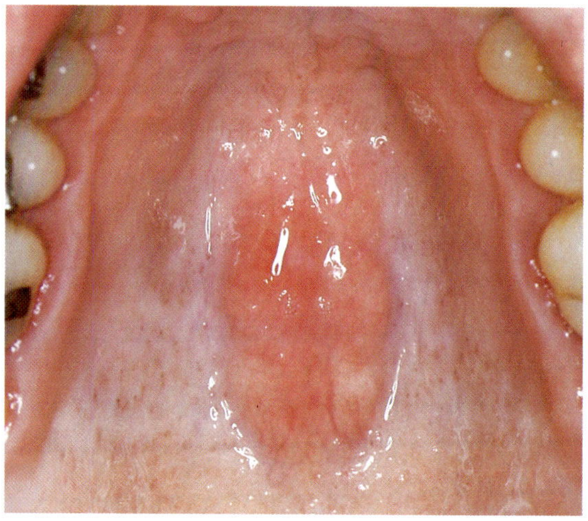

9.190

EXOSTOSES

Figure 9.191 It is fairly common to see exostoses at this site buccal to the maxillary posterior teeth.

Multiple jaw osteomas are occasionally a feature of Gardner's syndrome, which is an autosomal dominant trait characterized by colonic polyps (often pre-malignant), epidermoid cysts, desmoid tumours, pigmented ocular fundic lesions and impacted supernumerary teeth. These patients may also develop extra-colonic neoplasms.

STAFNE BONE CAVITY (*Latent bone cyst*)

Figure 9.192 A Stafne 'cyst' is not a cyst at all but a well-demarcated radiolucency at the lower border of the mandible, always below the inferior alveolar canal. It contains some normal submandibular salivary gland tissue. It is a developmental defect.

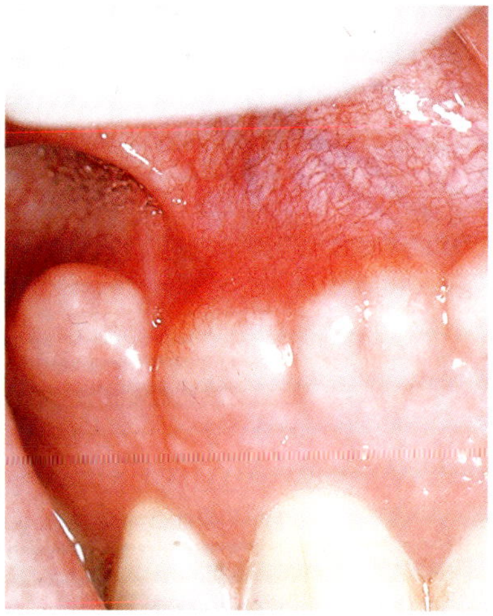

9.191

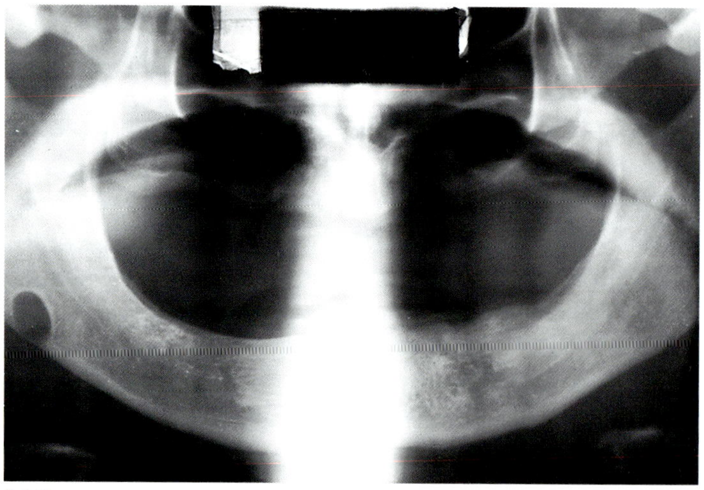

9.192

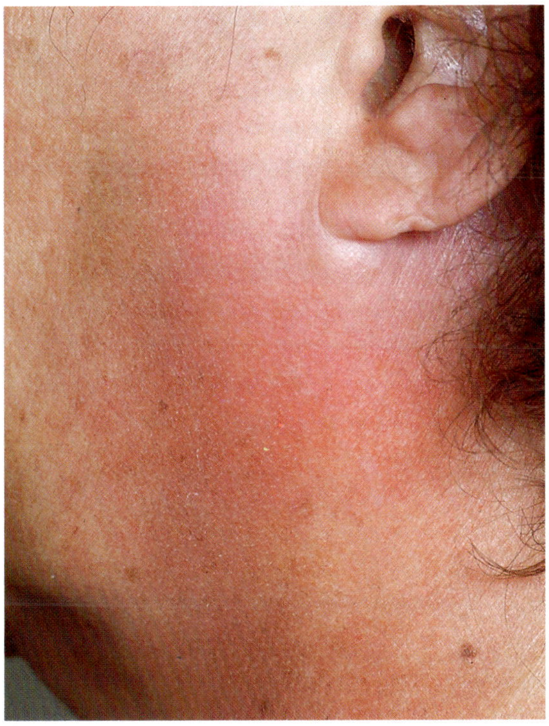

9.193

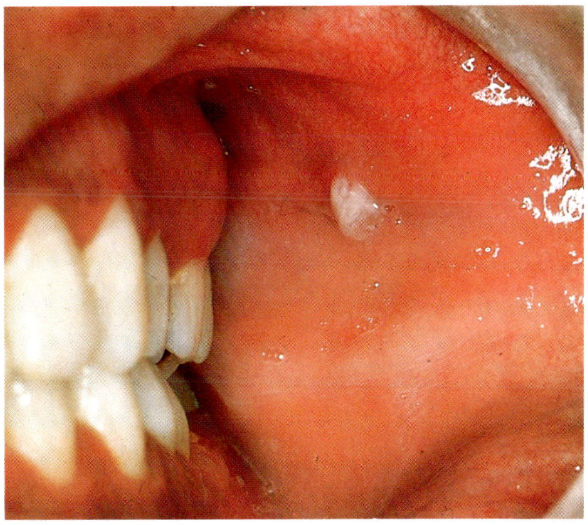

9.194

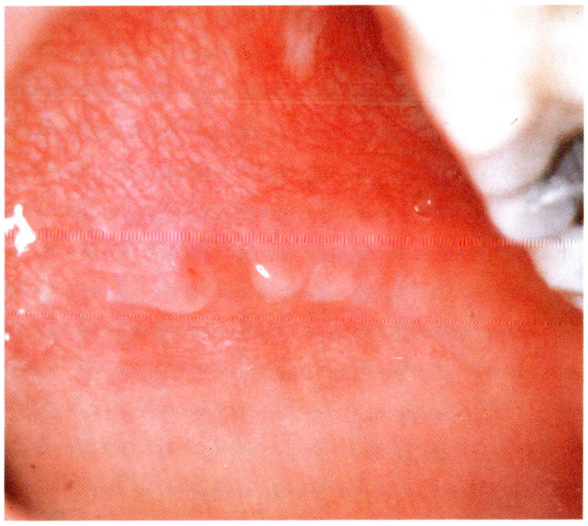

9.196

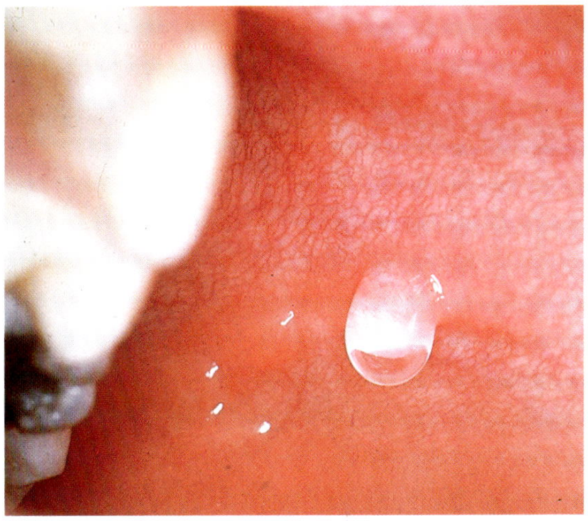

9.195

ACUTE BACTERIAL SIALADENITIS

Figure 9.193 This is almost invariably a mixed infection, often including penicillin-resistant *Staphylococcus aureus*, that ascends the duct because of xerostomia or a ductal anomaly. There is severe pain over the gland and often trismus if the parotid is affected, as here. There is erythema and swelling over the gland which is tender to palpation.

Enteric Gram-negative rods have a high oropharyngeal colonization in hospitalized persons and these rods and pseudomonads have been recently implicated in a few cases of sialadenitis.

Figure 9.194 Purulent saliva, as here, or frank pus may be expressed from the duct of the affected gland – in this case the parotid.

In children, there is a rare form of recurrent parotitis that is of uncertain aetiology, mainly seen in boys. It is characterized by recurrent painful swelling, usually unilateral. Peak incidence is between ages 3–6 years. The condition resolves spontaneously at puberty in most cases.

NORMAL PAROTID SALIVATION

Figure 9.195 This figure, for comparison with Figure 9.194, shows clear, watery, normal parotid saliva flowing from Stensen's duct.

SALIVARY FISTULA

Figure 9.196 Internal fistulae, as here, may be of congenital origin or acquired. They are inconsequential.

External fistulae usually follow trauma in an accident, assault, or after surgery, and are disconcerting and unpleasant for the patient.

SUBMANDIBULAR SIALOLITHIASIS

Figure 9.197 Salivary calculi are not uncommon and usually affect the submandibular duct. Sometimes asymptomatic, the typical presentation is pain in, and swelling of, the gland around mealtimes.

Figure 9.198 Calculi are usually yellow or white and can sometimes, as here, be seen in the duct (which has ulcerated), or may be palpable. Not all are radio-opaque.

Figure 9.199 Quite large submandibular calculi can form, and calculi may be multiple. Chronic sialadenitis may develop if a salivary obstruction is not removed.

PAROTID OBSTRUCTIVE SIALADENITIS

Figure 9.200 Stones are less common in the parotid and less often radio-opaque, but obstruction can also be caused by mucus plugs, strictures, or the oedema associated with ulceration of the parotid papilla. Rarely, salivary obstruction has other aetiologies.

SIALOLITH IN MINOR SALIVARY GLAND

Figure 9.201 Occasionally a stone forms in one of the minor salivary glands, here in the buccal mucosa.

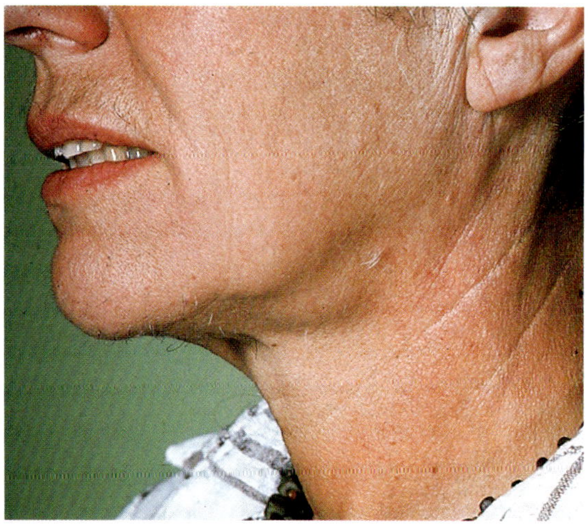

9.197

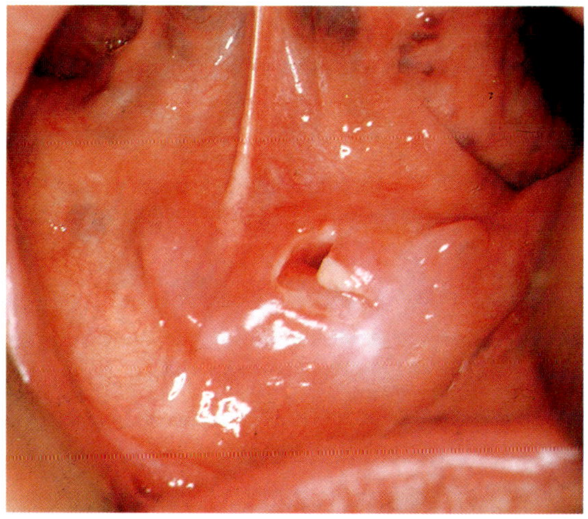

9.198

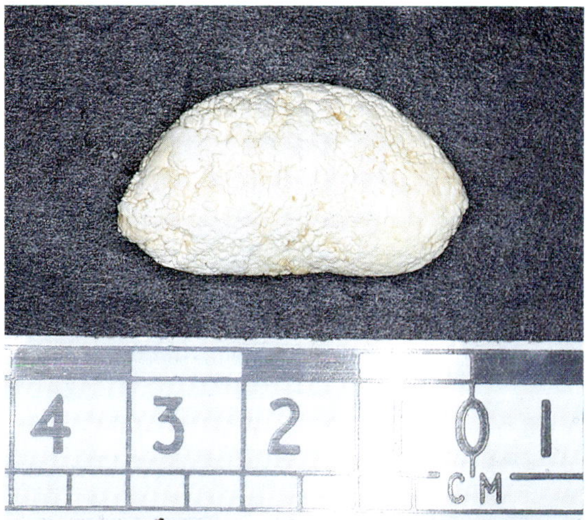

9.199

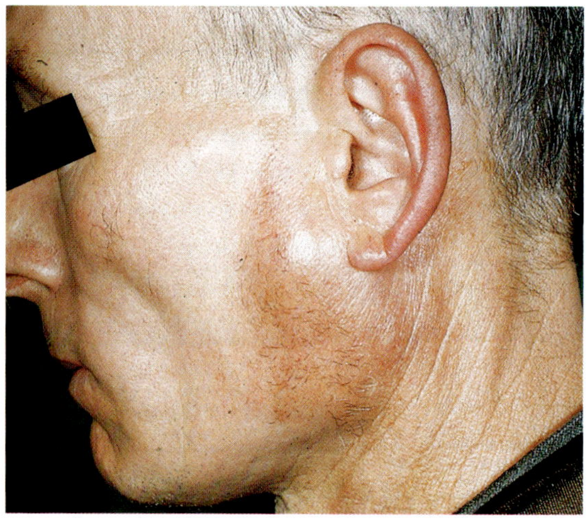

9.200

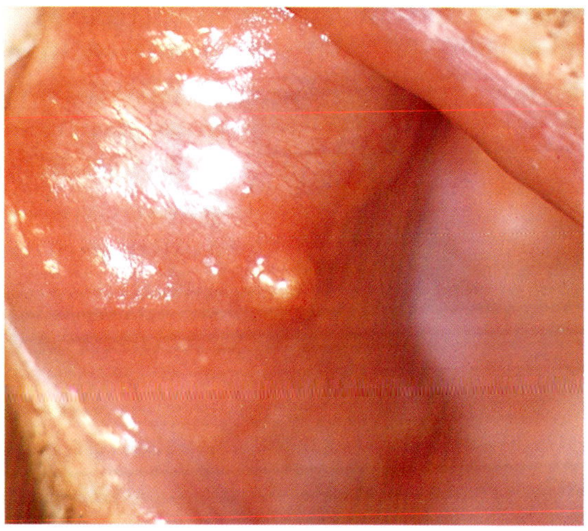

9.201

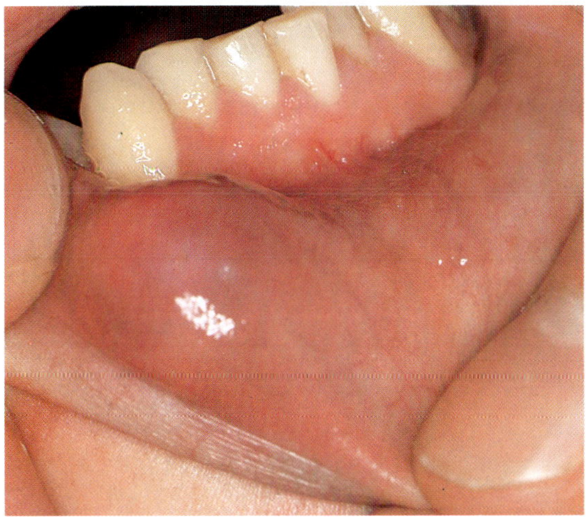

9.202

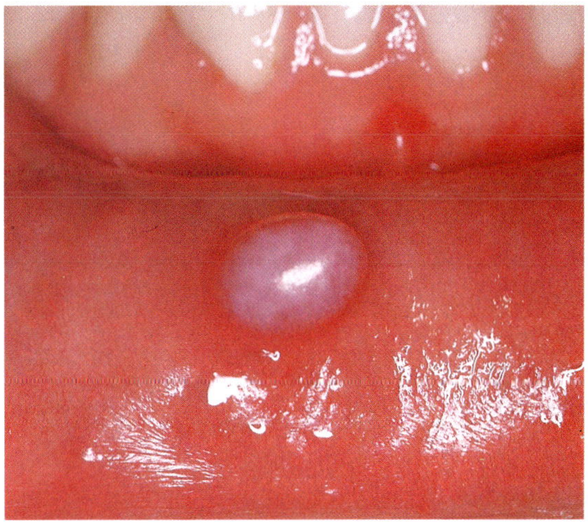

9.203

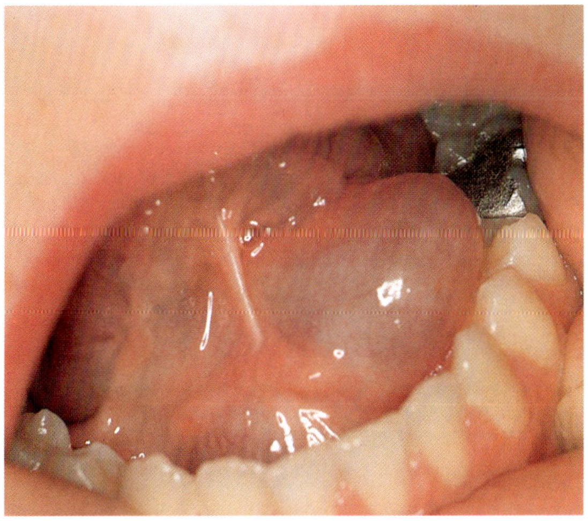

9.204

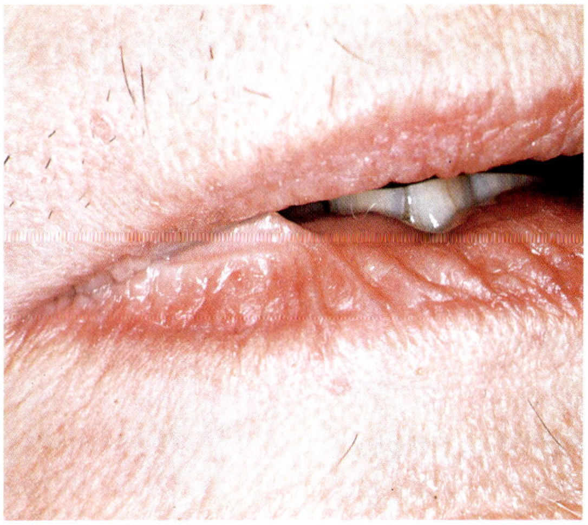

9.205

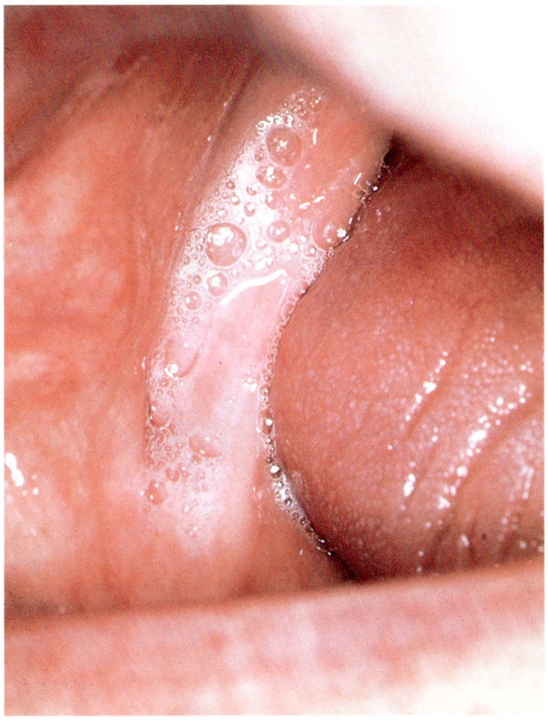

9.206

MUCOCELE

Figure 9.202 Most mucoceles are caused by saliva extravasating into the tissues from a damaged salivary duct. They are most common in the lower labial and ventral lingual mucosa. Occasional mucoceles are retention cysts.

Figure 9.203 The mucocele is a dome-shaped, fluctuant, bluish, non-tender, submucosal swelling with a normal overlying mucosa.

Cysts may occasionally develop within salivary neoplasms.

RANULA

Figure 9.204 Extravasation mucoceles arising from the sublingual gland are termed ranulas, because of their resemblance to a frog's belly. Rarely, a ranula extends through the mylohyoid muscle – a plunging ranula.

XEROSTOMIA

Figure 9.205 Many patients complain of a dry mouth and yet lack objective evidence of xerostomia. In true xerostomia, as here, the dry mucosa may become tacky and the lips adhere one to another. An examining dental mirror may often stick to the mucosa.

The main causes of dry mouth are drugs (those with anticholinergic or sympathomimetic activity), irradiation of the salivary glands, Sjögren's syndrome (see page 184), sarcoidosis and dehydration.

Figure 9.206 In true xerostomia there may be lack of salivary pooling in the floor of the mouth; any saliva present tends to be viscous and appear frothy, as here, and saliva flows poorly, if at all, from the ducts of the major glands on stimulation or palpation.

SIALOSIS (*Sialadenosis*)

Figure 9.207 Painless bilateral chronic swelling of the salivary glands, typically the parotids as here, without xerostomia, characterizes sialosis. There appears to be serous cell hypertrophy and striated duct atrophy.

Figure 9.208 Although sialosis is benign and usually idiopathic, it is important to exclude underlying causes such as drugs (eg, methyldopa), endocrinopathies (eg, diabetes mellitus and acromegaly), alcoholic liver cirrhosis or malnutrition.

Salivary glands, especially the submandibular, may also swell in cystic fibrosis and most affected children also have antral polyps.

NECROTIZING SIALOMETAPLASIA

Figure 9.209 Necrotizing sialometaplasia is a rare ulcerative lesion of unknown aetiology, seen especially in the hard palate in adult males. It may resemble a neoplasm clinically and histologically.

Figure 9.210 This chronic swelling of the palate ulcerated and then healed slowly over 1–2 months.

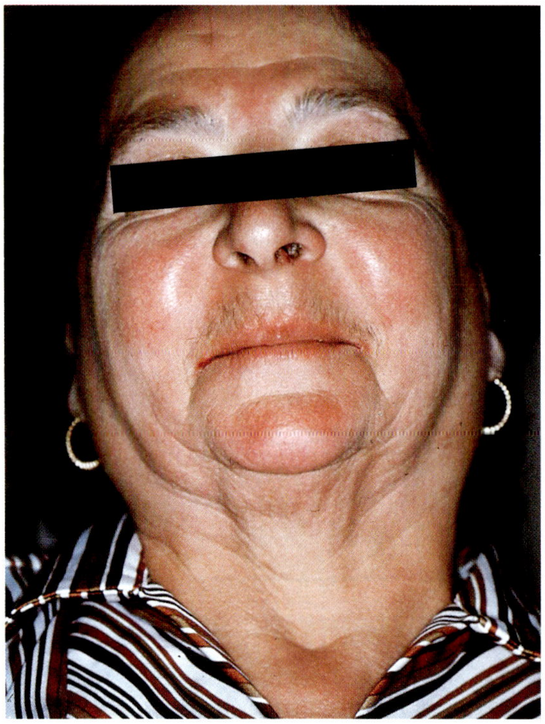

9.207

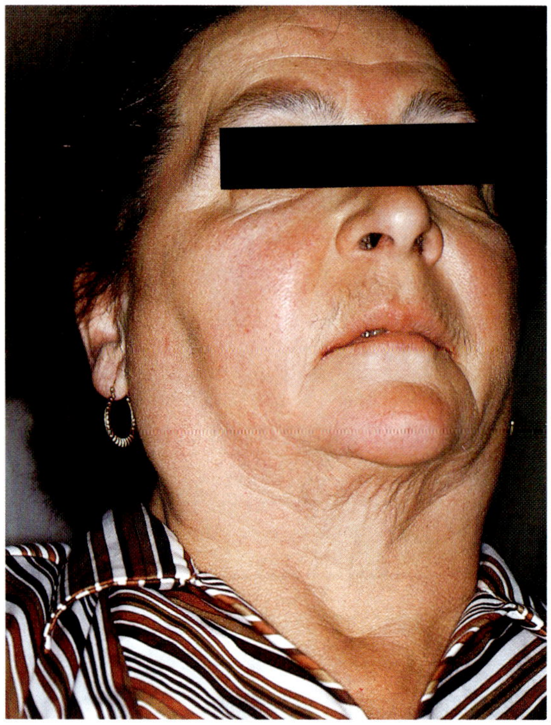

9.208

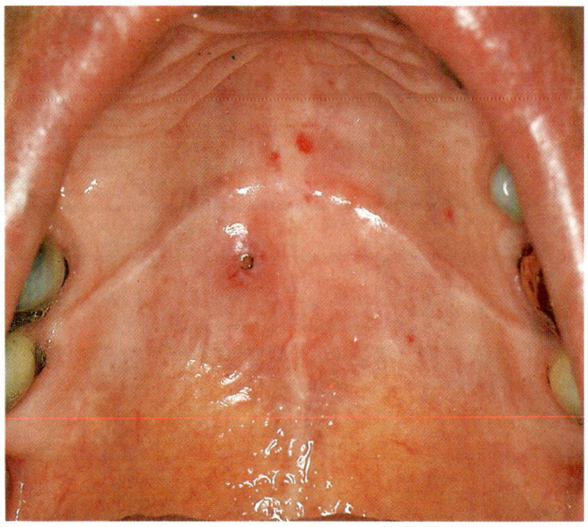

9.209

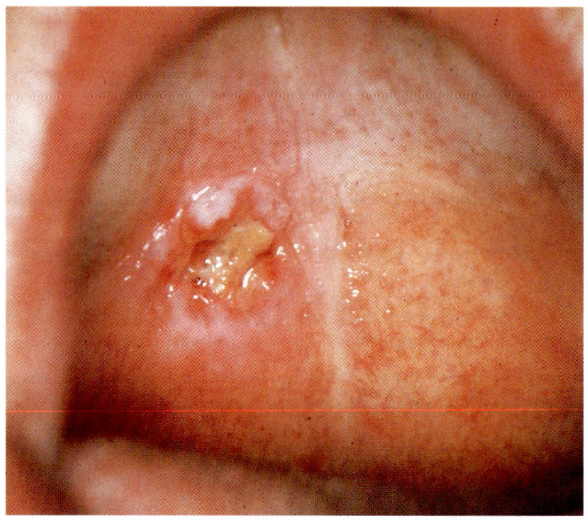

9.210

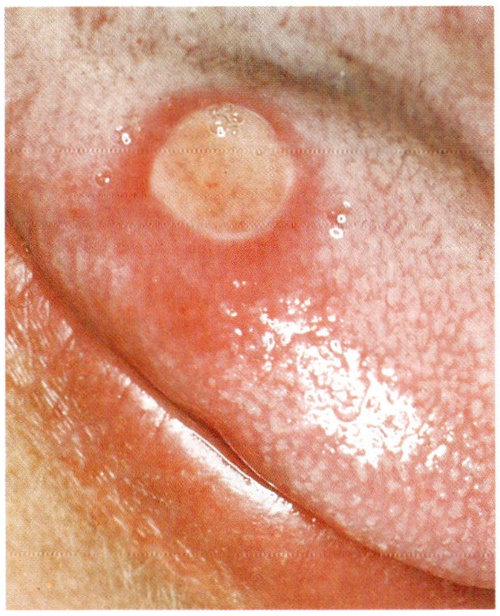

9.211

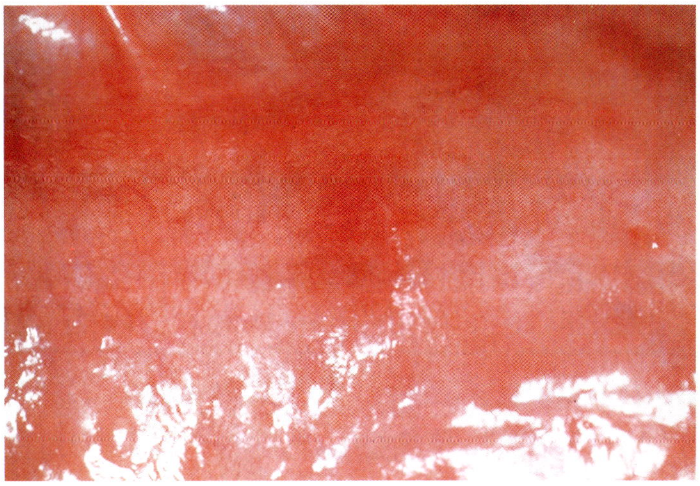

9.212

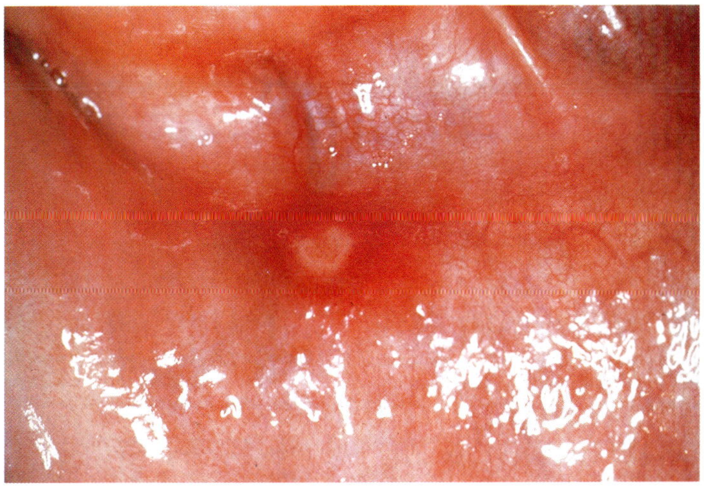

9.213

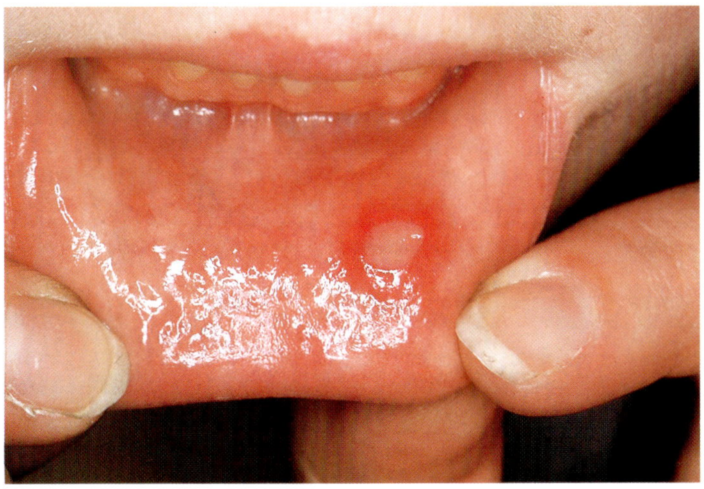

9.214

RECURRENT APHTHAE (*Recurrent aphthous stomatitis, RAS*)

Figure 9.211 Recurrent aphthae are typically ovoid or round ulcers with a yellowish floor and pronounced inflammatory halo. Episodes begin usually in childhood and the natural history is of spontaneous remission after some years. The aetiology is unknown.

Figure 9.212 Minor aphthae (Mikulicz aphthae) are small, 2–4 mm in diameter, last 7–10 days, tend not to be seen on gingiva, palate or dorsum of tongue, and heal with no obvious scarring. This is an early lesion.

Figure 9.213 This is the same patient as Figure 9.212, 24 hours later, showing an obvious ulcer. Most patients develop not more than six ulcers at any single episode.

Figure 9.214 This is a typical minor aphthous ulcer in a common site in a teenager.

Most patients with RAS are otherwise apparently well, but a significant proportion of those referred to a hospital clinic prove to be deficient in a haematinic such as iron, folate or vitamin B_{12}; 2–3 per cent have coeliac disease; and there are also occasional associations with menstruation, stress, food allergy and immunodeficiencies. Most patients with aphthae are non-smokers and others may develop aphthae for the first time on ceasing smoking.

Aphthae may occasionally be a manifestation of Behçet's syndrome (see page 137).

Aphthous-like ulcers may occasionally be a manifestation of cyclic neutropenia, or a similar recently-described syndrome with periodic fever and pharyngitis, but with no neutropenia.

RECURRENT APHTHAE
(continued)

Figure 9.215 Major aphthae are recurrent, often ovoid ulcers with an inflammatory halo, but are less common, much larger, more persistent than minor aphthae, and can affect the dorsum of tongue and soft palate as well as other sites.

Figure 9.216 Sometimes termed Sutton's ulcers or periadenitis mucosa necrotica recurrens (PMNR), major aphthae can be well over 1 cm in diameter and can take several months to heal. This ulcer is beginning to epithelialize.

Figure 9.217 This major aphtha has almost healed. At any one episode there are usually fewer than six ulcers present.

Figure 9.218 Major aphthae may leave obvious scars on healing, as here.

Figure 9.219 Herpetiform aphthae are so termed because the patients have a myriad of small ulcers that clinically resemble those of herpetic stomatitis. It is, however, a distinct entity, lacking the associated fever, gingivitis and lymph node involvement of primary herpetic stomatitis.

Figure 9.220 Pinpoint herpetiform aphthae enlarge and fuse to produce irregular ulcers, as here. These aphthae affect females more than males, present at a slightly later age (often from 30 years of age) than other forms of RAS, and affect any site in the mouth.

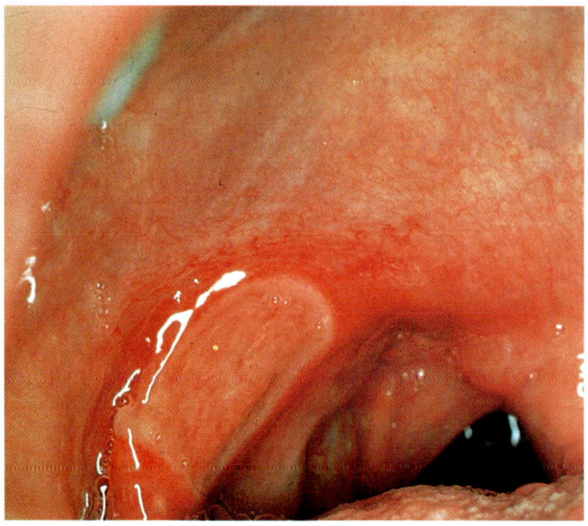
9.215

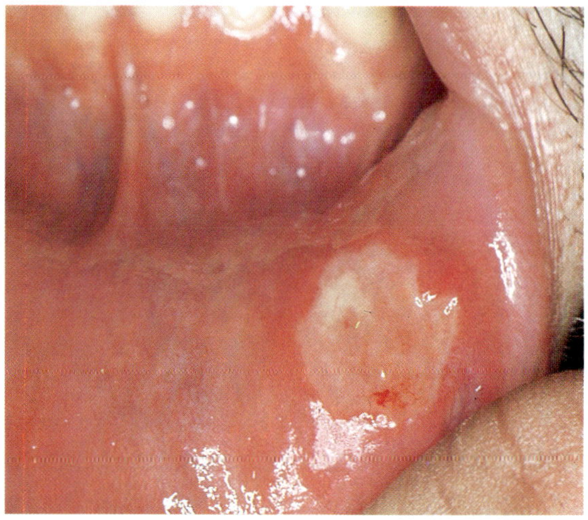
9.216

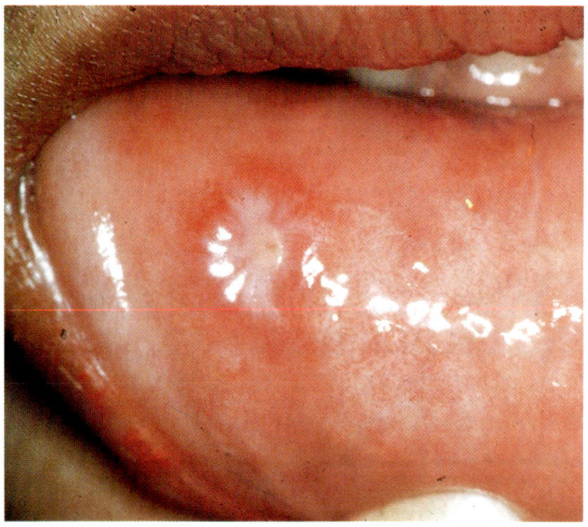
9.217

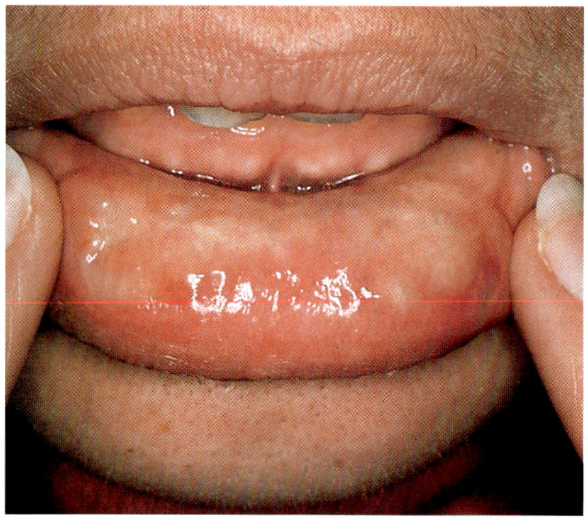
9.218

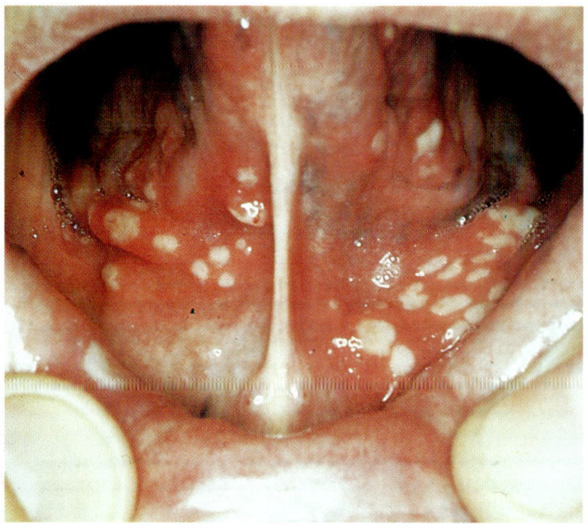
9.219

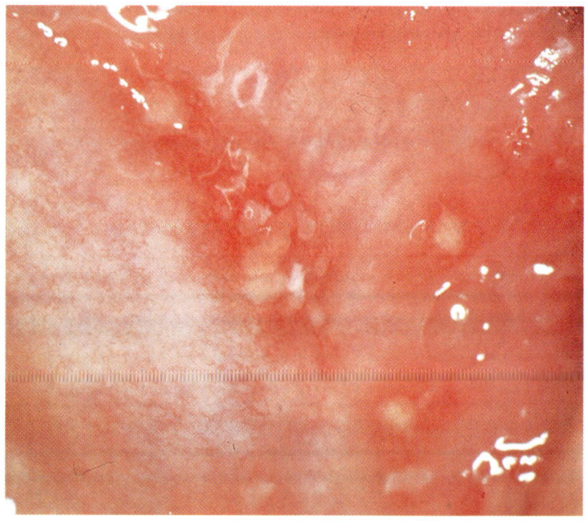
9.220

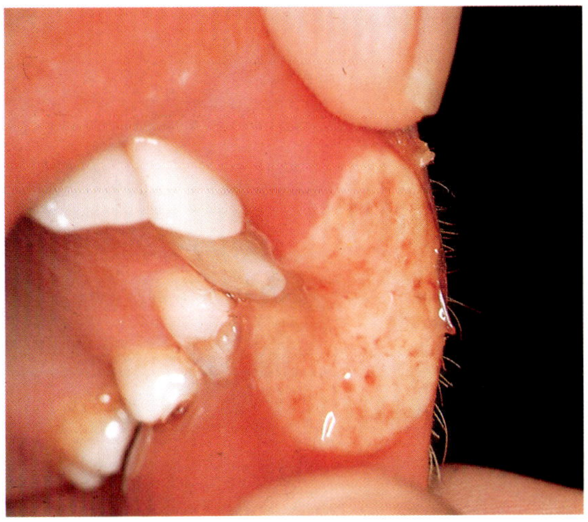

9.221

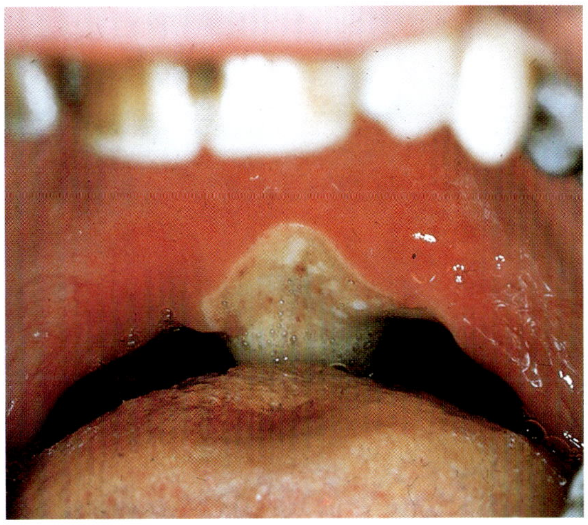

9.222

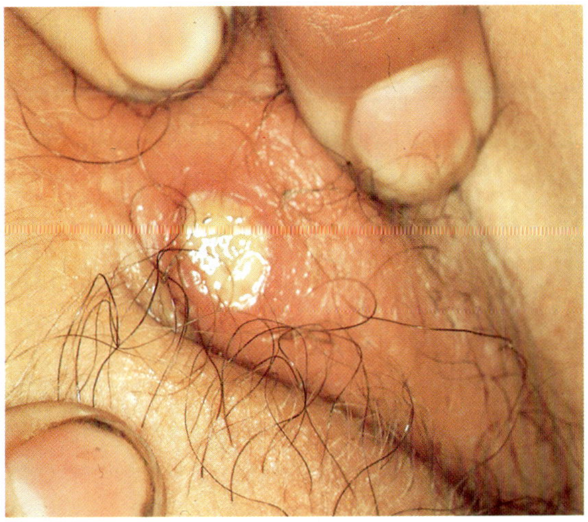

9.223

BEHÇET'S SYNDROME
(*Behçet's disease*)

Figure 9.221 Aphthae of any of the types previously described usually occur in isolation in apparently healthy persons. A minority are a manifestation of Behçet's syndrome, as here, where major aphthae were associated with genital ulcers and uveitis.

Figure 9.222 Behçet's syndrome is a multisystem disease affecting the mouth in most cases: this figure shows a major aphtha. Other sites commonly affected are genitals, eyes, skin and joints; but Behçet's syndrome is not the only cause of this constellation of lesions. Other causes, such as ulcerative colitis, Crohn's disease, mixed connective tissue disease, lupus erythematosus and Reiter's syndrome, should be excluded.

Figure 9.223 Behçet's syndrome is most common in Japan, China, Korea and the Middle East. Genital ulcers in Behçet's syndrome often closely resemble oral aphthae. This vulval ulcer is fairly typical.

BEHÇET'S SYNDROME
(continued)

Figure 9.224 Uveitis (posterior uveitis: retinal vasculitis) is one of the more important ocular lesions of Behçet's syndrome but anterior uveitis, as here, and other changes occur. The left pupil has been dilated for fundoscopy. Ocular and arthritic symptoms are more common in males. Neurological involvement may cause headache, psychiatric, motor or sensory manifestations.

Figure 9.225 Erythema nodosum can be a feature of Behçet's syndrome, particularly in females.

Figure 9.226 Of the various rashes seen in Behçet's syndrome, an acneiform pustular rash, as here, is common.

Patients with Behçet's syndrome may develop pustules at the site of vene-puncture (pathergy) but this feature is uncommon in British patients.

Although large joint arthropathy is not uncommon in Behçet's syndrome, an overlap syndrome with relapsing polychondritis has also been described (mouth and genital ulcers with inflamed cartilage (MAGIC) syndrome).

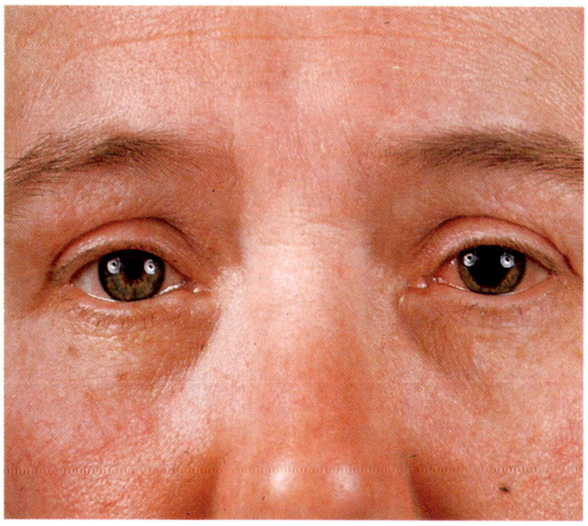

9.224

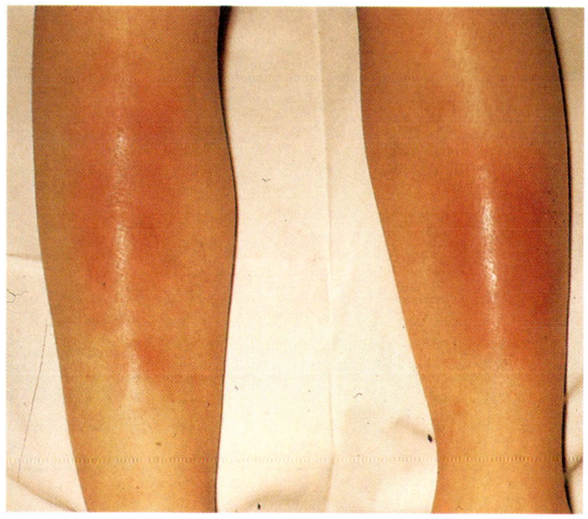

9.225

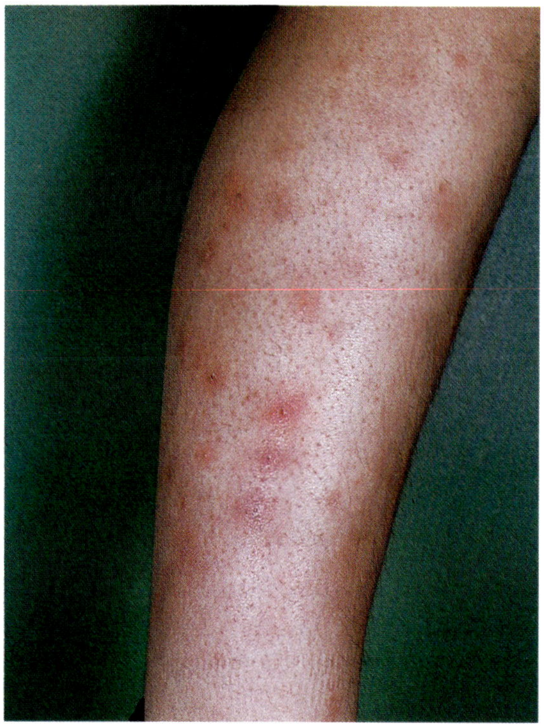

9.226

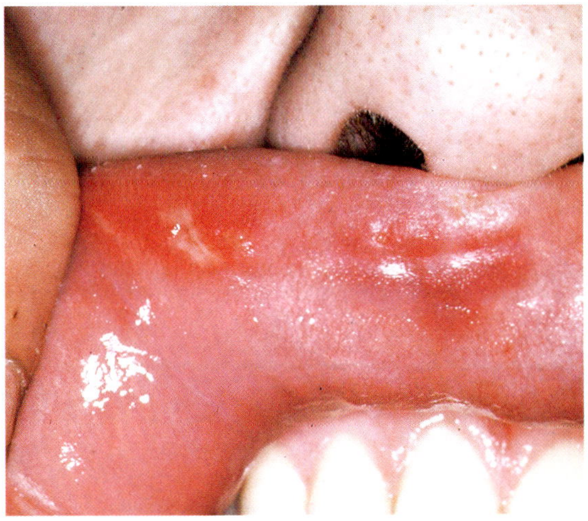

9.227

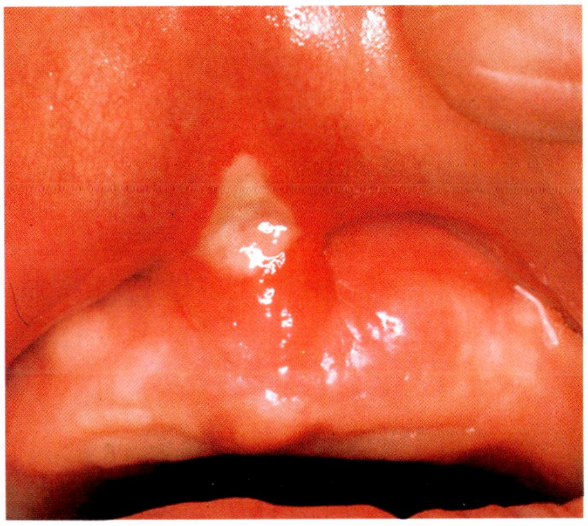

9.228

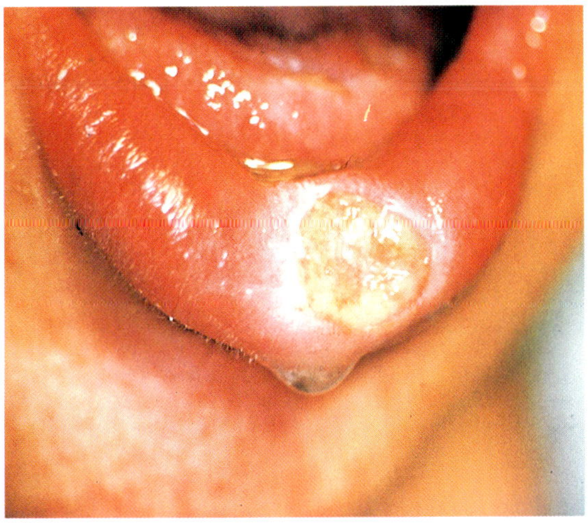

9.229

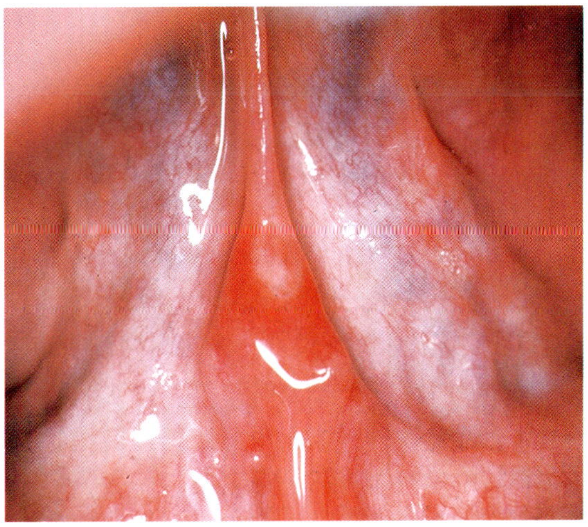

9.230

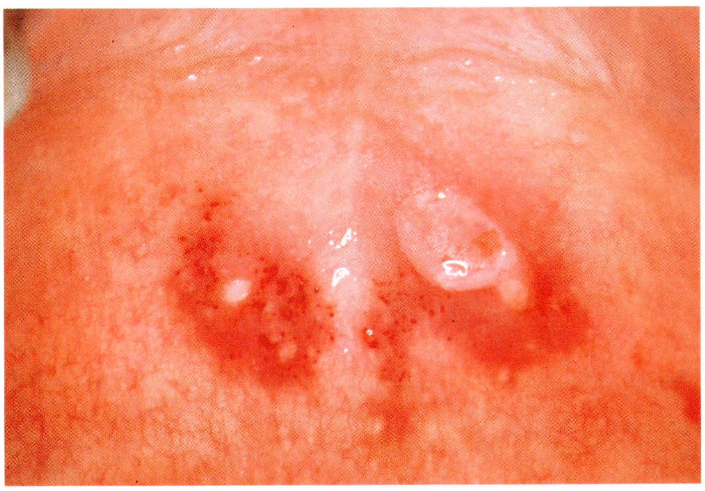

9.231

TRAUMATIC ULCERS

Figure 9.227 Traumatic ulcers and ecchymosis: traumatic ulcers are common, usually caused by accidental biting, hard foods, appliances such as dentures or orthodontic appliances, or following dental treatment. Less common causes are shown here. In this patient, small bruises and ulcers have followed a blow on the lip.

Figure 9.228 Child abuse syndrome (non-accidental injury): ulceration of the upper labial fraenum in a child may follow a traumatic fraenal tear, a feature of child abuse.

The mouth is often traumatized. Bruised and swollen lips, lacerated fraenae, and even subluxed teeth or fractured mandible can be features of child abuse.

Figure 9.229 Chronic self-induced traumatic ulcer: self-mutilation in a mentally handicapped or disturbed patient has caused a chronic ulcer with surrounding keratosis.

Figure 9.230 Cunnilingus tongue: the lingual fraenum has been traumatized by repeated rubbing over the lower incisor teeth. A similar lesion can be seen in children with recurrent bouts of coughing as in whooping cough, termed Riga-Fedes disease.

Figure 9.231 Fellatio palate: traumatic ulceration of the soft palate is fairly uncommon. Here, trauma from the erect penis together with oral suction have produced ulceration, bruising and petechiae.

Neonates occasionally develop an ulcer at a similar site (Bednar's ulcer) which is thought may be caused by trauma from the examining finger of the paediatrician.

DERMOID CYST

Figure 9.232 Dermoid cyst is an uncommon midline entity, often presenting with a slowly growing swelling beneath the chin.

Figure 9.233 Found in the floor of the mouth, the dermoid cyst sometimes resembles a ranula, as here.

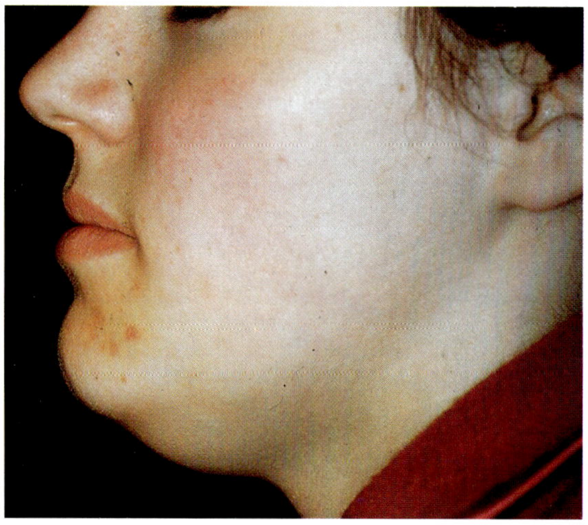

9.232

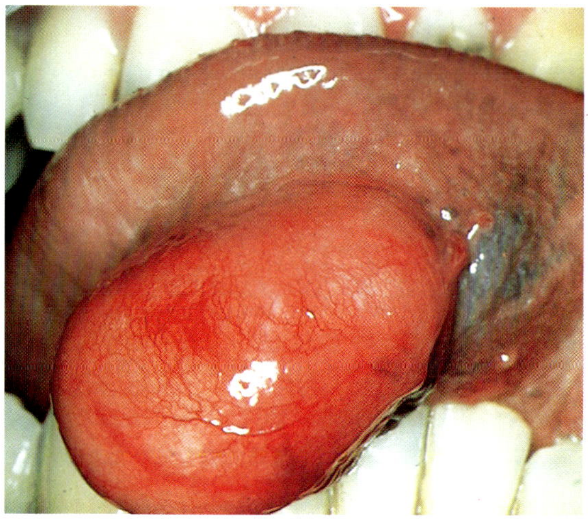

9.233

GINGIVAL CYSTS IN NEONATES

Figure 9.234 Small white nodules are extremely common on the alveolar ridge and midline palate of the newborn. Sometimes termed Epstein's pearls or Bohn's nodules, they usually disappear spontaneously by rupturing or involution within a month or so.

Figure 9.235 There may be an association of gingival cysts with milia (superficial epidermal inclusion cysts). This figure shows the same infant as in Figure 9.234.

Oral cysts are otherwise rare in neonates, although cysts may rarely be present at the base of the tongue where they can cause stridor.

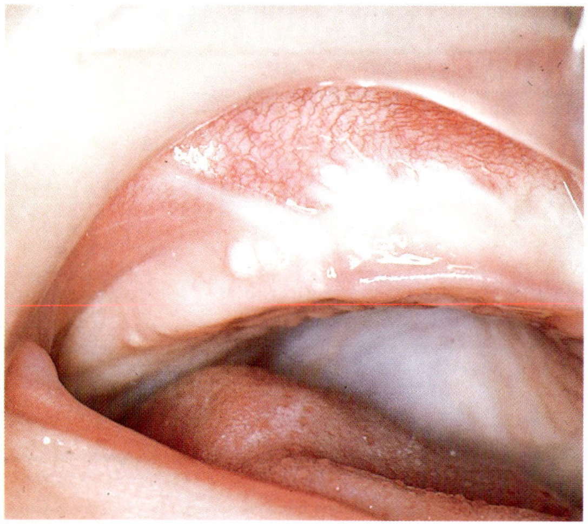

9.234

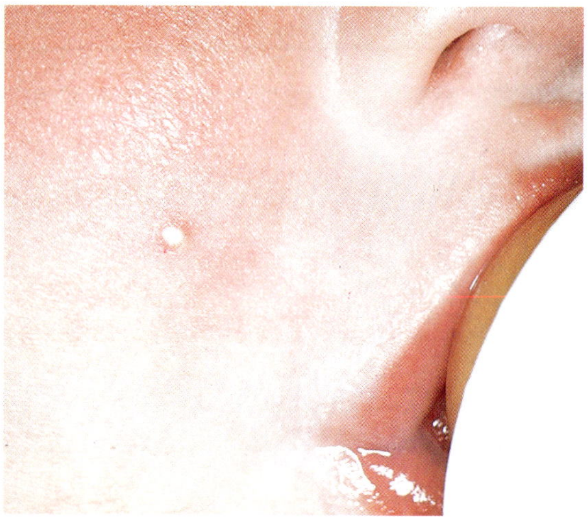

9.235

LYMPHOEPITHELIAL CYST

Figure 9.236 The lymphoepithelial cyst is a rare lesion associated with lymphoid tissue, usually seen as an asymptomatic small yellowish movable cystic swelling in the floor of the mouth or ventrum of tongue, and may represent simple oral lymphoid tissue.

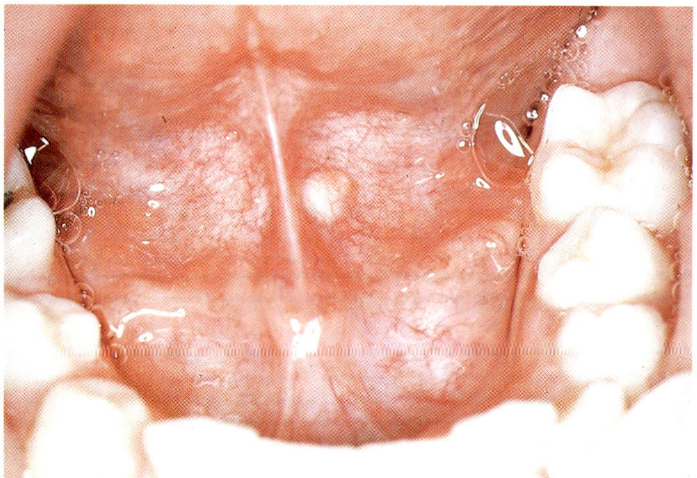

9.236

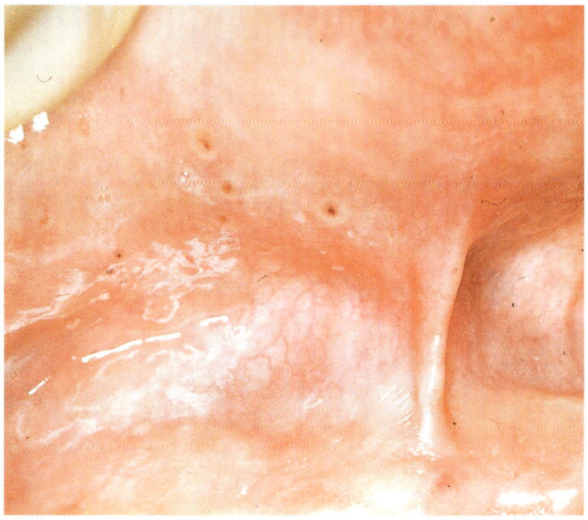

9.237

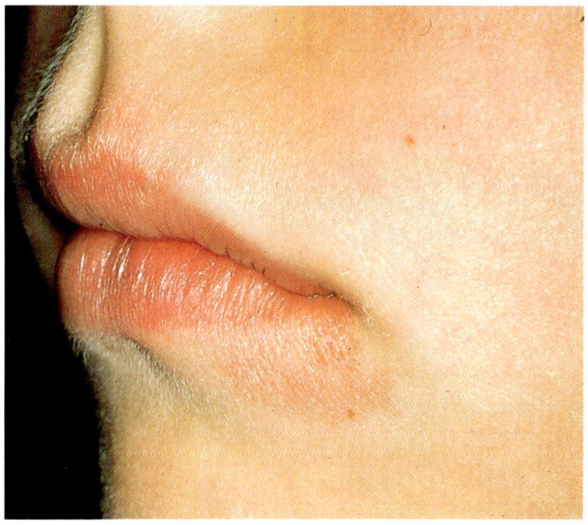

9.238

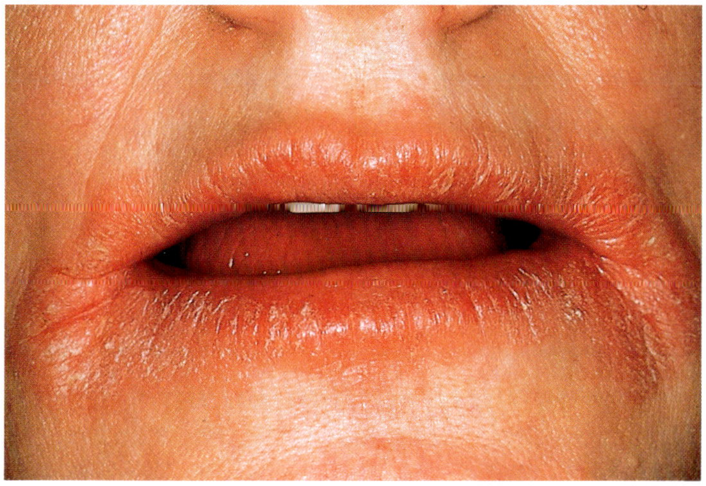

9.239

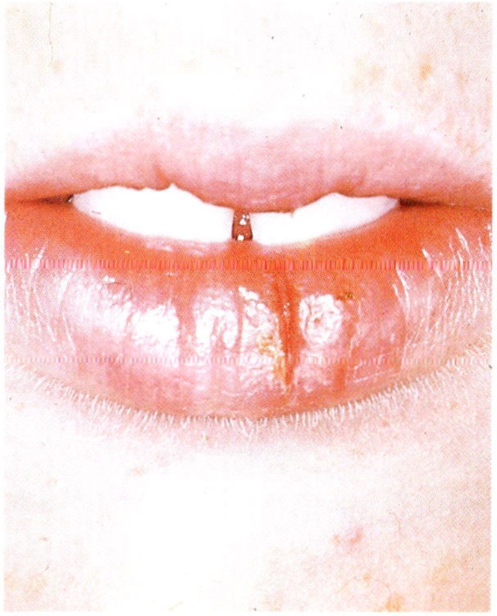

9.240

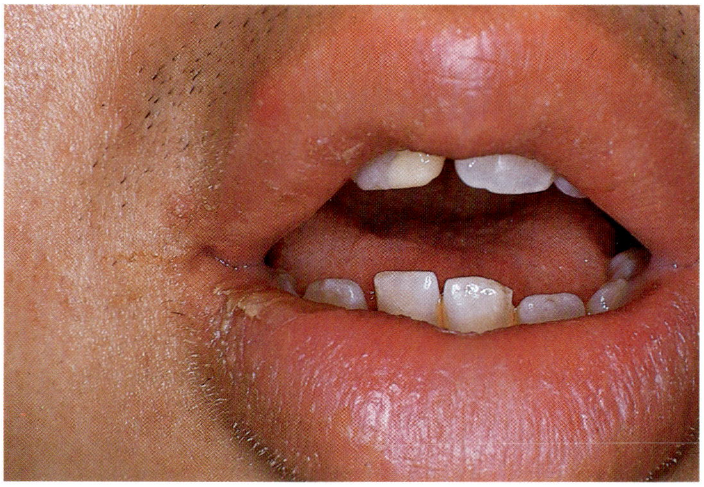

9.241

CHEILITIS

Figure 9.237 Cheilitis glandularis: the black puncta here, inside the upper lip, were associated with swelling and a thick mucinous exudate from the minor salivary glands. This lesion, of unknown aetiology, may be premalignant and usually affects the lower lip.

Figure 9.238 Cheilitis caused by lip-licking: children in particular may develop a habit of licking the lip and adjacent skin, leading to erythematous lesions such as shown. Candidosis may infect some of these lesions.

PERIORAL DERMATITIS

Figure 9.239 Perioral dermatitis is seen mainly in females and related to the use of cosmetics, corticosteroid creams or ointments.

Allergic reactions may follow contact with a variety of topical agents (especially essential oils); with various vegetables (especially artichokes and asparagus); with medicaments or dental materials (see page 220).

LIP FISSURE

Figure 9.240 A fissure may develop in the lip where a patient, typically a child, is mouth-breathing. Lip fissures are common in Down's syndrome. The lips may crack in this way if swollen, for example, in oral Crohn's disease.

EXFOLIATIVE CHEILITIS

Figure 9.241 Persistent scaling of the vermilion of the lips is seen mainly in adolescent or young adult females. It may have a somewhat cyclical nature but is of unknown, possibly factitious, aetiology. The lips scale and peel and can be covered with a shaggy yellowish coating.

KERATOSIS (*Leukoplakia*)

Figure 9.242 Hyperkeratosis in the mouth can present as a white lesion, as here in the buccal sulcus. Most keratoses are flat and smooth-surfaced (homogeneous), and benign.

Figure 9.243 This homogeneous leukoplakia of the lower lip was seen in a heavy smoker. Smoking and tobacco-related habits are, with friction, the most common identifiable causes of keratoses.

Figure 9.244 Homogeneous keratosis in the buccal mucosa, a common site.

Figure 9.245 Keratoses may be extremely pronounced, as in this lesion on the lateral border of tongue and the buccal mucosa.

Figure 9.246 This keratosis of the palate has two components: a diffuse overall keratosis with a more verrucous area centrally. Verrucous or nodular keratoses have a low premalignant potential but higher than that of homogeneous keratoses.

A recently described variant termed proliferative verrucous leukoplakia is seen especially in the buccal mucosa in older women and about one half develop carcinoma.

Figure 9.247 The lesion in the anterior part of this keratosis is somewhat nodular and developed into a carcinoma.

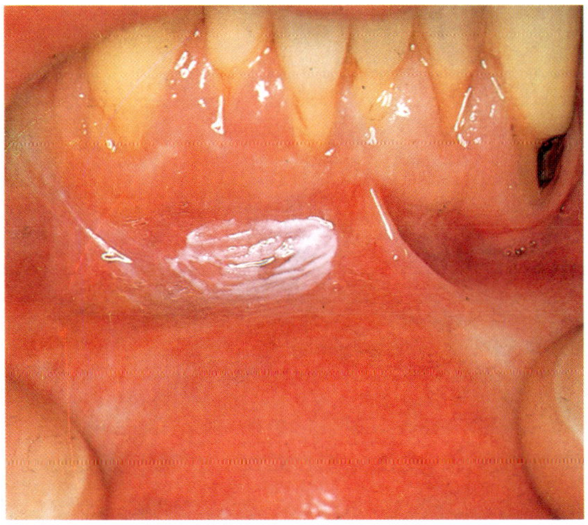

9.242

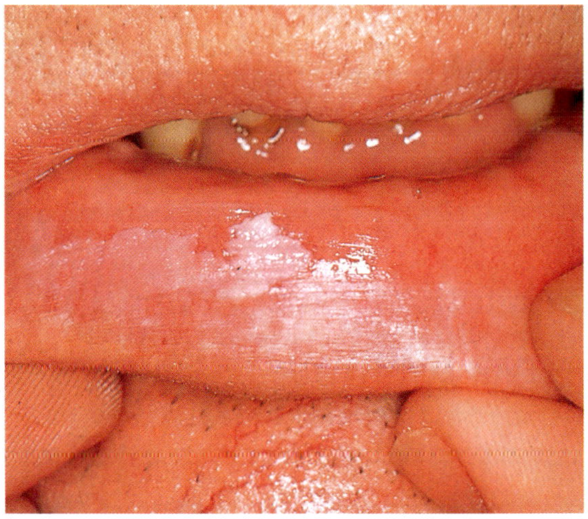

9.243

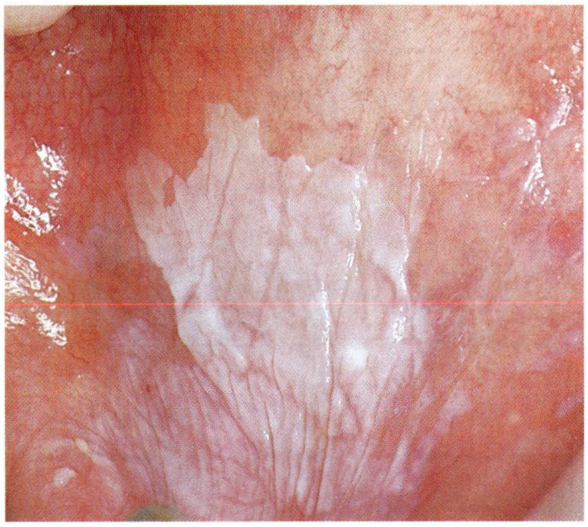

9.244

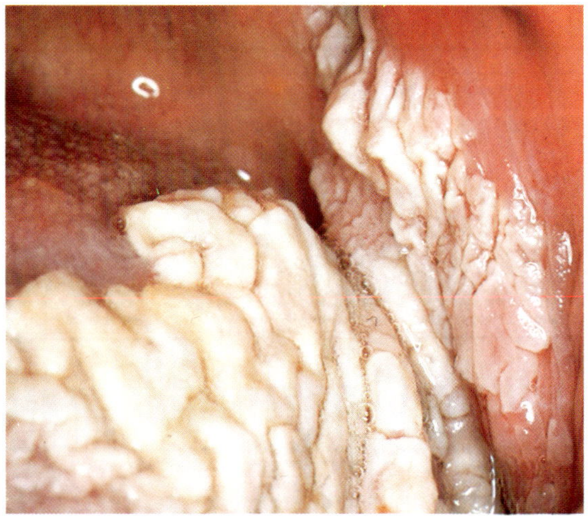

9.245

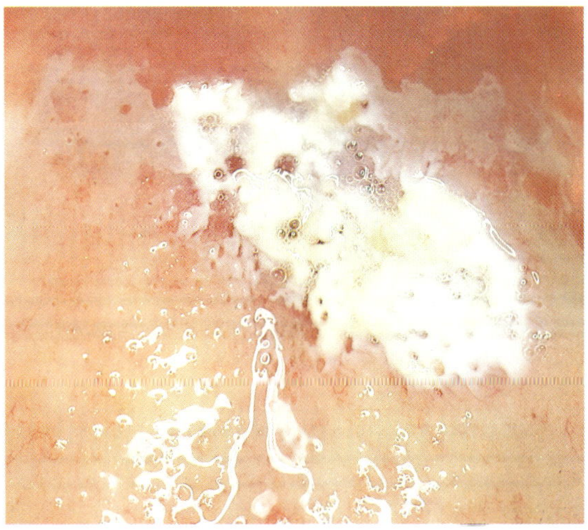

9.246

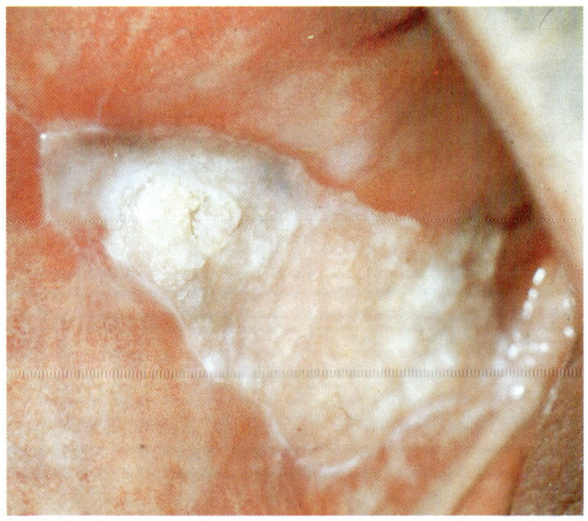

9.247

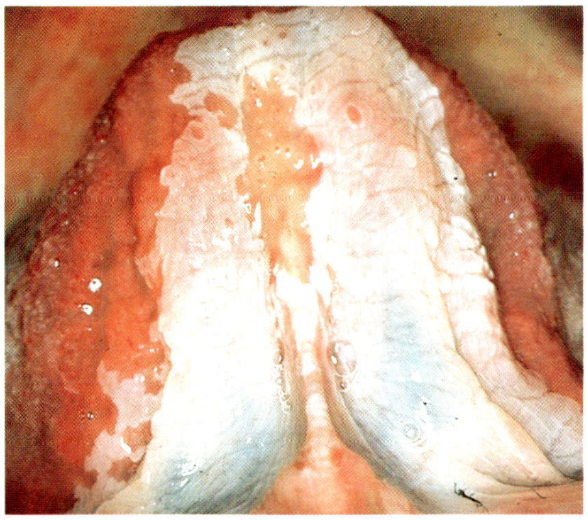

9.248

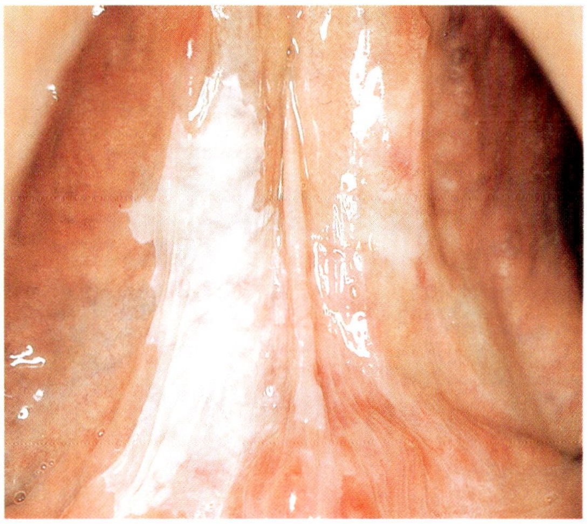

9.249

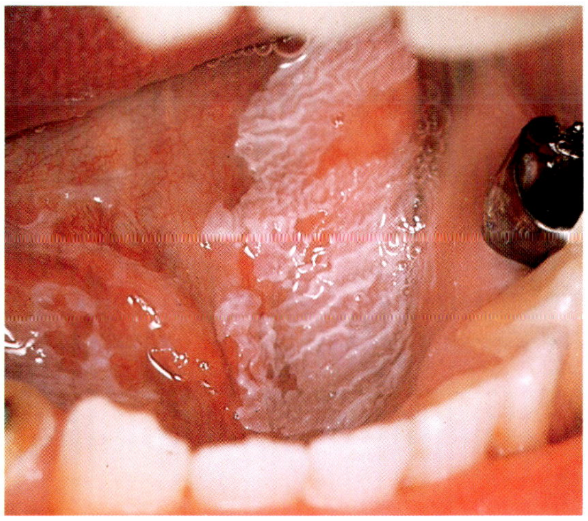

9.250

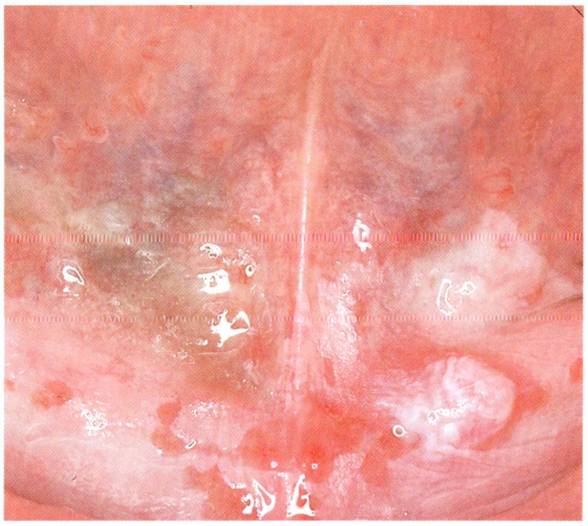

9.251

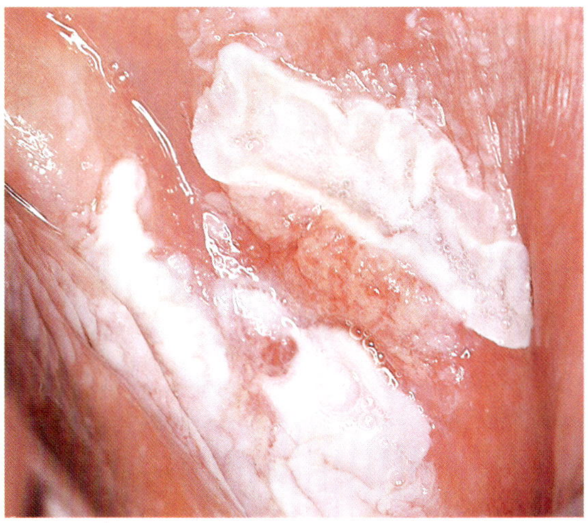

9.252

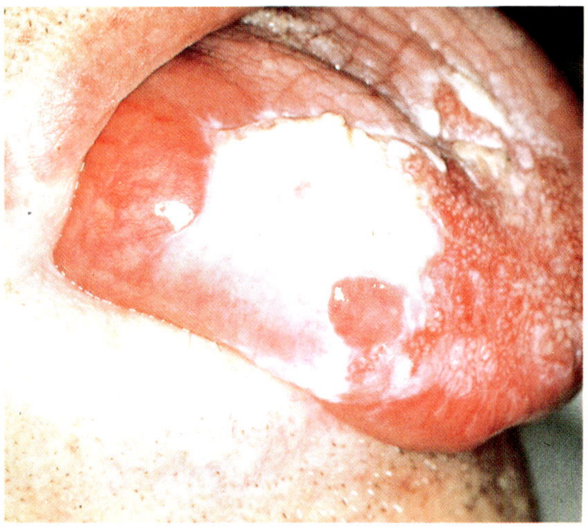

9.253

Figure 9.248 Keratosis on the ventrum of the tongue and floor of the mouth has a higher premalignant potential than similar lesions elsewhere.

Figure 9.249 Seen especially in middle-aged or older women, the sublingual keratosis is usually bilateral, but not invariably – as here.

Figure 9.250 The surface of the sublingual keratosis may have a so-called 'ebbing tide' appearance, resembling the appearance of sand on the beach as the tide ebbs.

Figure 9.251 The sublingual lesion may be a mixture of white and red lesions: a speckled leukoplakia. The red areas are most sinister.

Figure 9.252 Keratosis and carcinoma: keratoses must be examined clinically with care and biopsied. White lesions here flank a carcinoma.

Figure 9.253 Though the most obvious lesions here on the tongue are white, the more sinister is the red lesion (erythroplasia) on the lateral margin which showed severe epithelial dysplasia on histology. The patient has already had a carcinoma of the buccal mucosa excised and skin-grafted: he has widespread 'field changes' and may well develop another oral carcinoma.

Leukoplakia and glossitis on the dorsum of the tongue may sometimes have a syphilitic origin.

KERATOSIS (*continued*)

Figure 9.254 Speckled leukoplakias have the highest premalignant potential of the keratoses. Keratoses such as these may have a candidal association, although these are typically located at the commissures.

ERYTHROPLASIA (*Erythroplakia*)

Figure 9.255 Less common than leukoplakia, erythroplasia is characterized by epithelial atrophy and pronounced dysplasia. Erythroplasia is seen mainly in elderly males, in the buccal mucosa or palate.

STOMATITIS NICOTINA (*Smoker's palate*)

Figure 9.256 Stomatitis nicotina is a fairly common lesion, seen typically in middle-aged or elderly pipe smokers. The palate is diffusely white and the orifices of the minor salivary glands are obvious as red spots.

Figure 9.257 Close-up view of this smoker's keratosis shows the typical features and the heavily tobacco-stained teeth. Smoker's keratosis is usually a benign lesion that regresses if smoking is stopped (compare Figure 9.258).

Figure 9.258 If a denture is worn, as here, the mucosa is protected by the denture and appears normal in contrast to the non-denture bearing area. The obvious red area proved, however, to be dysplastic.

PAPILLOMATOSIS

Figure 9.259 Papillomatous lesions in the vault of the palate may occasionally result from obstructed ducts of minor salivary glands.

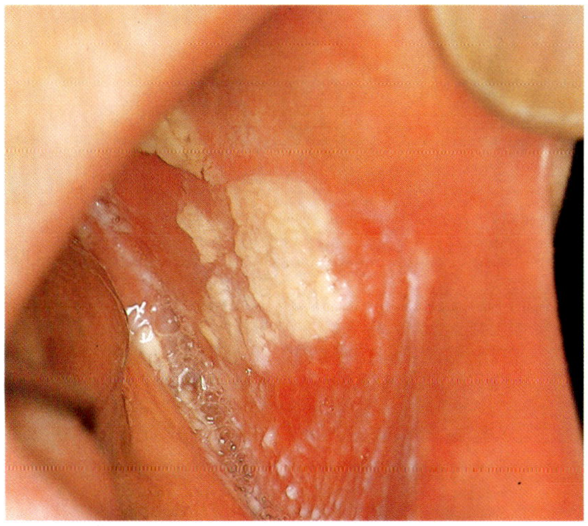

9.254

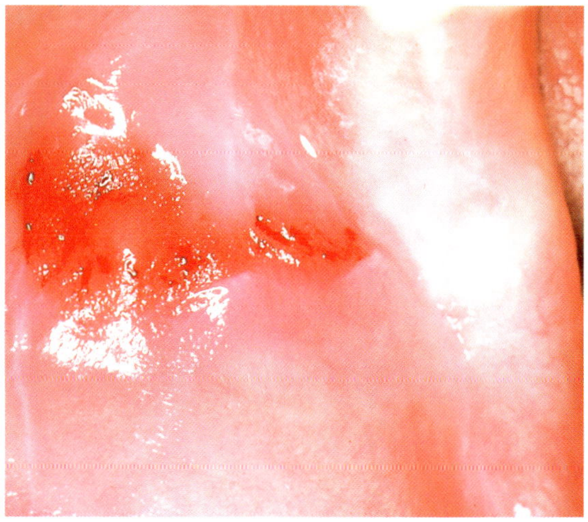

9.255

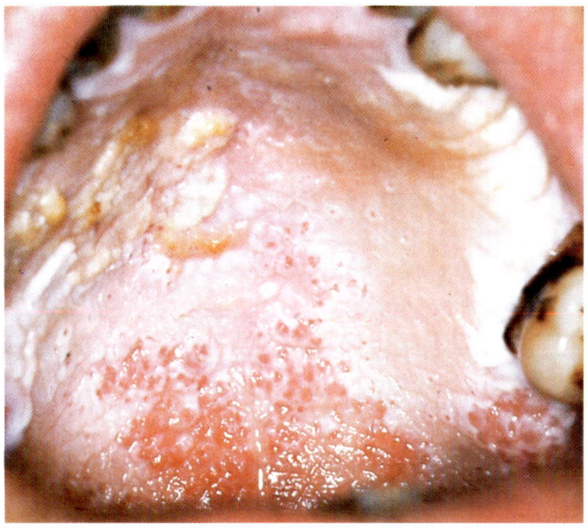

9.256

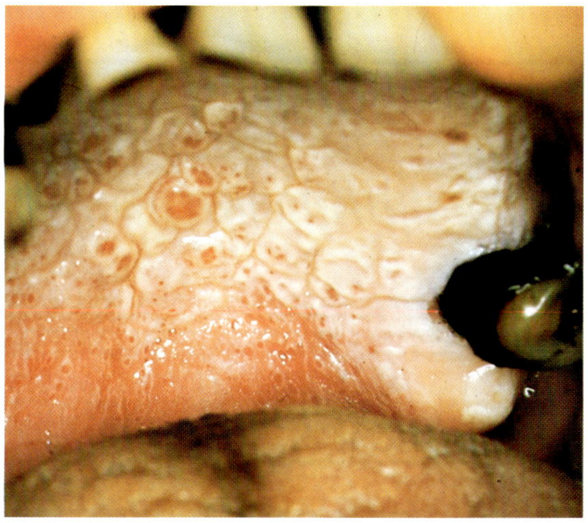

9.257

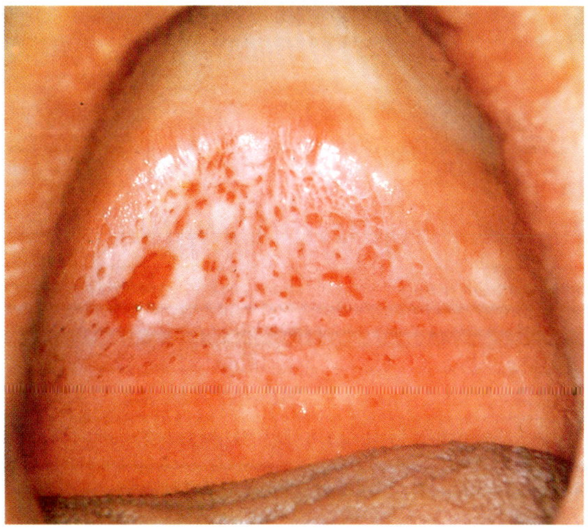

9.258

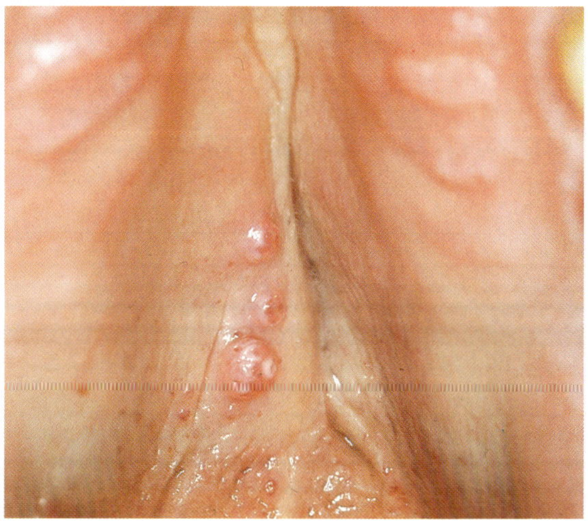

9.259

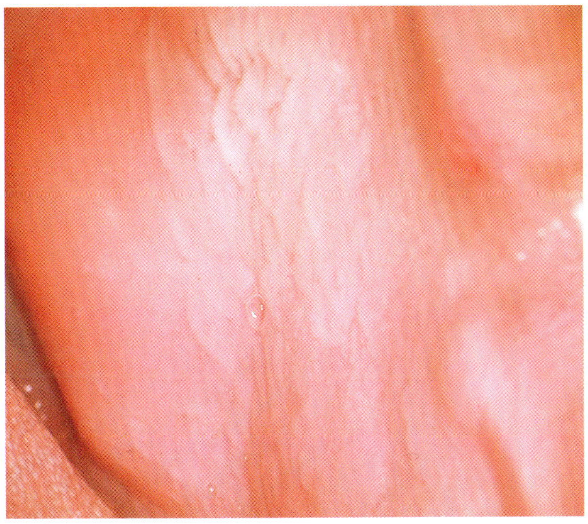

9.260

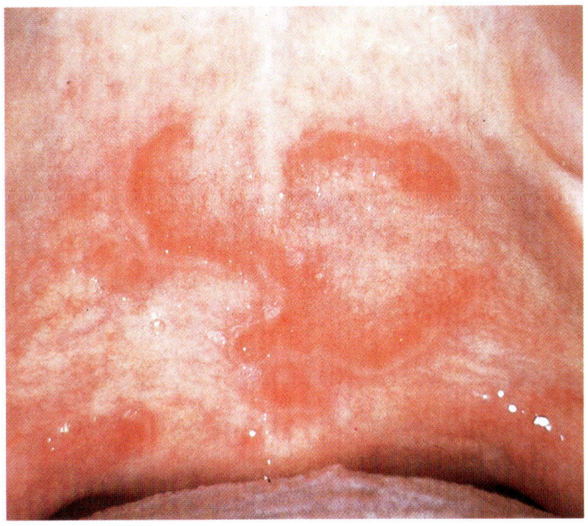

9.261

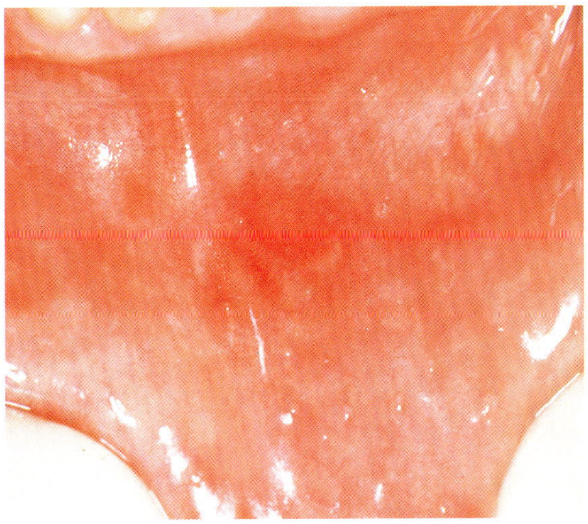

9.262

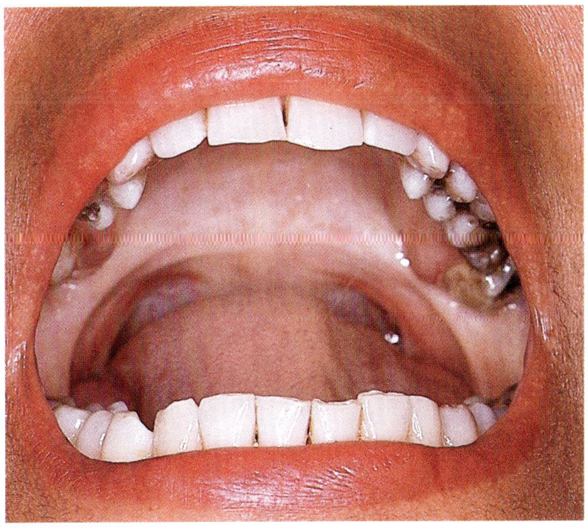

9.263

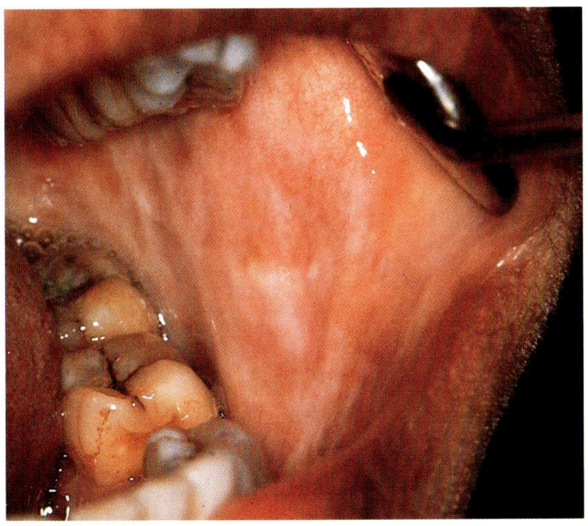

9.264

LEUKOEDEMA

Figure 9.260 Leukoedema is the term given to the clinical appearance of a milky whitish wrinkled film in the buccal mucosa (apparent anteriorly). It disappears if the mucosa is stretched when the cheek is pushed in from outside (as demonstrated posteriorly here).

ERYTHEMA MIGRANS (*Geographic or migratory stomatitis*)

Figure 9.261 Erythema migrans is common on the tongue but uncommon elsewhere. Often asymptomatic, the lesions are characterized by a somewhat serpiginous yellow-white lesion with surrounding erythema, which here simulated snailtrack ulcers (see also page 23).

Figure 9.262 A less pronounced lesion of erythema migrans. The lesions change in shape and site and are totally benign. They may represent a variant of psoriasis.

ORAL SUBMUCOUS FIBROSIS

Figure 9.263 Oral submucous fibrosis (OSMF) is a chronic disorder affecting the oral and sometimes pharyngeal mucosa, characterized by pain and the development of epithelial atrophy and fibrosis leading to stiffening of the mucosa and restricted mouth-opening, as here.

Figure 9.264 Seen in persons who use betel (*Areca catechu*) nuts, the lesions of OSMF appear to be due to constituents such as alkaloids, tannin and catechin. OSMF is seen mainly in Asians. There appears to be a genetic predisposition. The mucosa is pale, tight, with vertical submucosal fibrous bands and may develop carcinoma.

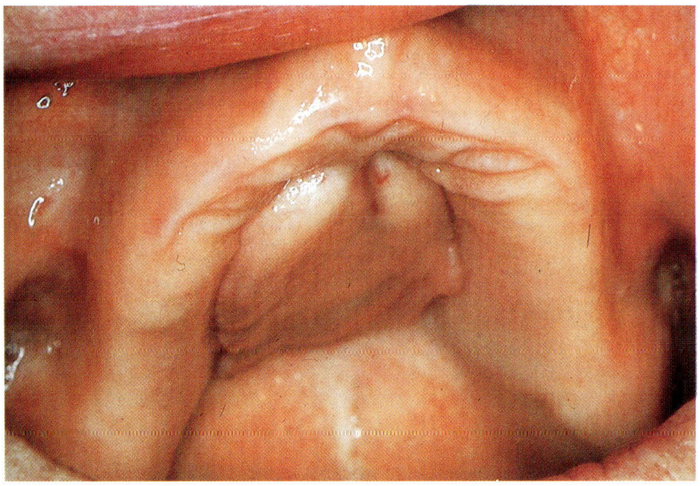

9.265

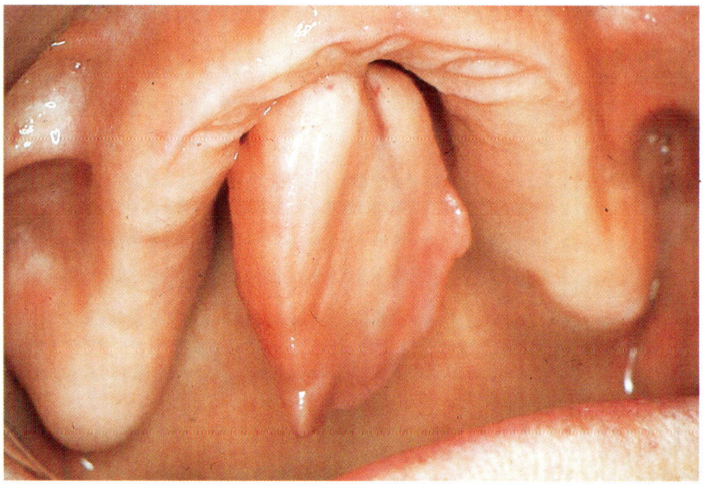

9.266

FIBROUS LUMP (*Fibroepithelial polyp*)

Figure 9.265 Fibrous lumps such as these may be related to irritation, but this is not always evident. This lesion was beneath a denture.

Figure 9.266 The lesion in Figure 9.265 is a so-called 'leaf fibroma', although it is not actually a true fibroma. It is totally benign.

Figure 9.267 Fibrous lumps on the margin of the tongue may also be benign, although biopsy is prudent.

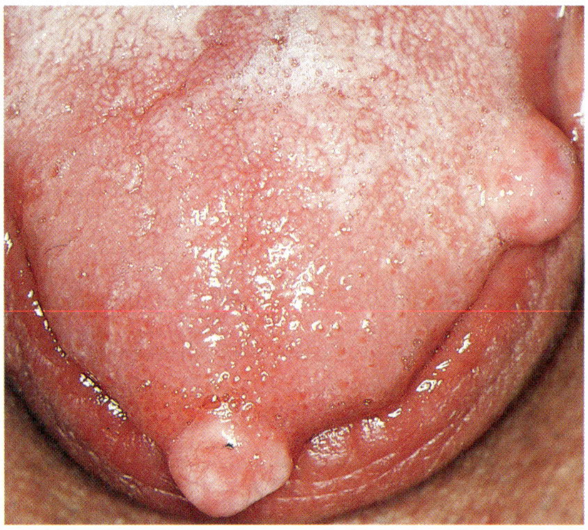

9.267

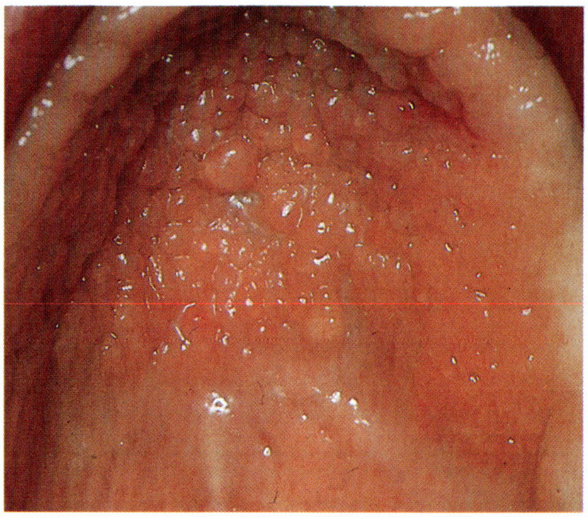

9.268

PAPILLARY HYPERPLASIA

Figure 9.268 Papillary hyperplasia of the palate is a benign condition of unknown aetiology, but is often more obvious where a denture is worn and where there is denture-induced stomatitis.

Figure 9.269 Papillary hyperplasia can also appear in the absence of dentures.

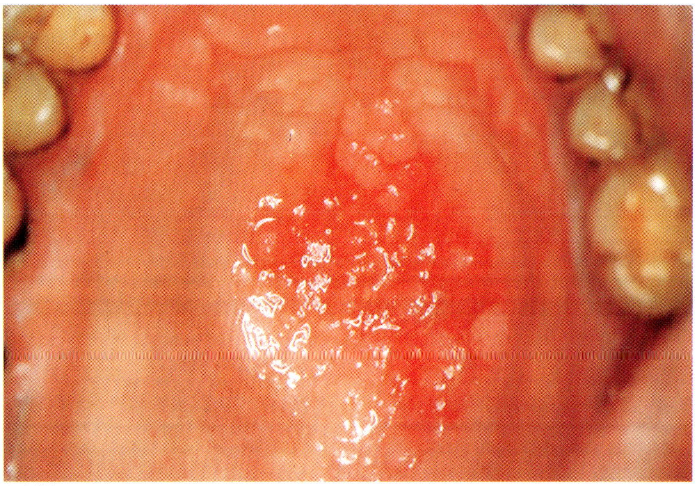

9.269

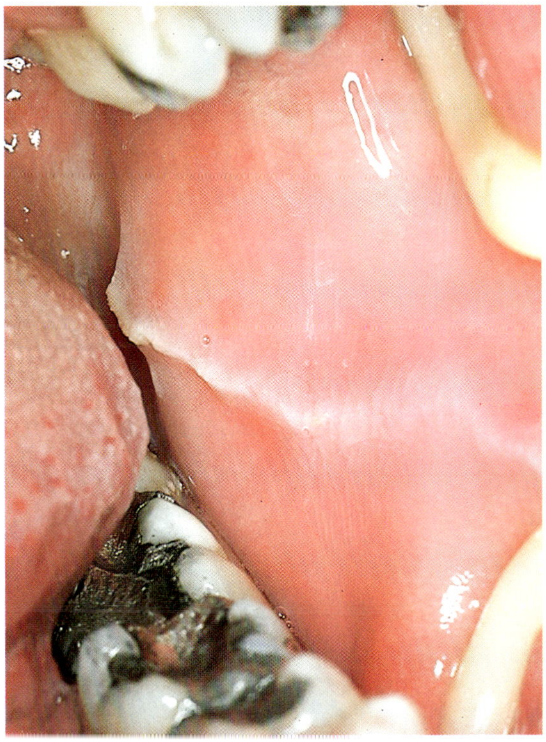

9.270

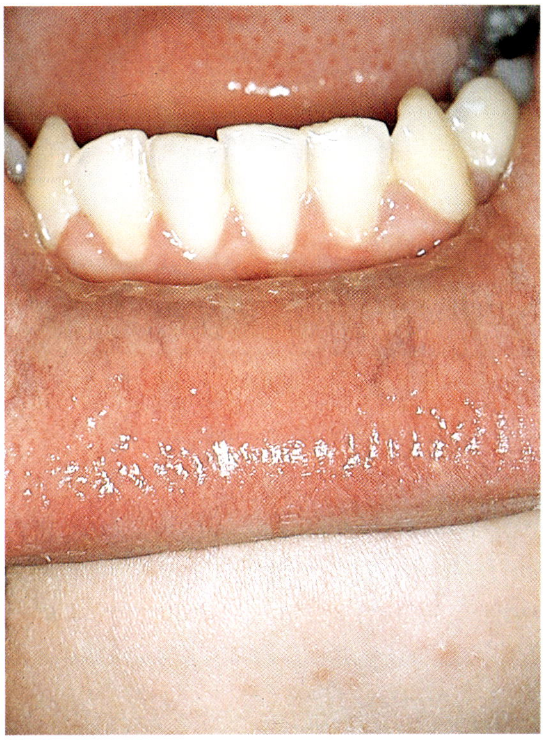

9.271

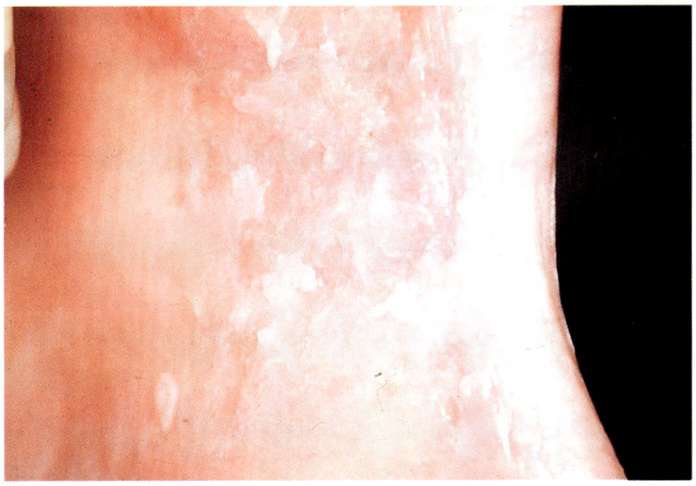

9.272

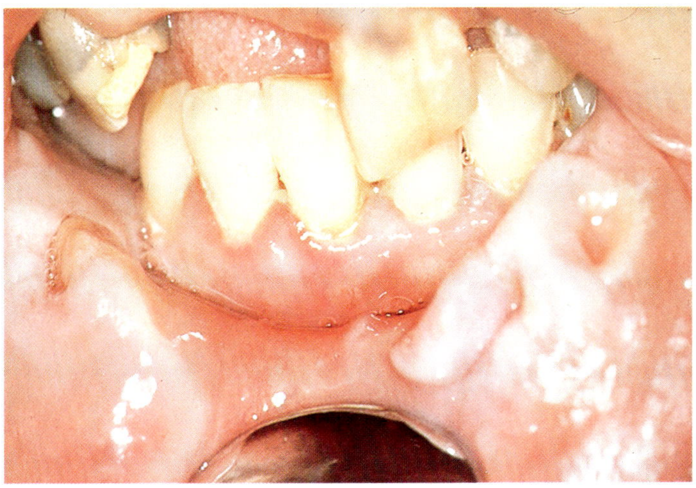

9.273

LINEA ALBA
(*Occlusal line*)

Figure 9.270 A horizontal whitish line at the level where the teeth occlude is a common benign lesion, more obvious in patients with parafunctional habits such as jaw clenching or tooth-grinding, and in those with temporomandibular pain-dysfunction syndrome.

LIP-BITING
(*Morsicatio buccarum*)

Figure 9.271 Lip-biting is a common habit, particularly in anxiety states, and may be associated with a few traumatic petechiae.

CHEEK-CHEWING

Figure 9.272 The mucosa is shredded with a shaggy white appearance similar to that of white sponge naevus (page 197) but restricted to areas close to the occlusal line.

Figure 9.273 An extreme example of self-induced lesions. This may be seen in disturbed psychiatric or mentally-handicapped patients.

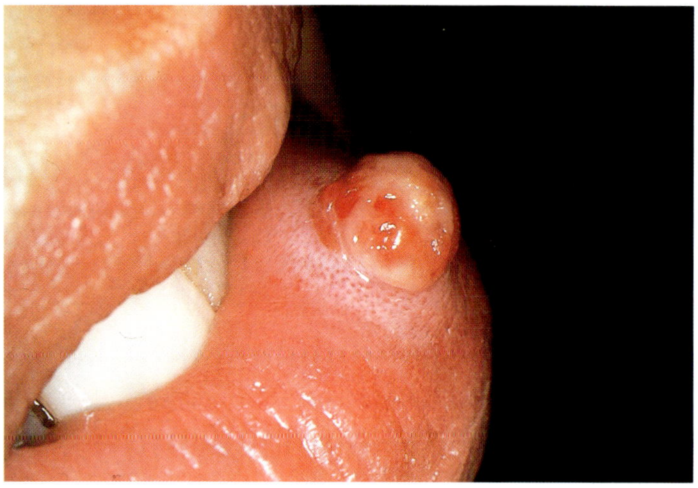

9.274

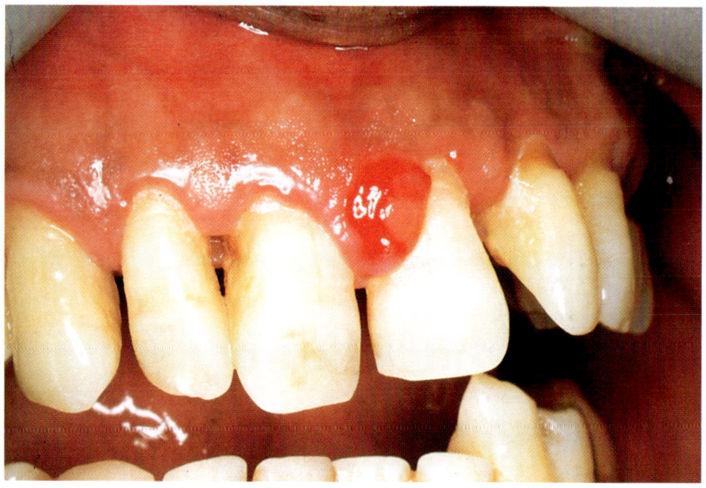

9.275

PYOGENIC GRANULOMA

Figure 9.274 Pyogenic granulomas are an exaggerated response to minor trauma. They tend to be soft, fleshy, rough-surfaced vascular lesions that bleed readily.

Figure 9.275 The gingiva is the most common site, the granuloma often arising on the buccal aspect from the interdental papilla and especially where there is a slight malocclusion leading to plaque accumulation, as here.

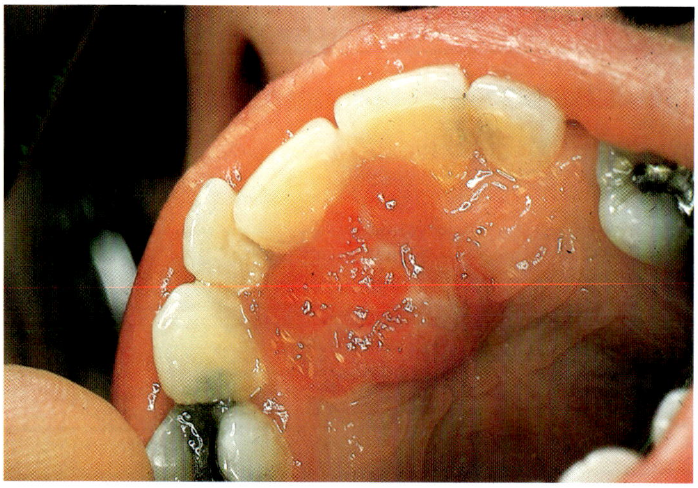

9.276

Figure 9.276 This pyogenic granuloma has arisen again at a site of tooth crowding. Most pyogenic granulomas are seen in the maxilla, anteriorly.

EOSINOPHILIC ULCER (*Eosinophilic granuloma of oral mucosa*)

Figure 9.277 Eosinophilic granuloma of the oral mucosa is a rare chronic lesion found typically on the tongue of males, and supposed to have a traumatic aetiology. Numerous eosinophils are seen on biopsy examination.

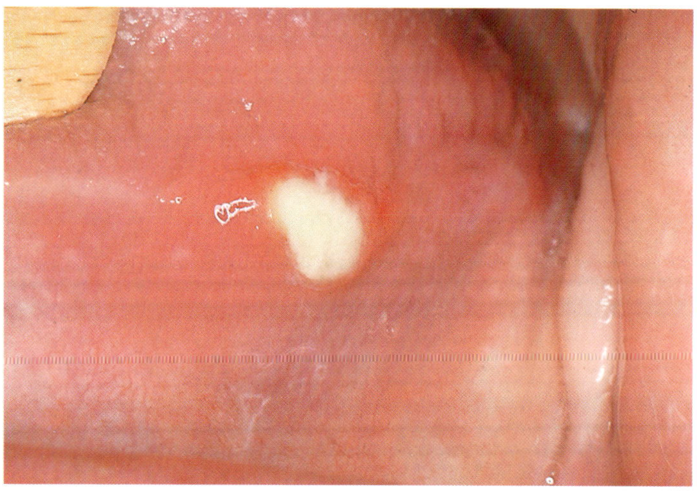

9.277

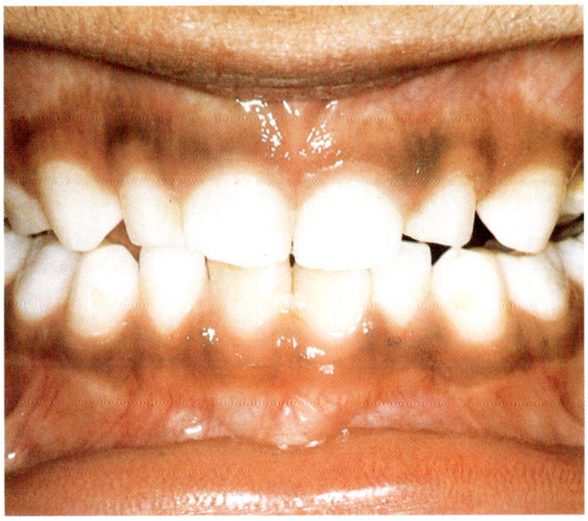

9.278

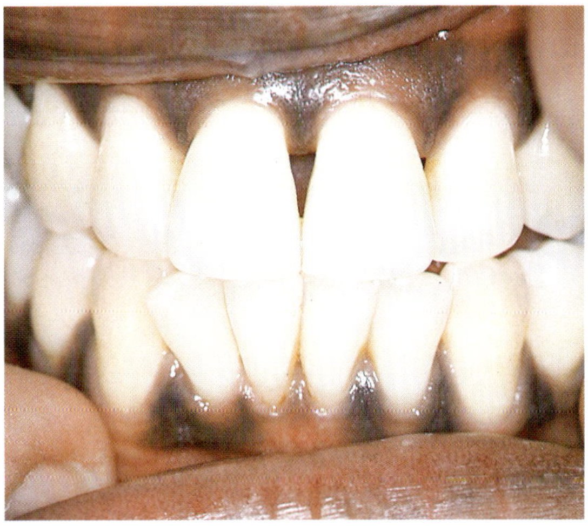

9.279

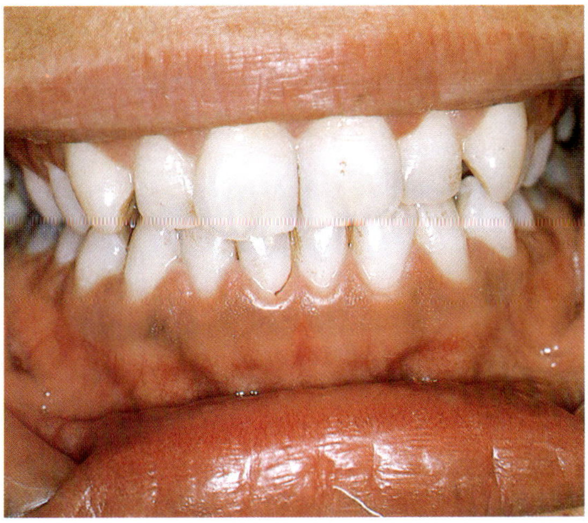

9.280

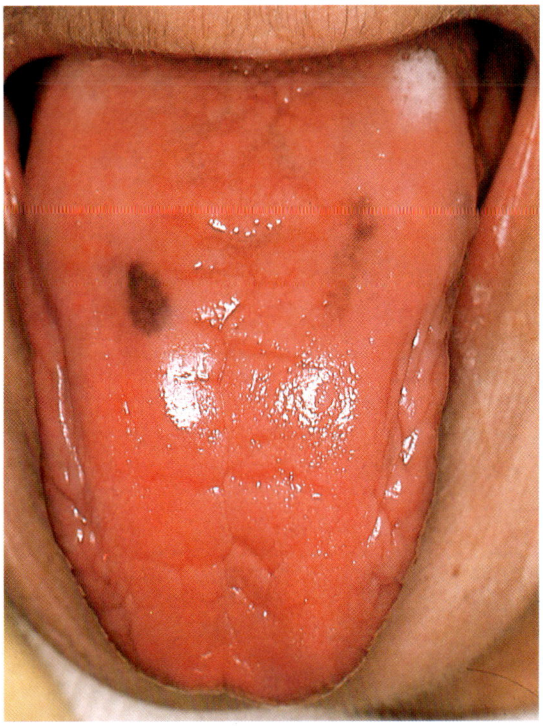

9.281

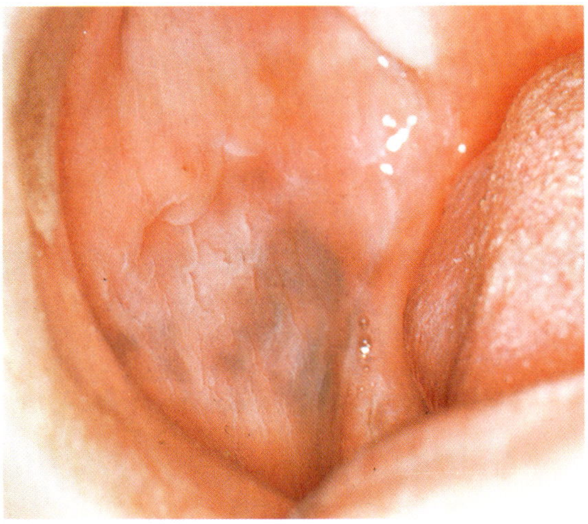

9.282

RACIAL PIGMENTATION

Figure 9.278 There is no direct correlation between skin colour and gingival pigmentation. Figures 9.278–80 show the range of racial pigmentation that may be seen. Pigmentation is clearly visible on the attached gingiva in this Asian child.

Figure 9.279 An adult negro with racial pigmentation on the gingiva.

Figure 9.280 Racial pigmentation may be seen in races such as those of southern European descent.

MELANOTIC MACULES

Figure 9.281 Oral melanotic macules are brown or black macules, seen typically on the lips and especially in females. They are benign and are unrelated to racial pigmentation.

PIGMENTARY INCONTINENCE

Figure 9.282 Pigmentary incontinence may rarely be seen in lichen planus and can persist after the lichen planus has resolved, as here (see also Figure 9.286).

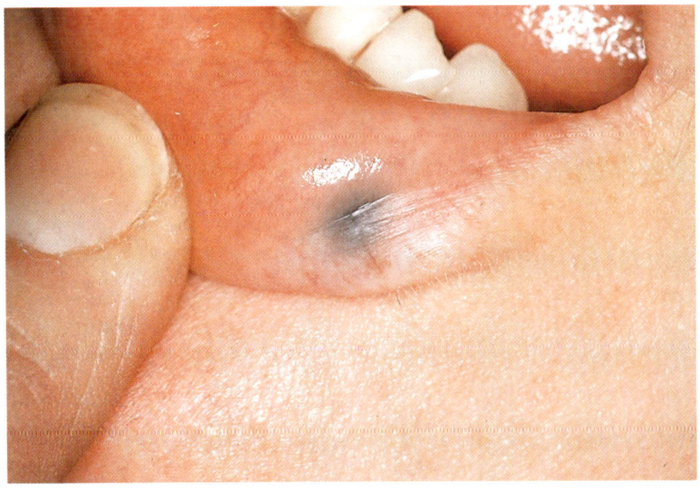

9.283

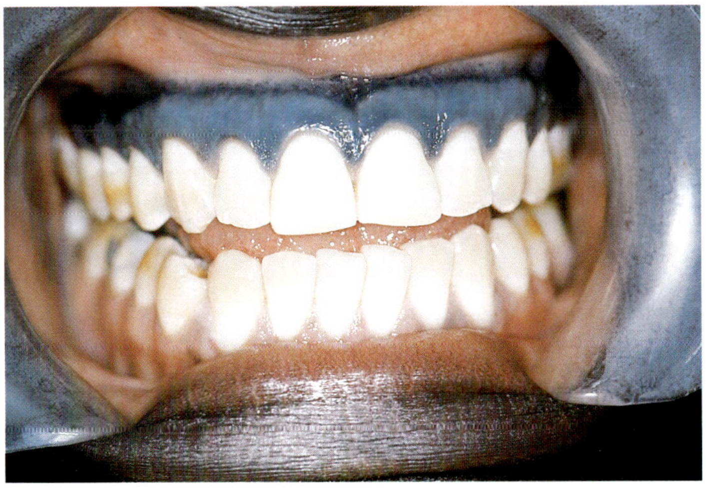

9.284

TATTOO

Figure 9.283 Foreign body tattoo: pigmentation after foreign material (metal) was left in the lip after an accident.

Figure 9.284 'Cosmetic' tattoo: tattooing of the upper gingiva as a tribal custom.

Figure 9.285 Deliberate tattoo: tattooing of the lower labial mucosa – perhaps a tribal custom.

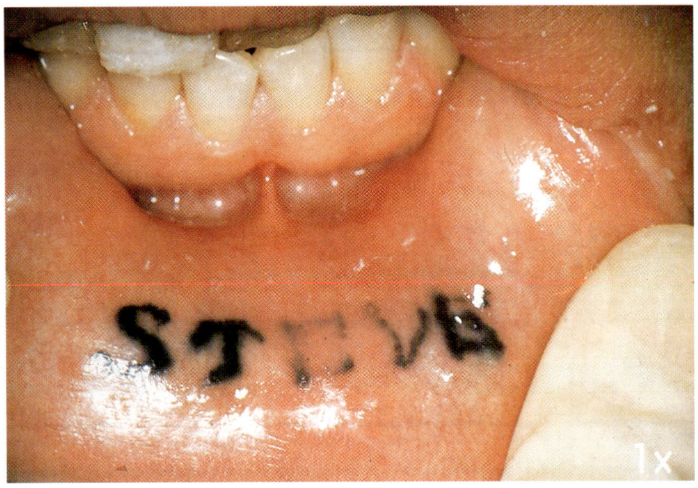

9.285

SMOKER'S MELANOSIS

Figure 9.286 Melanosis in a smoker (who also has keratosis) caused by pigmentary incontinence following chronic irritation.

Pigmentation of the soft palate may be seen in conditions with ectopic production of adrenocorticotrophic hormone, for example, bronchogenic carcinoma.

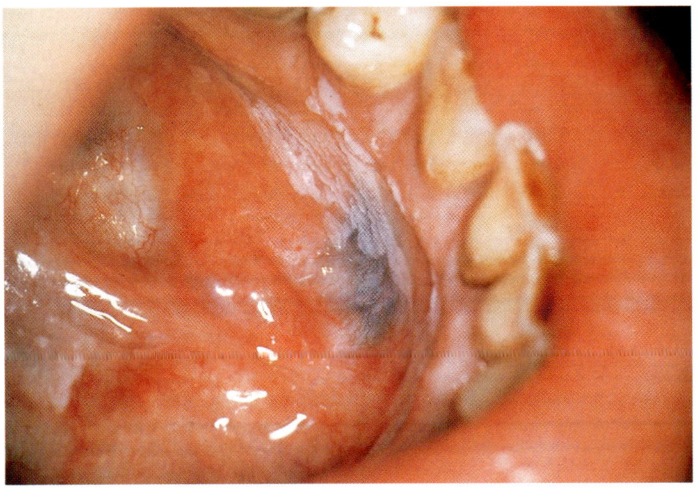

9.286

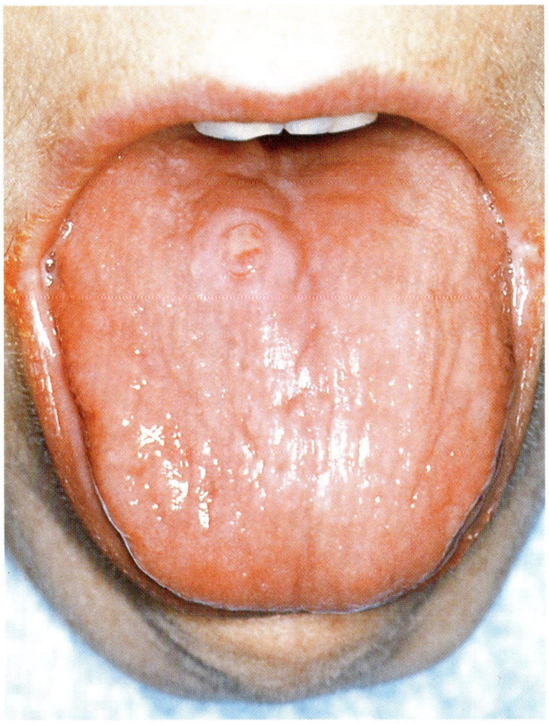

9.287

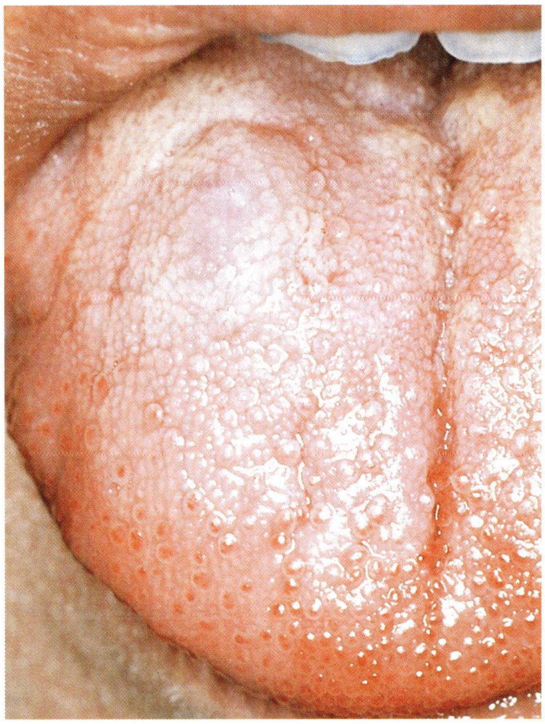

9.288

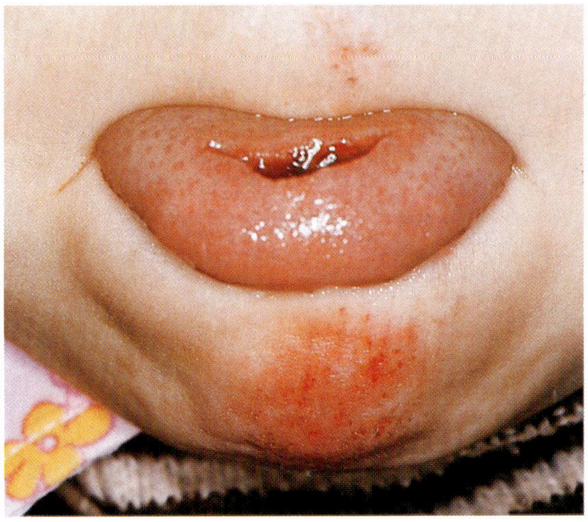

9.289

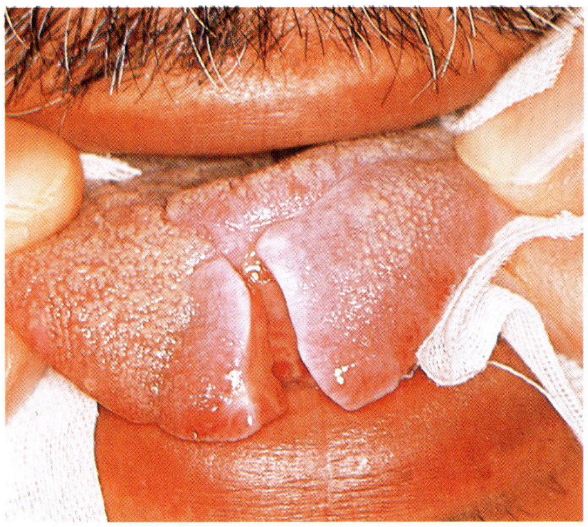

9.290

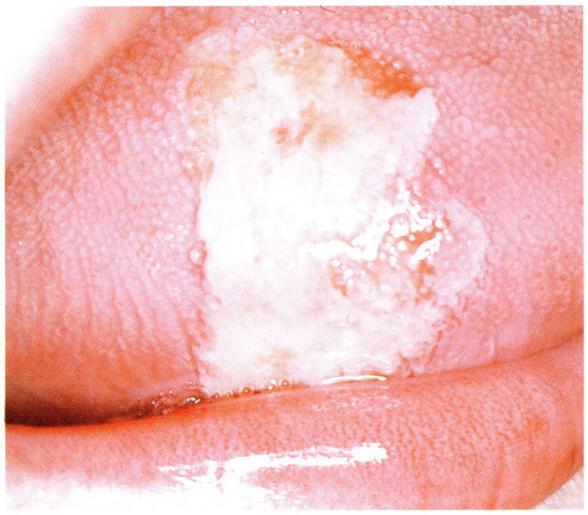

9.291

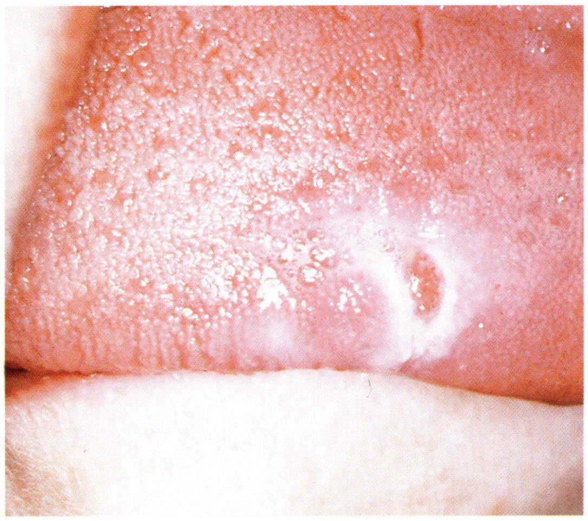

9.292

LINGUAL ABSCESS

Figure 9.287 Lingual abscesses are uncommon but may follow a penetrating injury, or infection of a lesion such as a neoplasm, cyst or haematoma.

LINGUAL HAEMATOMA

Figure 9.288 Trauma to the tongue, especially in a patient with a bleeding tendency, may produce a haematoma.

LINGUAL LACERATION

Figure 9.289 Laceration of the tongue by the teeth of a child who fell on his chin.

Figure 9.290 A laceration that was not sutured has resulted in the appearance of a false bifid tongue.

LINGUAL TRAUMATIC ULCER, SELF-INDUCED

Figure 9.291 An unusual ulcer on the tongue in a child that was self-induced.

Figure 9.292 Same patient as in Figure 9.291, after 2 weeks.

ERYTHEMA MIGRANS (*Geographic tongue, benign migratory glossitis*)

Figure 9.293 Erythema migrans is an extremely common benign condition, of unknown aetiology, in which the filiform papillae desquamate in irregular demarcated areas. Patients with a fissured (scrotal) tongue often have erythema migrans.

Figure 9.294 Same patient as in Figure 9.293 on the following day, showing the appearance of a second area of depapillation and change configuration of the initial lesion.

Figure 9.295 The next day the lesions seen in Figures 9.293 and 9.294 have enlarged and coalesced.

Figure 9.296 In this example, the yellowish serpiginous borders are more obvious than the areas of depapillation.

Figure 9.297 This example shows a single depapillated patch with yellowish margin.

Figure 9.298 If the tongue is furred, the lesions of erythema migrans appear quite pronounced.

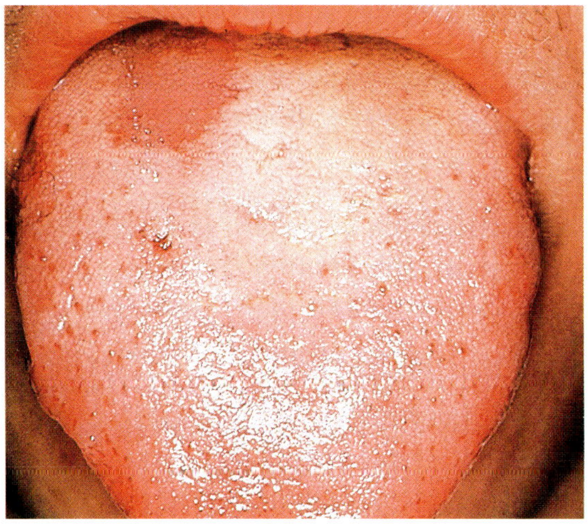

9.293

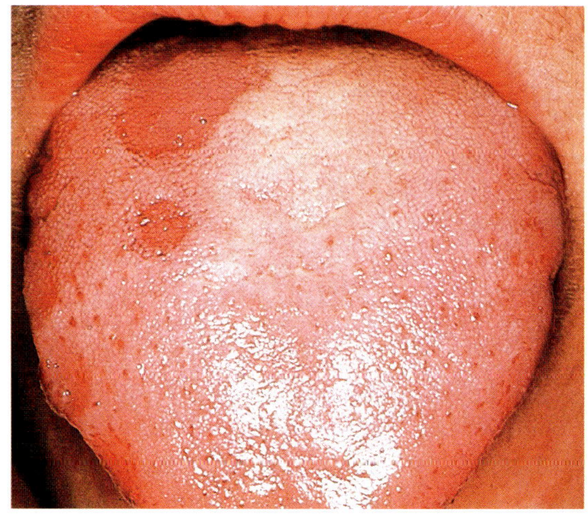

9.294

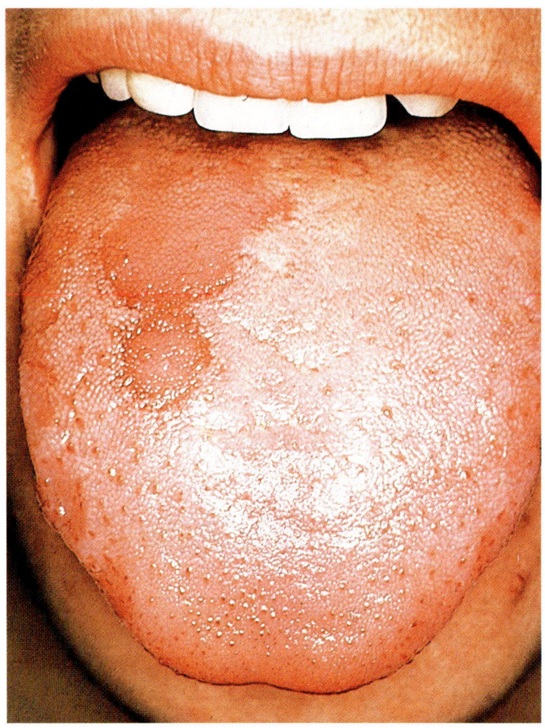

9.295

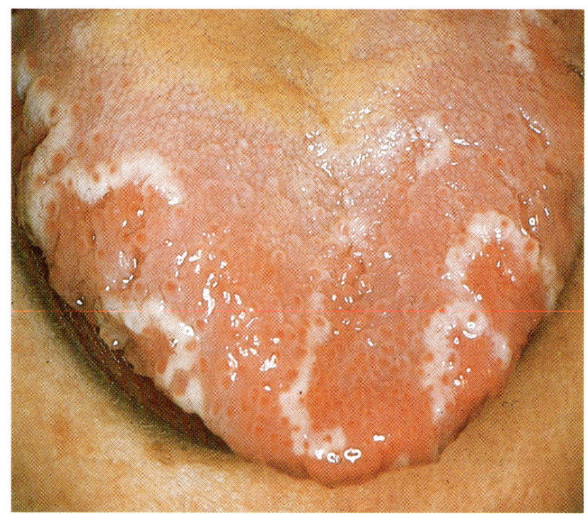

9.296

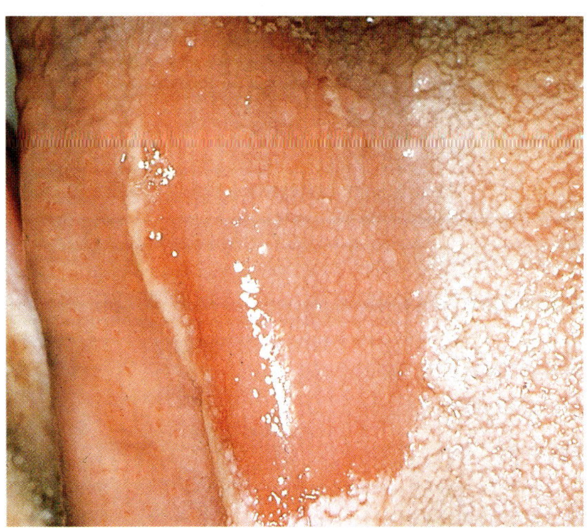

9.297

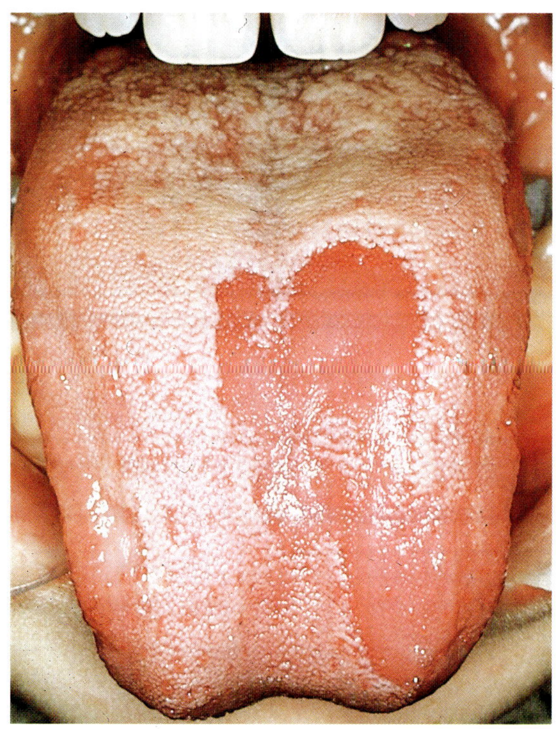

9.298

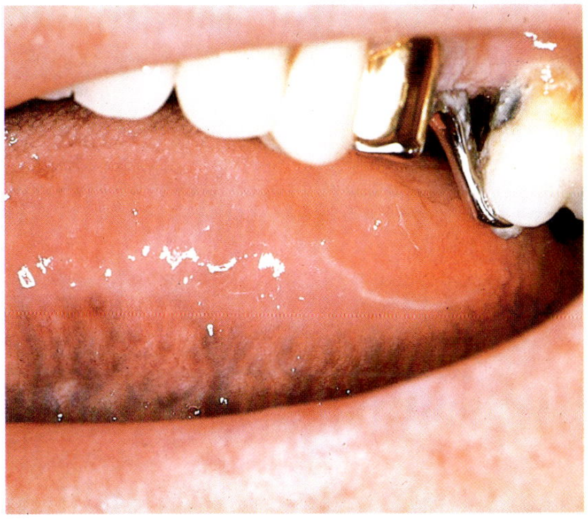

9.299

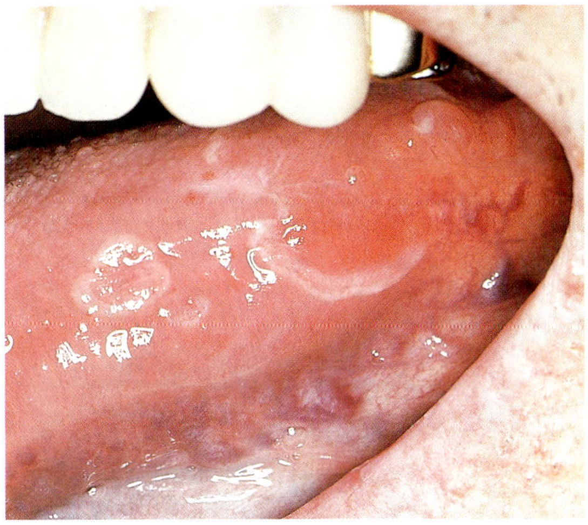

9.300

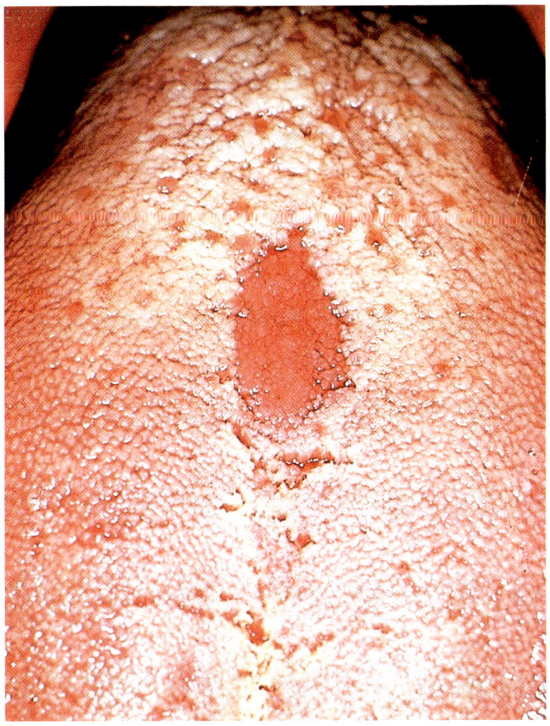

9.301

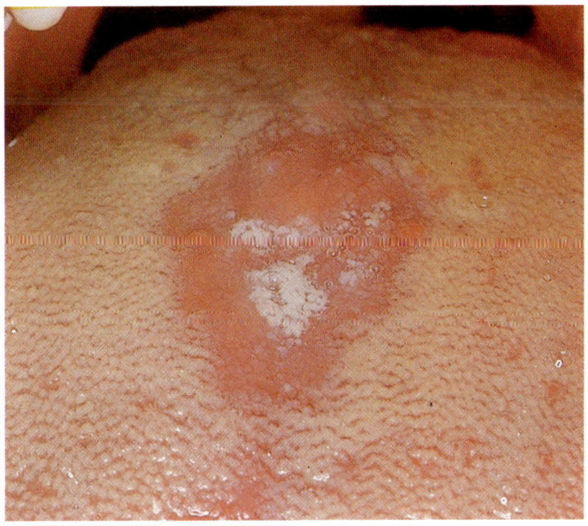

9.302

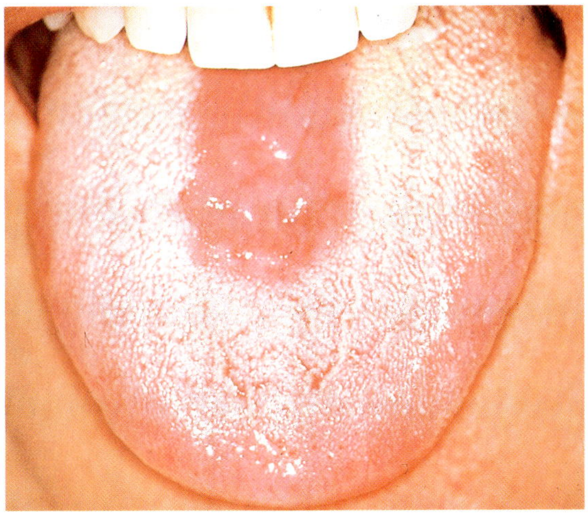

9.303

Figure 9.299 Though the configuration of the lesions can change over a few hours there are rare examples where the lesion is persistent and unchanging (erythema migrans perstans is the rather inappropriate term used).

Figure 9.300 This patient, also shown in Figure 9.299, has had a virtually identical lesion over 4 years: biopsy has confirmed this is erythema migrans.

MEDIAN RHOMBOID GLOSSITIS (*Central papillary atrophy*)

Figure 9.301 Median rhomboid glossitis is a rhomboidal red depapillated area in the midline of the dorsum of tongue, just anterior to the circumvallate papillae.

Figure 9.302 Median rhomboid glossitis was thought to be a development anomaly owing to persistence of the tuberculum impar, but is now thought to be related to localized candidosis, predisposed by smoking, the wearing of dentures, and diabetes. Occasionally, it is a mixed red and white lesion.

Figure 9.303 Median rhomboid glossitis is usually asymptomatic though it may cause slight discomfort. Some lesions may, as here, appear somewhat sinister. The finding of candida-induced pseudoepitheliomatous hyperplasia has caused some of these lesions to be misdiagnosed as carcinomas. Oral carcinoma is rare at this site.

A recent report of the isolation of *Neisseria gonorrhoea* from tongue lesions resembling median rhomboid glossitis has yet to be confirmed and may be coincidental, since the mouth can be a reservoir for this organism.

FURRED TONGUE

Figure 9.304 The tongue is rarely furred in a healthy child but may be lightly furred in a healthy adult, especially if the oral hygiene is poor, the patient smokes, wears full dentures, or the diet is soft. Any febrile illness may cause a furred tongue.

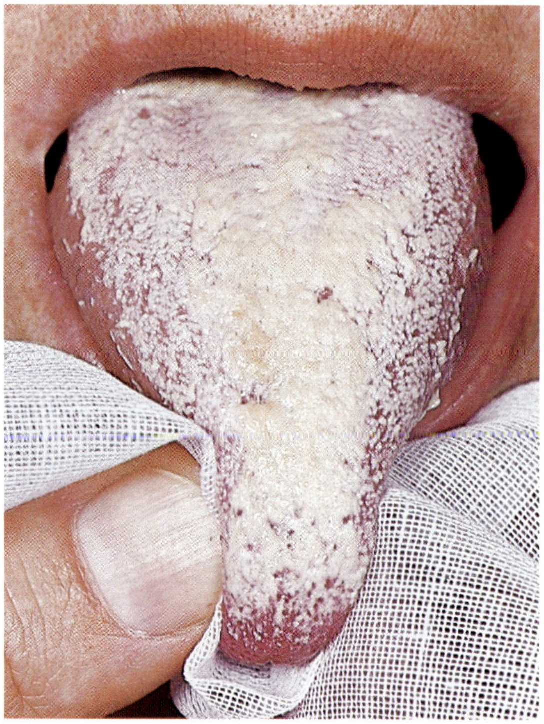

9.304

BROWN HAIRY TONGUE

Figure 9.305 Although often idiopathic, a brown hairy tongue may be seen for any of the reasons discussed above (Figure 9.304). Mouthwashes, antibiotics, smoking, or gastrointestinal disease may predispose.

White or coloured lesions of the tongue are also sometimes seen in immunocompromised patients. It is now evident that any of a range of microorganisms may become opportunistic pathogens in such patients. For example, a soil saprophytic fungus *Ramichloridium schulzeri* has been described as causing a 'golden' tongue.

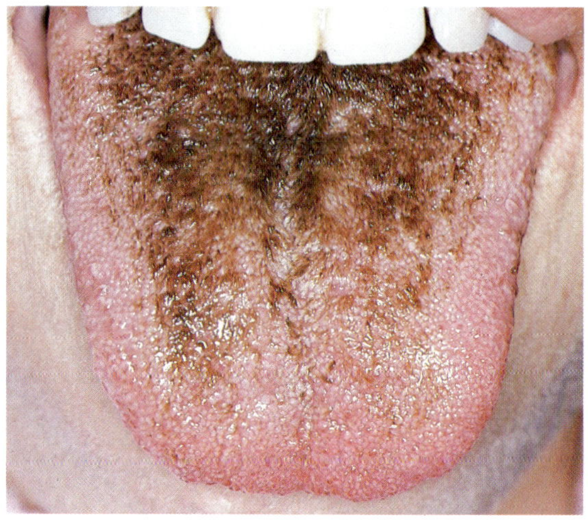

9.305

BLACK HAIRY TONGUE

Figure 9.306 Overgrowth of the filiform papillae, with proliferation of chromogenic bacteria may cause a black hairy tongue. This patient also incidentally has a cleft lip and palate.

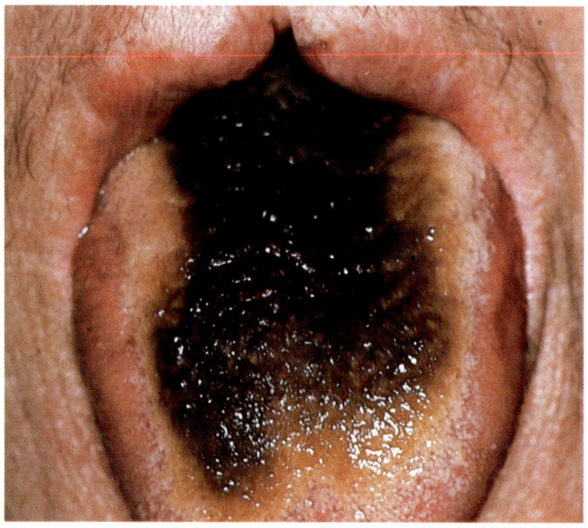

9.306

FOLIATE PAPILLITIS

Figure 9.307 The size and shape of the foliate papillae are variable and occasionally they swell if irritated mechanically or if there is an upper respiratory infection. Located at a site of high predilection for lingual carcinoma, they may give rise to anxiety about cancer.

Inflammation of the lingual tonsils may also give rise to concern as it may present with pain and dysphagia.

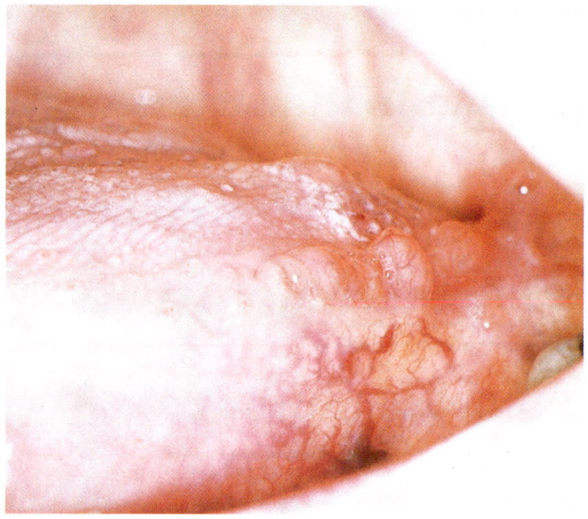

9.307

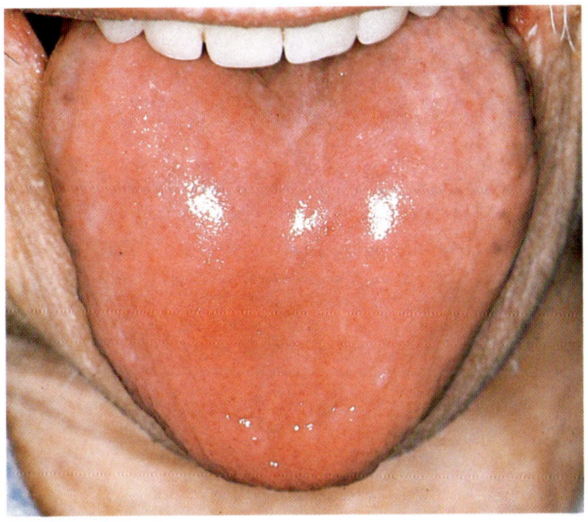

9.308

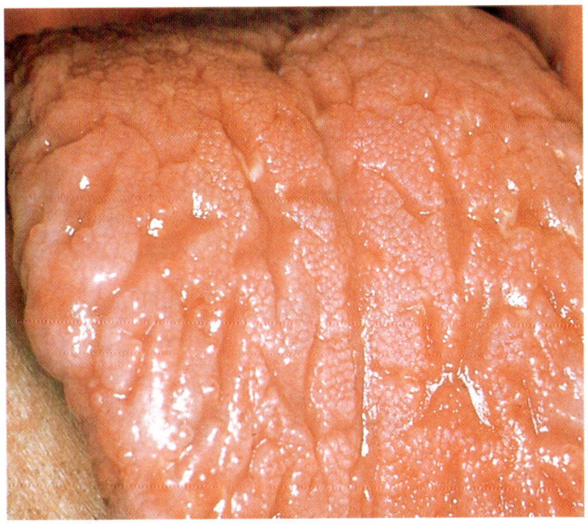

9.309

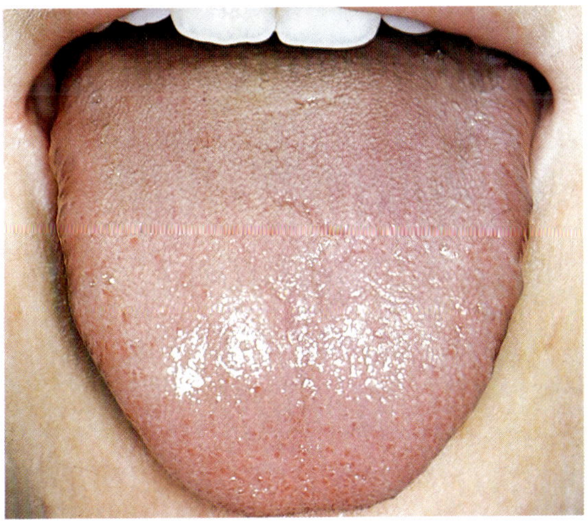

9.310

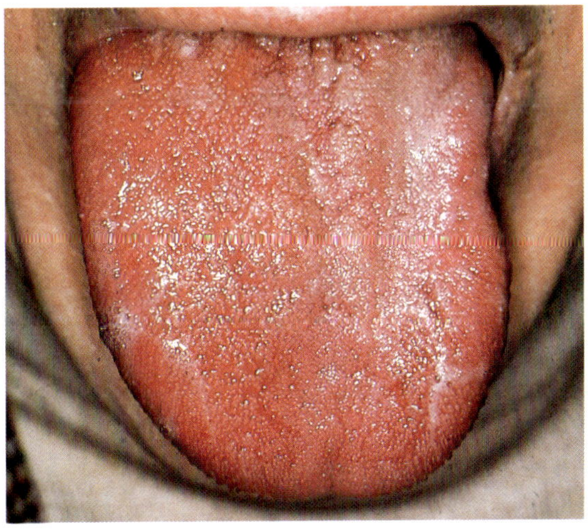

9.311

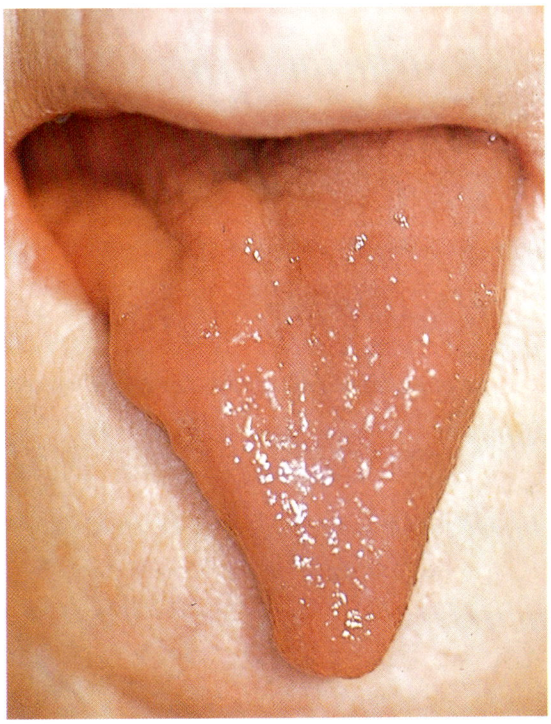

9.312

ATROPHIC GLOSSITIS

Figure 9.308 Lingual papillary atrophy is usually due to haematinic deficiency but atrophy may be seen after repeated ulceration, burns, or irradiation.

FISSURED TONGUE (*Scrotal or plicated tongue*)

Figure 9.309 Fissured tongue is a common developmental anomaly that may appear after puberty. It is of little significance, though often associated with erythema migrans. Fissured tongue is one feature of Melkersson-Rosenthal syndrome (see page 157) and is found more frequently than normal in Down's syndrome (see page 210) and psoriasis.

GLOSSODYNIA (*Glossopyrosis*)

Figure 9.310 Most patients with glossodynia have no identifiable organic lesion of the tongue and the discomfort has a psychogenic basis (see also page 74).

LINGUAL HEMIHYPERTROPHY

Figure 9.311 Hypertrophy of the right side of the tongue.

The whitish lines on the tongue are caused by strands of saliva, as this patient also has xerostomia.

LINGUAL HEMIATROPHY

Figure 9.312 A lower motor neurone hypoglossal nerve lesion has caused atrophy here.

CROHN'S DISEASE

Figure 9.313 Crohn's disease is a chronic inflammatory bowel disease of unknown aetiology, affecting mainly the ileum although any part of the gastrointestinal tract can be involved, including the mouth. Non-caseating granulomas are also seen in sarcoid and it is possible that oral Crohn's disease is actually a similar but distinct condition. Some use the term 'orofacial granulomatosis'. Swelling of the lips and angular stomatitis are common.

Figure 9.314 Swelling of the upper lip in a patient with gastrointestinal Crohn's disease. Biopsy of the lip showed lymphoedema and granulomas.

Figure 9.315 Facial swelling in this patient affects the right cheek and is less pronounced than the examples above.

Figure 9.316 Gingival swelling may be a feature. The majority of patients with 'oral Crohn's disease' do not have identifiable gastro-intestinal lesions and some seem to have lesions as a consequence of food 'allergy'

Figure 9.317 Persistent irregular ulcers, as here, or classic aphthae, are common features. Pyostomatitis vegetans (see page 158) may also be seen, but is usually associated with ulcerative colitis.

Figure 9.318 Swelling and persistent ulcers in the palate.

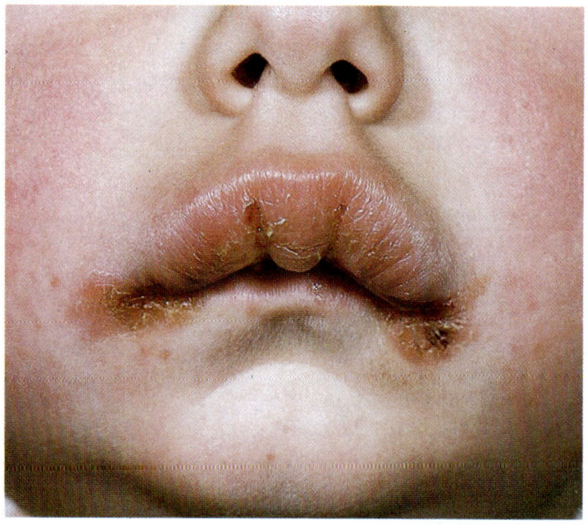

9.313

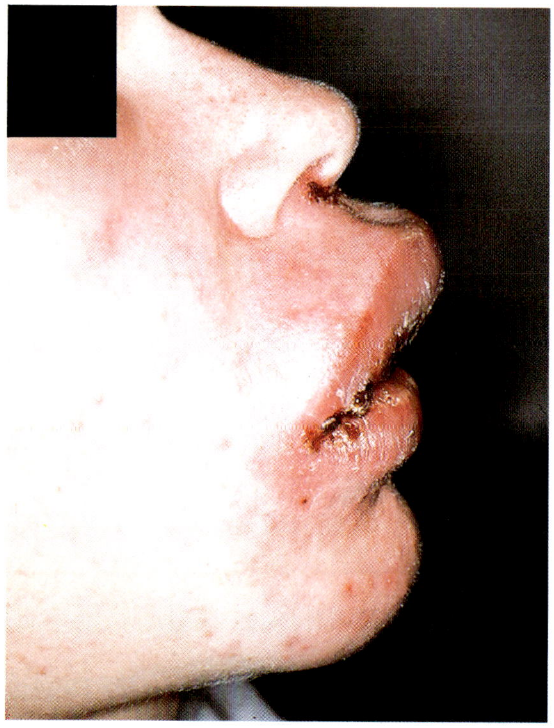

9.314

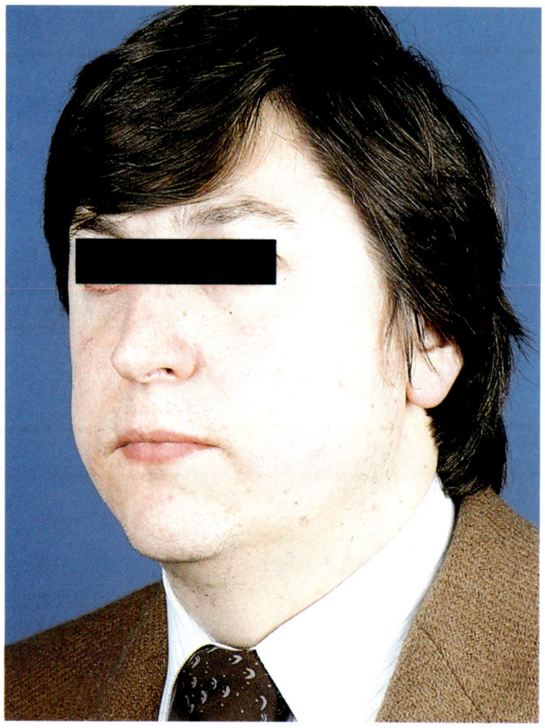

9.315

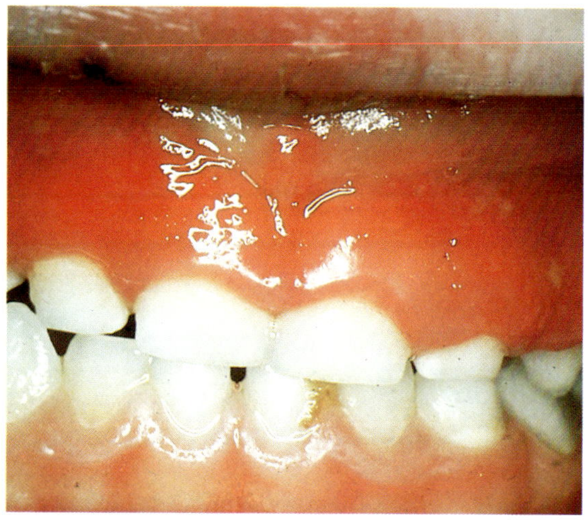

9.316

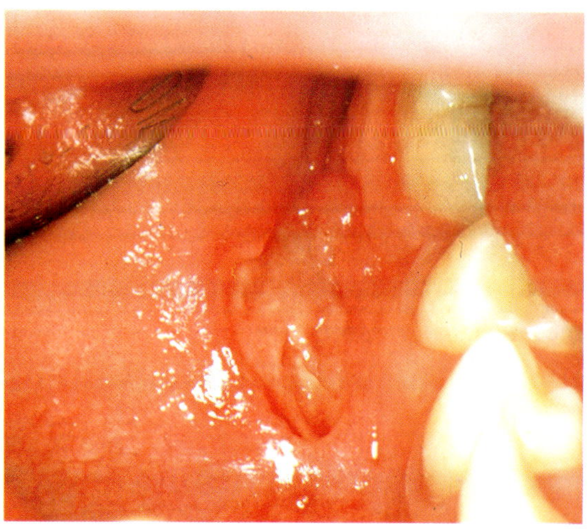

9.317

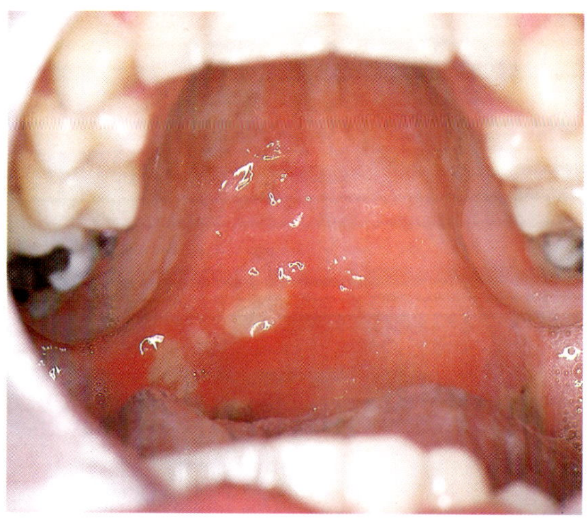

9.318

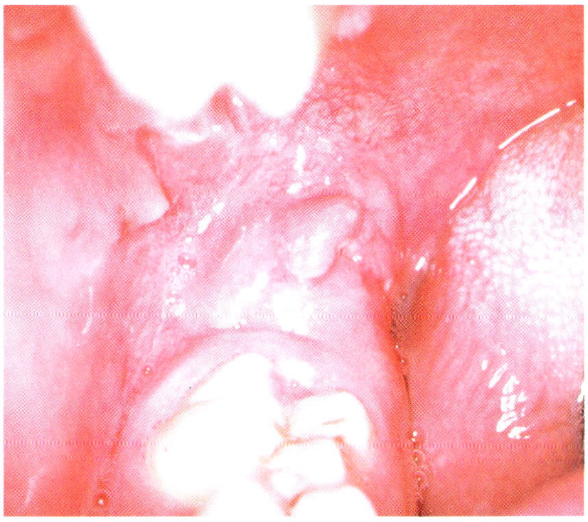

9.319

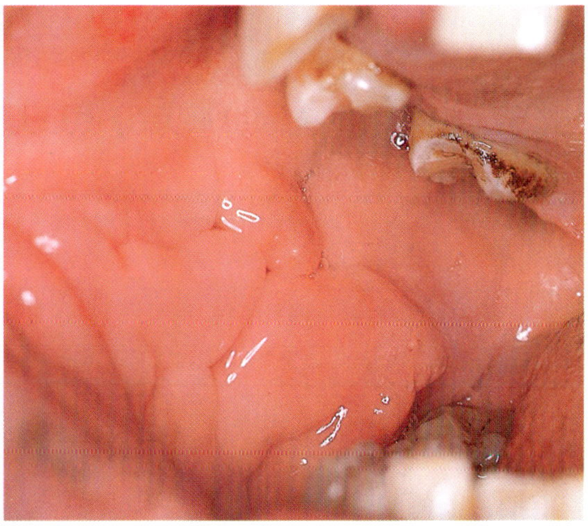

9.320

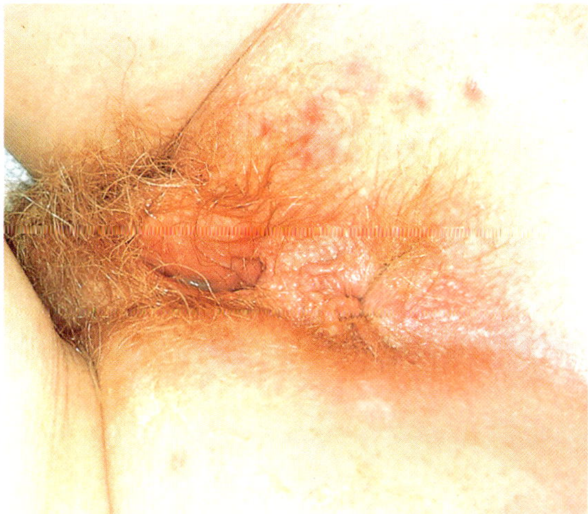

9.321

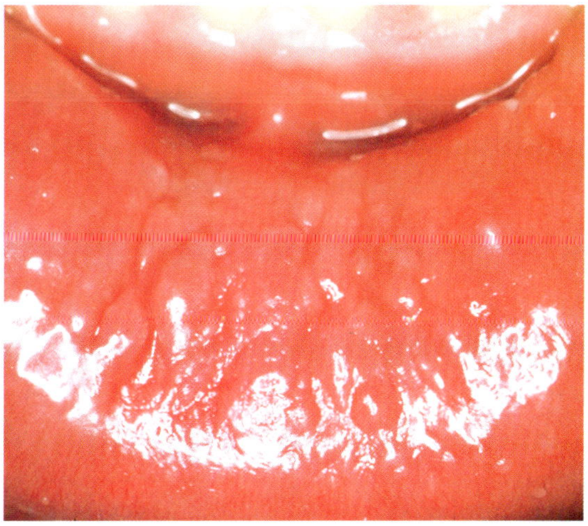

9.322

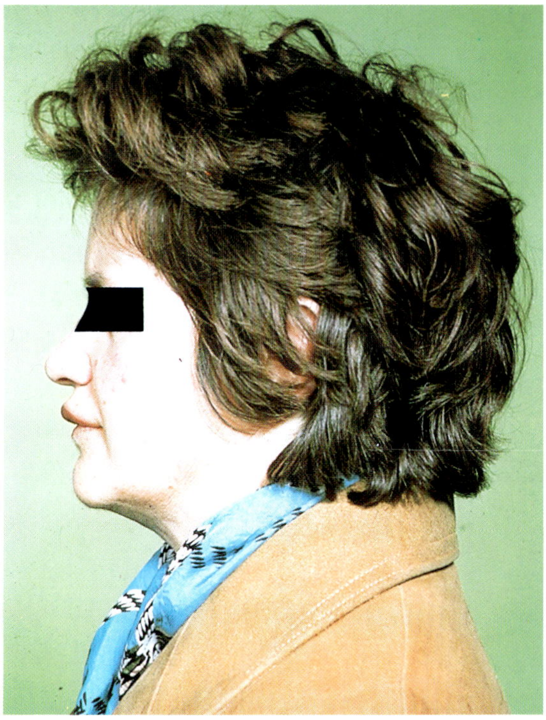

9.323

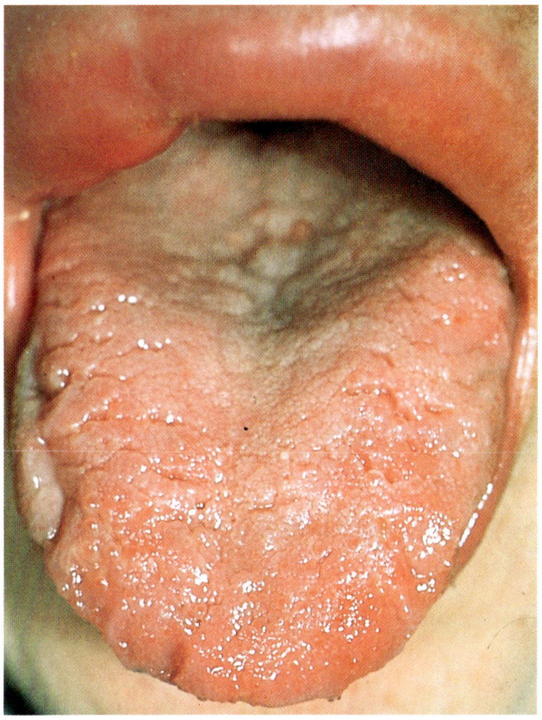

9.324

Figure 9.319 Mucosal tags are a feature in some patients.

Figure 9.320 Folding of the oral mucosa may lead of a 'cobblestone' appearance.

Figure 9.321 Perianal tags in Crohn's disease.

OROFACIAL GRANULOMATOSIS

Figure 9.322 The clinical features seen in Crohn's disease may be present in the absence of identifiable intestinal disease. This patient, for example, who had a somewhat swollen lower lip with a cobblestoned mucosa, proved to be reacting to cinnamon.

MELKERSSON-ROSENTHAL SYNDROME

Figure 9.323 Melkersson-Rosenthal syndrome is the association of orofacial swelling (here of the upper lip), fissured tongue and unilateral lower motor neurone facial palsy. It appears to be related to cheilitis granulomatosa, oral Crohn's disease, sarcoidosis and orofacial granulomatosis.

The swelling is non-tender and will not pit on pressure. Intraoral swelling may involve the buccal mucosa and gingiva.

Figure 9.324 This is the fissured tongue of the patient shown in Figure 9.323.

ULCERATIVE COLITIS

Figure 9.325 Oral lesions in ulcerative colitis include ulcers and pustules (pyostomatitis vegetans) which may also be found in Crohn's disease or overlap syndromes. This patient had severe ulcerative colitis: exacerbation of the oral ulceration preceded exacerbation of colitis.

Figure 9.326 Ulceration in the patient in Figure 9.325 was widespread and produced an unusual type of desquamative gingivitis. The tongue is only rarely ulcerated in ulcerative colitis.

Figure 9.327 Multiple small pustules on the gingiva.

Figure 9.328 Irregular ulceration which clinically resembled a 'snailtrack' ulcer, resulting from fusion of ulcerated pustules.

Figure 9.329 An aphthous type of ulcer that is probably a manifestation of pyostomatitis gangrenosum.

GLUTEN-SENSITIVE ENTEROPATHY (*Coeliac disease*)

Figure 9.330 Up to 3 per cent of patients seen as out-patients with aphthae prove to have coeliac disease, as in this patient.

See also page 135.

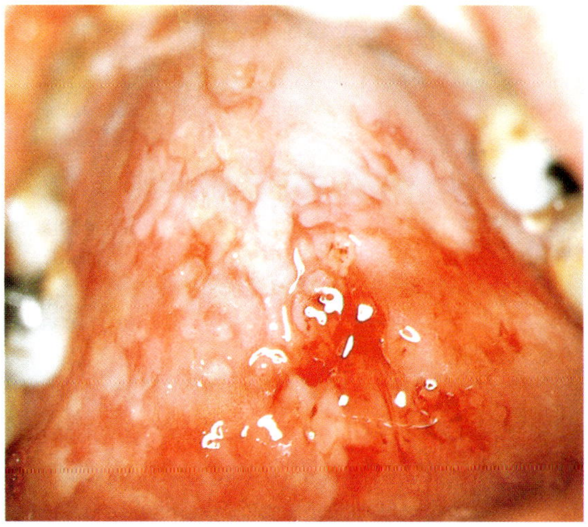

9.325

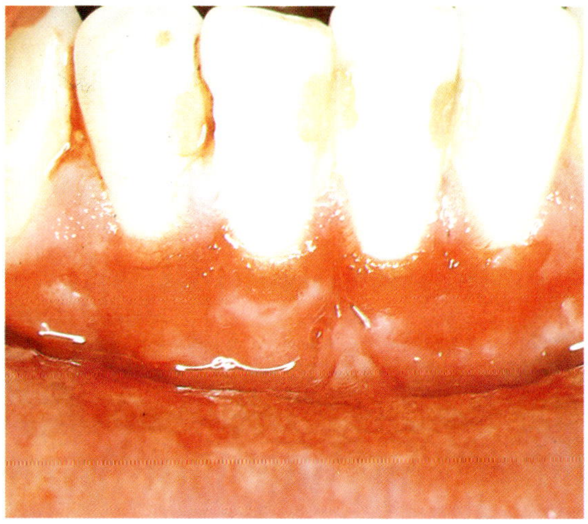

9.326

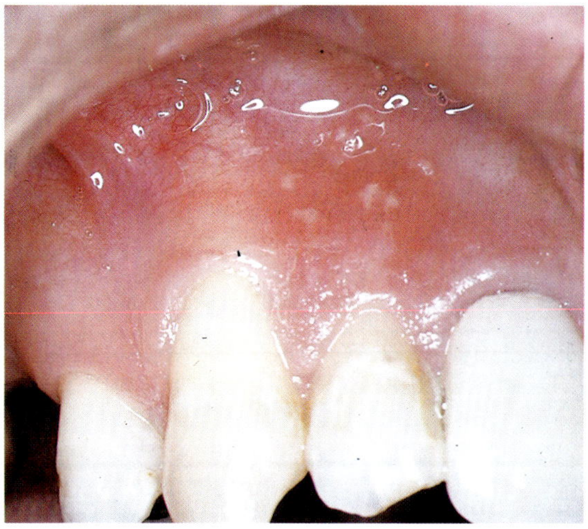

9.327

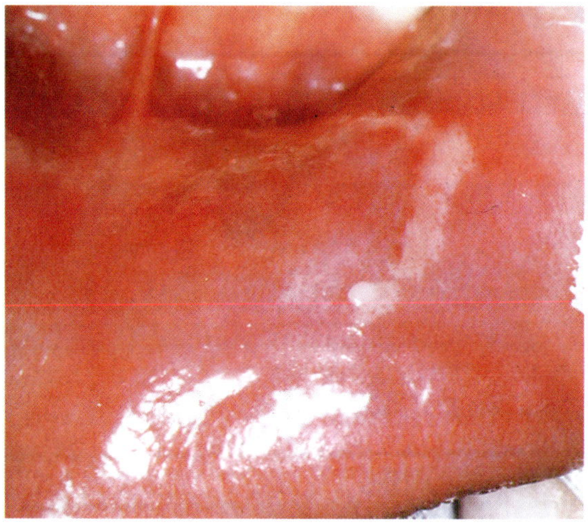

9.328

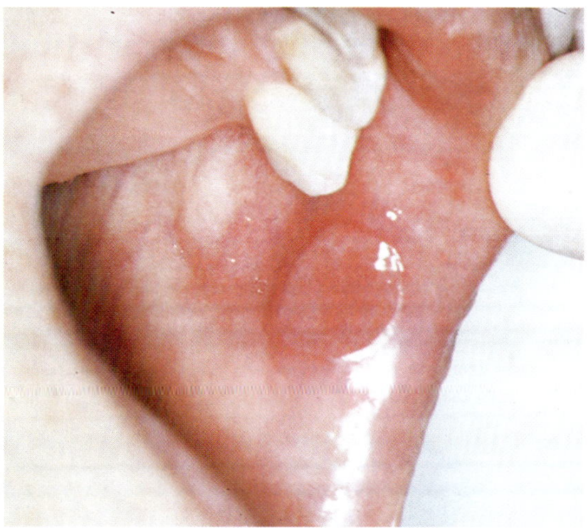

9.329

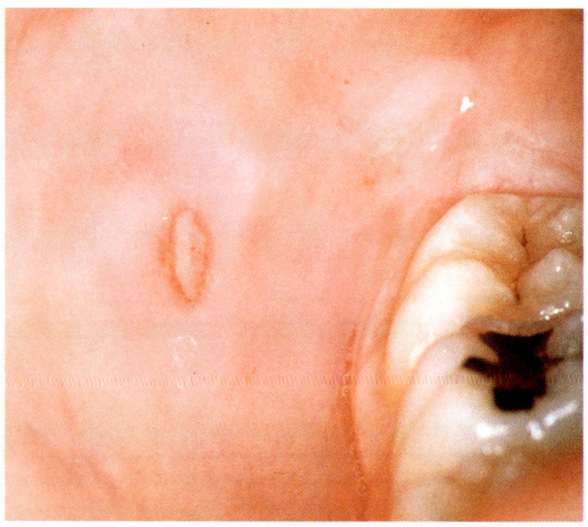

9.330

10

Diseases of the genito-urinary system

URAEMIC STOMATITIS

Figure 10.1 An unpleasant taste and dry mouth are common in chronic renal failure; other oral lesions may include ulcers and mixed bacterial plaques, as here, keratosis, candidosis and purpura.

Skeletal changes, which seem especially to affect the jaws in patients on haemodialysis, include changes in trabecular pattern and localized radiolucencies. The dental pulp chambers tend to narrow.

HYPOPHOSPHATAEMIA (*Vitamin D-resistant rickets, renal rickets*)

Figure 10.2 This is a sex-linked disorder characterized by a renal tubular defect of phosphate resorption due to end-organ resistance to vitamin D. Teeth may be hypoplastic as here. Incidentally, the upper lateral incisor is absent.

Figure 10.3 The condition may be genetically-linked: this is the brother of the patient in Figure 10.2.

The teeth may be hypoplastic and eruption retarded.

Figure 10.4 The teeth have large pulp chambers and abnormal dentine calcification.

Figure 10.5 Even minimal caries or attrition can produce pulpitis: multiple periapical abscesses are thus common. Here there is an abscess labial to the central incisor.

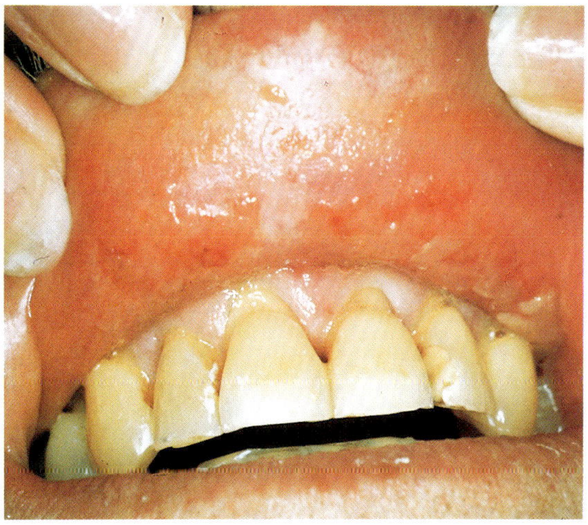

10.1

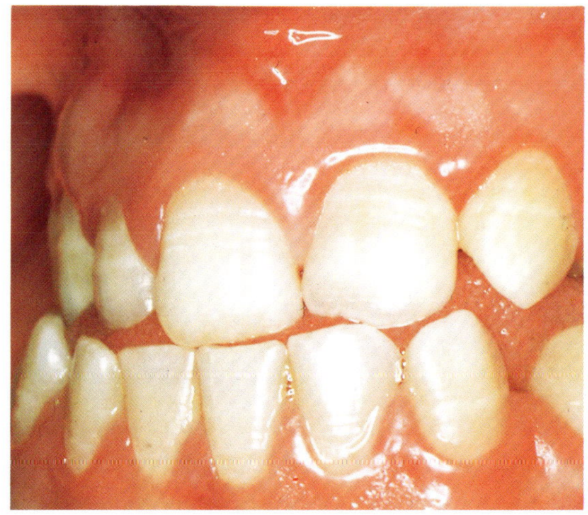

10.2

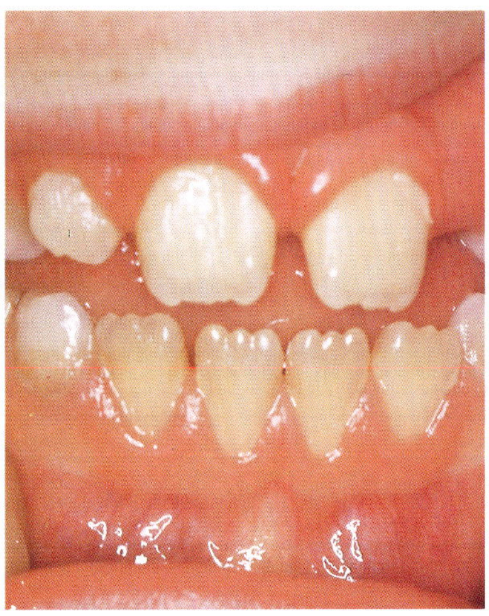

10.3

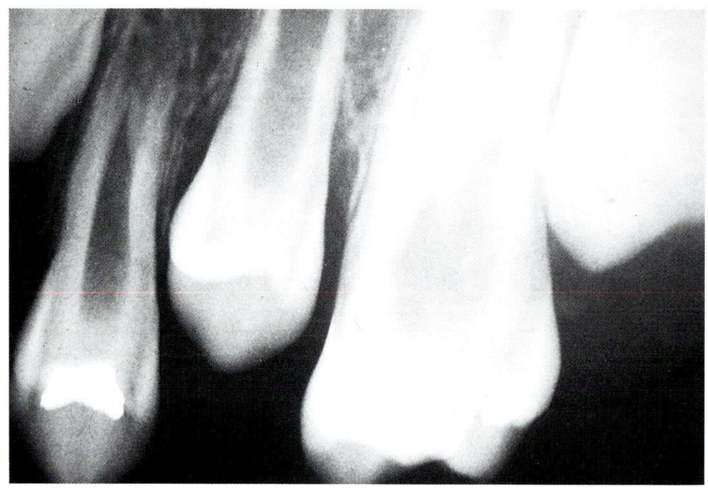

10.4

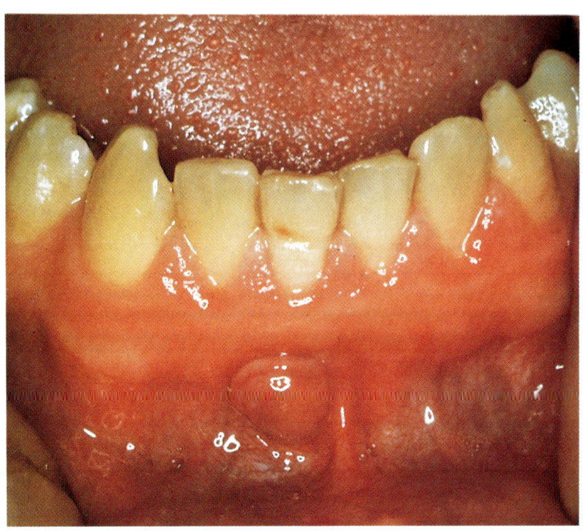

10.5

11

Complications of pregnancy, childbirth and the puerperium

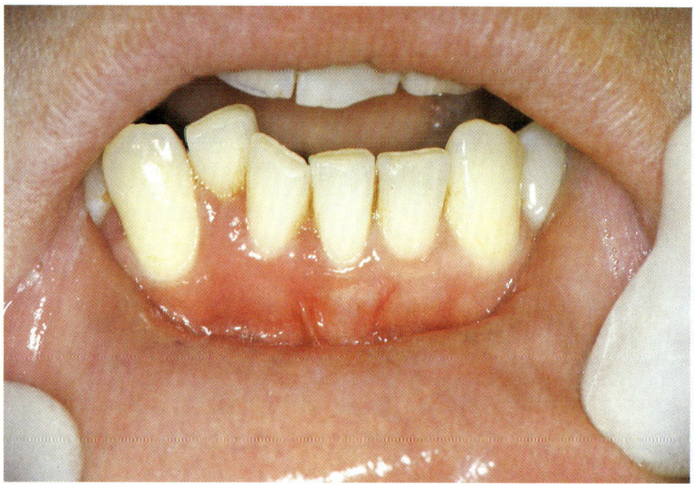

11.1

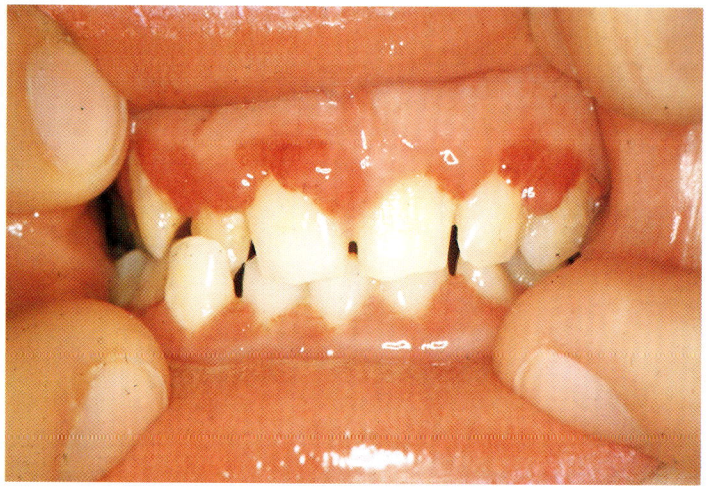

11.2

GINGIVITIS DURING MENSTRUATION

Figure 11.1 Where there is gingivitis, for example, as here, where plaque accumulates on the crowded teeth, there may be an exacerbation premenstrually.

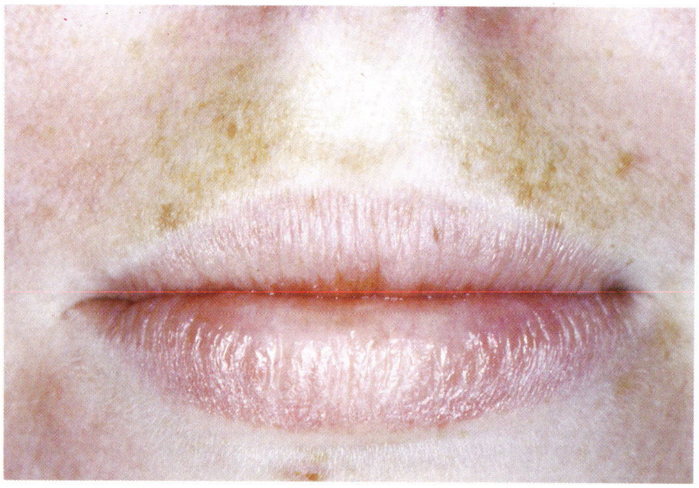

11.3

PREGNANCY GINGIVITIS

Figure 11.2 Gingivitis is most prevalent in pregnancy if oral hygiene is poor. A highly vascular marginal gingivitis appears at the second month of pregnancy, reaches maximum intensity by the eighth month, and then regresses.

CHLOASMA

Figure 11.3 Facial pigmentation in pregnancy.

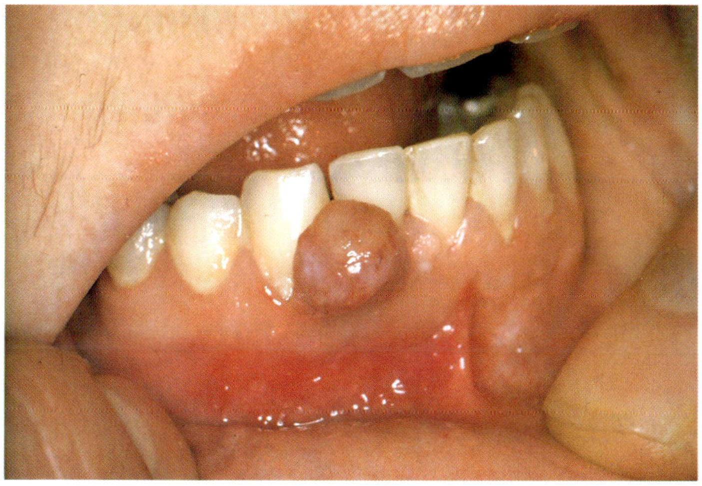

11.4

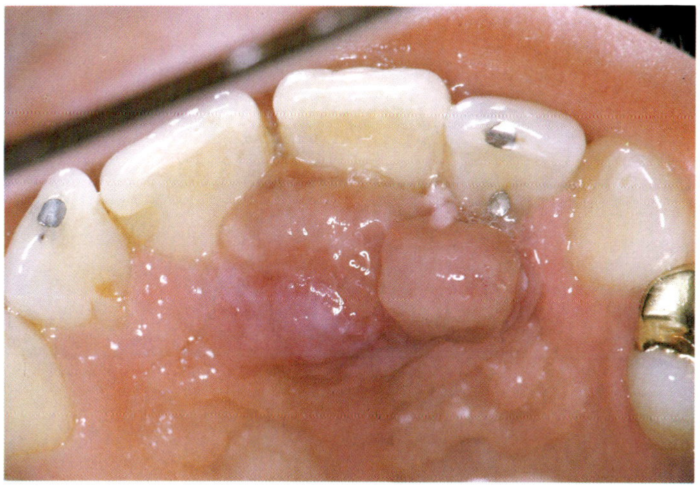

11.5

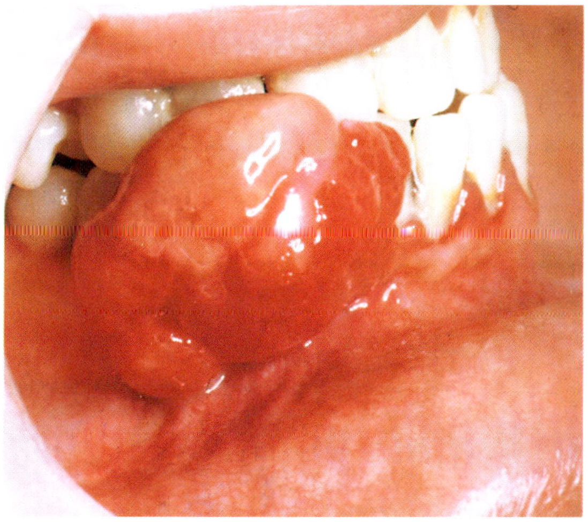

11.6

PREGNANCY EPULIS
(*Pregnancy granuloma*)

Figure 11.4 Pyogenic granulomas are common in pregnancy, when they are termed pregnancy epulis. They may bleed or be asymptomatic. They are benign.

Figure 11.5 A larger example, palatal to the upper incisors.

Figure 11.6 An extreme example of a pregnancy epulis.

12

Diseases of the skin and subcutaneous tissues

CARBUNCLE

Figure 12.1 Carbuncles are not seen in the mouth but may rarely affect the lip with tender red swelling and eventual suppuration.

Figure 12.2 Suppuration: same patient as shown in Figure 12.1.

Figure 12.3 An extreme example of a carbuncle of the lower lip.

LUDWIG'S ANGINA

Figure 12.4 Ludwig's angina is infection of the sublingual and submandibular fascial spaces, usually of odontogenic origin. It manifests with pain, submandibular swelling, dysphagia and fever and may be a hazard to the airway.

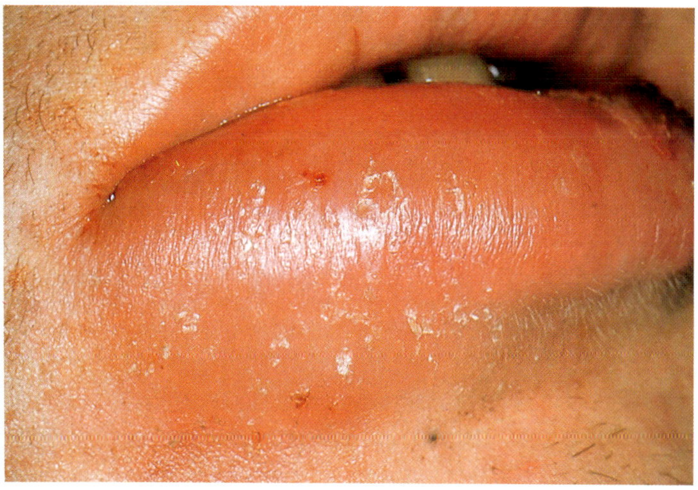

12.1

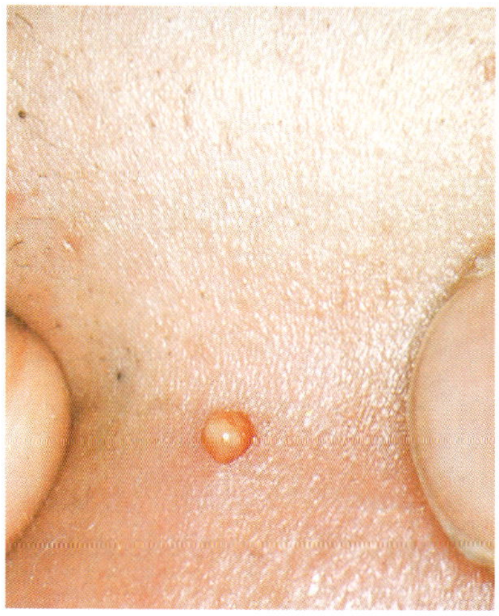

12.2

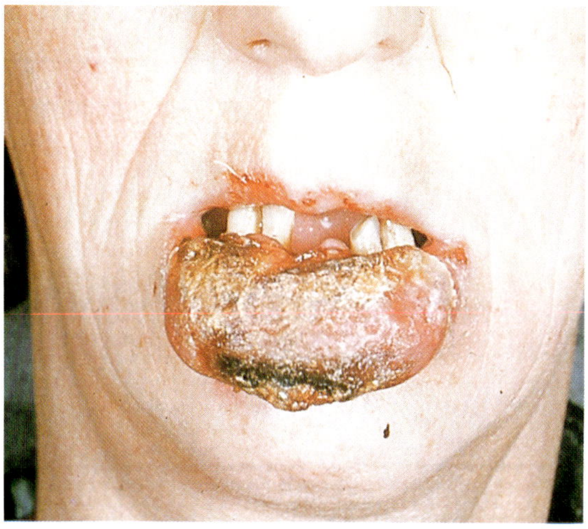

12.3

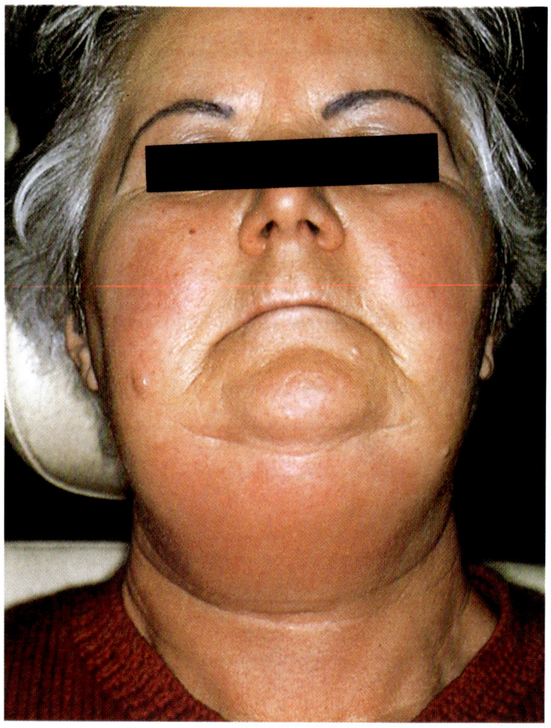

12.4

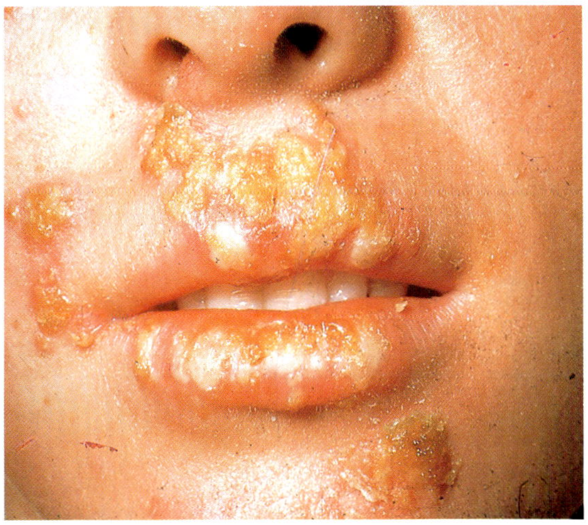

12.5

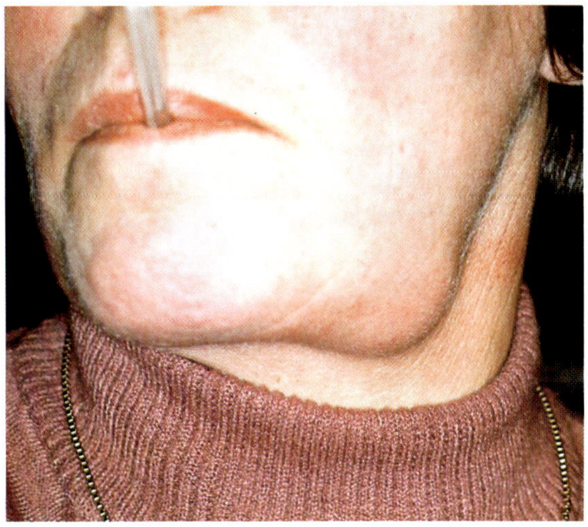

12.6

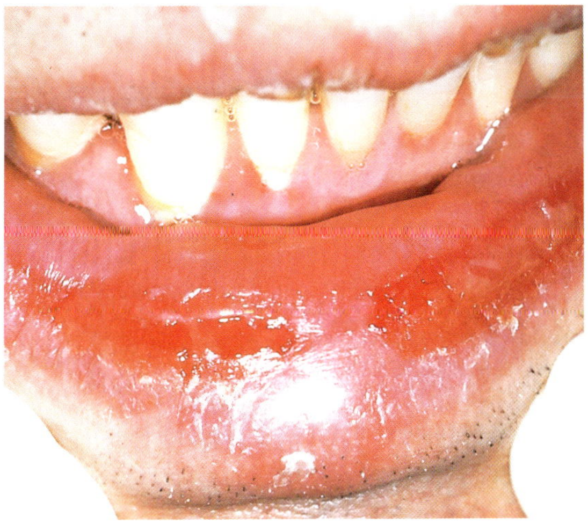

12.7

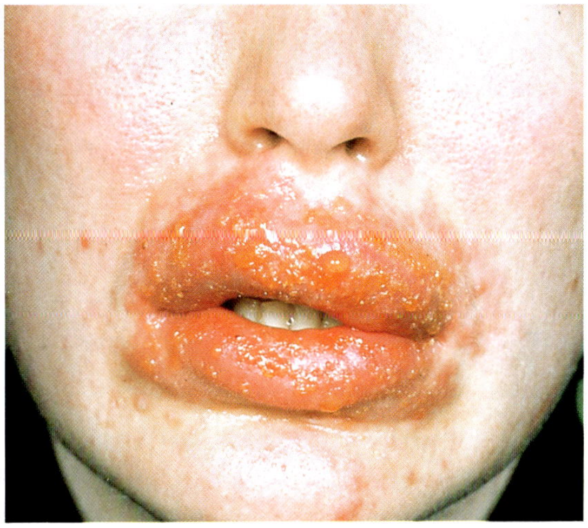

12.8

IMPETIGO

Figure 12.5 Perioral lesions such as herpes labialis or chickenpox may be secondarily infected with *staphylococci* or *streptococci*, resulting in impetigo as here. Alternatively, there may be a primary infection or spread of impetigo from elsewhere.

ACUTE LYMPHADENITIS

Figure 12.6 Lymphadenitis is usually a consequence of spread of infection from a focus in the drainage area. Occasionally a facial node (as here) or submandibular node is infected but the source unidentified. Such idiopathic submandibular abscesses are usually seen in pre-school children who are apparently healthy. *Staphylococcus aureus* is usually implicated and it is presumed that a small lesion in the nose or mouth is the focus.

Cervical lymph nodes may also be enlarged in the absence of an identifiable local infective lesion; in some systemic infections; in malignant disease; in connective tissue diseases; in sarcoid; and for other reasons.

ACTINIC CHEILITIS (*Solar elastosis*)

Figure 12.7 Outdoor workers, and others chronically exposed to sunlight, may develop ulcers and crusting, especially of the lower lip. Ultraviolet light appears to cause change of collagen into an elastic-like material. Actinic cheilitis may sometimes be followed by carcinoma.

ALLERGIC CHEILITIS

Figure 12.8 An allergic reaction to lipstick or other cosmetics is not uncommon. Swelling and sometimes blistering of the lips is seen.

DERMATITIS HERPETIFORMIS (*Duhring's disease*)

Figure 12.9 Dermatitis herpetiformis (DH) is an uncommon skin disease, often associated with gluten-sensitive enteropathy, and most common in adult males.

Oral lesions start as vesicles that rupture to leave non-specific ulcers – as here on the vermilion.

Figure 12.10 Superficial oral ulceration is one manifestation but some patients also have hyperkeratotic areas.

Figure 12.11 The typical rash is very itchy and consists of multiple, tense, vesicles on the elbows, shoulders and other extensor surfaces. This figure shows excoriated vesicles.

LINEAR IgA DISEASE

Figure 12.12 Linear IgA disease is a variant of DH in which the IgA deposits are linear rather than granular at the epithelial basement membrane zone. This patient had vesicles in the palate.

Chronic bullous dermatosis of childhood is a rare related disorder, seen in young children.

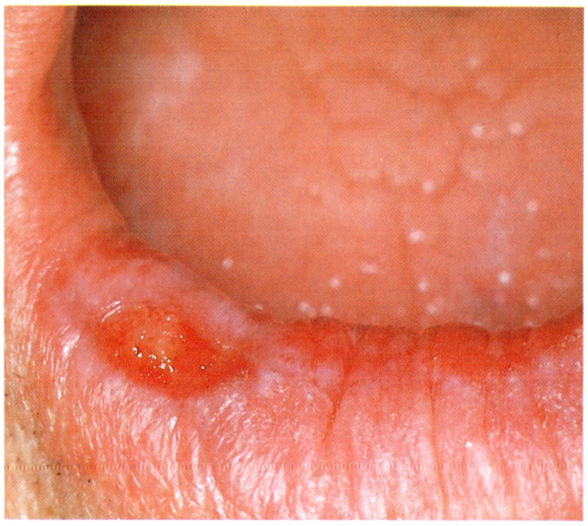

12.9

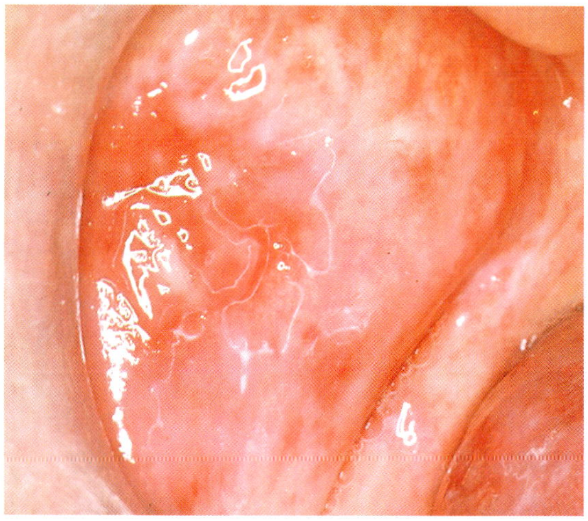

12.10

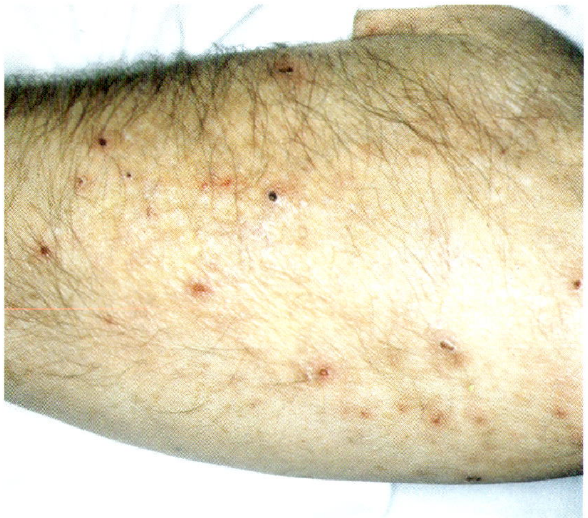

12.11

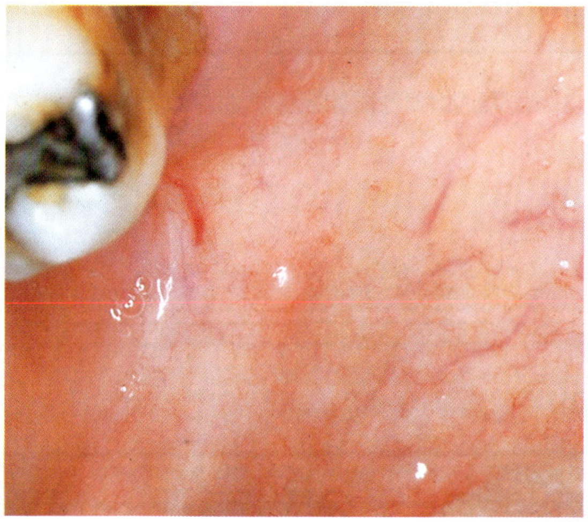

12.12

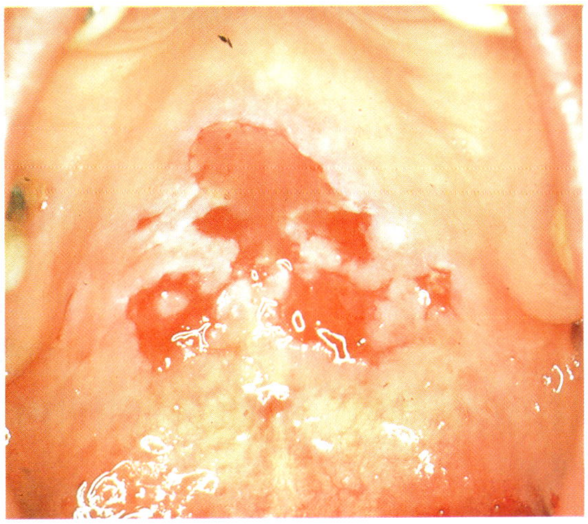

12.13

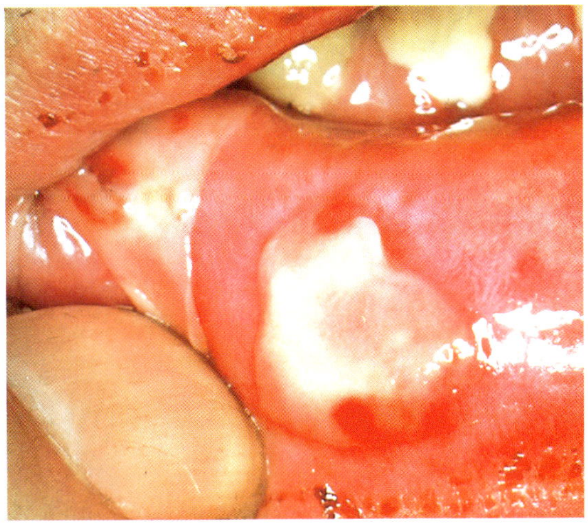

12.14

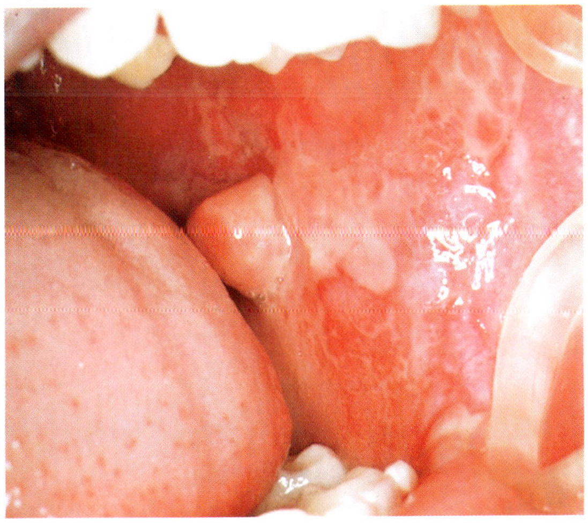

12.15

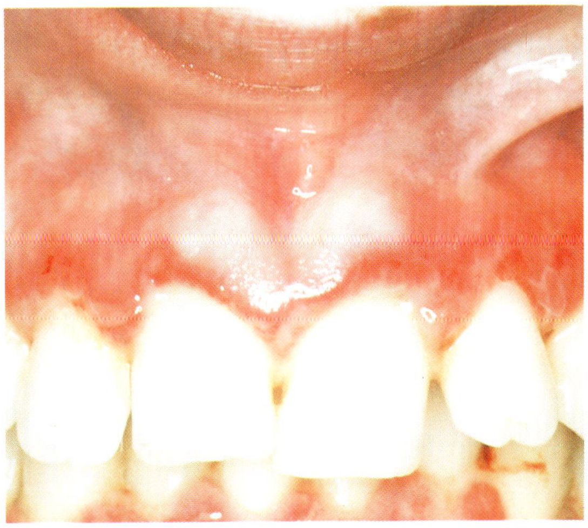

12.16

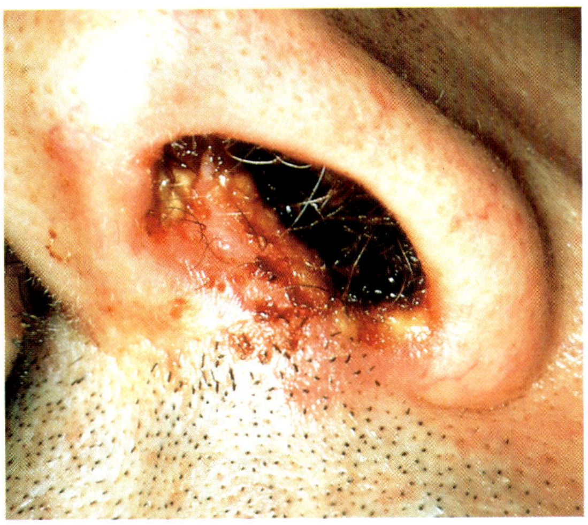

12.17

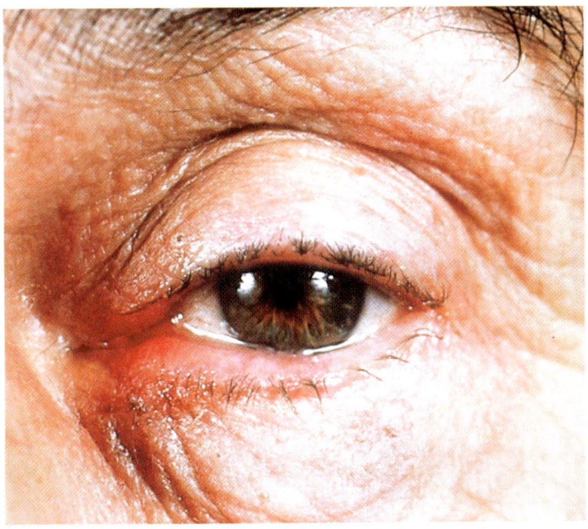

12.18

PEMPHIGUS

Figure 12.13 Pemphigus is a potentially lethal disorder characterized by autoantibodies directed against intercellular substance of stratified squamous epithelium, and seen especially in the middle-aged or elderly.

Pemphigus vulgaris is the most common type of pemphigus involving the mouth, although still an uncommon disease. Pemphigus vegetans may involve the mouth but oral lesions of the foliaceus and erythematosus types of pemphigus are very rare.

Occasional cases of pemphigus are drug-related (for example, to penicillamine or rifampicin).

PEMPHIGUS VULGARIS

Figure 12.14 Vesicles or blisters are rarely seen intact in the mouth as they break down rapidly to superficial irregular ulcers as here and in Figure 12.13. The ulcers may be covered with a fibrin slough.

Figure 12.15 Widespread erosions may be seen, especially where the mucosa is traumatized in the buccal mucosa, palate or gingiva. Oral lesions, as here, often precede skin manifestations.

Figure 12.16 Gingival involvement leads to one form of desquamative gingitivis.

Figure 12.17 Pemphigus can affect any stratified squamous epithelium: here the anterior nasal mucosa is affected.

Figure 12.18 Conjunctival involvement.

PEMPHIGUS VULGARIS
(continued)

Figure 12.19 Skin blisters tend to be flaccid, and appear at sites of trauma (Nikolsky sign). These lesions, on the anterior chest wall, were produced by the edge of a brassière.

Figure 12.20 Skin blisters break down to leave extensive scabbed lesions.

Figure 12.21 The axilla, shown here, and groin are often lesion sites.

Figure 12.22 Rarely, the nail beds are involved.

PEMPHIGUS VEGETANS

Figure 12.23 Pemphigus vegetans often presents initially in the mouth and, even in those with initial skin lesions, the mouth is usually eventually involved. White serpiginous lesions or sometimes vegetations, as here, are the main manifestations.

The Neumann type follows a similar course to pemphigus vulgaris, whereas the Hallopeau type is more benign. Oral lesions are, however, virtually invariable in both types.

Figure 12.24 The commissures are the sites most commonly affected, as shown here, and the tongue may be affected with white serpiginous lesions, and sometimes described as a 'cerebriform tongue'.

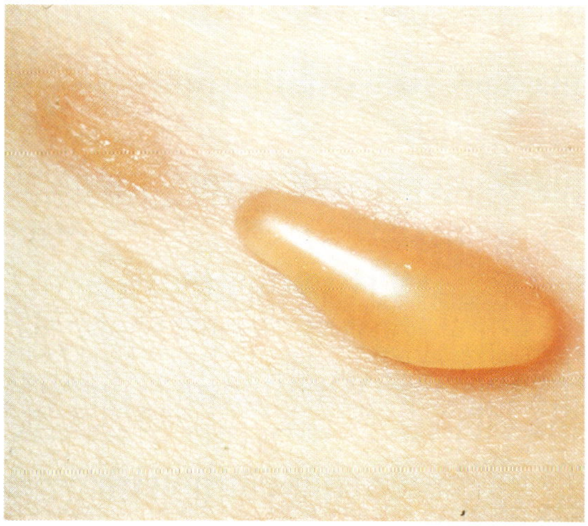

12.19

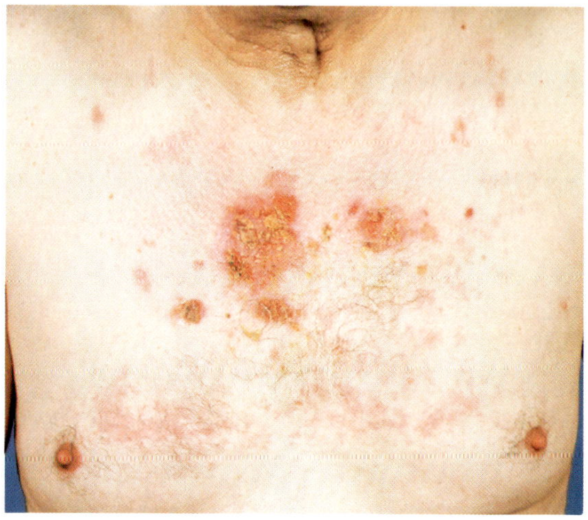

12.20

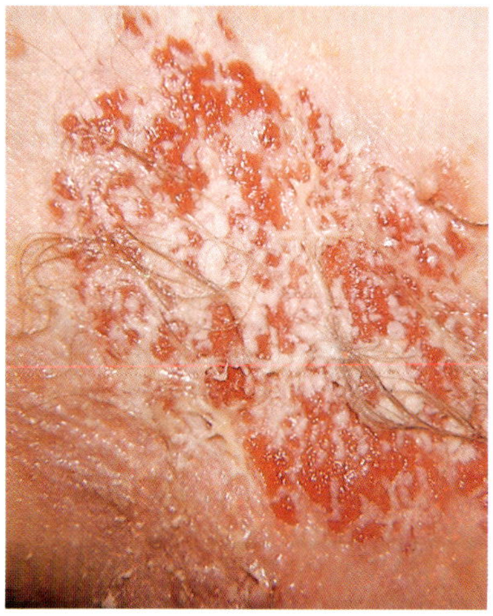

12.21

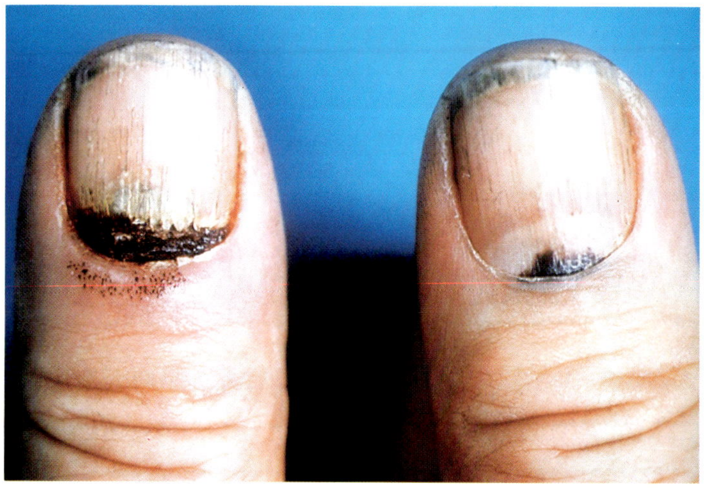

12.22

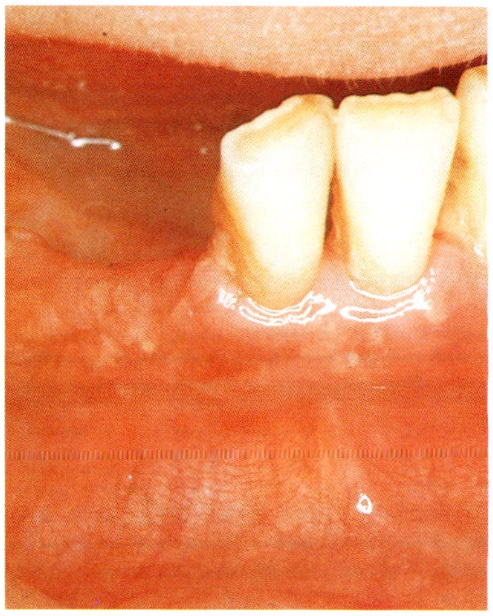

12.23

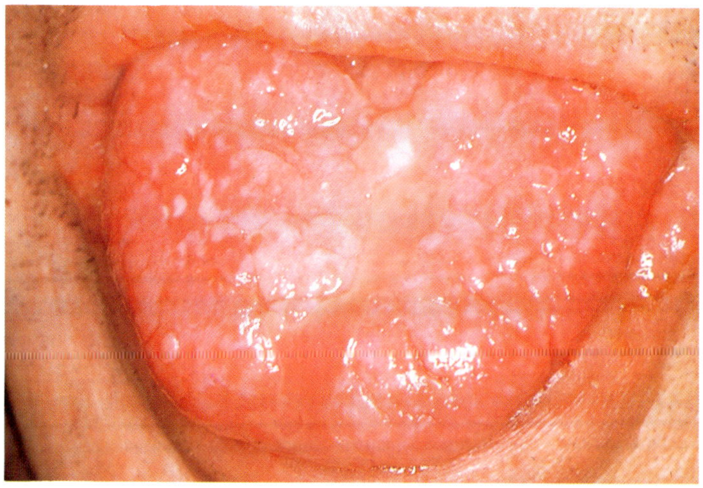

12.24

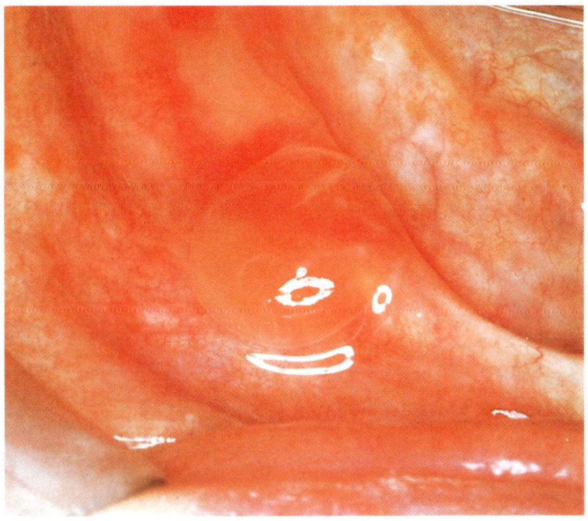

12.25

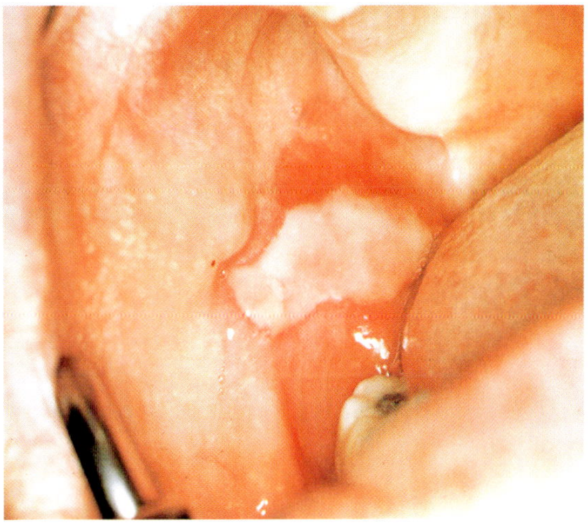

12.26

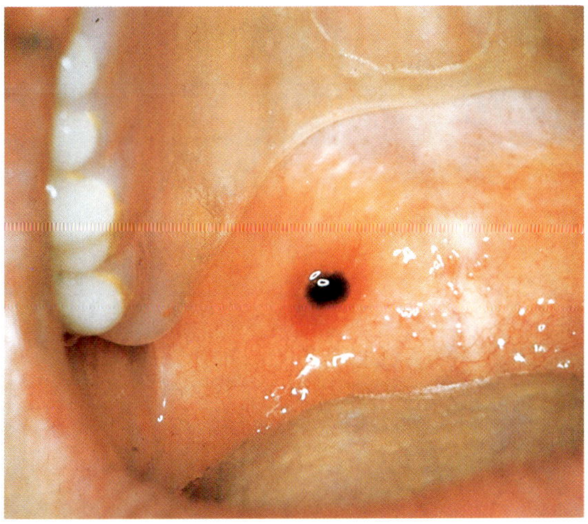

12.27

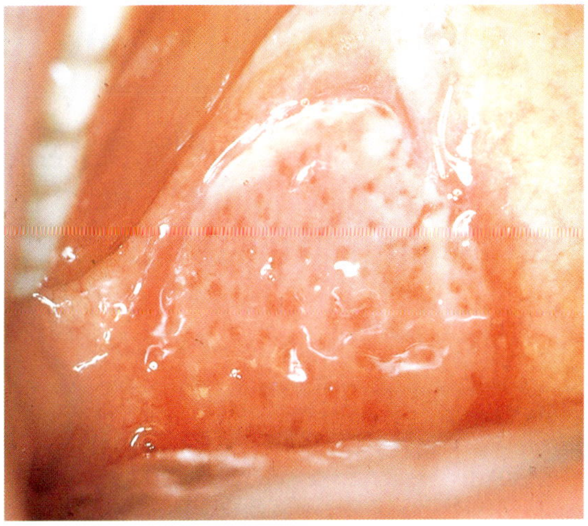

12.28

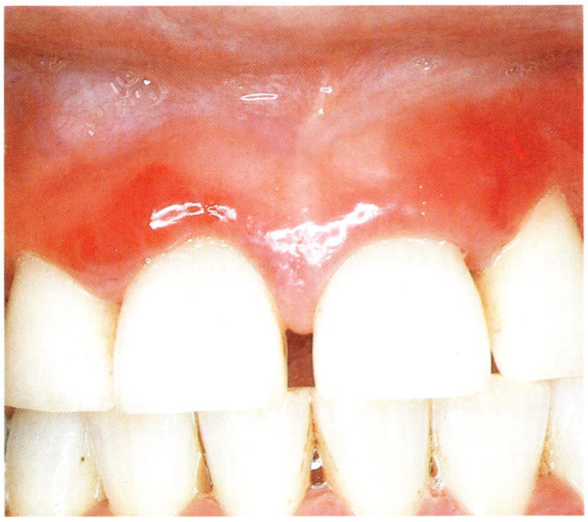

12.29

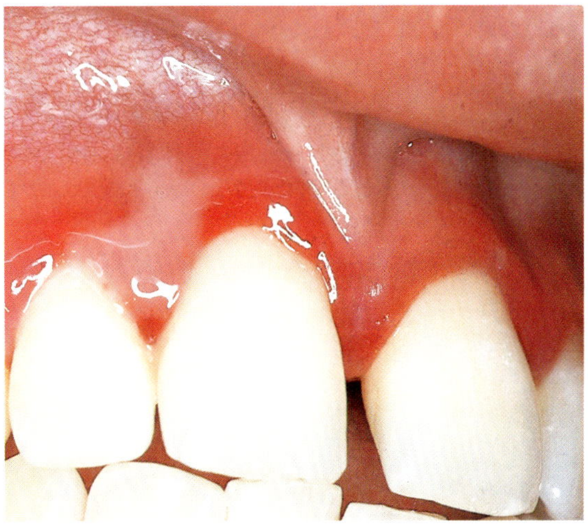

12.30

MUCOUS MEMBRANE PEMPHIGOID (*Cicatricial pemphigoid*)

Figure 12.25 Mucous membrane pemphigoid is a disorder of stratified squamous epithelia in which there are autoantibodies against epithelial basement membrane zone.

Mucous membrane pemphigoid often causes oral lesions; bullous pemphigoid rarely involves the mouth. An intact bulla is seen here over the lower alveolus.

Figure 12.26 Although intact vesicles or bullae may be seen, as in Figure 12.25, they eventually break down to leave irregular ulcers as here.

Figure 12.27 Lesions typically affect buccal mucosa, palate, and gingiva. Blisters are sometimes blood-filled.

Figure 12.28 The lesion shown in Figure 12.27 enlarged dramatically and broke down to leave this ulcer.

Figure 12.29 Mucous membrane pemphigoid is a frequent cause of desquamative gingivitis. Desquamation leads to patches of sore erythema. In contrast to marginal gingivitis, the interdental papillae and gingival margins may appear normal.

Figure 12.30 Occasionally there is frank gingival ulceration as well as superficial gingival desquamation.

MUCOUS MEMBRANE PEMPHIGOID *(continued)*

Figure 12.31 Conjunctiva and other squamous epithelia may be involved. Scarring may lead, as here, to symblepharon or, in the larynx, to stenosis. Skin lesions are uncommon.

Figure 12.32 Ocular involvement is potentially serious since it may, as here, culminate in blindness. The eyes are dry and the cornea becomes opaque.

BULLOUS PEMPHIGOID

Figure 12.33 Skin lesions are far more common than oral lesions in bullous pemphigoid. Oral vesicles, bullae and erosions may, however, be seen.

Figure 12.34 The skin vesicles and bullae of pemphigoid tend to be more tense than those of pemphigus and are seen most often on the abdomen, groin, axillae and flexures. Bullous pemphigoid is occasionally drug-induced, or secondary to ultraviolet light exposure. Brunsting-Perry disease is a mild variant of bullous pemphigoid.

LOCALIZED ORAL PURPURA (*Angina bullosa haemorrhagica*)

Figure 12.35 Localized oral purpura is a common condition that mimics pemphigoid, although it is unassociated with an immunopathogenesis. Patients present with blood blisters, typically on the soft palate, often after eating.

Figure 12.36 There is subepithelial vesiculation and an ulcer eventually forms. This type of ulcer has been described as a 'sunburst ulcer'.

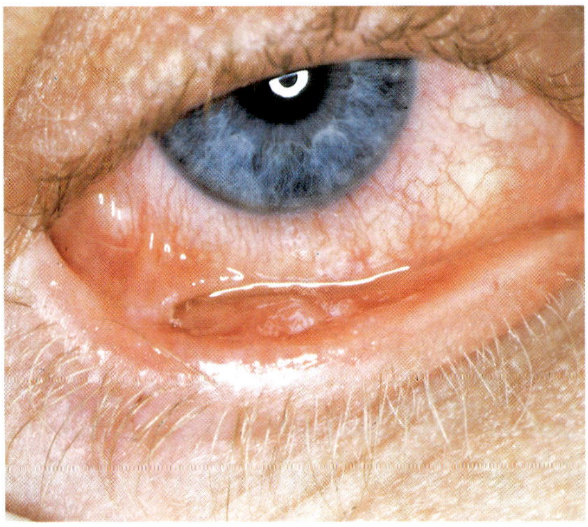

12.31

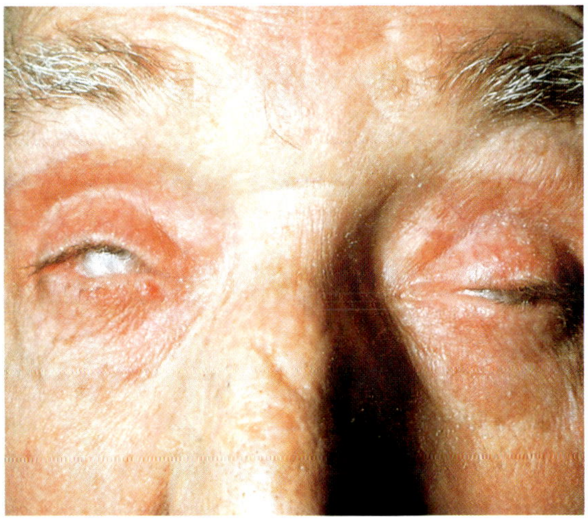

12.32

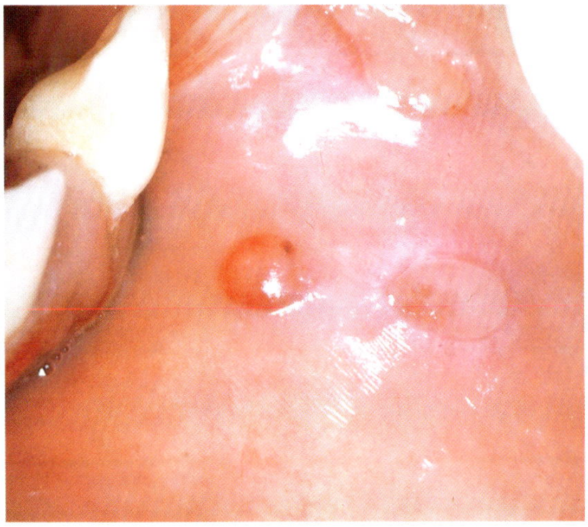

12.33

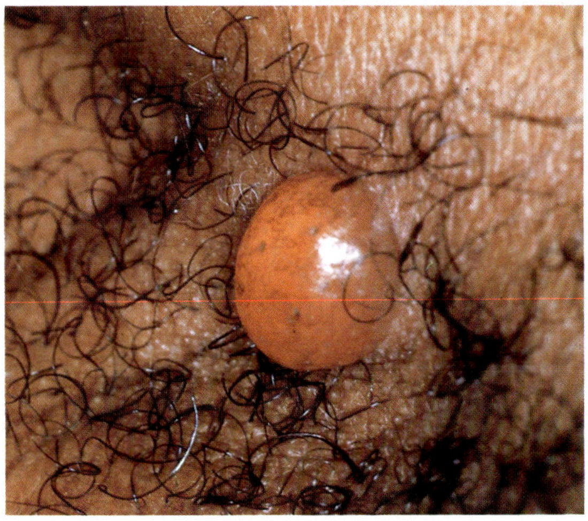

12.34

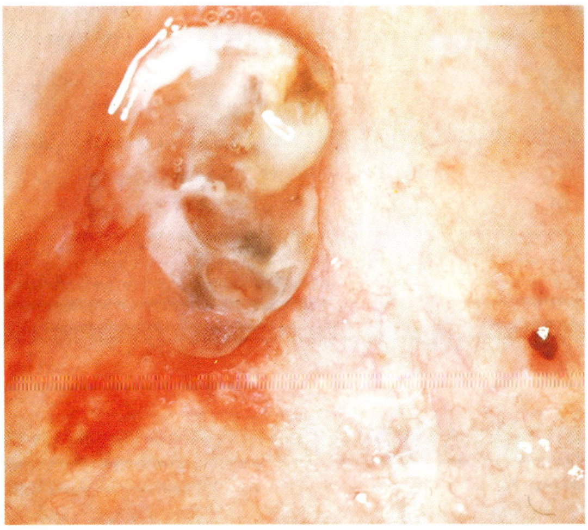

12.35

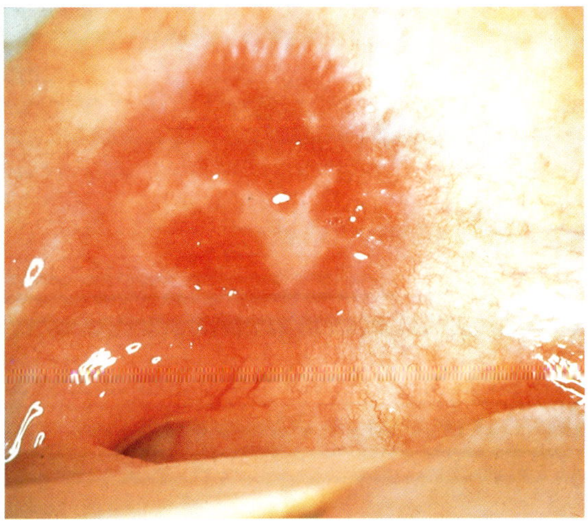

12.36

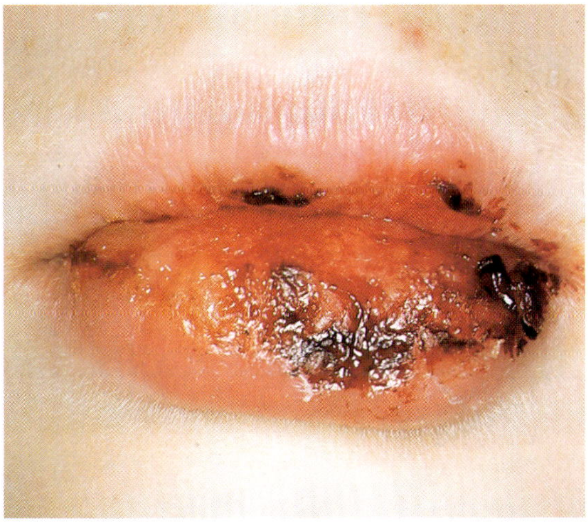

12.37

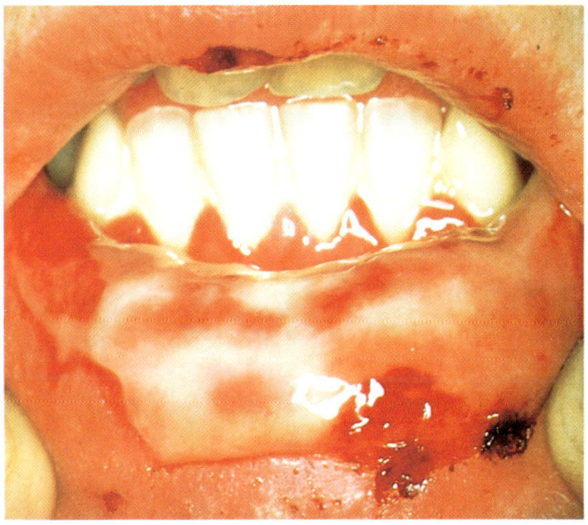

12.38

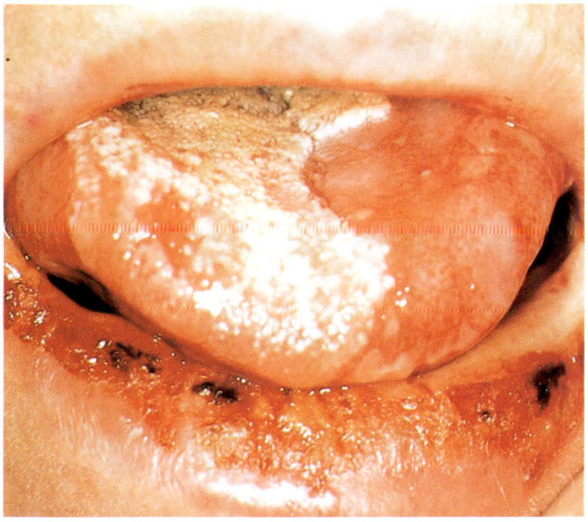

12.39

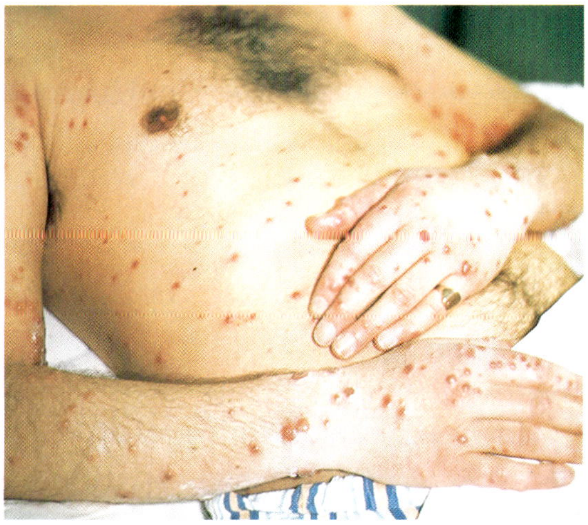

12.40

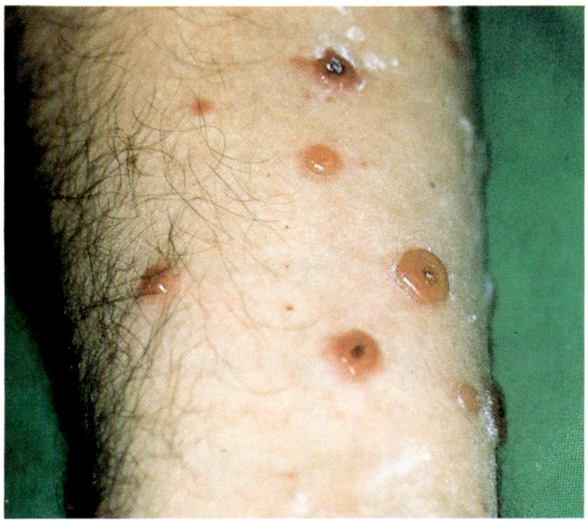

12.41

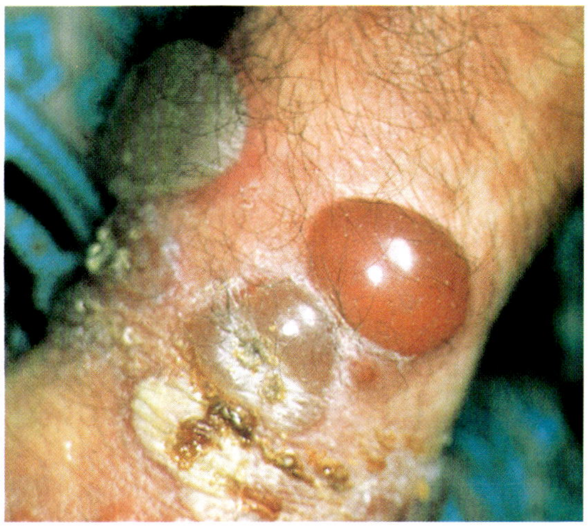

12.42

ERYTHEMA MULTIFORME

Figure 12.37 The virtually pathognomonic feature of erythema multiforme is swollen, blood-stained or crusted lips. Most patients are males, typically adolescents or young adults, and there are periods of remission from the disease.

Figure 12.38 Oral lesions progress through macules to blisters and ulceration, typically most pronounced in the anterior parts of the mouth.

Figure 12.39 Extensive oral ulceration may be seen.

Although the aetiology is unclear in most patients, in some the disorder is precipitated by infections (such as herpes simplex or mycoplasma), by drugs (sulphonamides, barbiturates, hydantoins and others) or by a range of other triggers, even menstruation.

Figure 12.40 Most patients have oral lesions only but, in some, other squamous epithelia are involved. Rashes of various types (hence 'erythema multiforme') are seen.

Figure 12.41 Close-up of the same patient as in Figure 12.40, showing a vesiculo-bullous rash: the blisters are collapsed and scabbed centrally.

Figure 12.42 More pronounced blisters in erythema multiforme, resembling pemphigoid.

ERYTHEMA MULTIFORME *(continued)*

Figure 12.43 The characteristic rash consists of 'target' or 'iris' lesions in which the central lesion has a surrounding ring of erythema.

Figure 12.44 Later stage of target lesions showing darkening and loss of distinction.

STEVENS-JOHNSON SYNDROME (*Erythema multiforme exudativum*)

Figure 12.45 Conjunctivitis, stomatitis and rash in the acute phase of Stevens-Johnson syndrome. The ocular changes resemble those of mucous membrane pemphigoid: dry eyes and symblepharon may result.

Figure 12.46 The patient shown in Figure 12.45 upon recovery.

Figure 12.47 Oral lesions (stomatitis) may be seen with conjunctivitis, genital and cutaneous lesions. Balanitis, urethritis and vulval ulcers are the typical genital lesions.

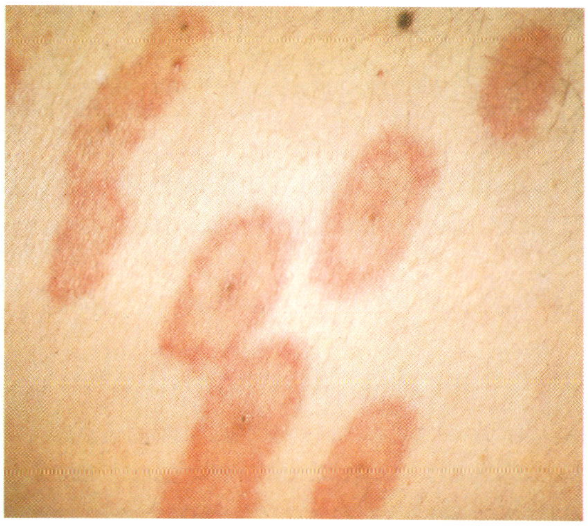

12.43

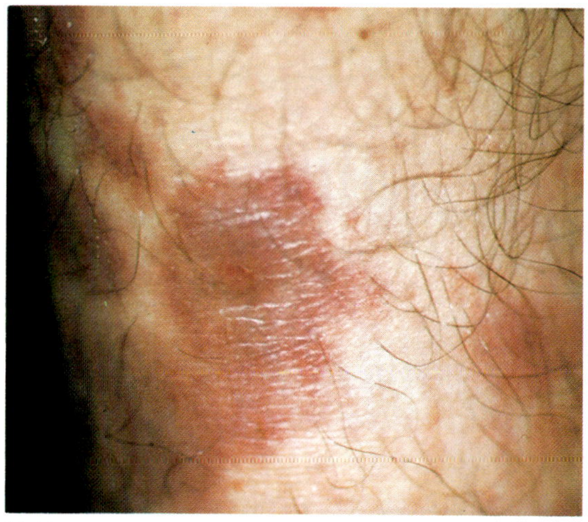

12.44

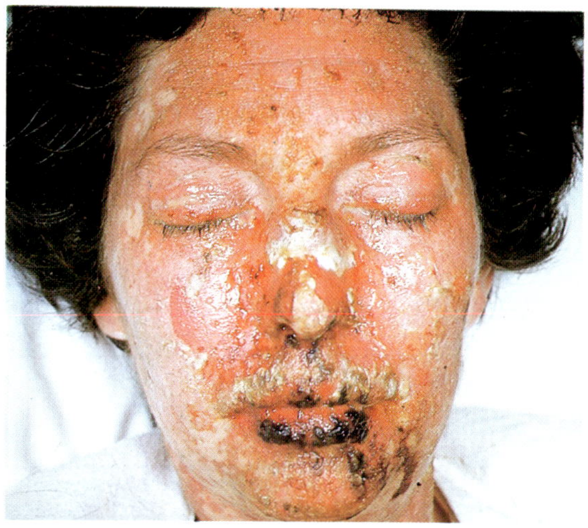

12.45

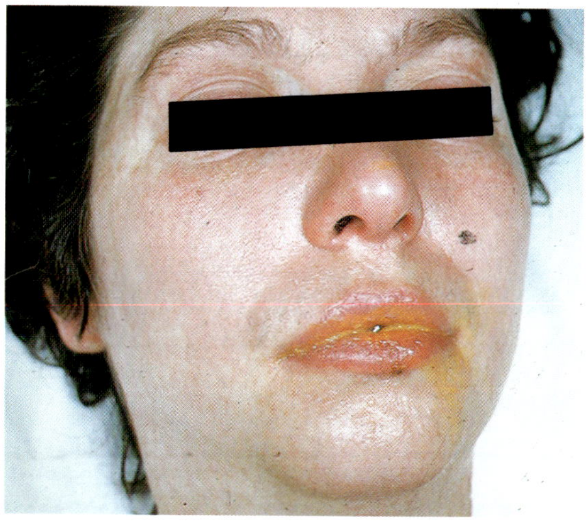

12.46

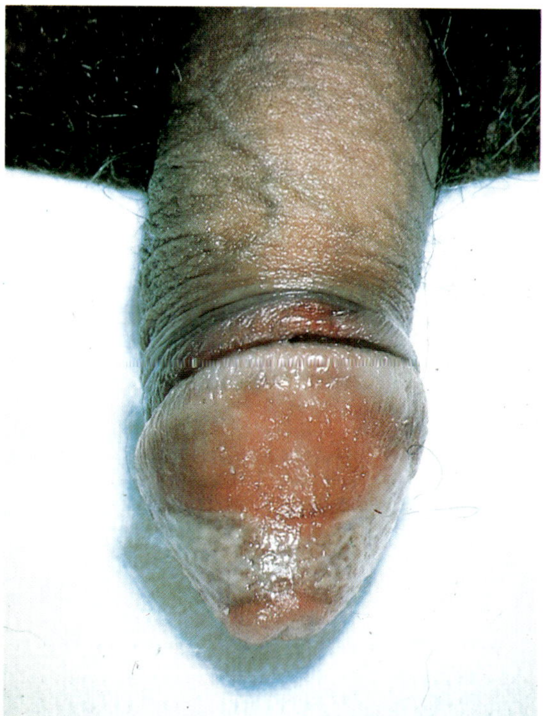

12.47

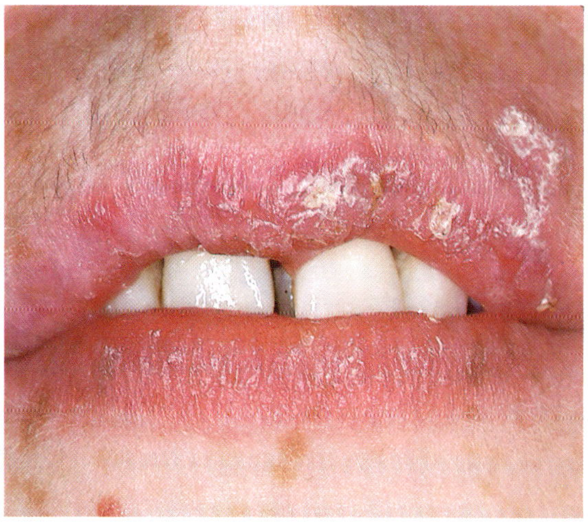

12.48

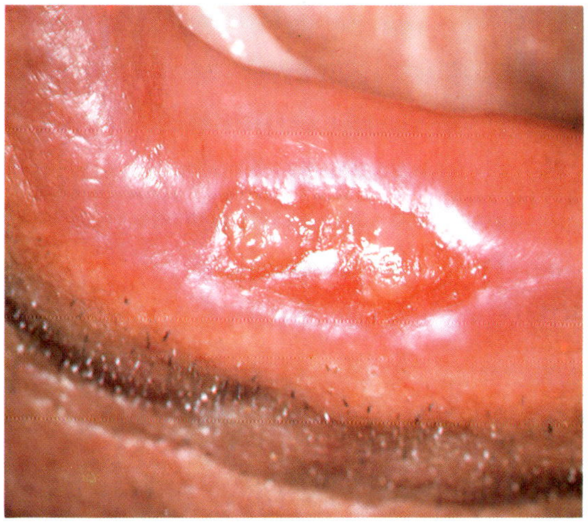

12.49

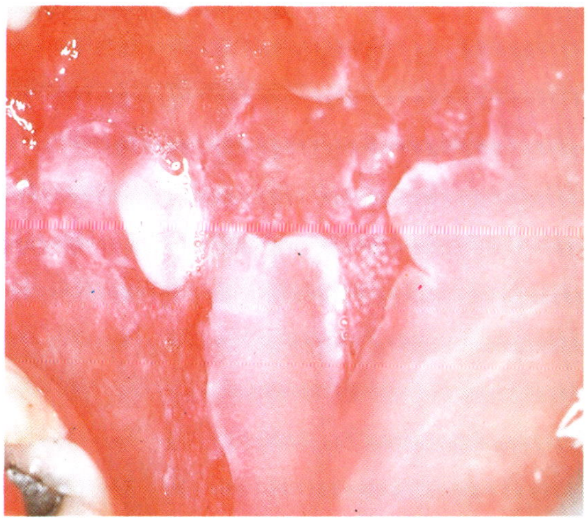

12.50

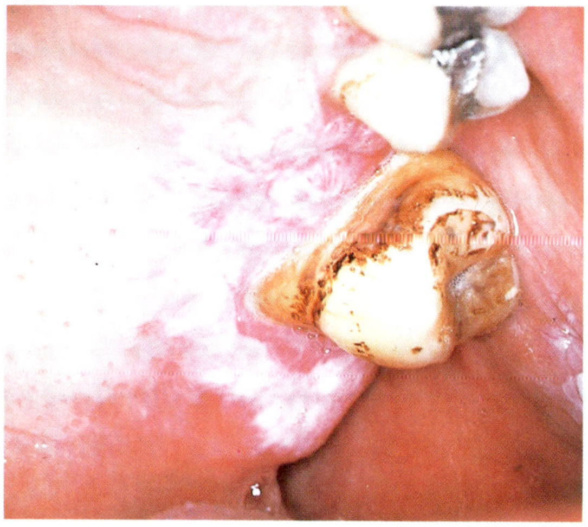

12.51

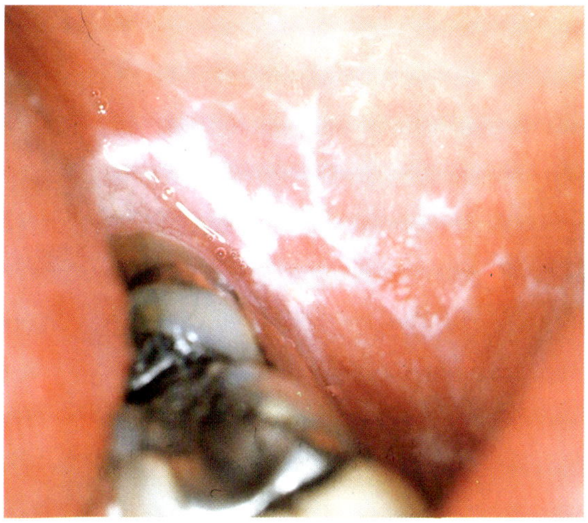

12.52

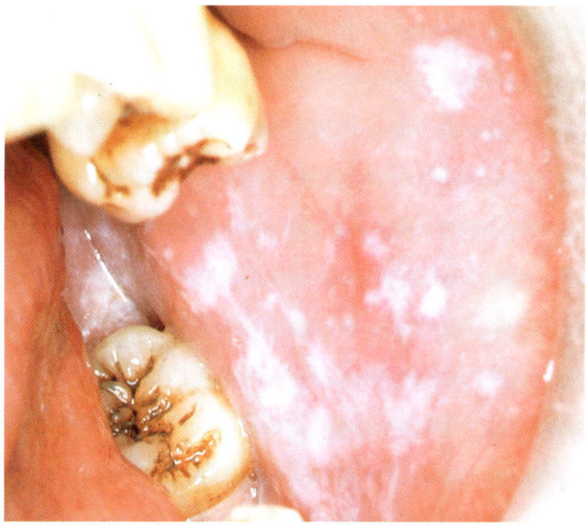

12.53

DISCOID LUPUS ERYTHEMATOSUS

Figure 12.48 Discoid lupus erythematosus is an immunologically-mediated disorder characterized by a rash on face, scalp, ears and hands, consisting of red patches with scaling and follicular plugging. Here there are scaly lesions on the vermilion, and perioral skin. The pigmented lesions (freckles) are unrelated.

Figure 12.49 Lesions may ulcerate, as here. There is a premalignant predisposition, especially in males with lesions on the lip.

Figure 12.50 The typical oral lesions have an irregular white border with telangiectasia, surrounding a central atrophic area in which there are small white papules.

Figure 12.51 Palatal lesions are far more common in lupus erythematosus than in lichen planus – the oral lesions of which can be difficult to differentiate clinically from lupus erythematosus.

LICHEN PLANUS

Figure 12.52 White lesions in the mouth are the typical feature of lichen planus and although often distinct from lupus erythematosus, as here, are by no means invariably so.

Figure 12.53 Papular type: oral lichen planus (LP) is common, mostly idiopathic and often asymptomatic. Of the many types described on the following pages, papular LP is the most common. White papules are seen typically in the buccal mucosa bilaterally.

LICHEN PLANUS
(continued)

Figure 12.54 Circinate type: white rings in the buccal mucosa. Lichen planus lesions are typically bilateral. In this patient, similar lesions were present in the other buccal mucosa.

Figure 12.55 Reticular type: a network of white lesions, again in the buccal mucosa. Oral lesions of LP are often persistent and patients may have lesions for many years.

Figure 12.56 Mixed papular and reticular: the clinical lesions in LP are not necessarily of one type alone.

Figure 12.57 Plaque type: lichen planus, especially in smokers, can give rise to confluent white patches difficult to distinguish clinically from keratoses (leukoplakia).

Figure 12.58 Confluent type: although the buccal mucosa is the common site for LP, lesions may also involve the dorsum and lateral margins of the tongue.

Figure 12.59 Plaque and atrophic types: the white lesion on the left side of the tongue is LP. On the right side is an atrophic depapillated lesion of LP.

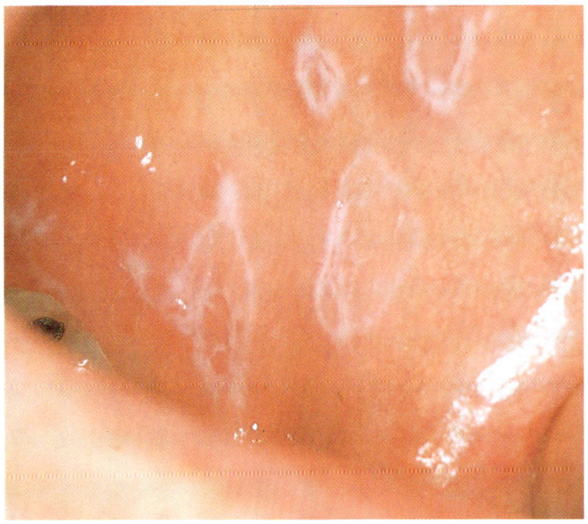

12.54

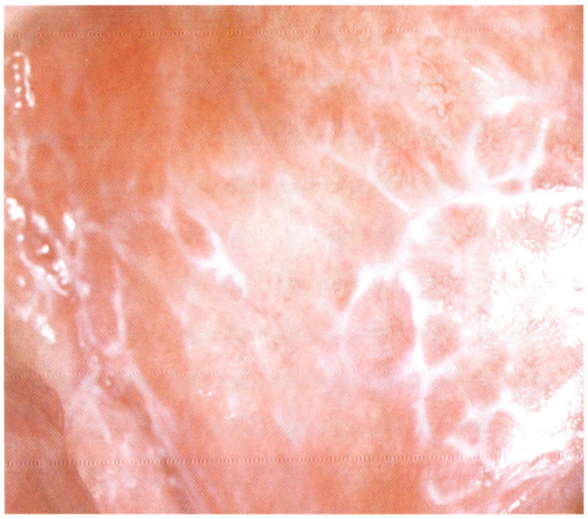

12.55

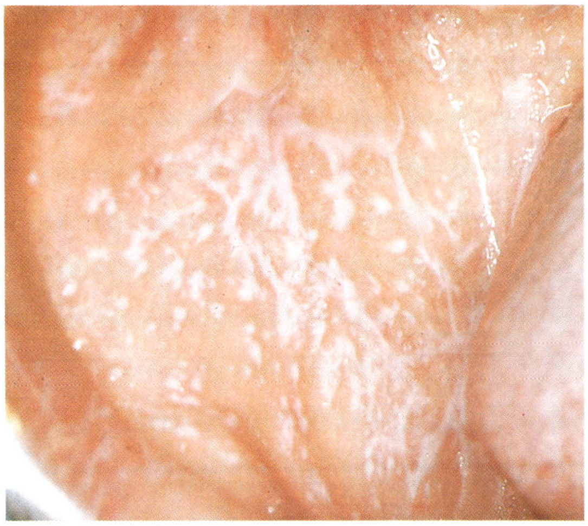

12.56

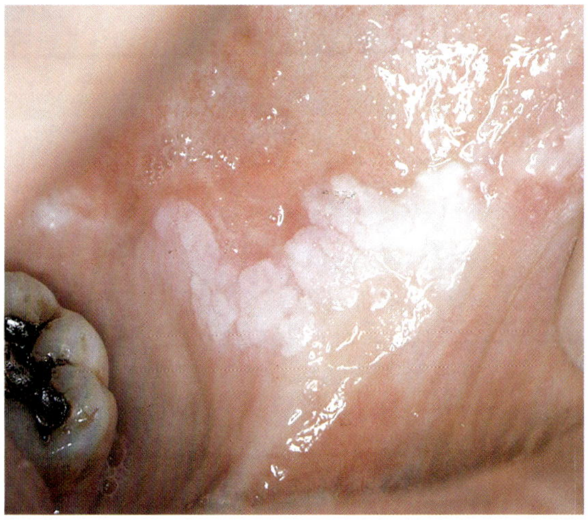

12.57

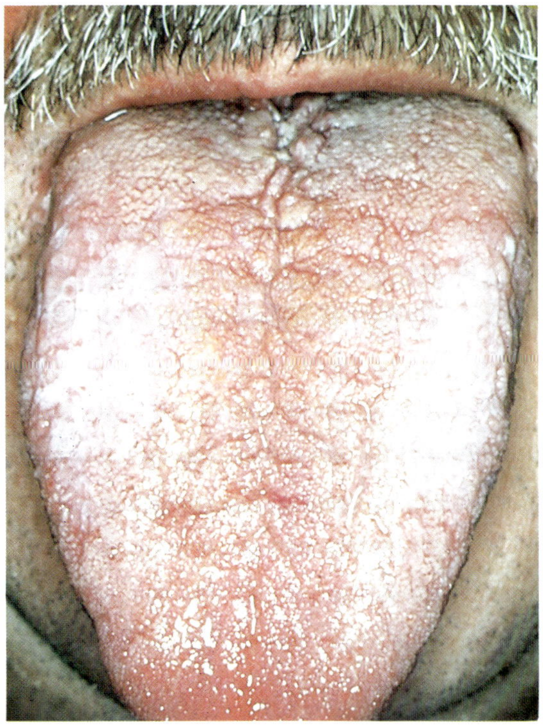

12.58

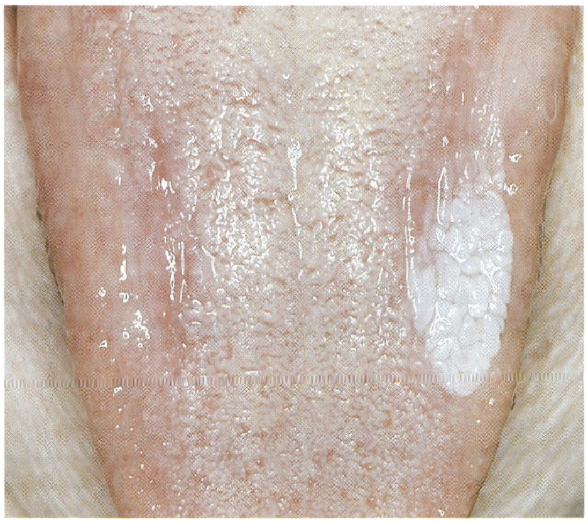

12.59

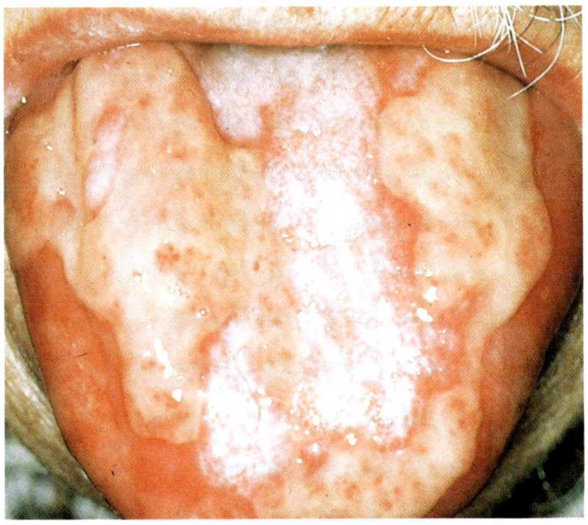

12.60

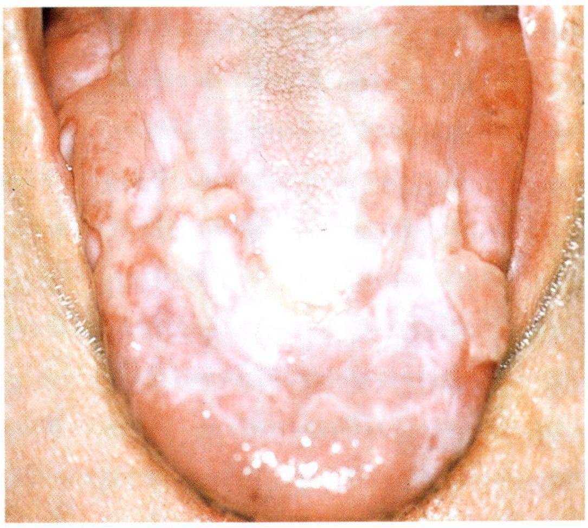

12.61

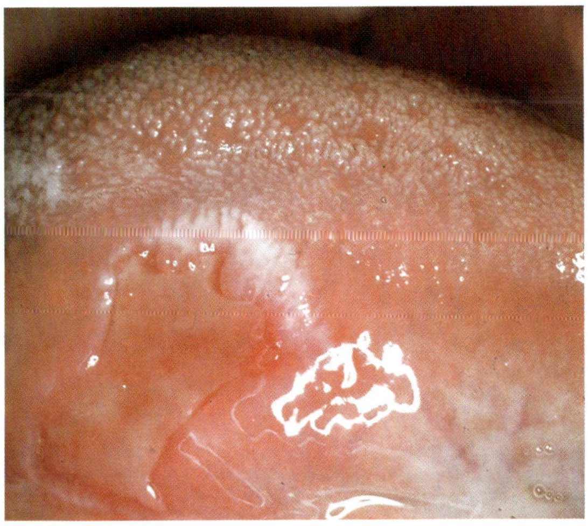

12.62

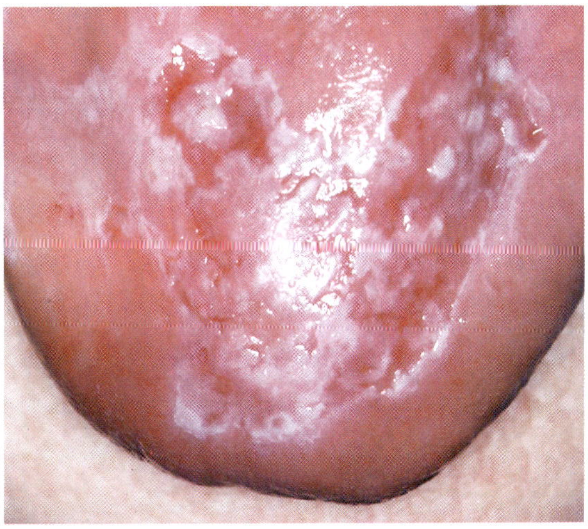

12.63

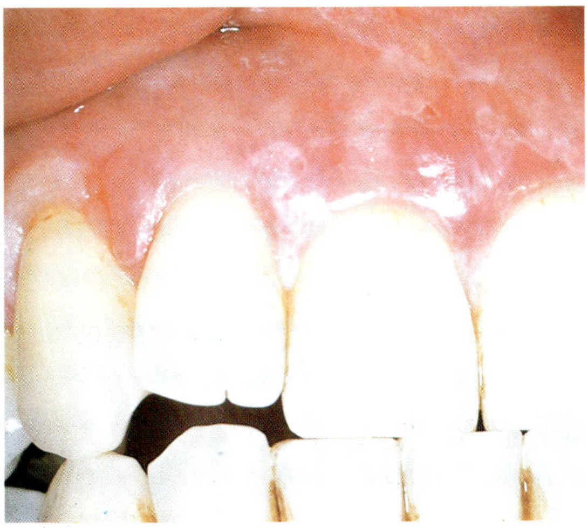

12.64

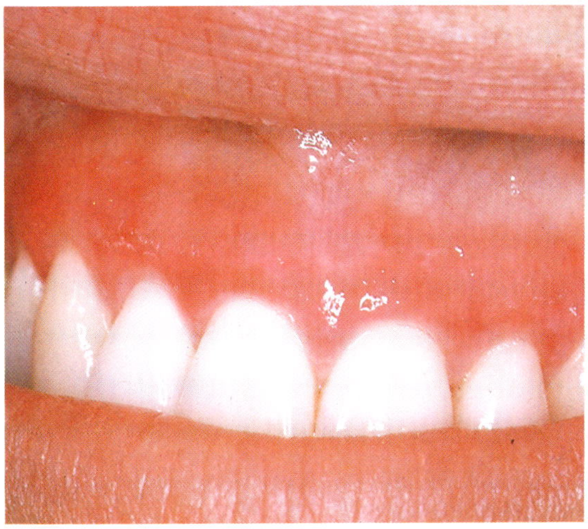

12.65

Figure 12.60 Erosive LP can cause pronounced discomfort. Erosions are irregular, often widespread, in the buccal and lingual mucosa, and persistent.

Figure 12.61 Erosive and atrophic forms of LP may be premalignant in less than 1 per cent of cases though these may represent associated erythroplasia.

Figure 12.62 The erosions may be irregular, often shaped like the leaf of a holly tree, and there may be associated white lesions, as here.

Figure 12.63 Atrophic type: atrophic erythroplastic lesions preceded the development of squamous carcinoma in this patient.

Figures 12.64 and 12.65 Lichen planus is a fairly common cause of desquamative gingivitis.

LICHEN PLANUS (*continued*)

Figure 12.66 Lichenoid eruption: lesions that resemble LP clinically and histologically may be induced by various identifiable factors. These lichenoid lesions may be caused by anti-hypertensives, oral hypoglycaemics, non-steroidal anti-inflammatory agents and a range of other drugs.

Lichenoid lesions may also appear in relation to metal restorative materials used in dentistry, and are a frequent complication of graft-versus-host disease.

Lichen planus has occasional associations with other diseases, especially with diabetes mellitus and autoimmune disorders.

Figure 12.67 Pigmentary incontinence: hyper-pigmentation may be seen in older lesions of oral LP but not as frequently as in cutaneous LP.

Figure 12.68 Cutaneous lesions if present are typically purple, polygonal, pruritic, papules on the flexor surfaces of the wrists.

Figure 12.69 White striae may be seen on the surfaces of the papules (Wickham's striae).

Figure 12.70 Wickham's striae.

Figure 12.71 Cutaneous lesions may be widespread and cause extreme itching.

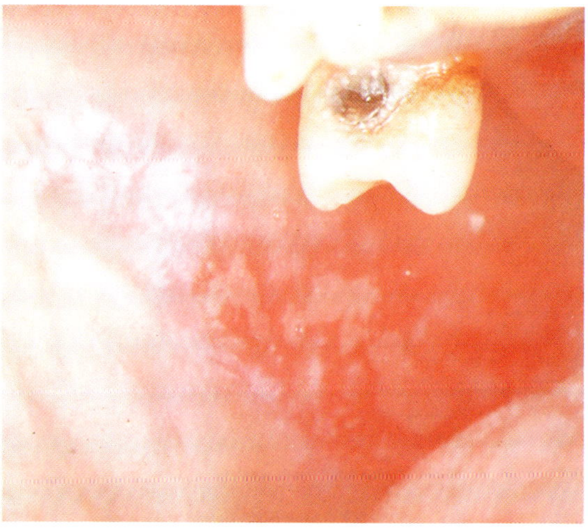

12.66

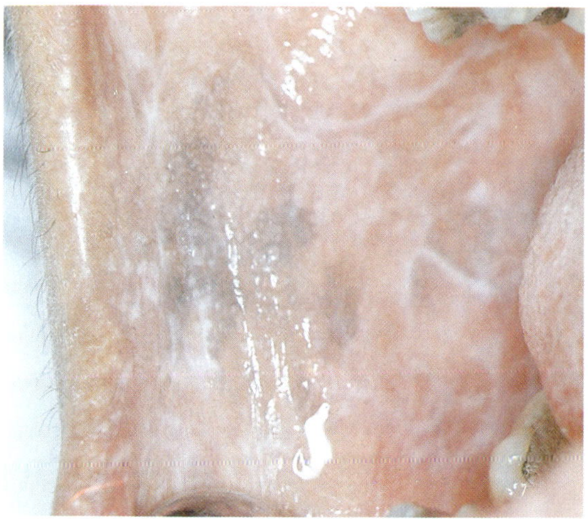

12.67

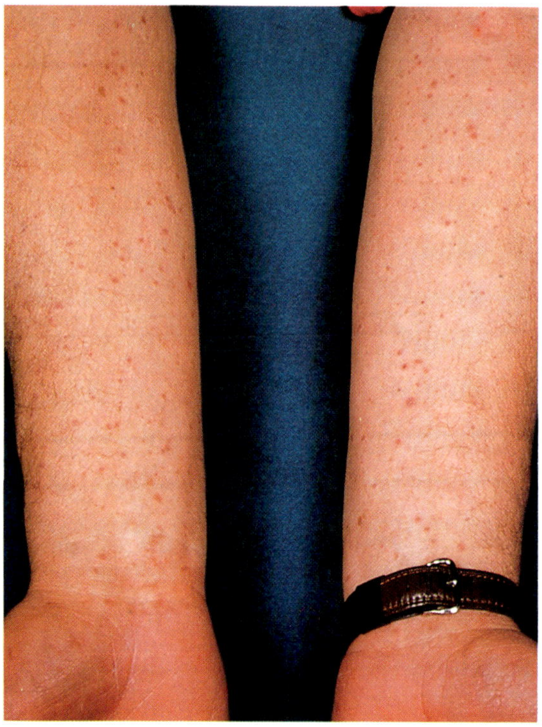

12.68

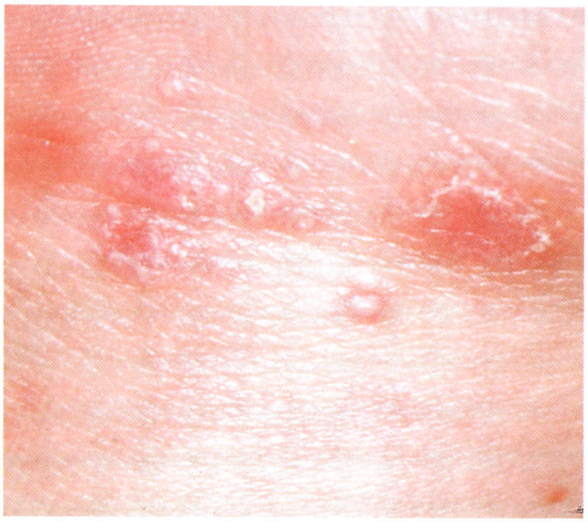

12.69

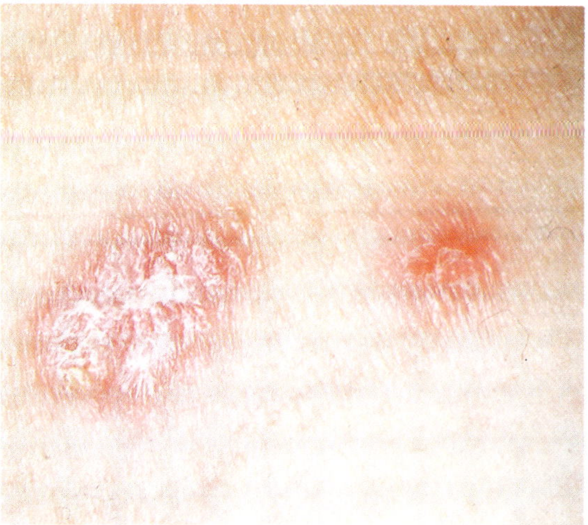

12.70

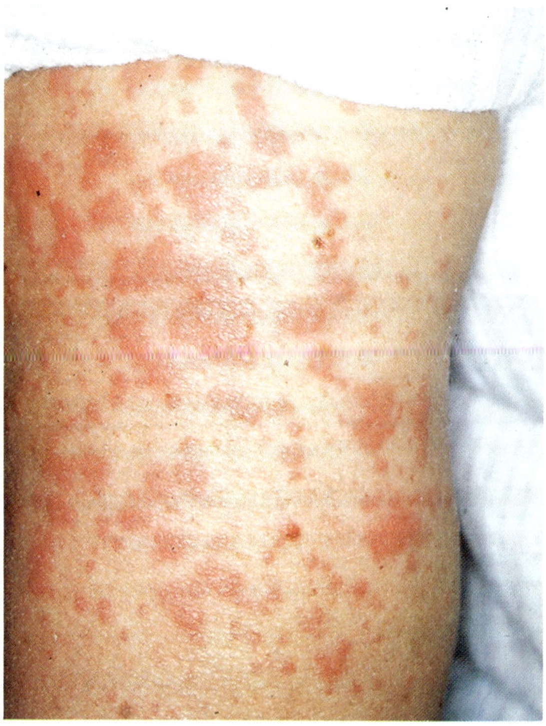

12.71

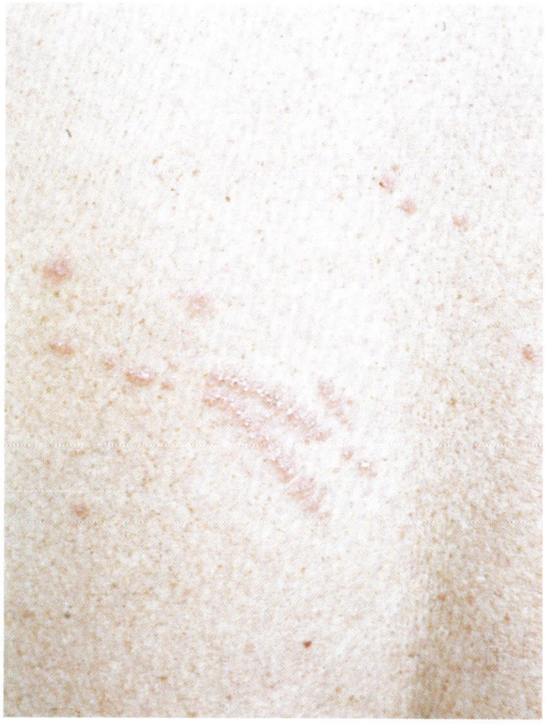

12.72

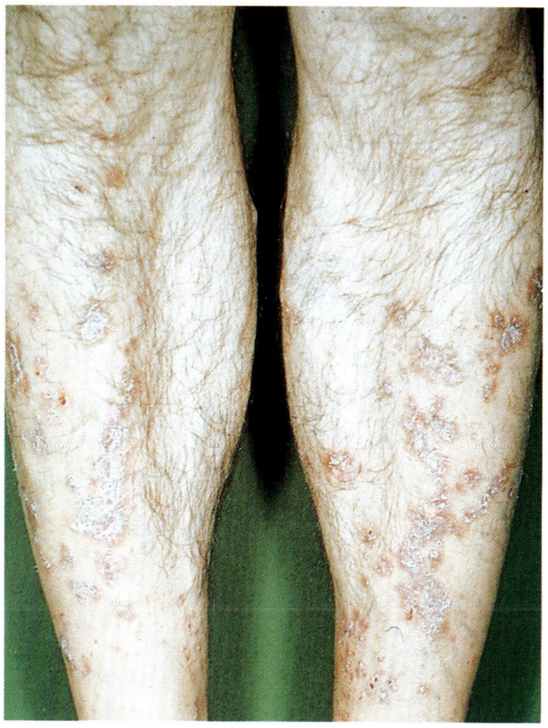

12.73

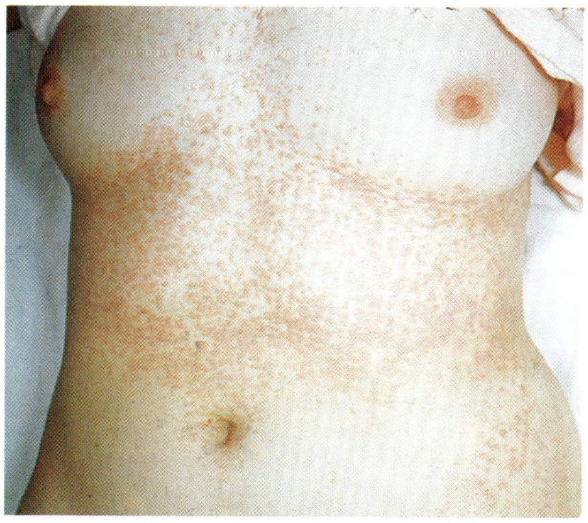

12.74

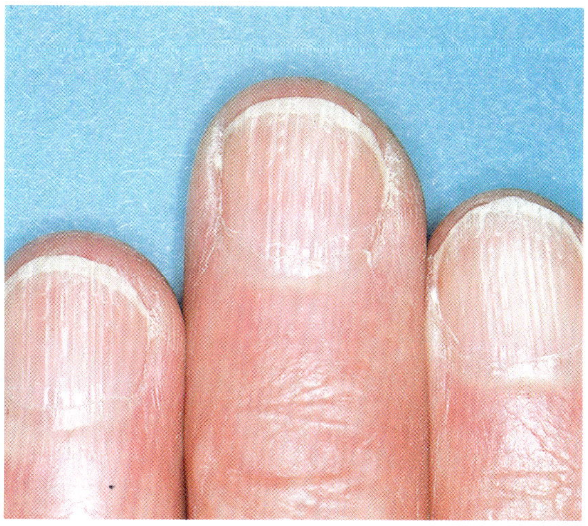

12.75

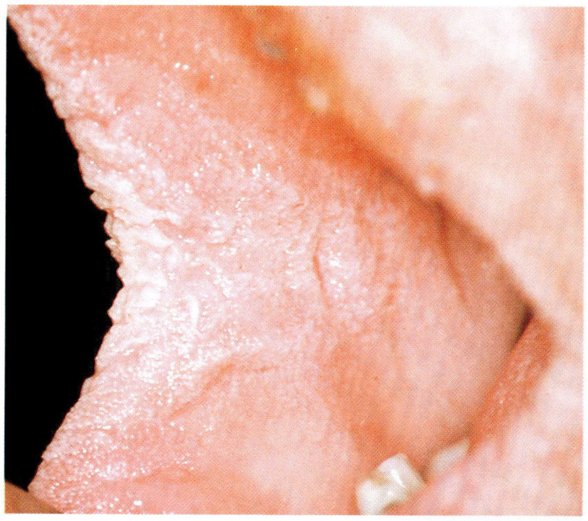

12.76

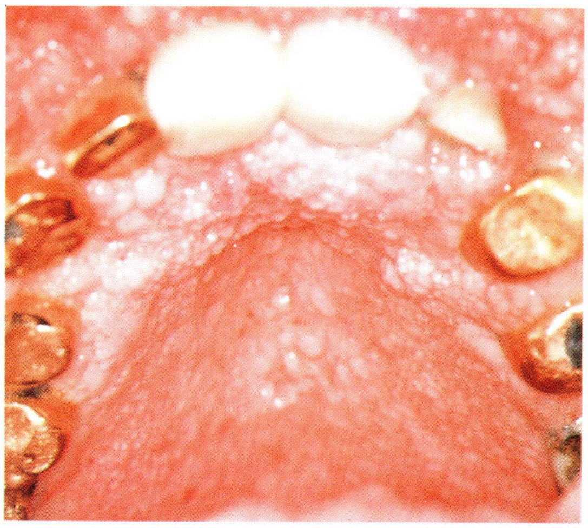

12.77

Figure 12.72 Rubbing or scratching the skin may produce a row of lesions, termed the Koebner phenomenon.

Figure 12.73 Lesions are common over the shins.

Figure 12.74 Skin lesions may also be seen elsewhere but are rare on the face. Alopecia may be seen.

Figure 12.75 Nail involvement may produce longitudinal ridging, as here.

ACANTHOSIS NIGRICANS

Figure 12.76 Acanthosis nigricans is a rare disorder characterized by hyperkeratosis and pigmentation. The so-called 'malignant type' precedes accompanies, or follows the detection of an internal malignancy, especially a stomach adenocarcinoma.

Figure 12.77 The lips and tongue are most frequently involved. Thickening of the mucosa with a papilliferous surface characterizes acanthosis nigricans. Typical cutaneous lesions are brown, velvety macules, especially in axillae, neck, inguinal and other flexural areas.

Acanthosis nigricans can be inherited (autosomal dominant), drug-induced (diethylstilboestrol, nicotinic acid), or associated with insulin-resistance and other endocrinopathies or various other rare disorders.

13

Diseases of the musculoskeletal system and connective tissue

SYSTEMIC LUPUS ERYTHEMATOSUS

Figure 13.1 Systemic lupus erythematosus (SLE) is a multisystem immune complex-mediated disorder affecting in particular the skin, blood and kidneys. The classic rash is over the bridge of nose and cheeks ('butterfly' or 'malar' rash).

Systemic lupus erythematosus is also associated with photosensitivity, arthritis, serositis, anaemia, leukopenia and multiple autoantibodies, as well as non-specific features such as malaise or fever.

Figure 13.2 Oral lesions include petechiae and persistent irregular red lesions, sometimes with keratosis. The palate is a common site. Sjögren's syndrome may be associated.

SYSTEMIC SCLEROSIS (*Scleroderma*)

Figure 13.3 Systemic sclerosis is an immunologically-mediated multisystem disorder. Rare cases are drug-induced (bleomycin, tryptophan or carbidopa), associated with graft-versus-host disease or occupational (PVC, silicosis). Affecting predominantly the skin, respiratory and gastrointestinal tract, the most common manifestation is Raynaud's phenomenon. The skin becomes tight, waxy and eventually hidebound, and the face smooth with a 'Mona Lisa' appearance. Skin pigmentation is also increased, as here.

Figure 13.4 The lips tighten with radiating furrows – the so-called 'tobacco pouch' mouth – and oral opening is restricted not only by the tight skin but also by pseudoankylosis of the temporomandibular joint. The condyles or zygomatic arches are, rarely, resorbed.

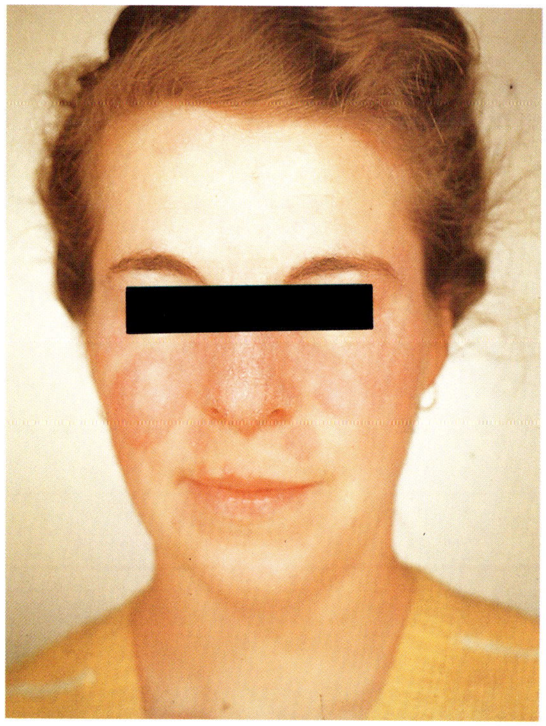

13.1

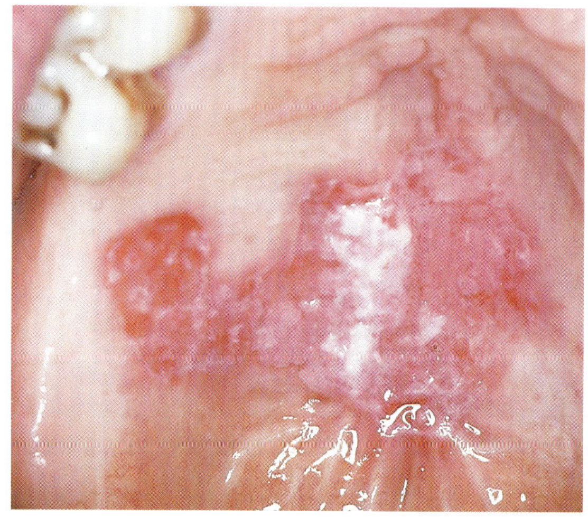

13.2

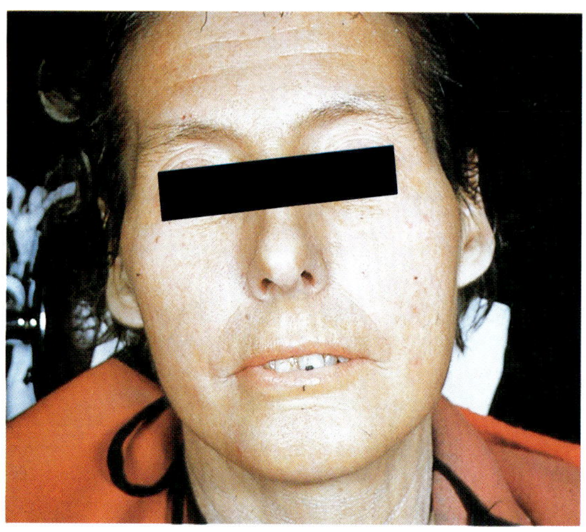

13.3

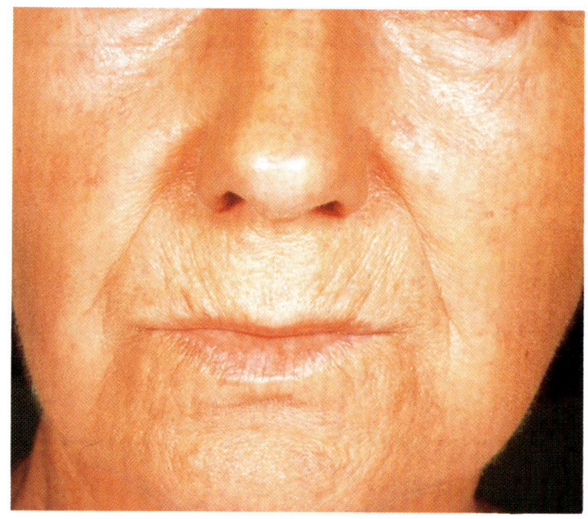

13.4

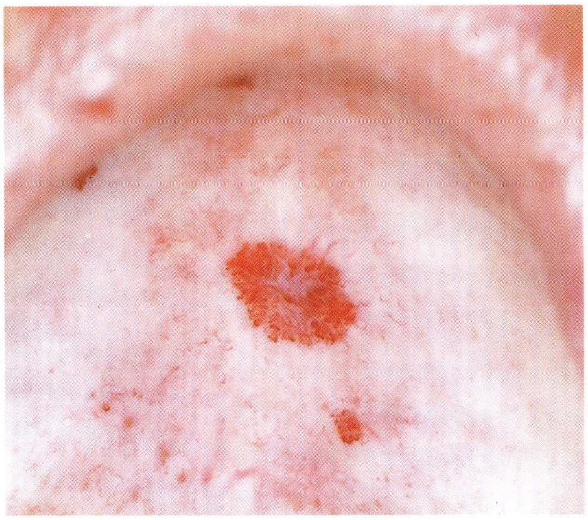

13.5

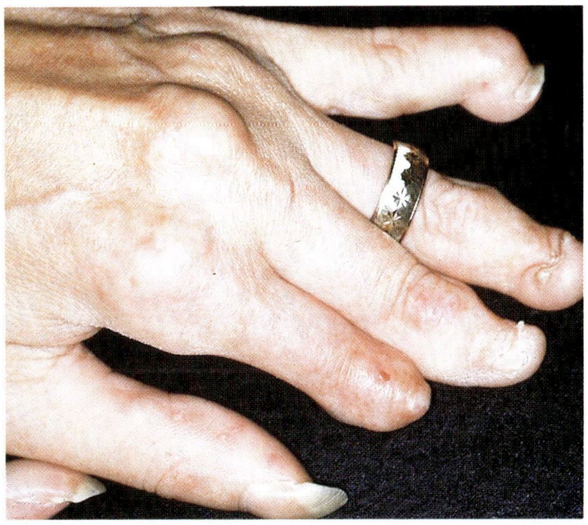

13.6

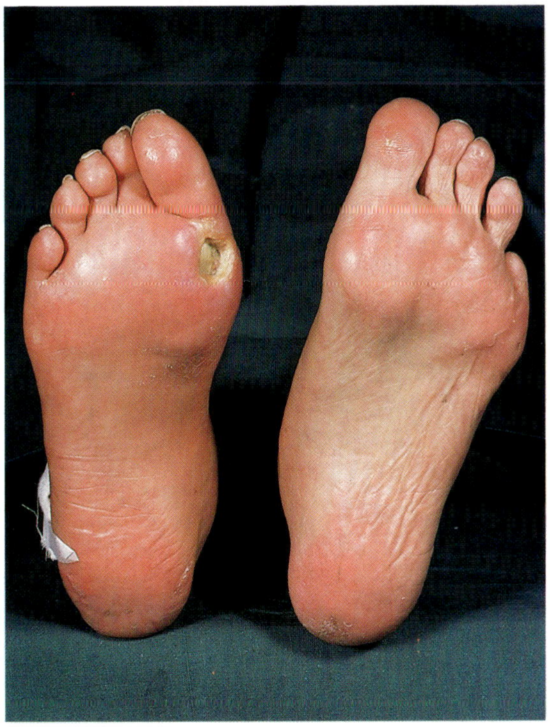

13.7

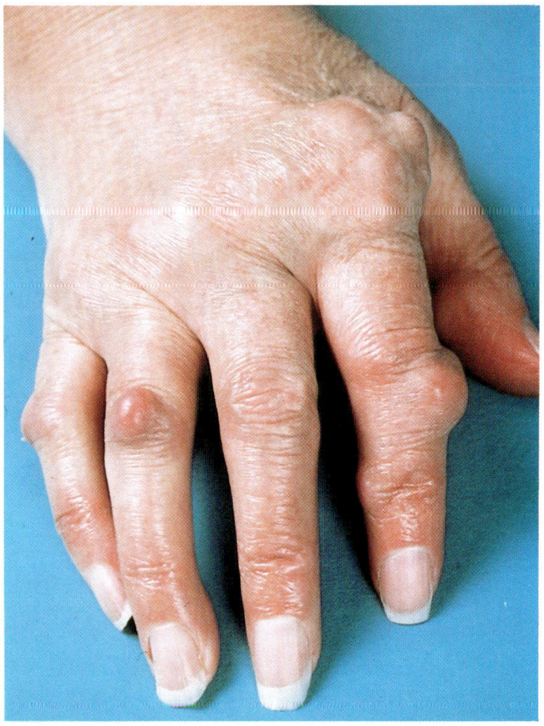

13.8

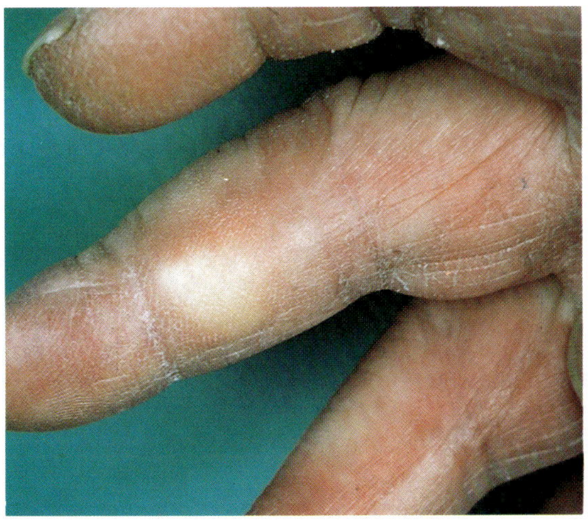

13.9

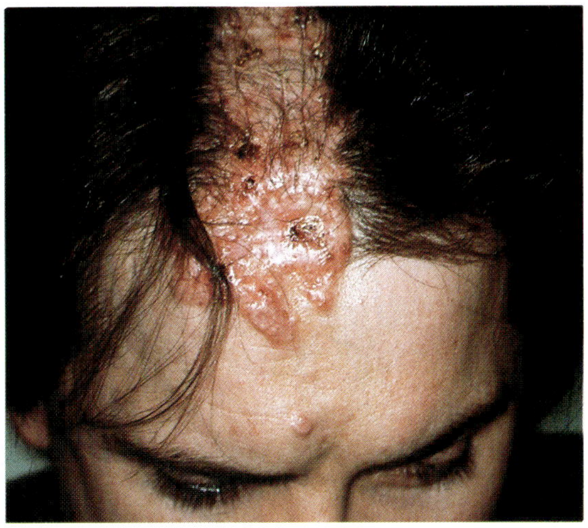

13.10

Figure 13.5 Telangiectasia may appear in the mouth and periorally, especially in the CRST variant (see Figure 13.8). Widening of the periodontal ligament is seen radiographically in some patients.

Figure 13.6 Raynaud's phenomenon is common in systemic sclerosis and can lead to digital wasting and necrosis.

Figure 13.7 Ulceration of the sole following Raynaud's phenomenon has exposed the tendon of the flexor hallucis longus here.

Systemic manifestations of systemic sclerosis include pulmonary fibrosis in most patients, hypomobile gastrointestinal tract, pulmonary hypertension, pleurisy and pericarditis.

CRST OR CREST SYNDROME

Figure 13.8 Calcinosis may be associated with Raynaud's phenomenon, scleroderma, oesophageal immobility and telangiectasia in the CRST or CREST syndrome. Calcinosis is shown here.

Figure 13.9 The calcific deposits are evident in the fingers here, but there may also be widespread calcification of internal organs.

LOCALIZED SCLERODERMA (*Morphoea*)

Figure 13.10 'Coup de sabre' appearance of morphoea.

SJÖGREN'S SYNDROME

Figure 13.11 Sjögren's syndrome is the association of dry eyes (keratoconjunctivitis sicca) with dry mouth (xerostomia). Alone these are termed primary Sjögren's syndrome (SS-1), but if a connective tissue disorder such as rheumatoid arthritis is present, the condition is termed secondary Sjögren's syndrome (SS-2). Dry mouth is obvious here.

Figure 13.12 Dry eyes lead to keratoconjunctivitis.

Figure 13.13 Rheumatoid arthritis is the most common connective tissue disease associated with SS-2, but there are common associations with primary biliary cirrhosis, systemic lupus erythematosus, systemic sclerosis, and other disorders.

Figure 13.14 Dry mouth predisposes to oral infections, especially candidosis, and caries as here. Incidentally, the black lesion in the lower vestibule is an amalgam tattoo after a previous apicetomy.

Figure 13.15 The salivary glands swell in up to one-third of patients with Sjögren's syndrome. The parotid glands most commonly enlarge.

Figure 13.16 Acute bacterial sialadenitis may be a complication in Sjögren's syndrome. Here there is pus exuding from Stensen's duct.

Sjögren's syndrome is a multisystem disorder affecting many exocrine glands. Respiratory, vaginal, and gastrointestinal secretions are impaired. There may also be neuropathy, renal tubular acidosis and interstitial pneumonitis. Rare complications of Sjögren's syndrome include lymphomas and other lymphoproliferative disorders.

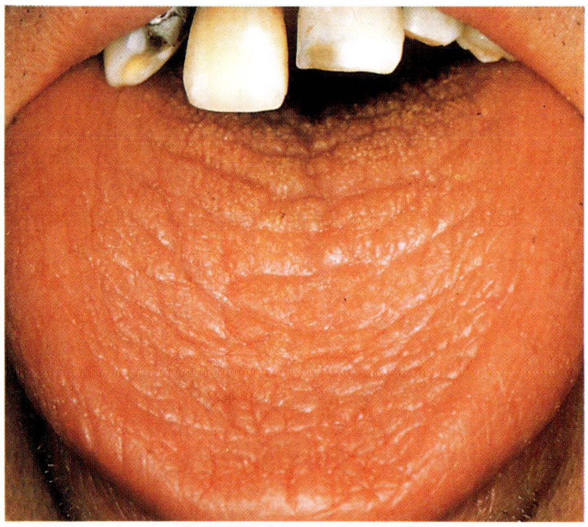

13.11

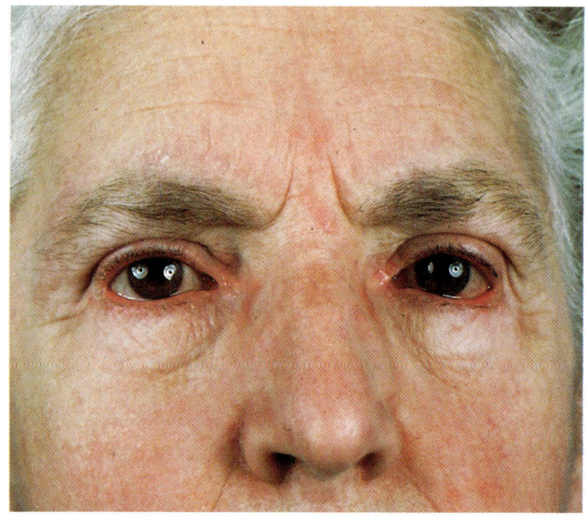

13.12

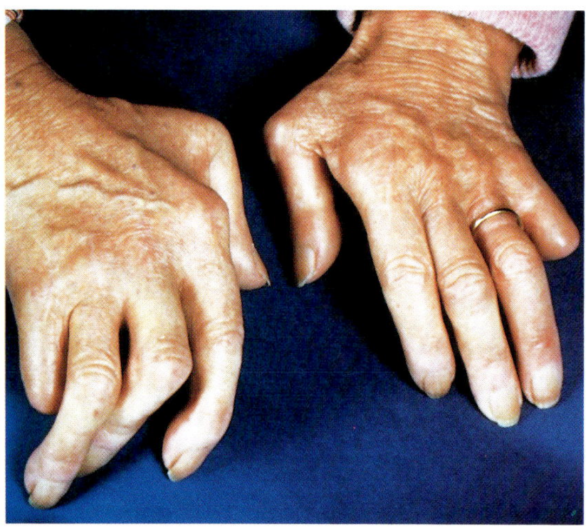

13.13

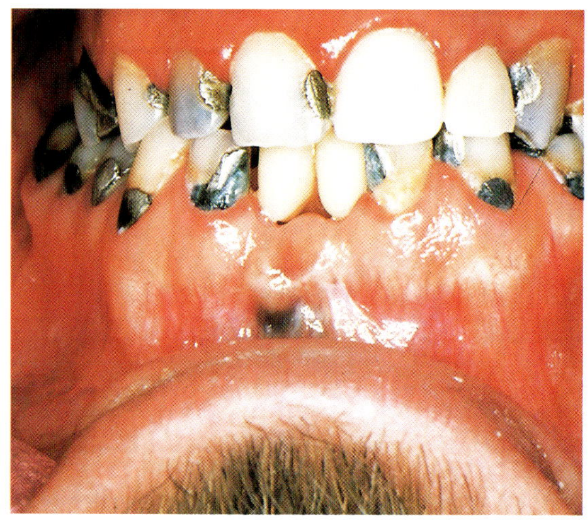

13.14

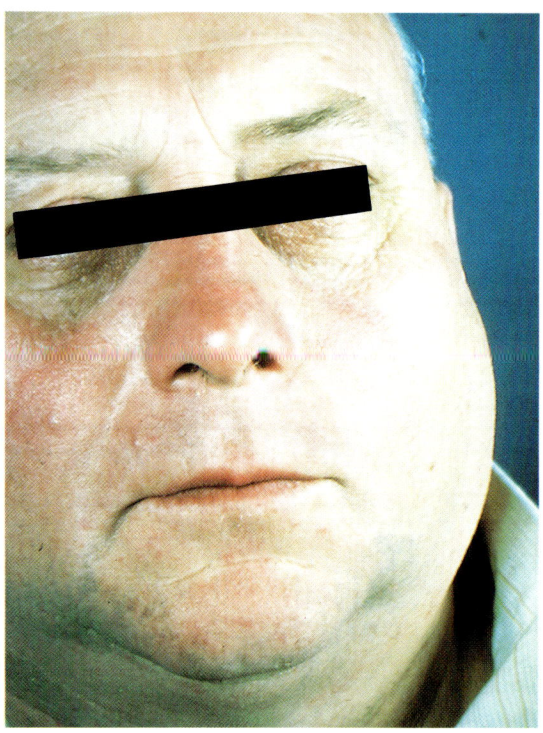

13.15

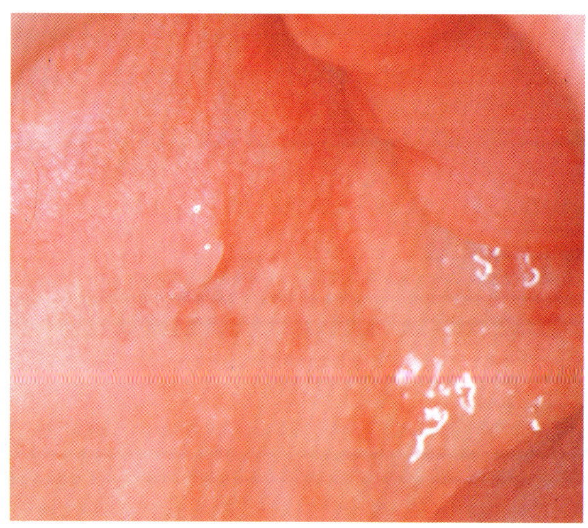

13.16

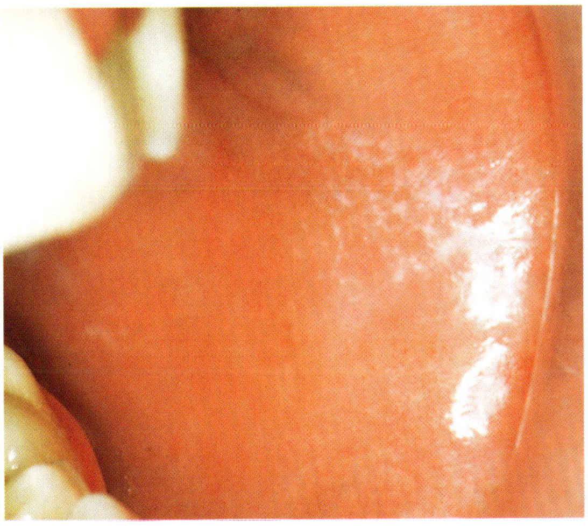

13.17

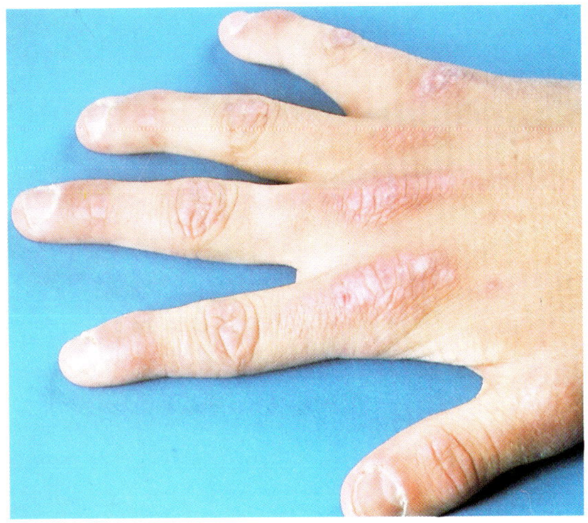

13.18

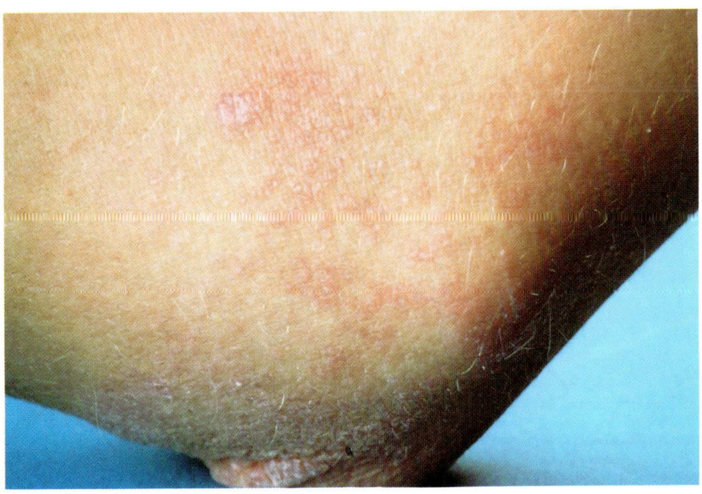

13.19

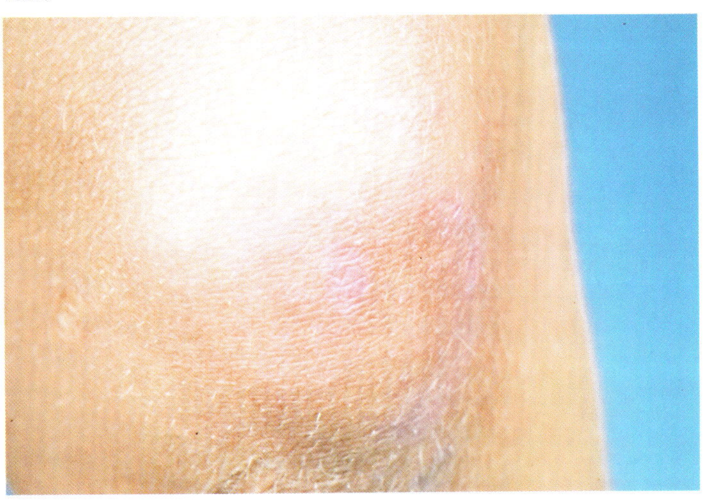

13.20

DERMATOMYOSITIS

Figure 13.17
Dermatomyositis and polymyositis are part of a group of immunologically-mediated inflammatory disorders of skeletal muscle. All have symmetric weakness of proximal muscles. Primary idiopathic dermatomyositis presents mainly in the middle-aged or elderly, with difficulty in climbing stairs, getting out of a chair or raising the head from the pillow.

Oral lesions may, as here, resemble lichen planus, or may show a dark red or bluish colour. There is also oedema of the gingiva.

Sjögren's syndrome, or other connective tissue disorders, may be seen in some patients with dermatomyositis.

Figure 13.18
Dermatomyositis is characterized by localized or diffuse erythema of the skin, a maculopapular rash, eczematoid dermatitis, or an almost pathognomonic lilac-coloured (heliotrope) change, especially over the eyelids, midface, around the nails and over the knuckles.

Figure 13.19 Skin lesions over the elbow. Skin changes precede, accompany or follow a proximal muscle weakness resembling polymyositis.

Figure 13.20 Skin lesions over the knee, another typical site.

Dermatomyositis is occasionally (about 10 per cent) associated with internal malignancy (lung, ovary, breast or stomach) or induced by drugs such as penicillamine or by Coxsackie viruses.

Childhood dermatomyositis is distinguished by vasculitis, arthritis, Raynaud's phenomenon and calcinosis.

PYOGENIC ARTHRITIS

Figure 13.21 Pyogenic arthritis of the temporomandibular joint (TMJ) is rare but may follow a penetrating injury; may result from contiguous infection; or may be haematogenous, for example, gonococcal. Infection may result in ankylosis.

RHEUMATOID ARTHRITIS

Figure 13.22 Rheumatoid arthritis (RA) is a chronic relapsing inflammatory arthritis. It usually affects many diarthrodial joints and is characterized by morning stiffness of the joints which, in advanced disease, become severely deformed.

Juvenile rheumatoid arthritis (20 per cent of which is Still's syndrome, with systemic disease) may interfere with mandibular growth, as shown here, and cause ankylosis. Sjögren's syndrome, however, is the most common oral complication of rheumatoid arthritis.

Figure 13.23 Involvement of the TMJ is common in rheumatoid arthritis but symptoms are rare. Osteoporosis, flattening of the mandibular condyle, marginal irregularities and limited movement may be seen. There may be restricted oral opening. The condyle may necrose in a patient on corticosteroids, leading to a slight anterior open bite, as here.

Osteoarthrosis may also affect the TMJ but, unlike RA, virtually never causes ankylosis.

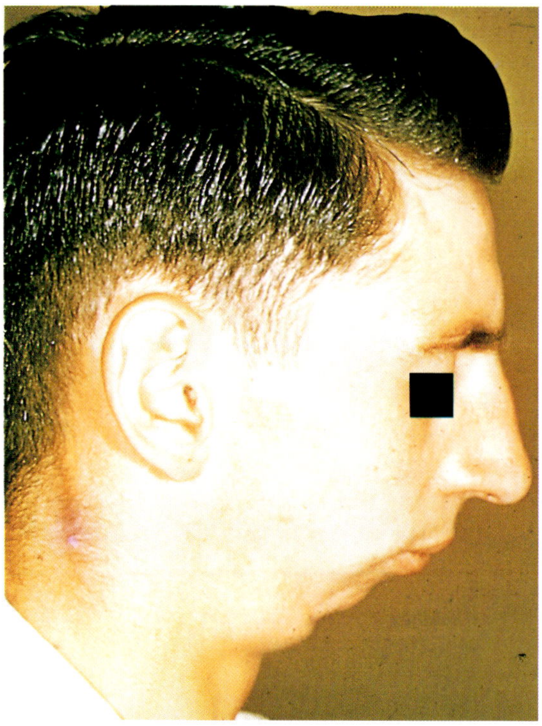

13.21

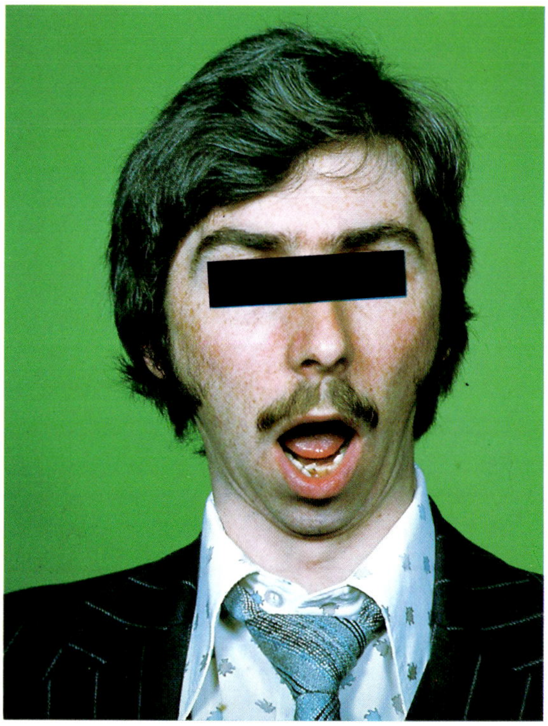

13.22

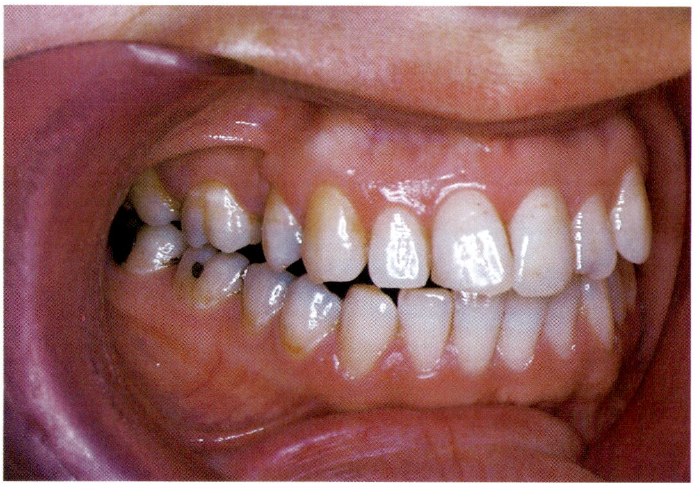

13.23

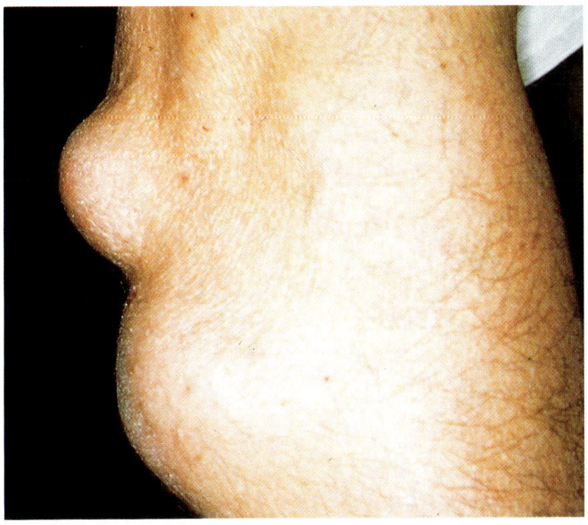

13.24

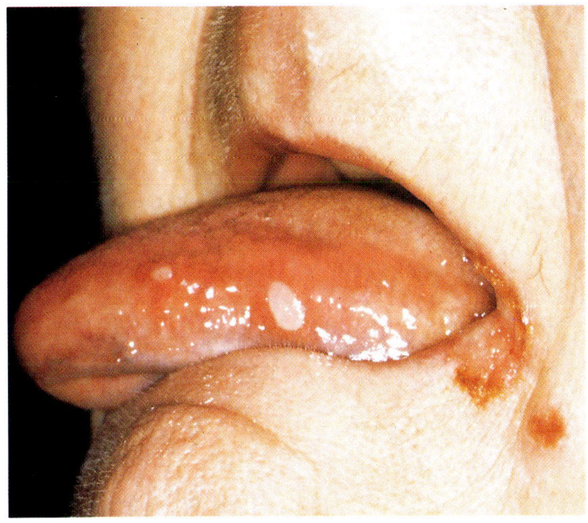

13.25

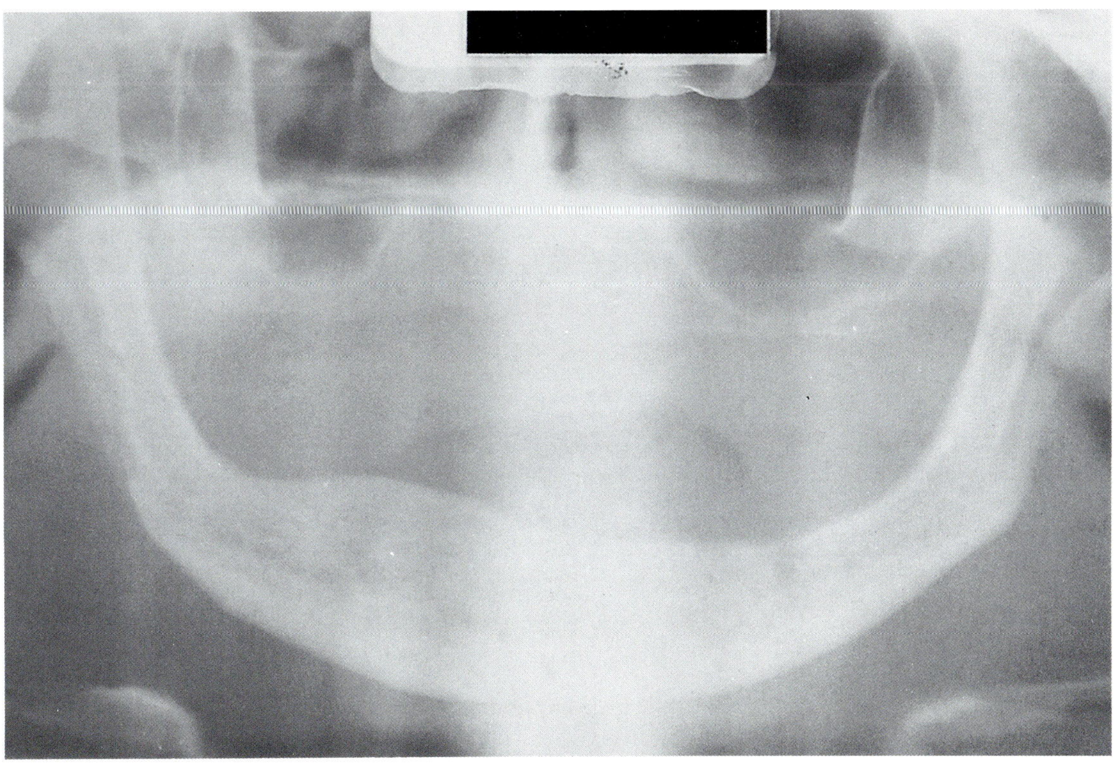

13.26

Figure 13.24 Rheumatoid nodules. Extra-articular features of RA include these subcutaneous nodules, nail-bed vascular loops, pleurisy, pulmonary fibrosis, pericarditis, scleritis and episcleritis, nerve entrapment syndromes and vasculitic skin ulcers.

FELTY'S SYNDROME

Figure 13.25 Felty's syndrome is the association of rheumatoid arthritis with splenomegaly and neutropenia, manifesting with recurrent infections. Patients with Felty's syndrome have a higher incidence of episcleritis, leg ulcers, pleurisy and neuropathy than do those with classical RA. Oral ulceration may be seen, either herpetic or, as here, non-specific

POLYVINYL CHLORIDE ACRO-OSTEOLYSIS

Figure 13.26 Occupational exposure to polyvinyl chloride may rarely cause a scleroderma-like disorder, sometimes with destruction of the mandibular condyle, as here, or resorption of the zygomatic arches.

MASSETERIC HYPERTROPHY

Figure 13.27 The masseter hypertrophies especially where there are parafunctional habits such as jaw-clenching.

Figure 13.28 Computed tomography scan showing thickened masseters.

TEMPOROMANDIBULAR JOINT SUBLUXATION

Figure 13.29 Some patients are able to sublux their TMJ deliberately. Subluxation is especially liable to occur in hypermobility syndromes, such as Ehlers–Danlos syndrome.

TEMPOROMANDIBULAR PAIN-DYSFUNCTION SYNDROME (*Facial arthromyalgia*)

Figure 13.30 A common complaint is of discomfort, and/or clicking and/or locking of the TMJ. Seen predominantly in young adult females the aetiology is unclear but may include psychogenic and/or occlusal factors. Clinical features include normal radiographic findings but discomfort on palpation of the TMJ and masticatory muscles, sometimes crepitus, and limitation of mandibular movements. This girl has caused erythema on the face by repeatedly rubbing the painful area.

Pain-dysfunction syndrome of the TMJ may be associated with migraine and other disorders which have a psychogenic element.

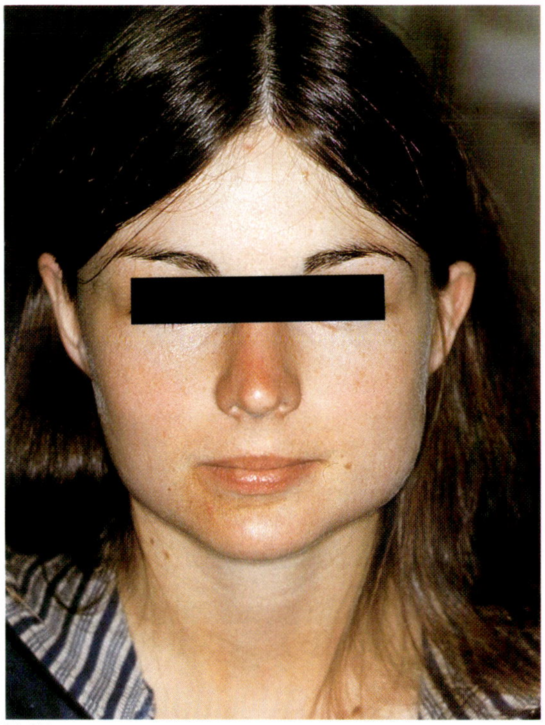

13.27

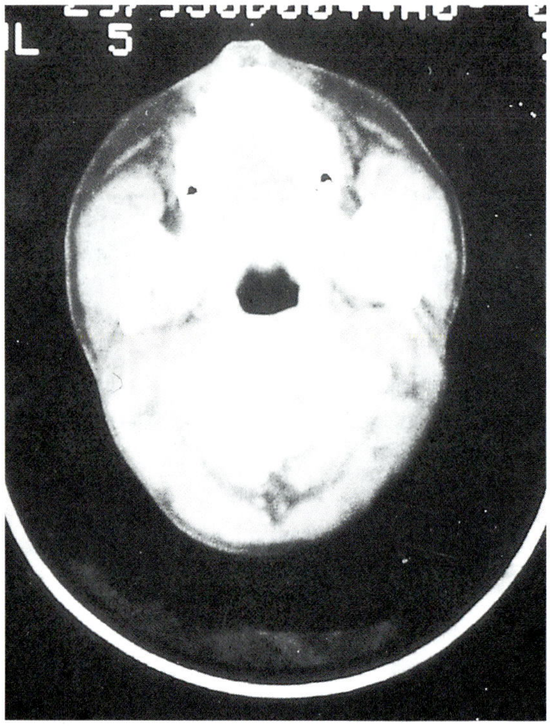

13.28

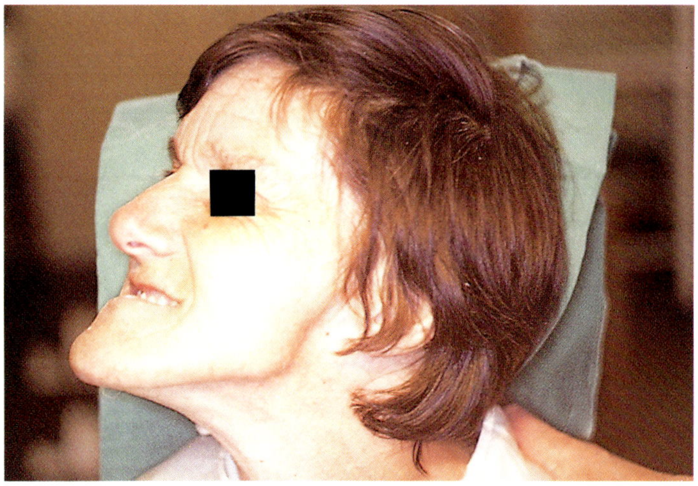

13.29

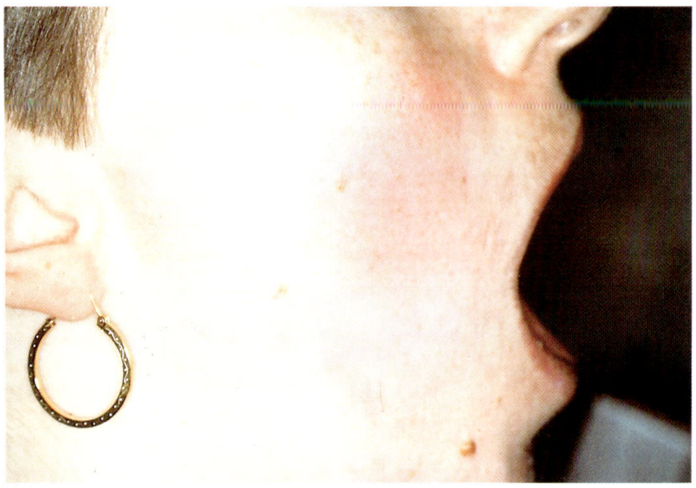

13.30

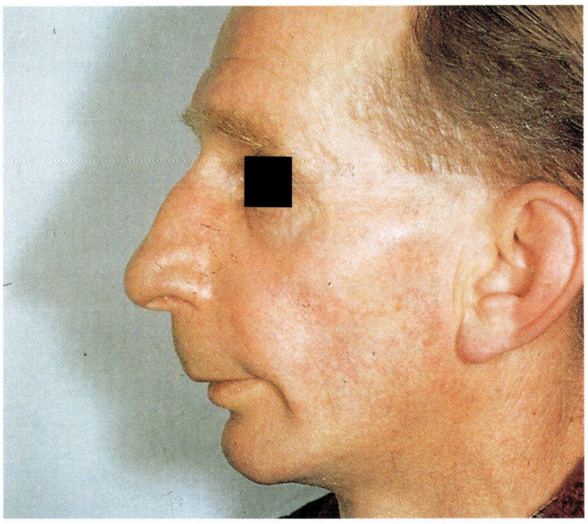

13.31

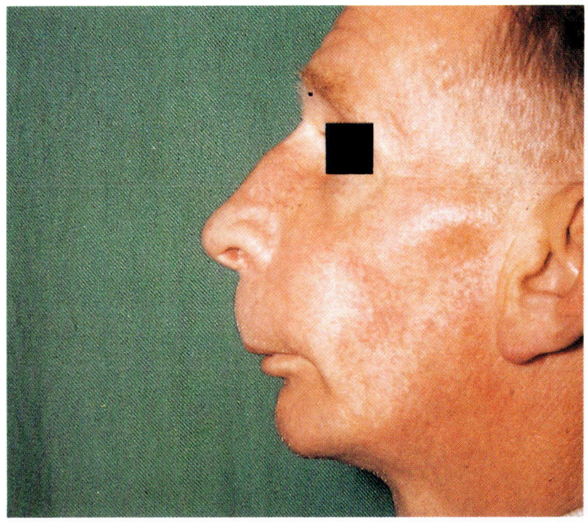

13.32

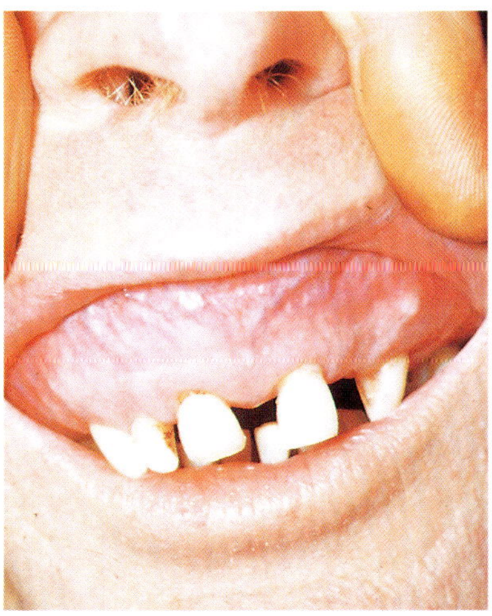

13.33

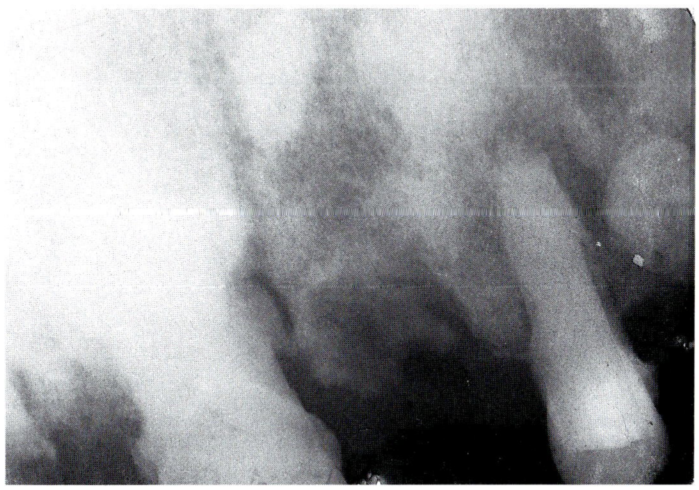

13.34

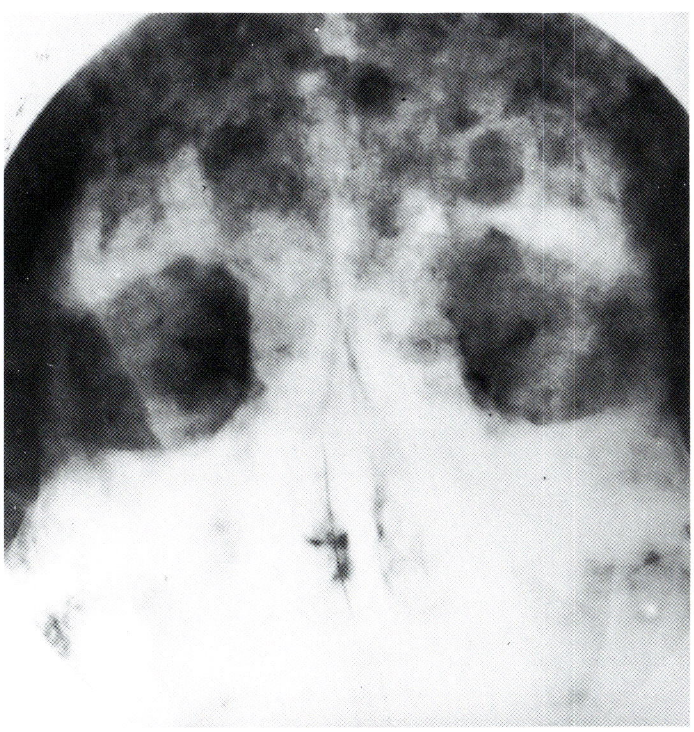

13.35

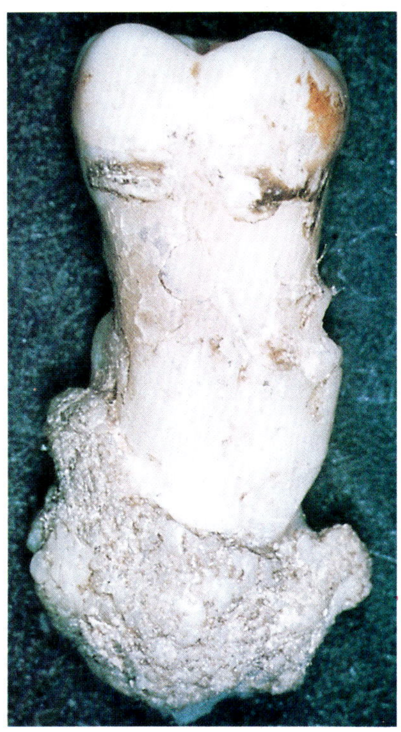

13.36

PAGET'S DISEASE (*Osteitis deformans*)

Figure 13.31 Paget's disease is common in Western countries, particularly the United Kingdom, in males aged over 50 years. Of unknown aetiology, possibly viral, the disease usually presents with swelling, often of skull bones.

Swelling of the maxilla (leontiasis ossea) is seen here in Paget's disease. The calvarium thickens in about one-half of the patients with clinical Paget's disease.

Figure 13.32 Same patient as in Figure 13.33, after 4 years, showing increase in maxillary swelling.

Figure 13.33 Maxillary swelling and spacing of teeth. The skull or jaws, especially the maxilla, are often affected in Paget's disease.

Figure 13.34 'Cotton wool' appearance of bone.

Figure 13.35 The skull bones are thickened and show a 'cotton wool' appearance on radiography. There may be overgrowth at the base.

Figure 13.36 Hypercementosis is a common feature of Paget's disease affecting the jaws.

PAGET'S DISEASE (*continued*)

Figure 13.37 The sacral and lumbar vertebrae, pelvis, tibiae and femur are commonly involved. The affected bones soften and bend as here.

Figure 13.38 Lytic areas are seen in long bones in the early phase of Paget's disease. The bone shows an irregularly widened cortex and sometimes perpendicular radiolucent lines (cortical infractions), or fractures.

Figure 13.39 Pelvic changes include bone resorption and new bone formation and a thickening of the pelvic brim. Here there is mainly innominate and ilial involvement.

Figure 13.40 Osteosarcoma is a rare complication of Paget's disease and is particularly unusual in the jaws (as here).

Other complications of Paget's disease include pathological fractures, spinal compression, arteriovenous shunts that may lead to high-output cardiac failure, calcific aortic valve disease, cranial nerve palsies and post-extraction haemorrhage or infection.

A rare disorder that may be a juvenile form of Paget's disease has been described with skull and maxillary enlargement and bowing of the legs (hyperostosis corticalis deformans juvenilis).

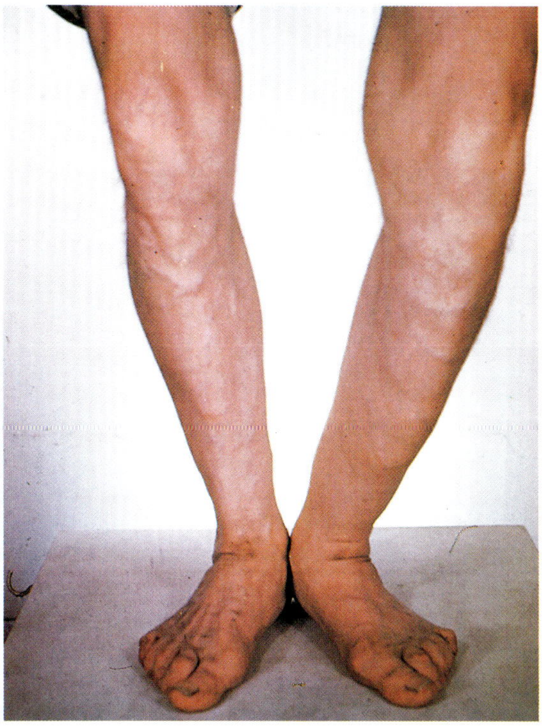

13.37

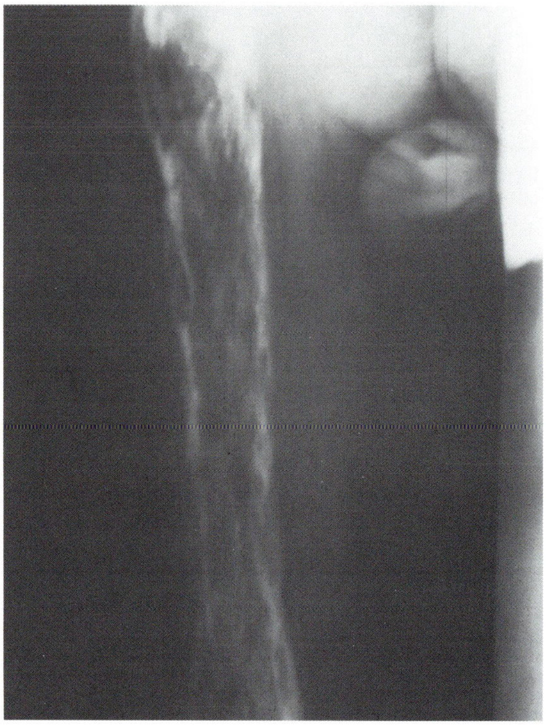

13.38

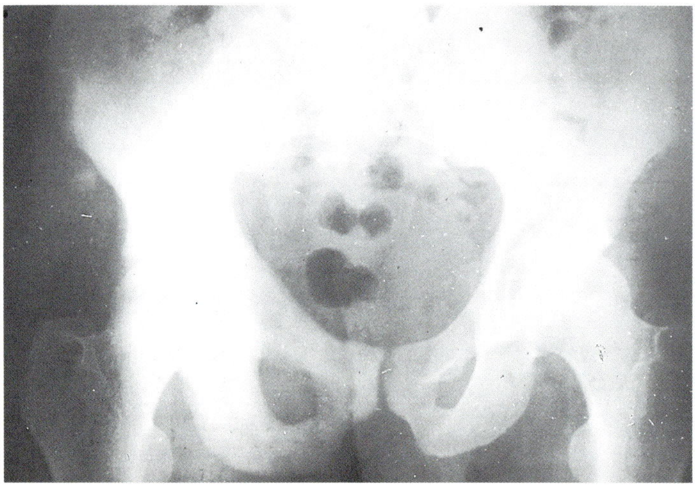

13.39

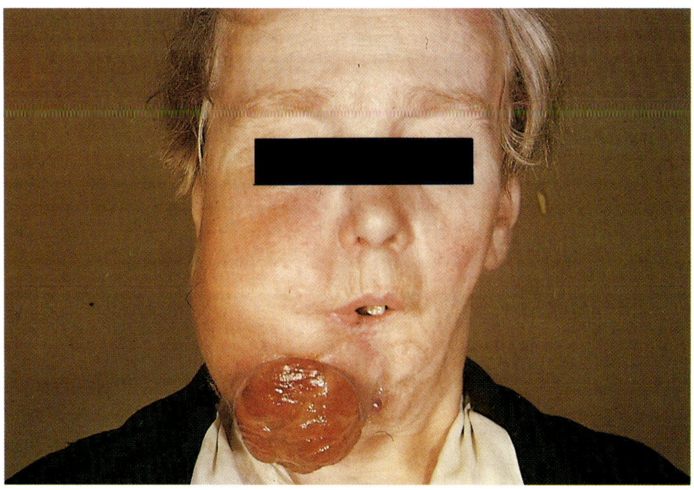

13.40

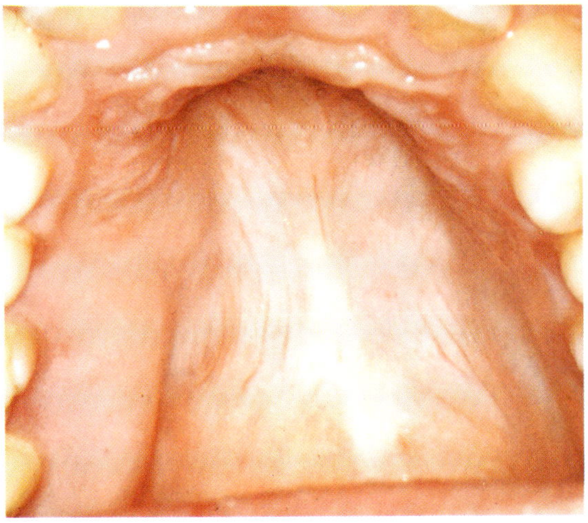

13.41

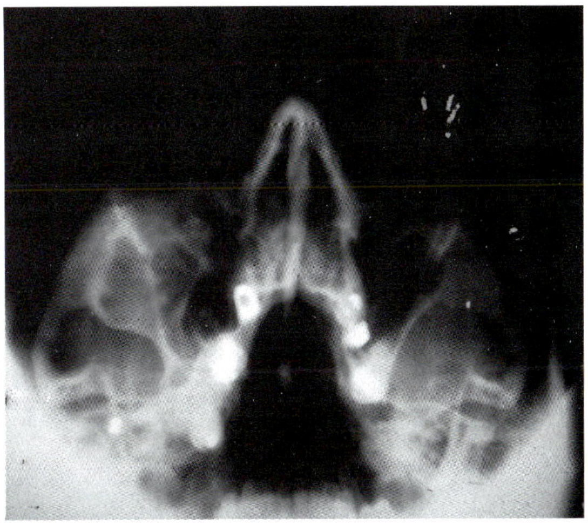

13.42

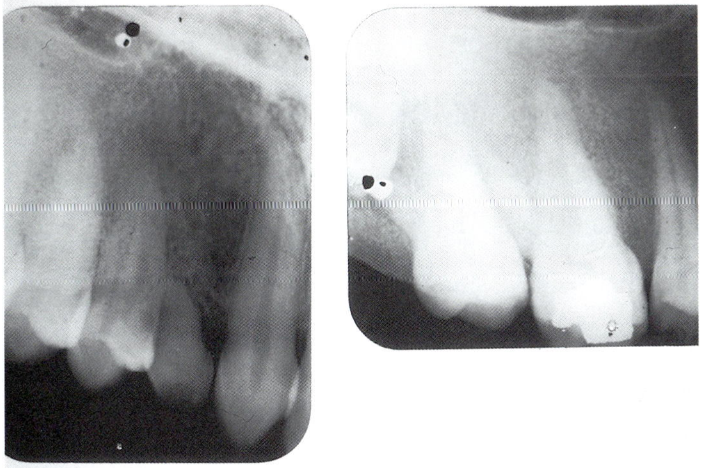

13.43

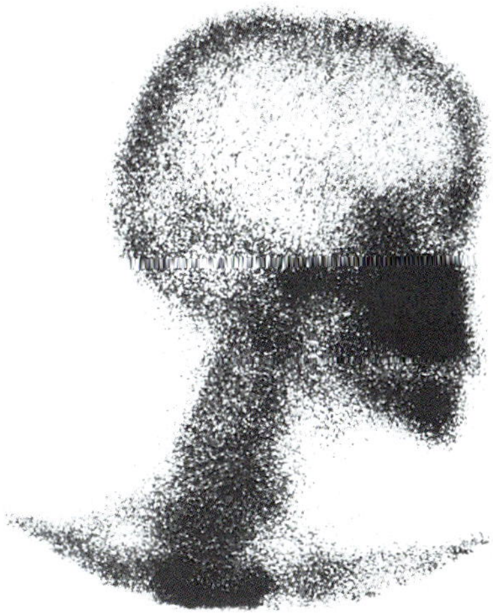

13.44

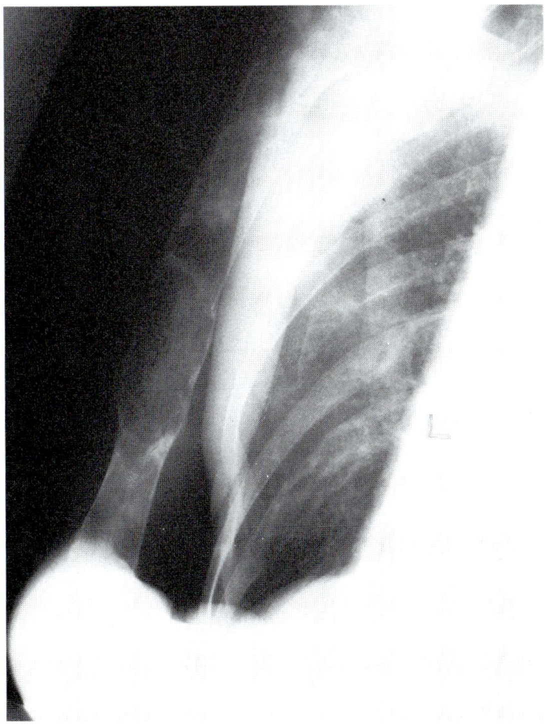

13.45

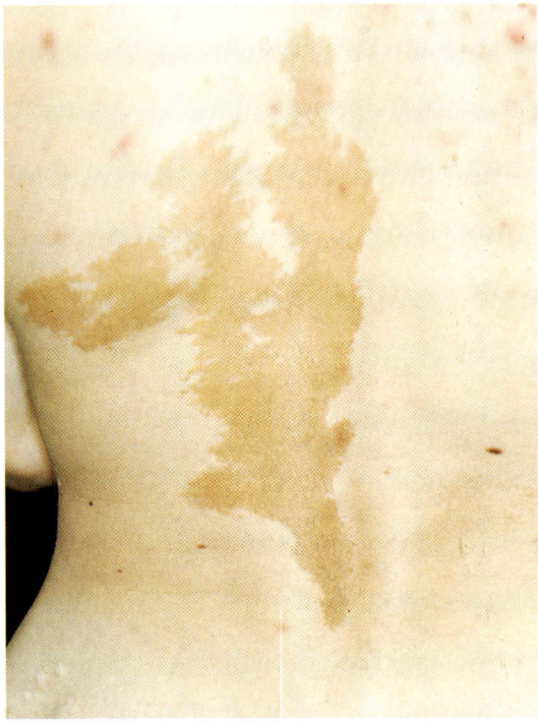

13.46

FIBROUS DYSPLASIA

Figure 13.41 Fibrous dysplasia is an uncommon benign fibro-osseous lesion, of unknown aetiology, often affecting only one bone, as here, where the maxilla is enlarged. The swelling is painless and typically ceases to grow at the time of skeletal maturity.

Four subgroups of fibrous dysplasia have been described: monostotic, polyostotic, polyostotic fibrous dysplasia of Albright's syndrome and a form confined to the craniofacial complex (craniofacial fibrous dysplasia).

Figure 13.42 Radiography shows fibrous dysplasia on the right maxilla alone in monostotic fibrous dysplasia.

Figure 13.43 The typical appearance on radiography is of a 'ground glass' pattern.

Figure 13.44 Bone scan using technetium diphosphonate shows increased uptake of radionuclide in fibrous dysplasia of the maxilla.

Figure 13.45 Several bones may be affected: the humerus is involved in this patient with polyostotic fibrous dysplasia.

ALBRIGHT'S SYNDROME (*McCune–Albright syndrome*)

Figure 13.46 Albright's syndrome is the association of polyostotic fibrous dysplasia with cutaneous hyper-pigmentation, precocious puberty and occasionally other endocrine disorders.

CHERUBISM (*Familial fibrous dysplasia*)

Figure 13.47 Cherubism is the term given to a familial type of fibrous dysplasia which typically affects the angles of the mandible to produce a cherubic appearance.

Figure 13.48 Cherubism is an autosomal dominant trait, pictured here in the brother of the patient shown in Figure 13.48. Cherubism is seen especially in males and presents usually after the age of 4–5 years.

Figure 13.49 The radiograph shows multilocular mandibular radiolucencies, expansion of the mandible and absent second molar, features common to cherubism.

The swellings increase in size and then usually regress, at least partially, at puberty. Occasionally the maxillae are involved.

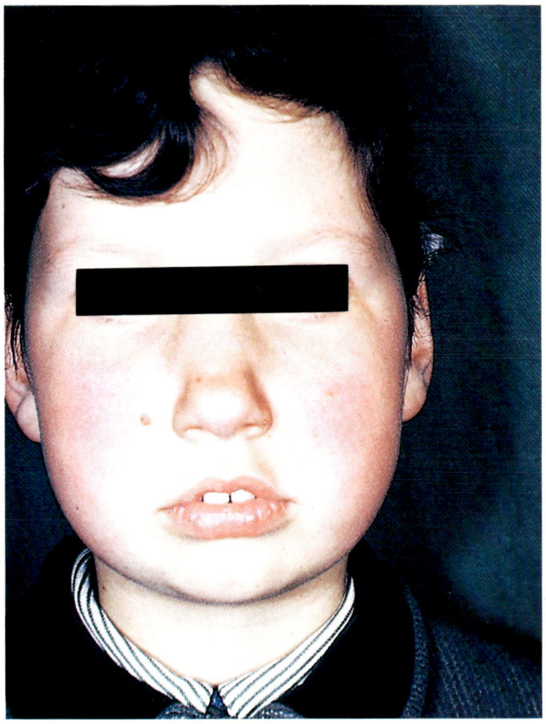

13.47

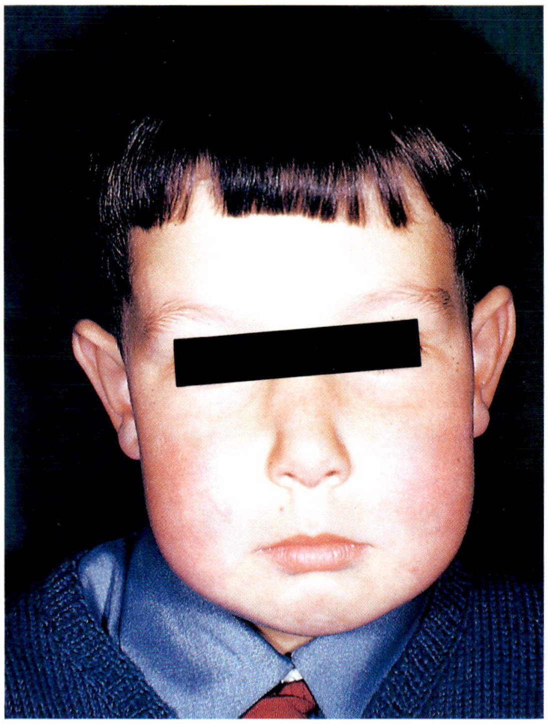

13.48

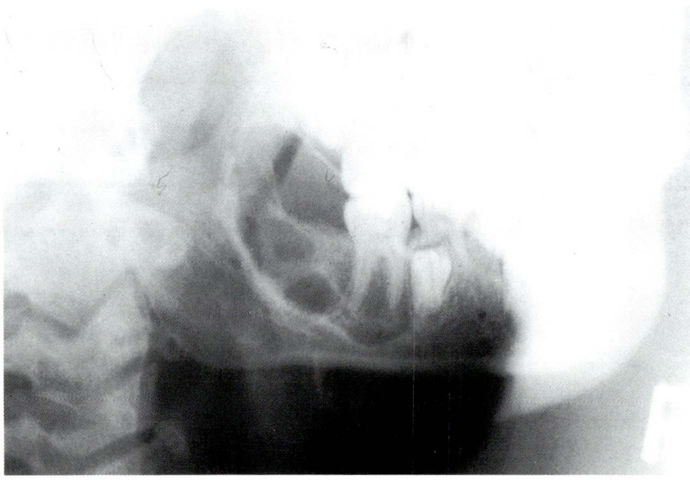

13.49

14

Congenital anomalies

BRANCHIAL CYST

Figure 14.1 A branchial cyst is a painless, developmental fluctuant swelling on the lateral aspect of the neck.

CYSTIC HYGROMA

Figure 14.2 Cervical cystic hygroma is a lymphangioma extending from the tongue down into the neck. A developmental anomaly, cystic hygroma usually presents at birth and virtually always in the first 2 years of life. Some cause dysphagia or respiratory embarrassment. A minority extend into the base of the tongue and some extend into the mediastinum.

TETRALOGY OF FALLOT

Figure 14.3 Tetralogy of Fallot is one of the most frequent of the cyanotic congenital heart diseases. Central cyanosis is seen in lips, tongue and other mucosae and the teeth are milky white in contrast. There is an increased prevalence of fissured and geographic tongue in children with cyanotic heart disease.

Figure 14.4 Ventricular septal defect, pulmonary stenosis, right ventricular hypertrophy and an aorta that overrides both ventricles are the features of the tetralogy. This patient, incidentally, has a prognathic mandible. Note the central cyanosis.

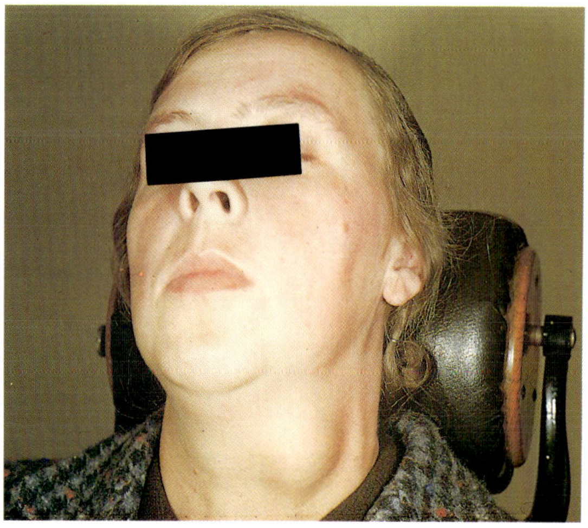

14.1

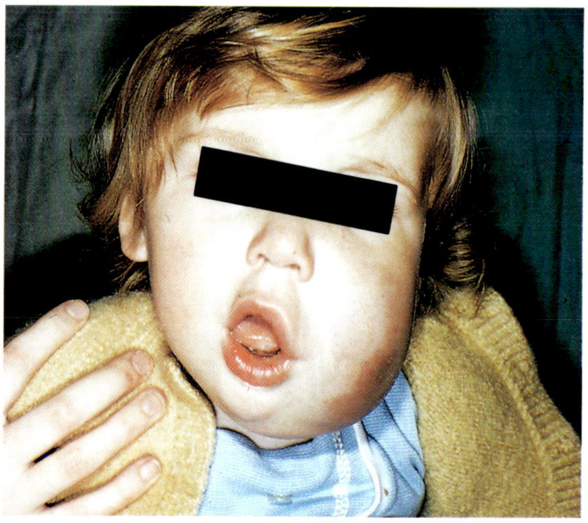

14.2

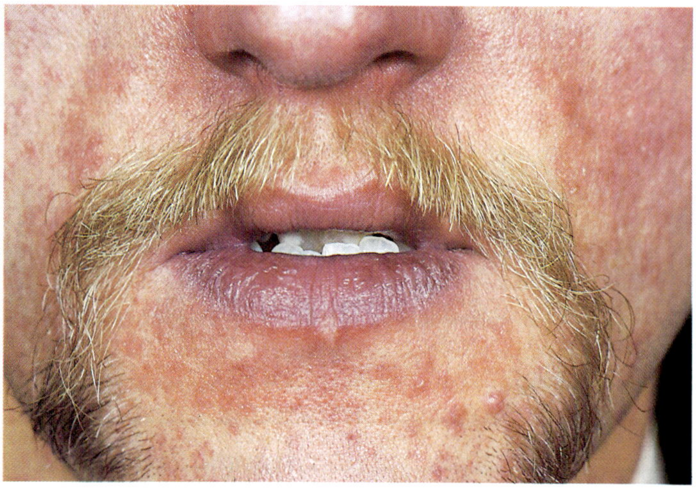

14.3

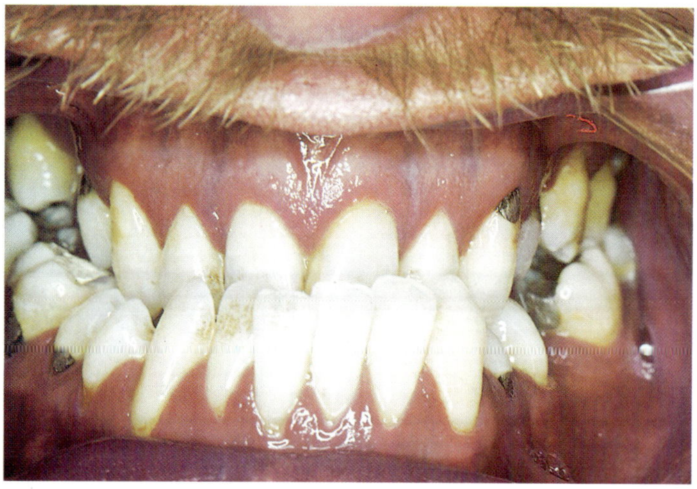

14.4

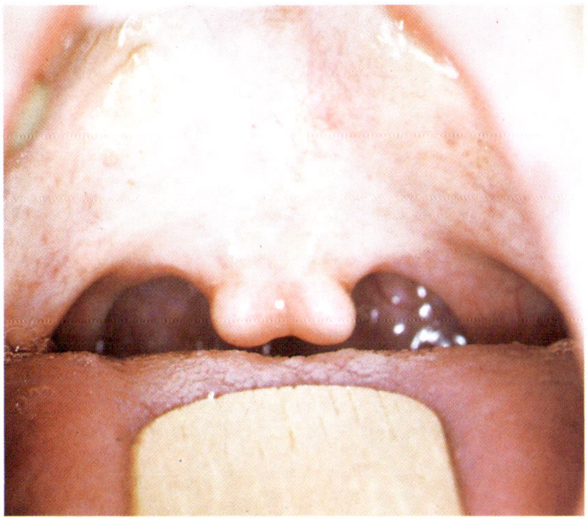

14.5

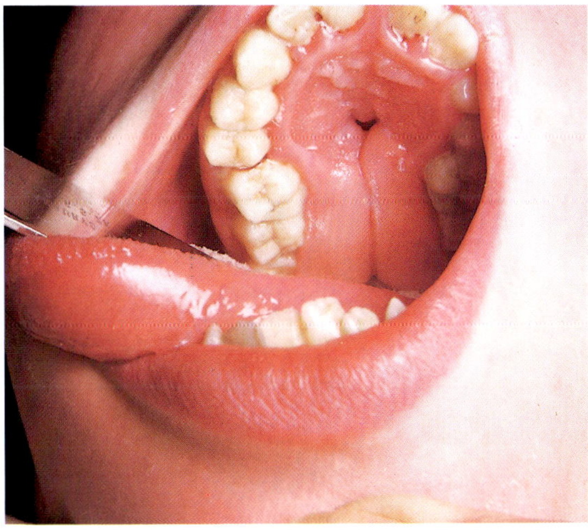

14.6

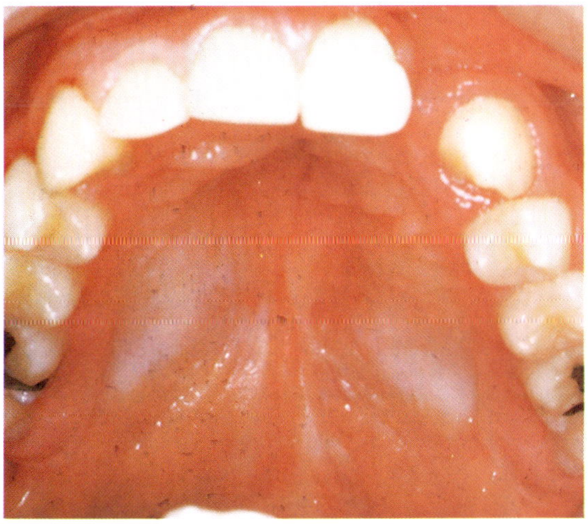

14.7

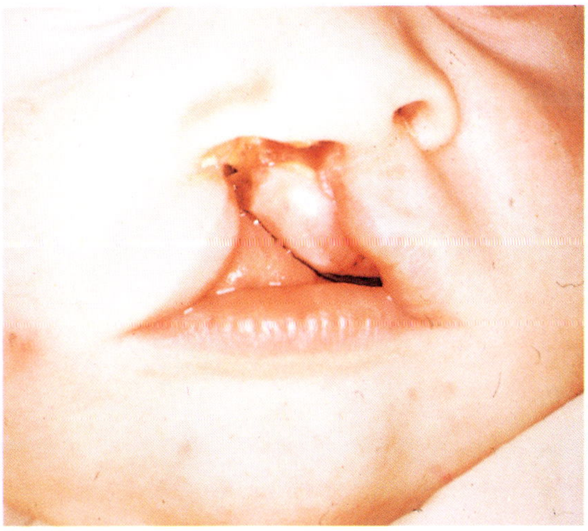

14.8

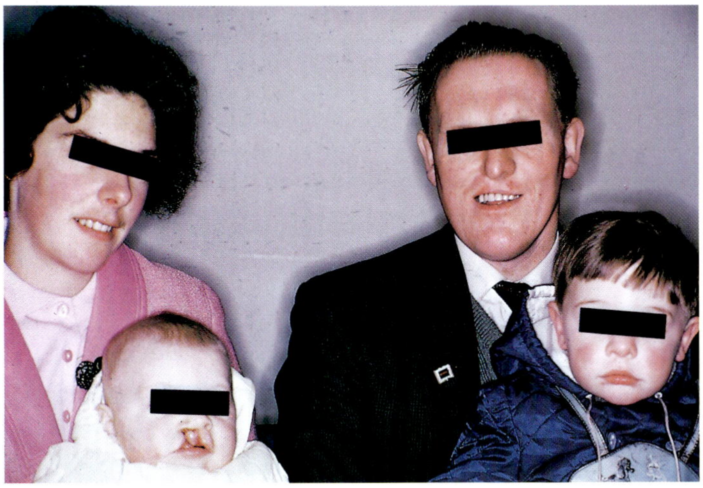

14.9

BIFID UVULA (*Cleft uvula*)

Figure 14.5 Bifid or cleft uvula is a fairly common minor manifestation of cleft palate but of little consequence.

CLEFT PALATE

Figure 14.6 Cleft of the secondary palate.

Figure 14.7 Complete unilateral cleft palate and lip after repair.

CLEFT LIP AND PALATE

Figure 14.8 Cleft lip and palate are more common together than is cleft lip alone. Though the lip is cleft here on the right, the cleft is on the left in over 60 per cent of patients. The cleft may be bilateral.

Figure 14.9 There is a familial tendency as illustrated here: when one parent is affected, the risk to a child is about 10 per cent.

Cleft lip and palate are, in about 20 per cent of cases, associated with anomalies of head and neck, extremities, genitalia or heart.

Isolated cleft palate is especially associated with Down's syndrome, Pierre-Robin syndrome, Treacher Collins' syndrome and Klippel-Feil syndrome.

TONGUE-TIE (*Ankyloglossia*)

Figure 14.10 Ankyloglossia is usually a congenital anomaly of little consequence. There is no evidence that ankyloglossia interferes with speech.

The eruption of lower permanent incisors lingual to the deciduous incisors is normal.

Figure 14.11 The main consequence of ankyloglossia is difficulty in using the tongue to cleanse food away from the teeth and vestibules.

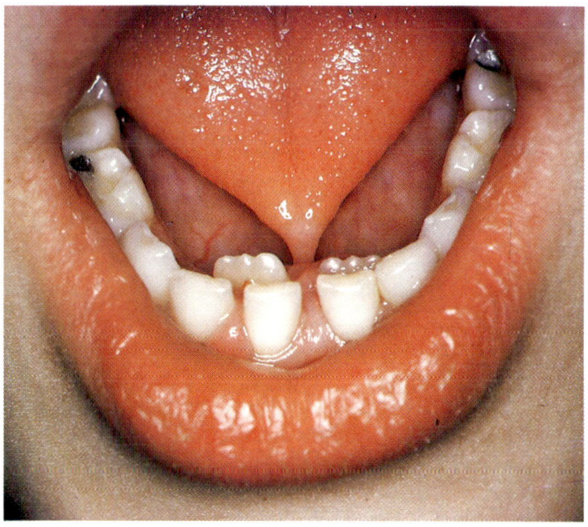

14.10

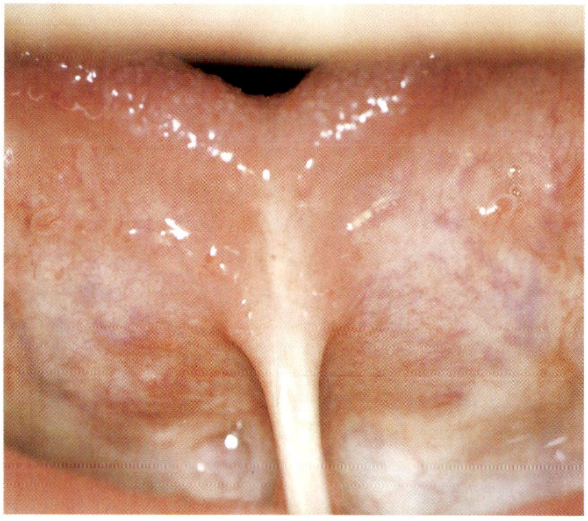

14.11

LIP PIT

Figure 14.12 Commissural lip pits are blind epithelial-lined developmental anomalies of no consequence.

Pits may also be paramedian on the vermilion and may exude mucus.

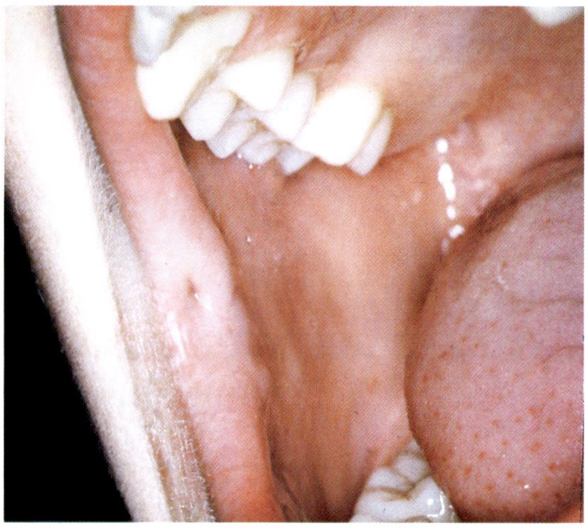

14.12

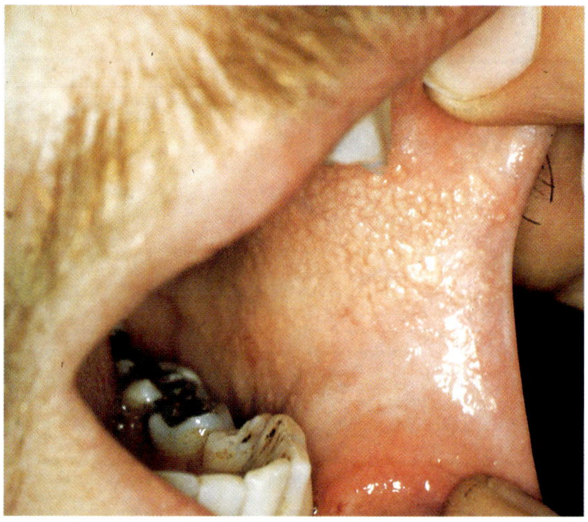

14.13

FORDYCE SPOTS

Figure 14.13 Fordyce spots are sebaceous glands in the vermilion of the lip (mainly the upper lip), and in the oral mucosa, especially in the anterior buccal mucosa, as here. Fordyce spots are of no consequence, but appear to be increased in patients with rheumatic disorders, especially Reiter's syndrome.

Figure 14.14 Often few in number, Fordyce spots are found in about 80 per cent of the population and become increasingly obvious with age. The retromolar region is often affected as here.

Figure 14.15 Fordyce spots are common in the upper lip and may cause the patient to complain because of their appearance.

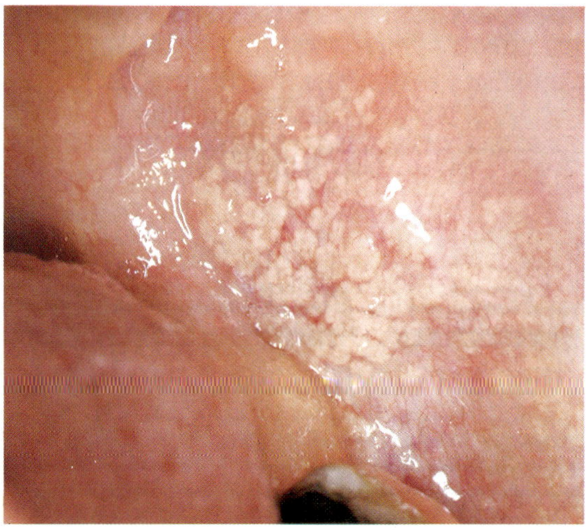

14.14

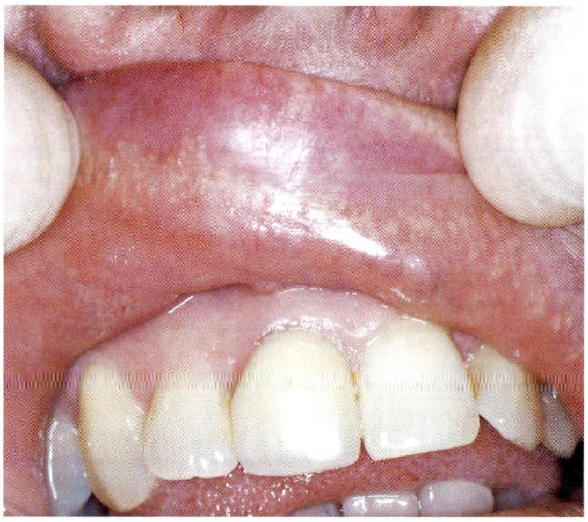

14.15

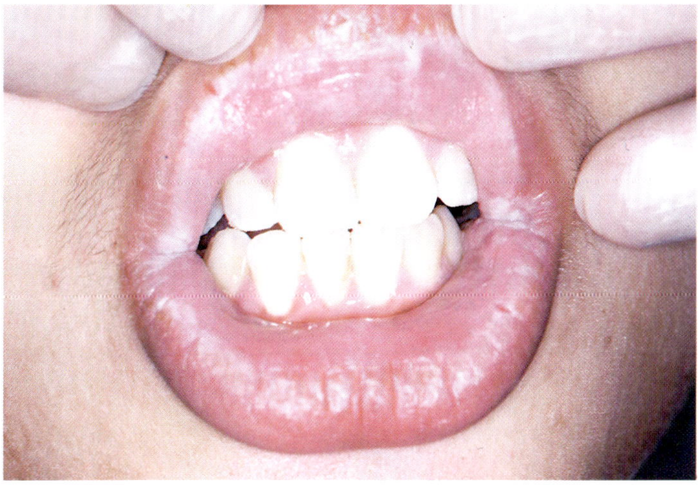

14.16

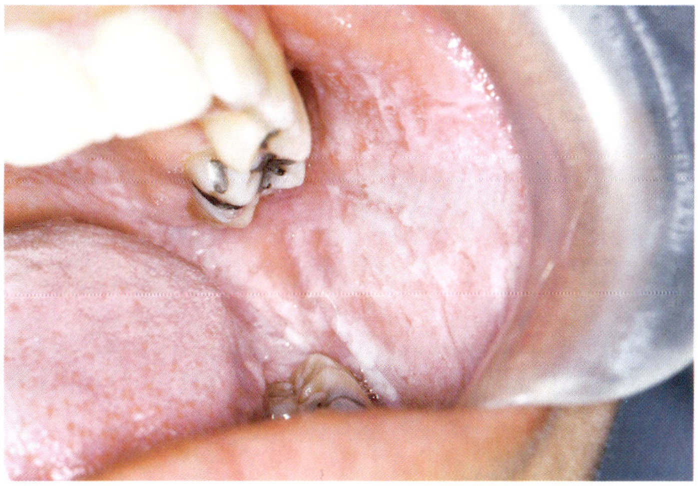

14.17

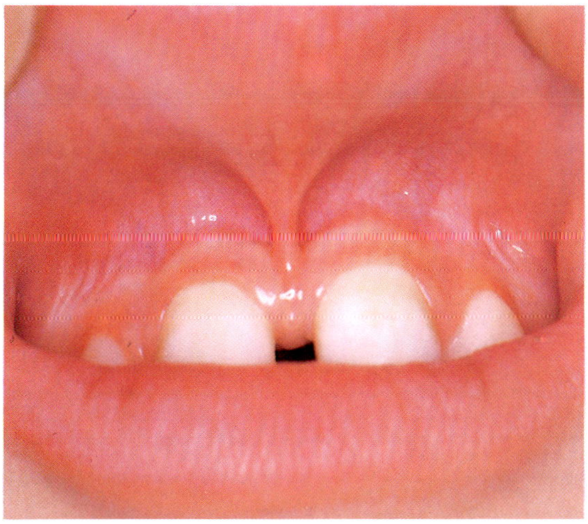

14.18

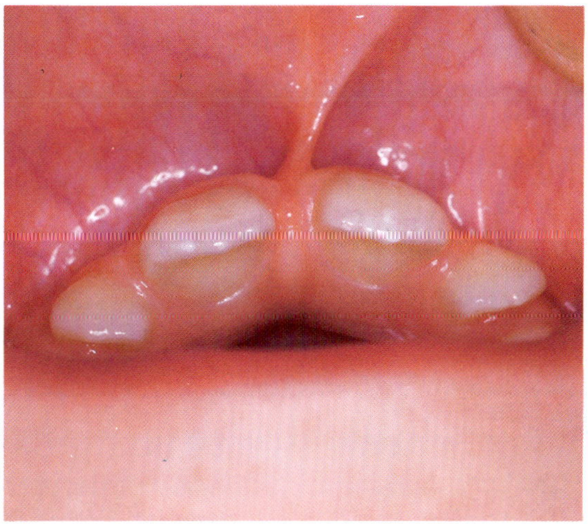

14.19

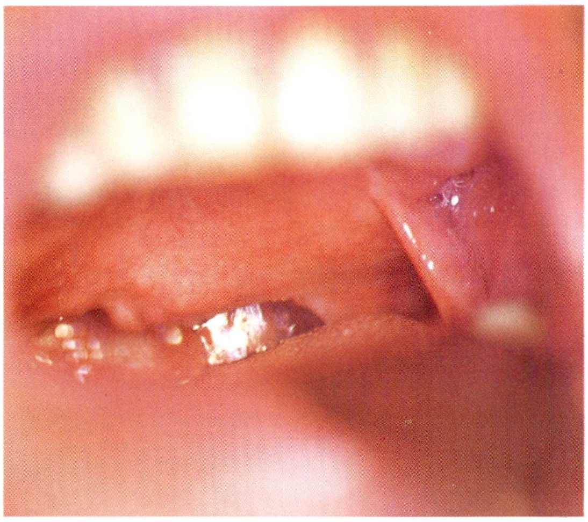

14.20

WHITE SPONGE NAEVUS (*Familial white folded gingivostomatosis*)

Figure 14.16 White sponge naevus is a symptomless inconsequential autosomal dominant condition which manifests from infancy. The oral mucosa is thickened, folded, spongy and white or grey.

Figure 14.17 Lesions are bilateral in the oral mucosa and can affect vaginal or anal mucosa.

ABNORMAL LABIAL FRAENUM

Figure 14.18 A labial maxillary fraenum may occasionally be associated with spacing between the central incisors – a maxillary median diastema.

Figure 14.19 The same patient as shown in Figure 14.18, showing the palatal attachment of the fraenum.

ABSENT UVULA

Figure 14.20 The uvula is rarely absent and then usually as a result of trauma or surgery. The uvula may be hypoplastic in Cowden's syndrome.

CLEIDOCRANIAL DYSPLASIA (*Cleidocranial dysostosis*)

Figure 14.21 Cleidocranial dysplasia is an inherited defect of membrane bones, often an autosomal dominant trait. Defects involve mainly the skull and clavicles. Persistence of the metopic suture gives rise to a vertical midline furrow in the forehead with frontal bossing.

Figure 14.22 The sutures are still open and multiple wormian bones evident in the occipito-parietal region. The midface is hypoplastic.

Figure 14.23 The clavicles are hypoplastic or aplastic. Here the right clavicle is aplastic, the left hypoplastic.

Figure 14.24. When the patient attempts to bring his shoulders forward and together, he can almost approximate them.

Figure 14.25 Radiography shows absence of the clavicles in the patient shown in Figure 14.24.

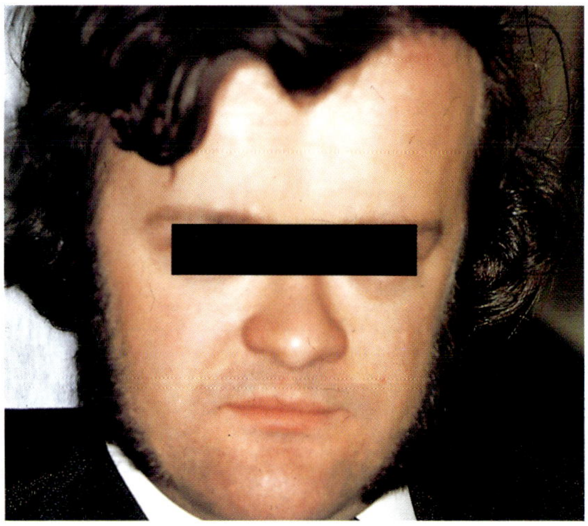

14.21

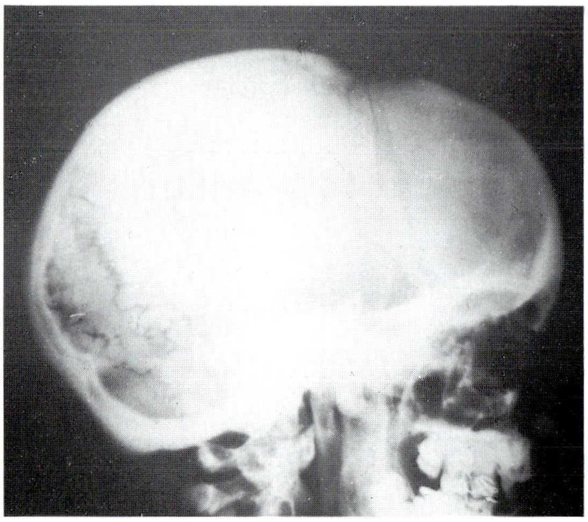

14.22

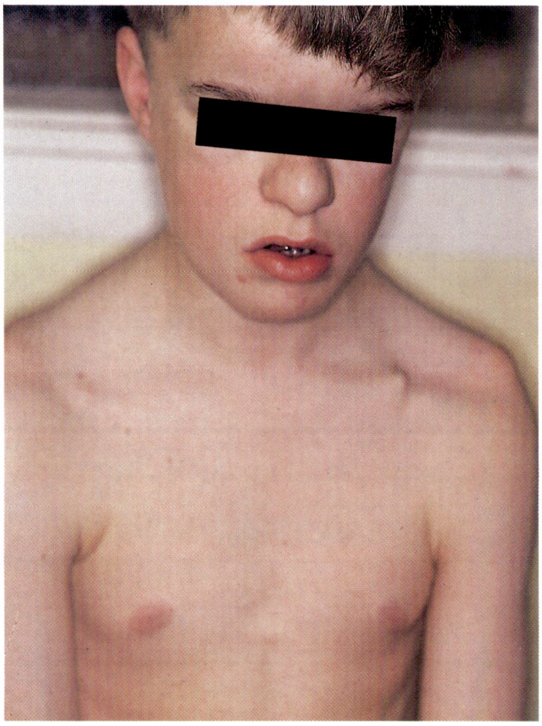

14.23

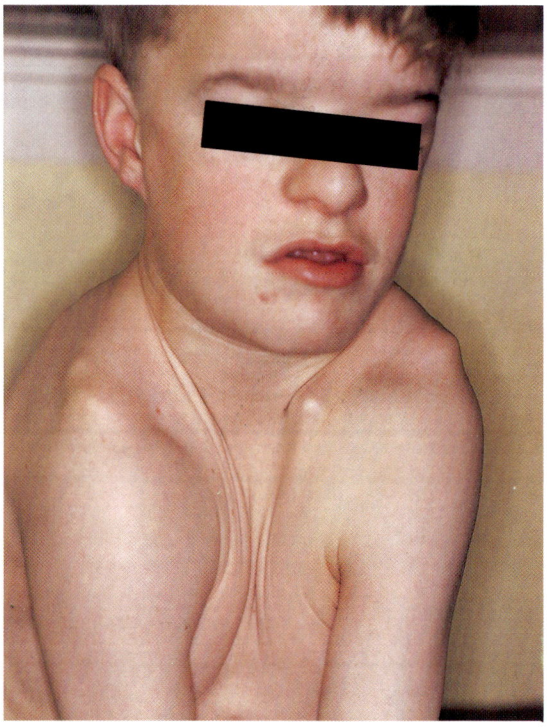

14.24

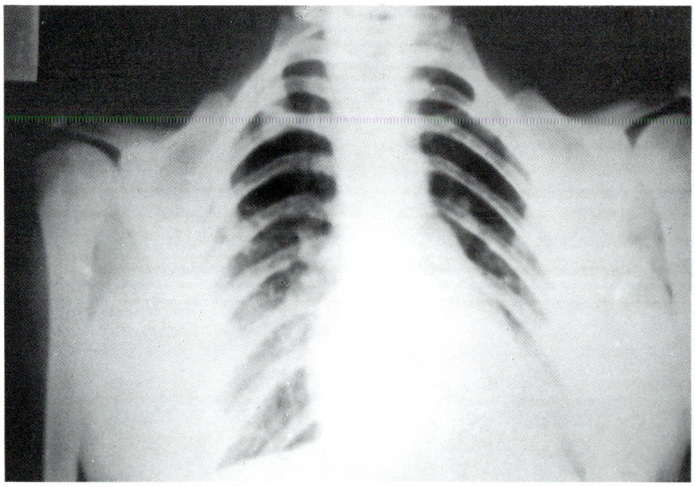

14.25

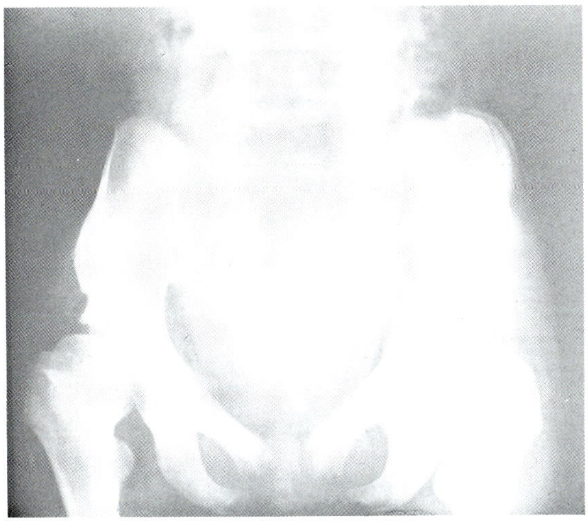

14.26

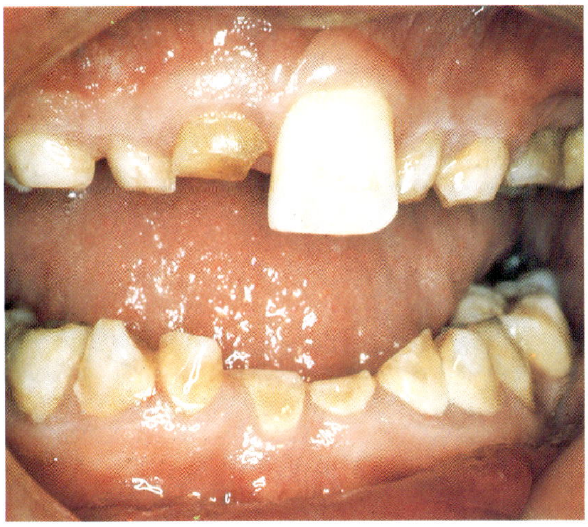

14.27

Figure 14.26 Pelvic anomalies may be seen and kyphoscoliosis is common.

Figure 14.27 The dentition may be disrupted because of multiple supernumerary teeth and impactions.

Figure 14.28 Radiography shows multiple unerupted and impacted teeth. Dentigerous cysts commonly form.

Figure 14.29 Several unerupted teeth and a dentigerous cyst.

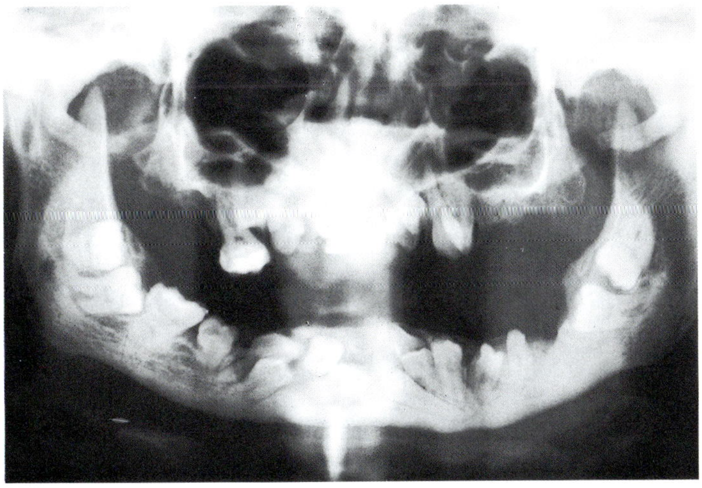

14.28

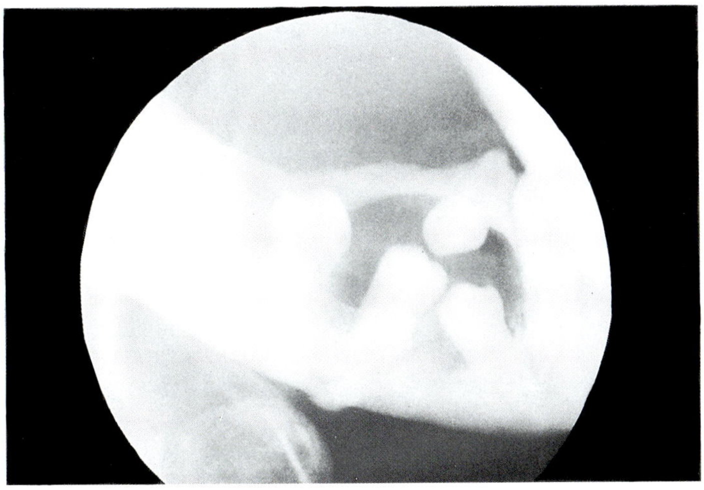

14.29

APERT'S SYNDROME
(*Acrocephalosyndactyly*)

Figure 14.30 Craniosynostosis, a high steep forehead, ocular hyperteleorism and antimongoloid slope to the eyes are characteristics of Apert's and Crouzon's syndromes.

Figure 14.31 Apert's syndrome involves progressive synostosis of bones in the hands, feet and vertebrae as well as ankylosis of joints.

Figure 14.32 Palatal anomalies are common, and one-third of patients have cleft palate. Maxillary hypoplasia is seen.

CROUZON'S SYNDROME
(*Craniofacial dysostosis*)

Figure 14.33 Craniosynostosis, ocular hyperteleorism and proptosis are characteristics of Crouzon's syndrome. Teeth may be missing, peg-shaped or enlarged.

Figure 14.34 Radiography shows craniosynostosis and abnormal skull morphology and pronounced digital impressions ('copper-beaten skull').

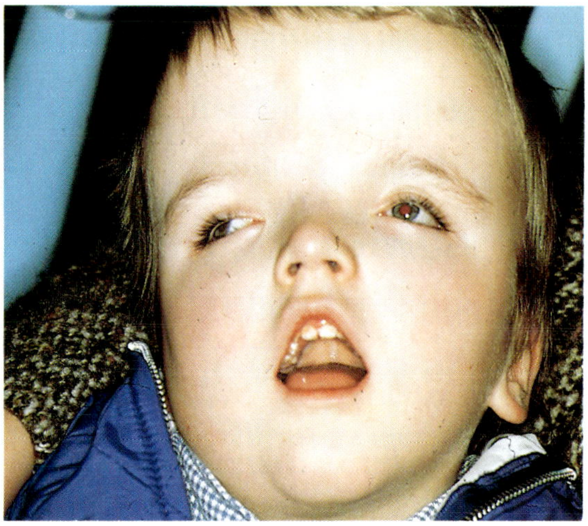

14.30

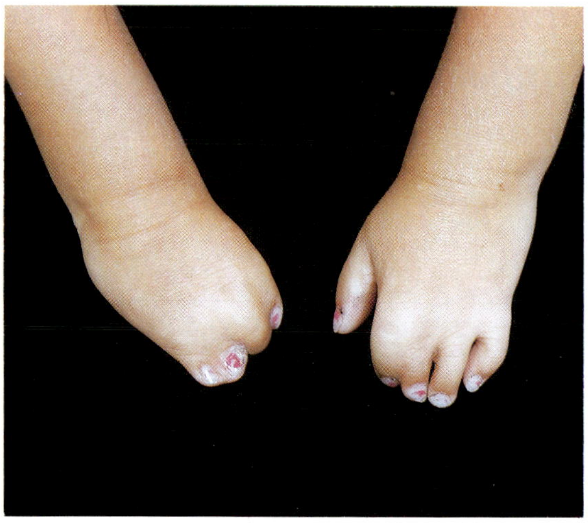

14.31

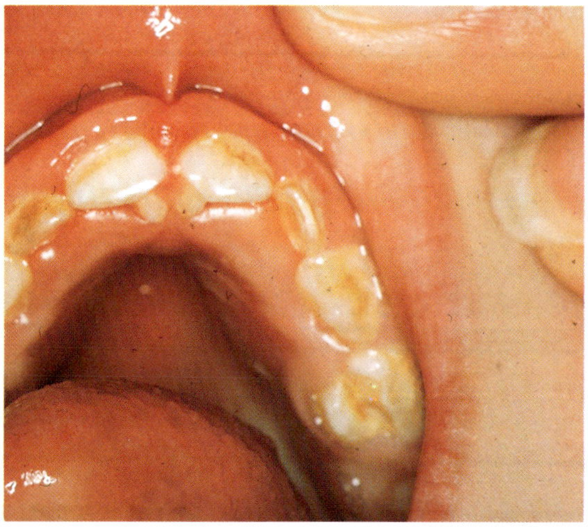

14.32

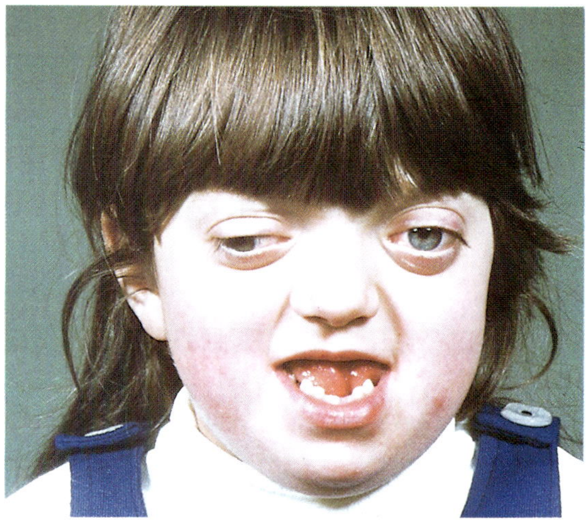

14.33

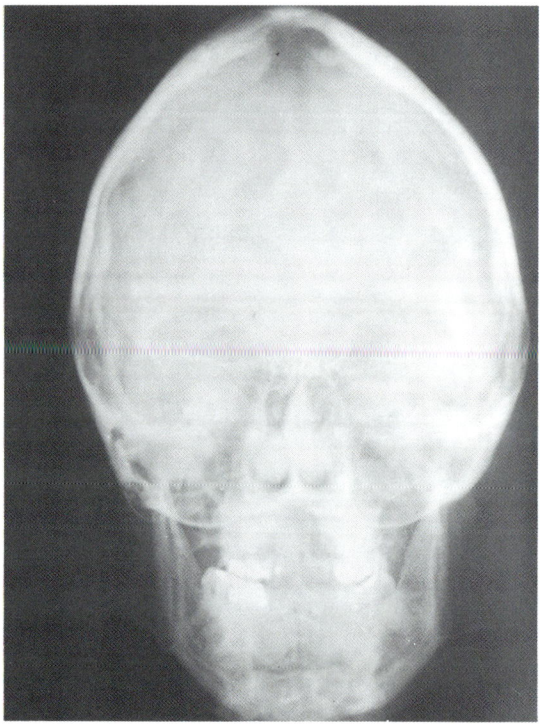

14.34

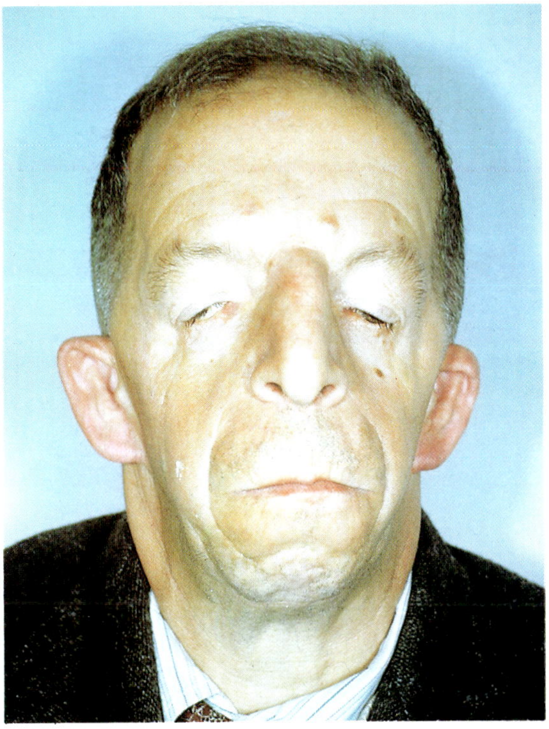

14.35

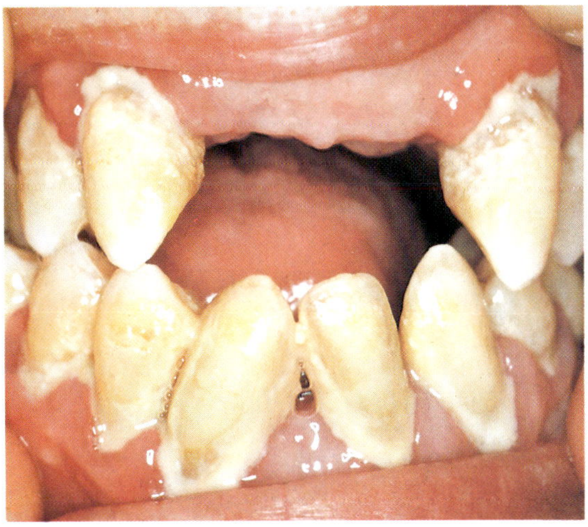

14.36

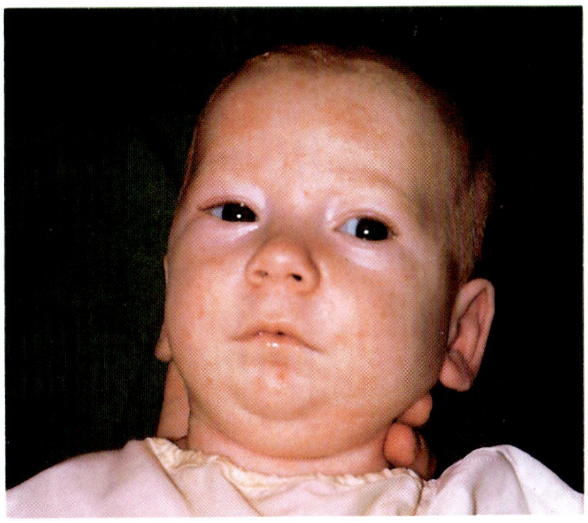

14.37

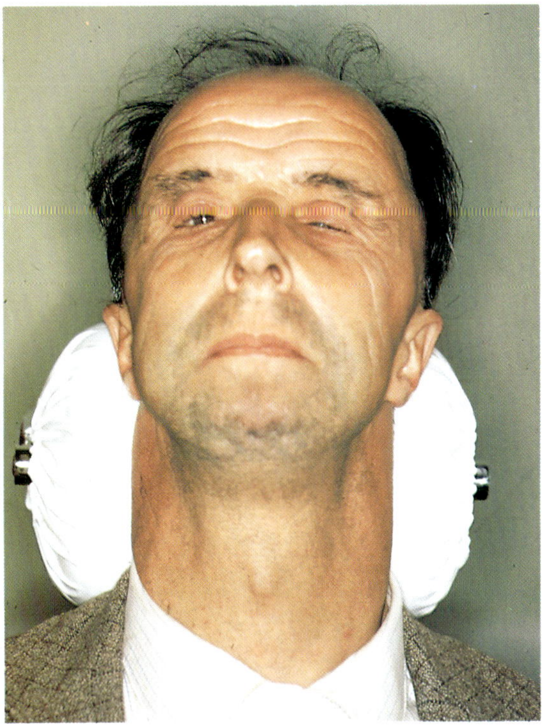

14.38

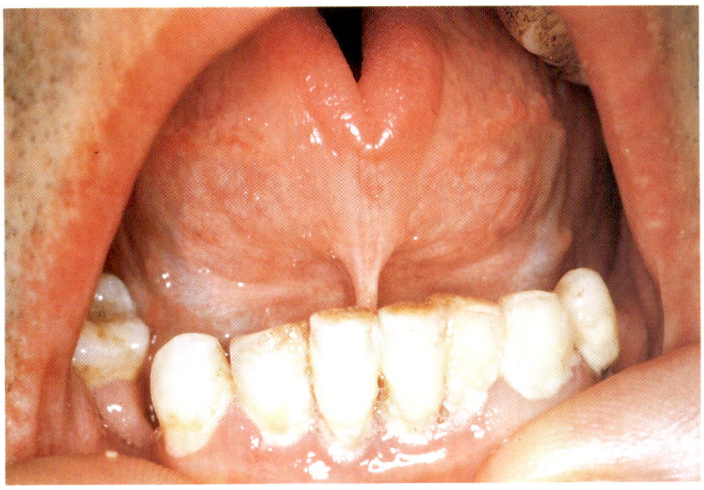

14.39

TREACHER COLLINS' SYNDROME (*Mandibulofacial dysostosis*)

Figure 14.35 The face in Treacher Collins' syndrome is characteristic, with pronounced antimongoloid slanting of the eyes, zygomatic and mandibular hypoplasia and low-set malformed ears. It is an autosomal dominant condition, often with deafness, caused by a first branchial arch anomaly.

Figure 14.36 Malocclusion is common, as here. Cleft palate is seen in about one-third of patients.

PIERRE ROBIN SYNDROME

Figure 14.37 In severe congenital micrognathia with a cleft palate there may be glossoptosis and respiratory embarrassment. Periodic dyspnoea is often evident from birth. There may also be congenital cardiac anomalies and mental handicap.

HALLERMANN-STREIFF SYNDROME (*Oculo-mandibulo dyscephaly*)

Figure 14.38 Zygomatic and mandibular hypoplasia, hypotrichosis and microphthalmia with blue sclerae and cataracts are the main features.

Figure 14.39 Teeth may be supernumerary, as here, or malformed or absent. Natal teeth may sometimes be seen in affected infants.

CHONDROECTODERMAL DYSPLASIA (*Ellis-van Creveld syndrome*)

Figure 14.40 Dwarfism, polydactyly, ectodermal dysplasia affecting nails and teeth (lateral incisors are missing here), multiple fraenae and hypoplastic teeth characterize this syndrome.

Figure 14.41 Polydactyly.

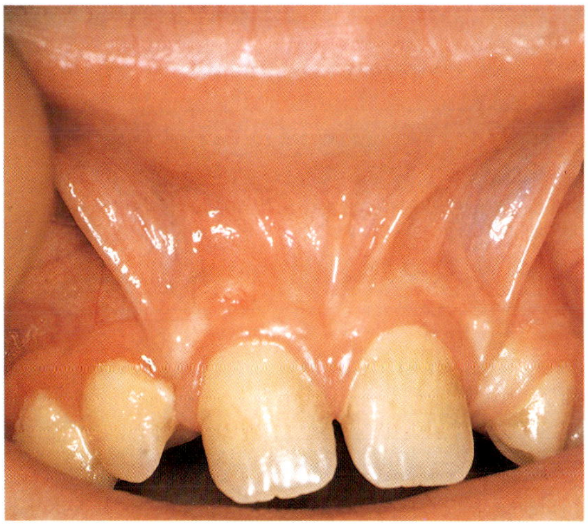

14.40

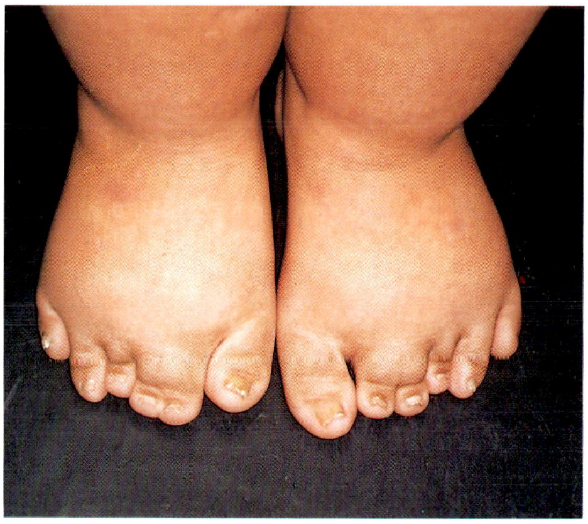

14.41

OSTEOGENESIS IMPERFECTA (*Fragilitas ossium*)

Figure 14.42 Osteogenesis imperfecta is a group of rare disorders in which a defect in type 1 collagen leads to fragile bones that fracture with minimal trauma. There are several subtypes varying in severity and in features such as otosclerosis, blue sclerae (seen here), hypermobile joints, cardiac valve defects (mitral valve prolapse or aortic incompetence) and dentinogenesis imperfecta.

Autosomal dominant and recessive types have been described.

Figure 14.43 The primary dentition may be affected by dentinogenesis imperfecta in some types of osteogenesis imperfecta. The permanent dentition is often unaffected.

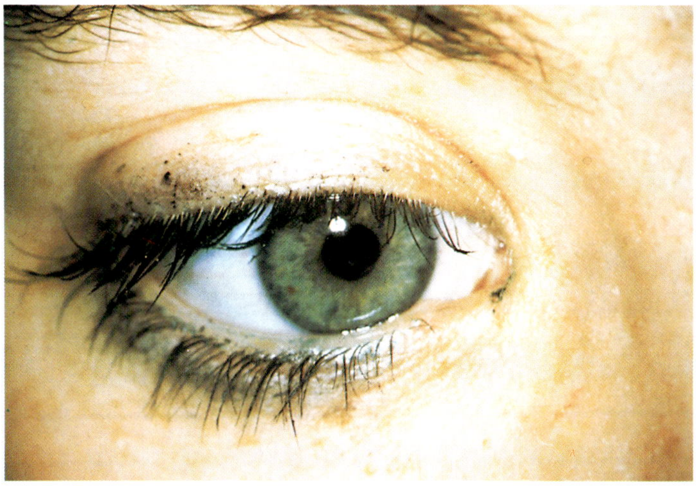

14.42

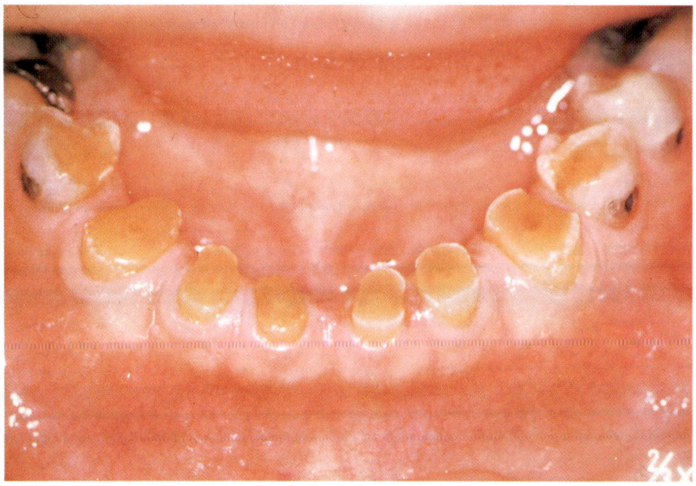

14.43

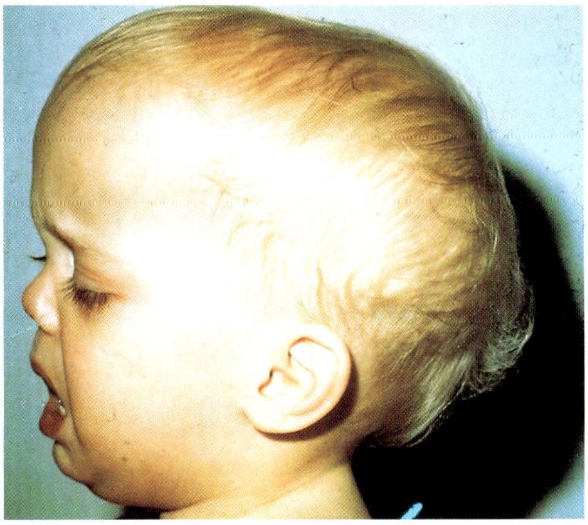

14.44

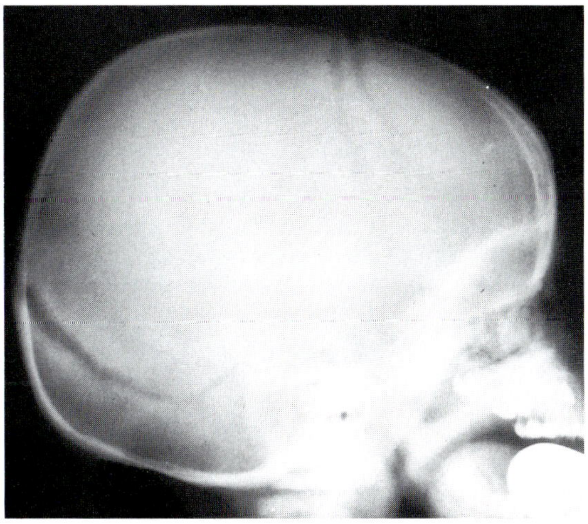

14.45

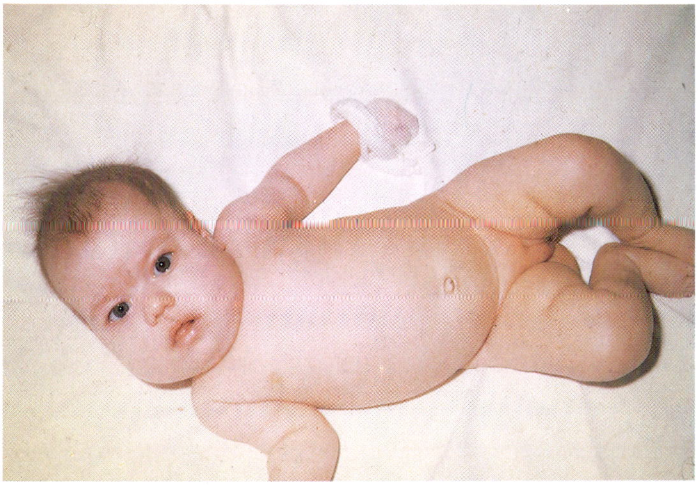

14.46

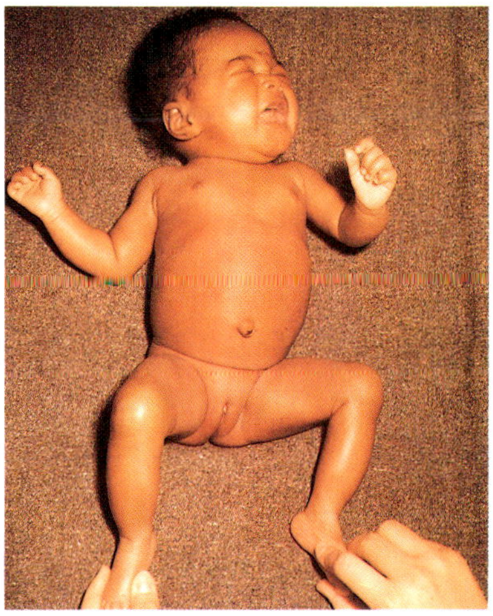

14.47

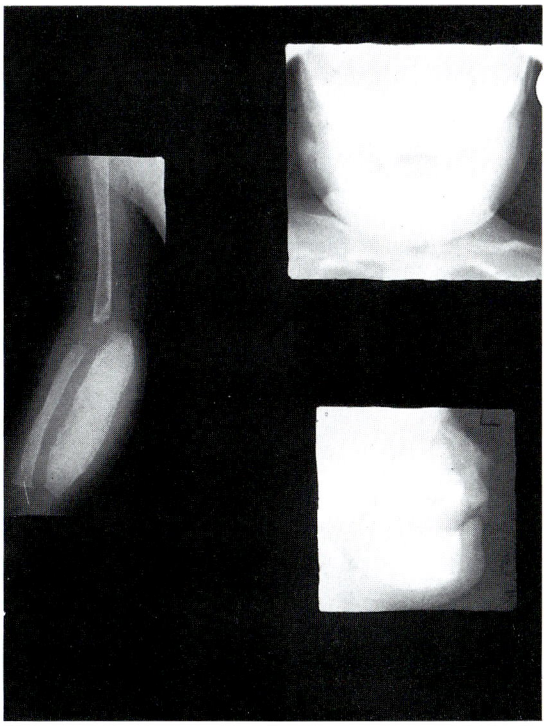

14.48

OSTEOPETROSIS (*Albers-Schoenberg syndrome*)

Figure 14.44 Osteopetrosis is a rare inherited disorder of bone. The autosomal recessive malignant type is lethal in early life but the autosomal dominant type is compatible with life. The maxilla is hypoplastic and sinuses obliterated.

Figure 14.45 The bones are extremely dense; teeth often have short roots and may erupt late or not at all. The dense bone causes a predisposition to osteomyelitis.

Generalized osteosclerosis with hyperostosis of calvaria, mandible and clavicles, syndactyly and facial palsy are seen in van Buchem's disease (sclerosteosis).

CAFFEY'S DISEASE (*Infantile cortical hyperostosis*)

Figure 14.46 This is a rare, possibly autosomal dominant condition, that presents often with swellings around the eyes or over the mandible, as here. The condition resembles cherubism but appears at 2–4 months of age. The teeth are neither hypoplastic nor delayed in eruption.

Figure 14.47 There are tender, soft tissue swellings over the tibiae, with fever, anaemia and irritability. These features are extremely similar to those seen in child abuse, or osteomyelitis.

Figure 14.48 Radiographs show periosteal new bone formation.

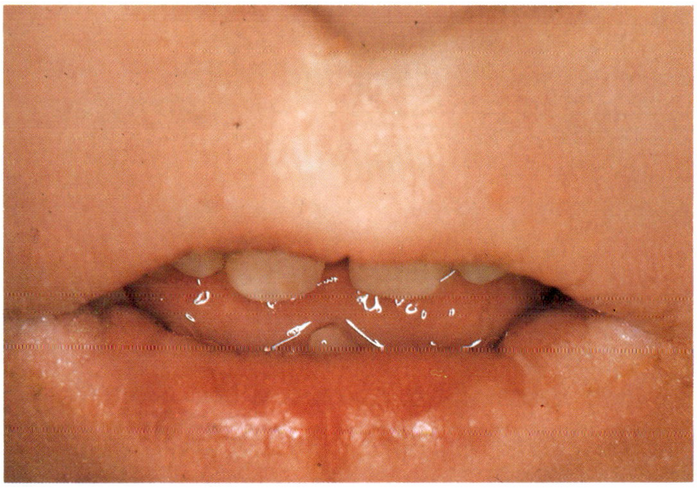

14.49

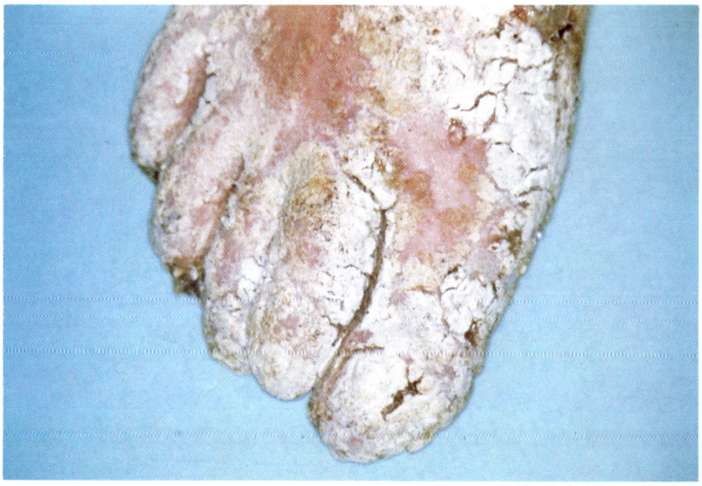

14.50

CONGENITAL ICHTHYOSIS

Figure 14.49 Ichthyoses are a group of conditions in which there is scaling of the skin. Perioral involvement is not uncommon and there may be enamel hypoplasia, delayed tooth eruption, periodontal disease and caries. Hyperkeratotic plaques have been described on the tongue.

Figure 14.50 Scales may involve many sites, depending on the type of ichthyosis. The most common is ichthyosis vulgaris, which is an autosomal dominant condition affecting the extremities in particular.

Figure 14.51 Nail involvement in ichthyosis.

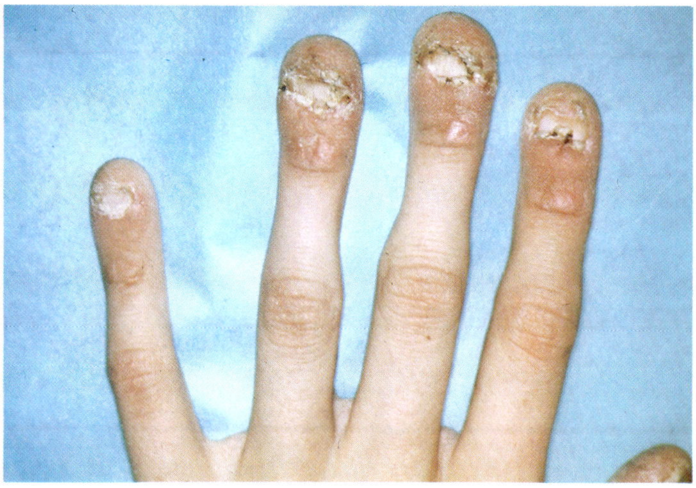

14.51

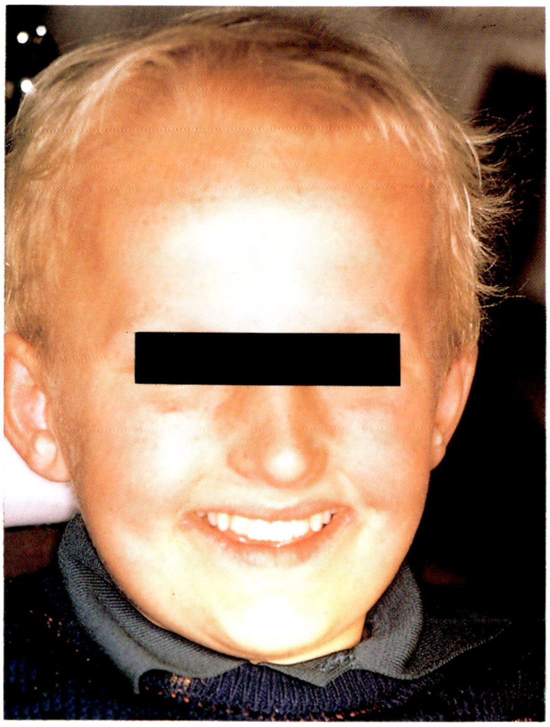

14.52

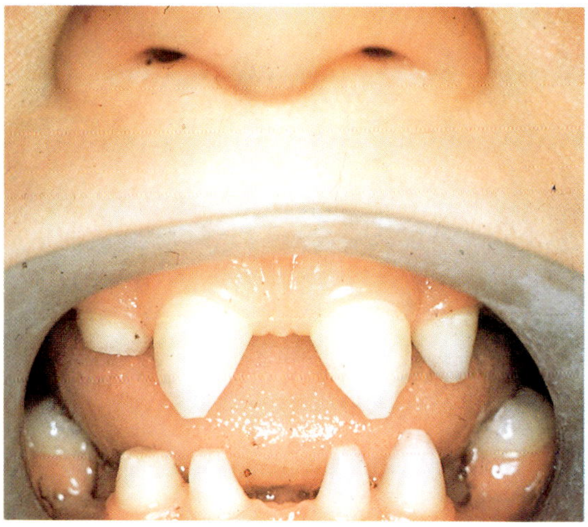

14.53

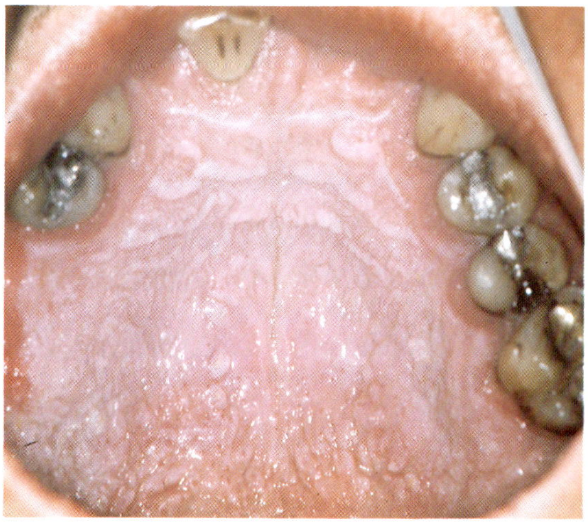

14.54

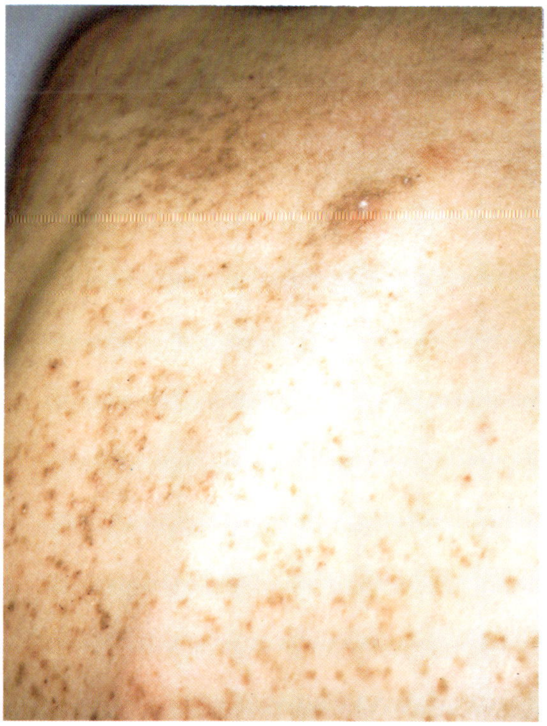

14.55

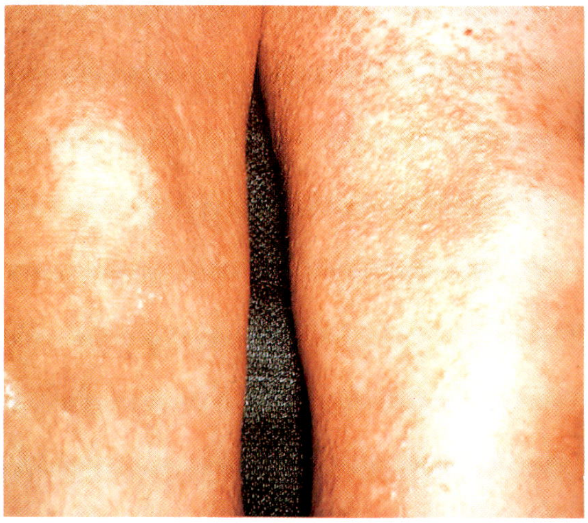

14.56

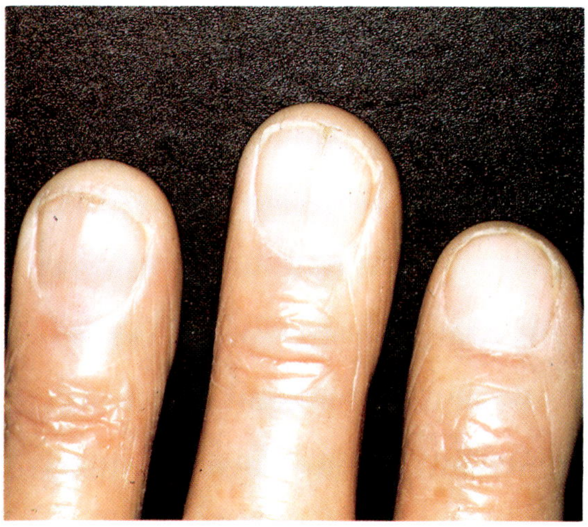

14.57

ECTODERMAL DYSPLASIA

Figure 14.52 Hypohidrotic ectodermal dysplasia is a genetic disorder, usually sex-linked, characterized by sparse hair (hypotrichosis), absent sweat glands (hypohidrosis) and consequent fever, respiratory infections, absent teeth (hypodontia) and sometimes frontal bossing. Patients are otherwise well and mentally normal. This patient has anodontia but is here wearing a denture.

Figure 14.53 There is usually hypodontia rather than anodontia, and the few teeth that are present often are of simple conical shape and erupt late. Dry mouth predisposes to caries.

Rare varieties include an autosomal dominant variety (the 'tooth and nail' type) characterized by hypodontia and hypoplastic nails, and a subtype in which teeth are normal (hypohidrotic ectodermal dysplasia with hypothyroidism).

DARIER'S DISEASE (*Dyskeratosis follicularis*)

Figure 14.54 Darier's disease is a rare autosomal dominant skin disorder characterized by multiple papules seen especially over the shoulders and upper arms. Oral lesions are common, starting as red papules that turn to white pebbly lesions seen especially in the palate, gingiva and dorsum of tongue.

Figure 14.55 Papules over shoulders and back.

Figure 14.56 Papules over knees.

Figure 14.57 Nail defects include longitudinal splits and fragility such that nails tend to be wider than long.

EHLERS-DANLOS SYNDROME

Figure 14.58 Ehlers-Danlos syndrome is a group of inherited disorders of collagen. Most types are inherited as autosomal dominant traits.

Hypermobility of joints is common, the skin is soft, extensible and fragile, purpura is common and there may be other defects, such as mitral valve prolapse. The teeth may be small with abnormally-shaped roots and, as here, multiple pulp stones.

Type VIII Ehlers-Danlos syndrome is associated with early onset periodontal disease.

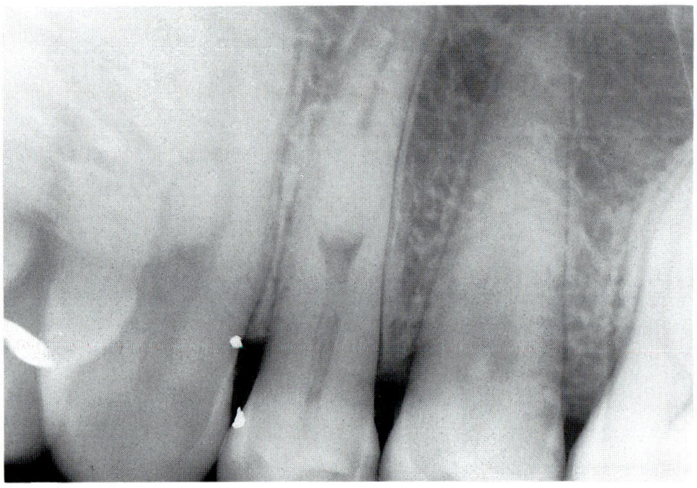

14.58

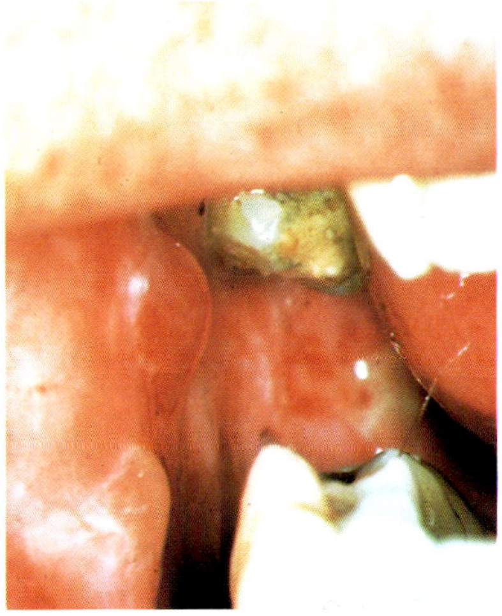

14.59

EPIDERMOLYSIS BULLOSA

Figure 14.59 Epidermolysis bullosa is a group of rare inherited disorders of skin and mucosa, mostly characterized by vesiculation at the epithelial basement membrane zone in response to minor trauma, and consequent scarring. In most forms, bullae may be seen in the mouth, as here. Oral lesions are seen rarely in the non-scarring simplex type of epidermolysis bullosa, in which the vesiculation is intra-epithelial.

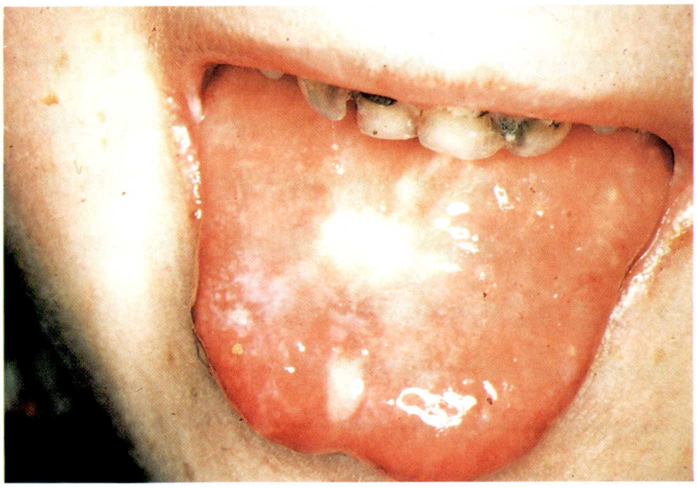

14.60

Figure 14.60 The tongue has become depapillated and scarred. Bullae appear early in life, often precipitated by suckling, and break down to persistent ulcers that eventually heal with scarring. Milia have been described intraorally in epidermolysis bullosa.

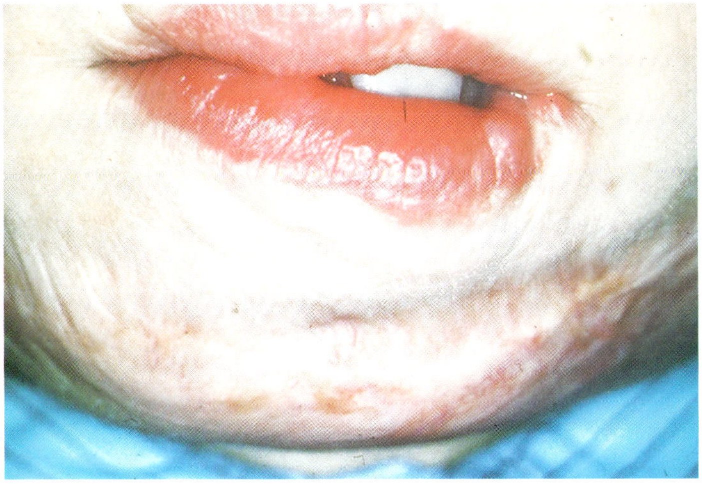

14.61

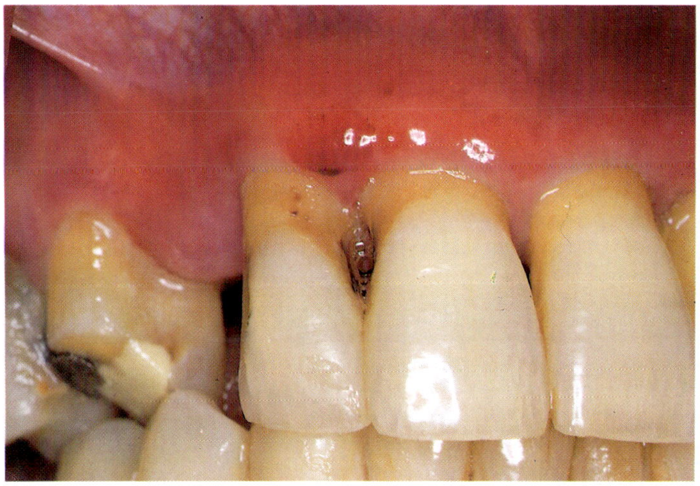

14.62

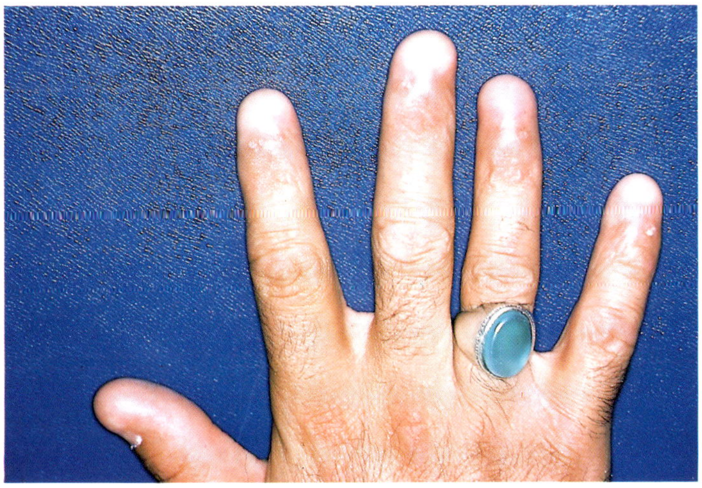

14.63

Figure 14.61 In this patient, scar formation has distorted the lower lip. Enamel hypoplasia may be seen and, in view of the fragility of mucosa, oral hygiene tends to be neglected with subsequent caries and periodontal disease. Squamous cell carcinoma is a rare complication.

Figure 14.62 Blister formation on the gingiva.

Figure 14.63 Scarring with the dystrophic form, affecting the extremities including the nails.

An acquired form of epidermolysis bullosa (epidermolysis bullosa acquisita) is a chronic blistering disease of skin and mucosa with autoantibodies to type VII procollagen of epithelial basement membrane.

INCONTINENTIA PIGMENTI (*Bloch-Sulzberger disease*)

Figure 14.64 This is a rare dominant disorder that is either sex-linked or lethal to males. Virtually all surviving patients are female. Pigmented, vesicular or verrucous skin lesions are seen, as here, often with mental handicap and visual defects.

Figure 14.65 Most patients have dental anomalies and both dentitions may exhibit anomalies. Hypodontia, conical teeth and delayed eruption are the usual features. Incontinentia pigmenti is a type of ectodermal dysplasia.

Figure 14.66 Teeth are often, as here, missing.

PACHYONYCHIA CONGENITA

Figure 14.67 In this autosomal dominant condition, the nails become thickened, hard and yellow, there is palmar and plantar hyperhidrosis and hyperkeratosis, and oral white lesions clinically resembling those of white sponge naevus. The dorsum of tongue is the common site, although other sites may be affected, as here. Natal teeth may be seen in affected neonates.

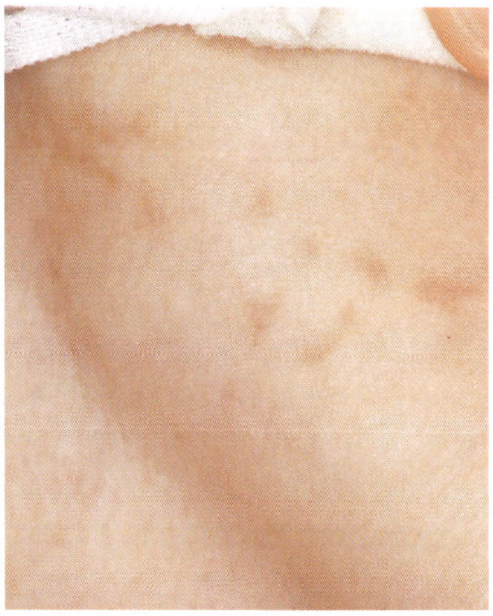

14.64

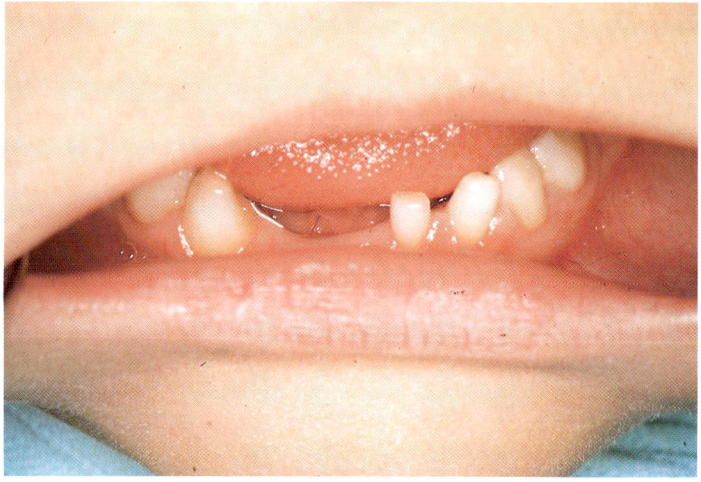

14.65

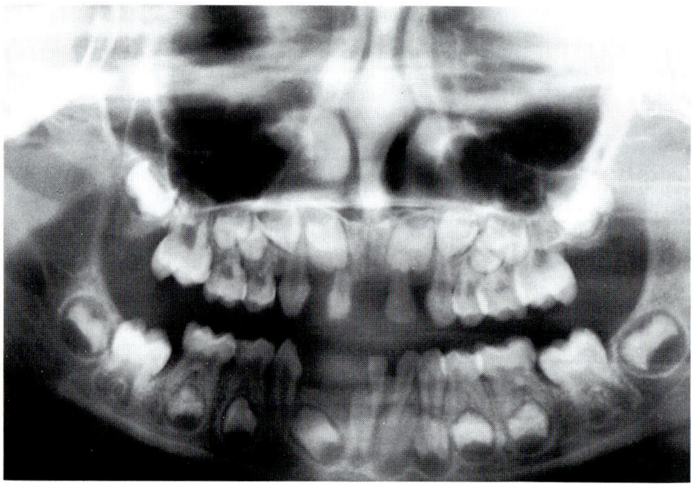

14.66

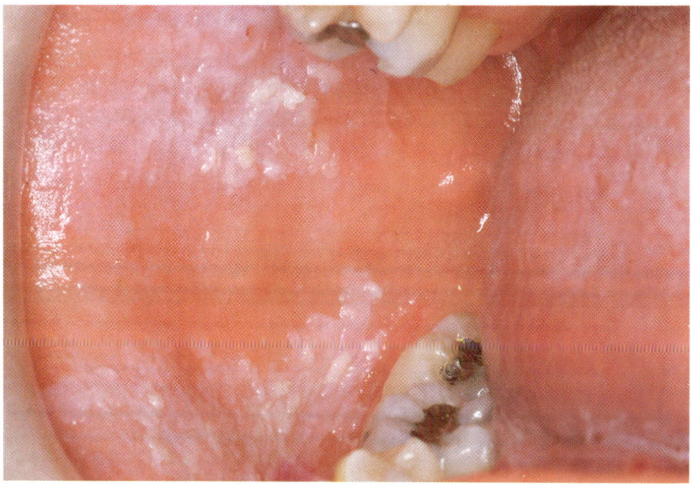

14.67

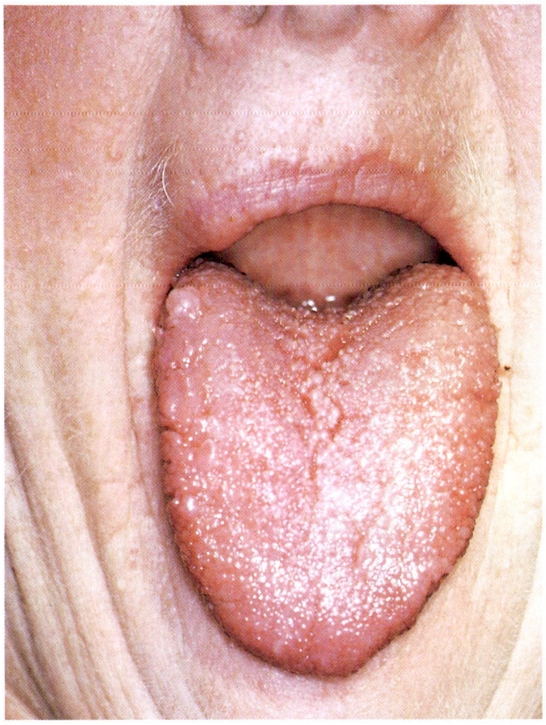

14.68

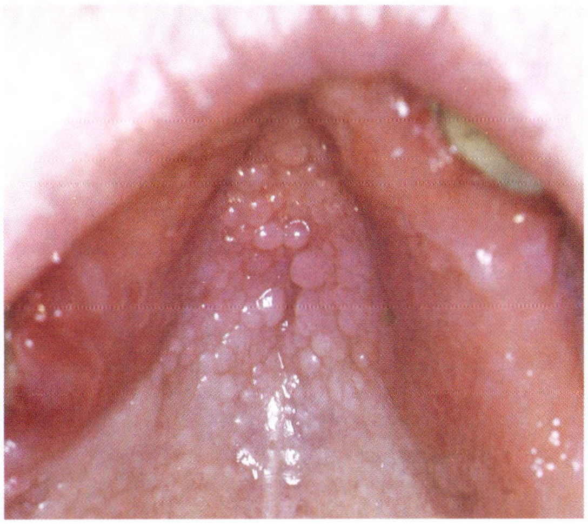

14.69

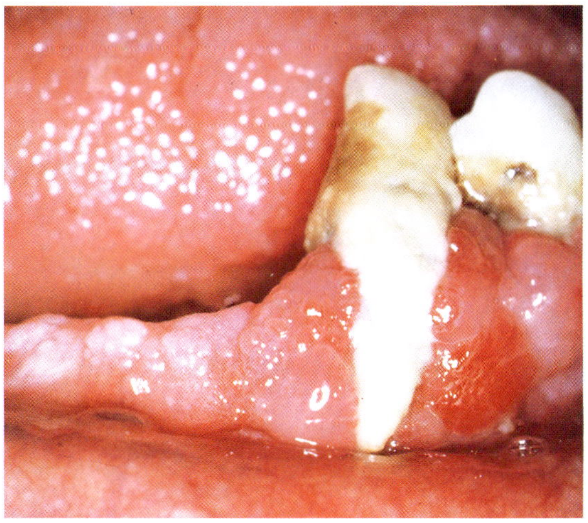

14.70

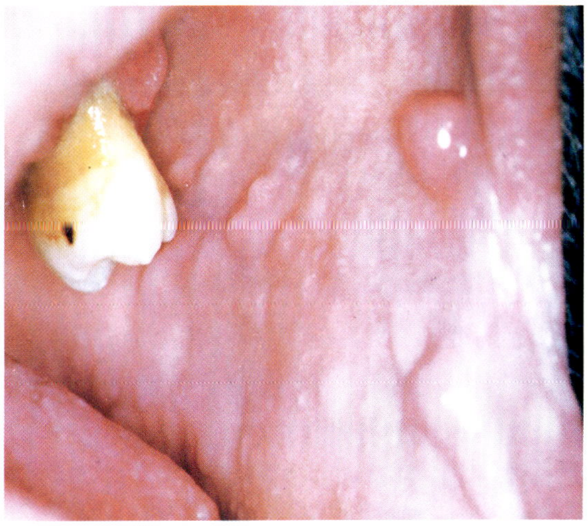

14.71

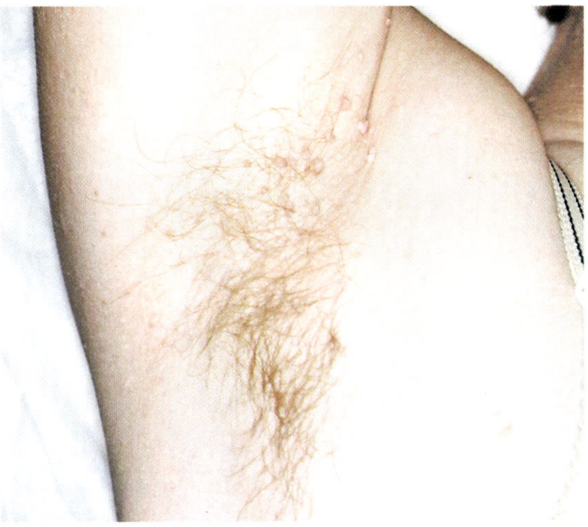

14.72

COWDEN'S SYNDROME (*Multiple hamartoma and neoplasia syndrome*)

Figure 14.68 This is an autosomal dominant condition of multiple hamartomas, with a predisposition to tumours, particularly carcinomas of breast, thyroid and colon. Papular oral lesions are common.

Figure 14.69 Papular lesions on palate. Mucocutaneous lesions often precede the appearance of malignant disease elsewhere.

Figure 14.70 Papular lesions on gingiva.

Figure 14.71 Papular lesions in buccal mucosa. Other oral lesions may include fissured tongue, hypoplasia of the uvula, and maxillary and mandibular hypoplasia.

Figure 14.72 Large numbers of papillomatous lesions are seen on the skin especially over the neck, nose and ear.

Other manifestations of Cowden's syndrome may include small keratoses on the palms and soles; mental handicap and motor incoordination.

DOWN'S SYNDROME

Figure 14.73 Down's syndrome is a trisomic chromosome anomaly in most instances, affecting children of elderly mothers. There is a typical mongoloid appearance.

Figure 14.74 Brachycephaly and short stature are prominent features of Down's syndrome. There are anomalies of many organs and virtually all patients are mentally handicapped.

Figure 14.75 A fairly characteristic, though not pathognomonic feature is the presence of white spots (Brushfield spots) around the iris.

Figure 14.76 Another feature is a single palmar crease (simian crease) and clinodactyly of the fifth finger.

Figure 14.77 Patients with Down's syndrome have multiple immune defects. Blepharitis and keratitis are common.

Figure 14.78 Upper respiratory infections are common. The dry mouth here is a consequence of mouth-breathing because of nasal obstruction.

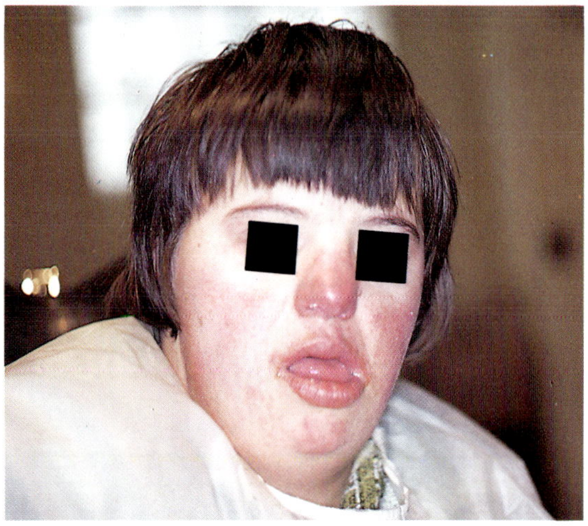

14.73

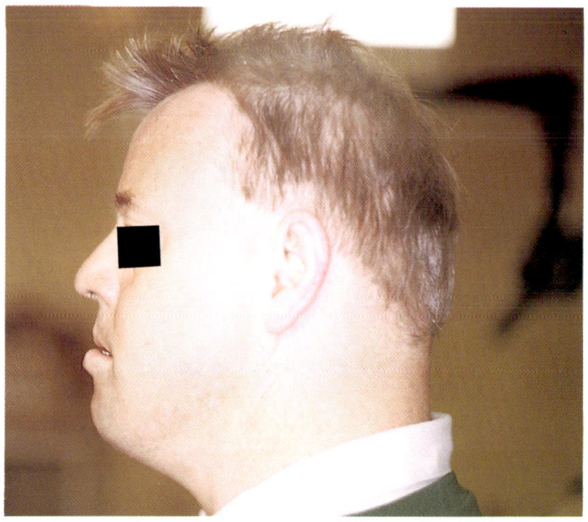

14.74

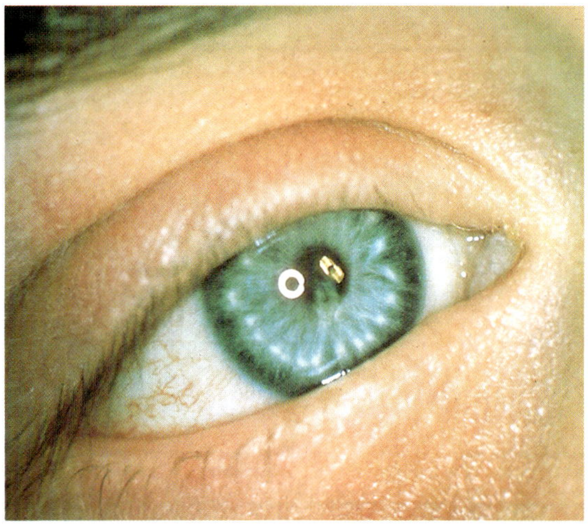

14.75

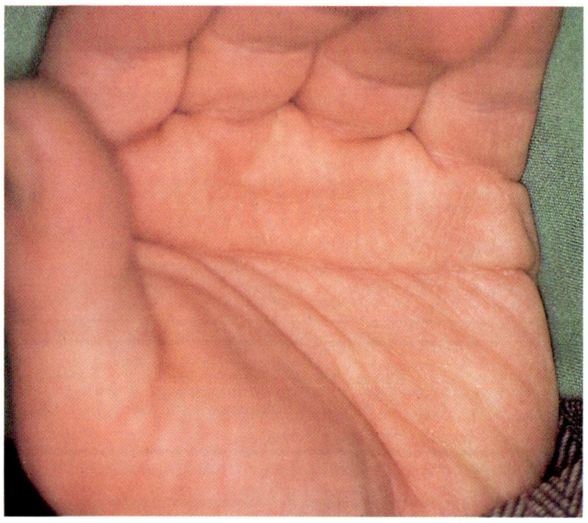

14.76

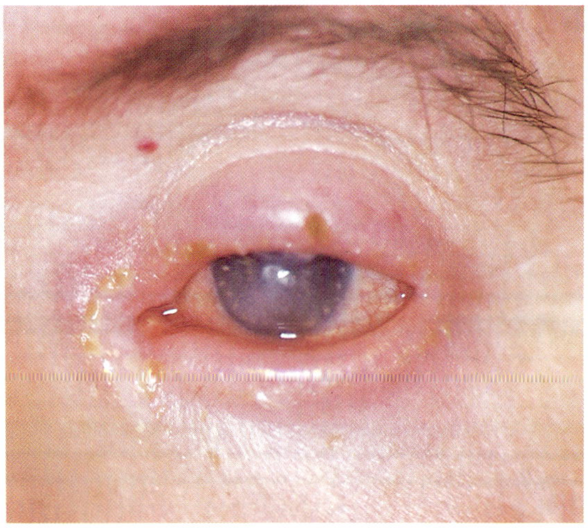

14.77

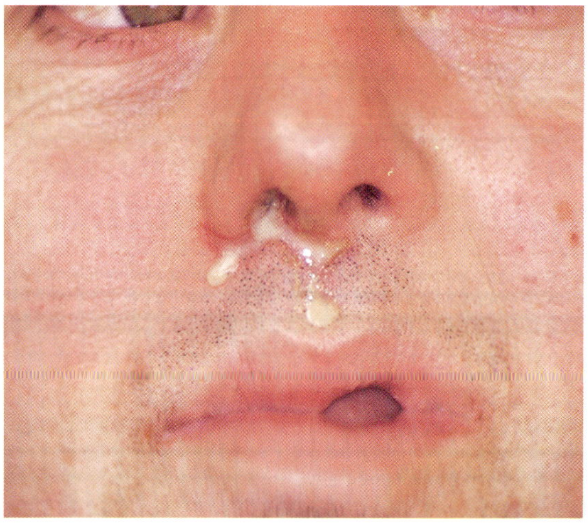

14.78

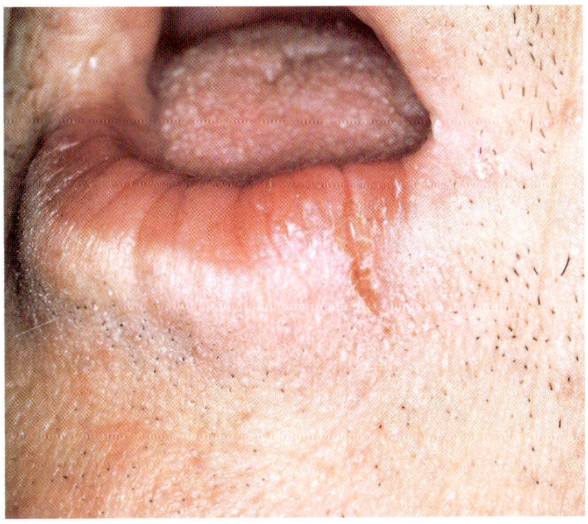

14.79

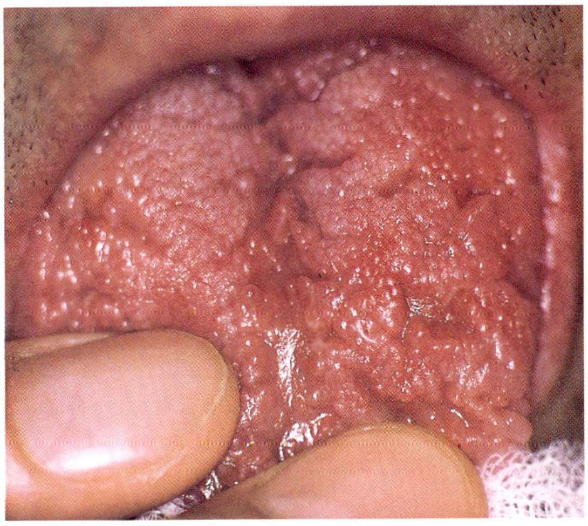

14.80

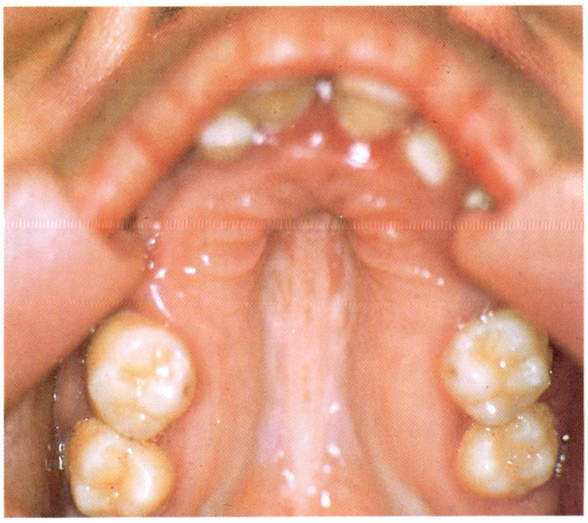

14.81

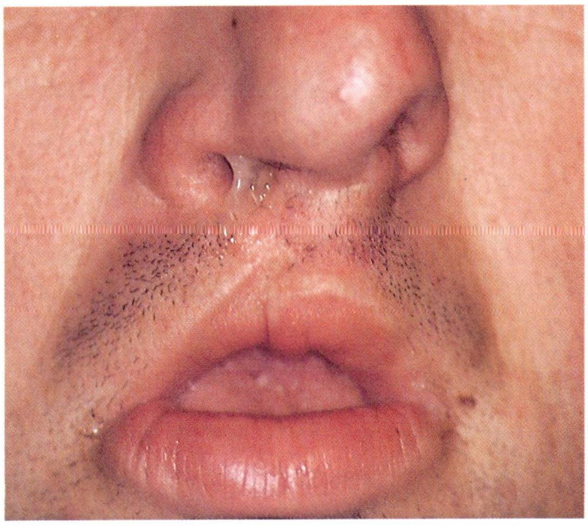

14.82

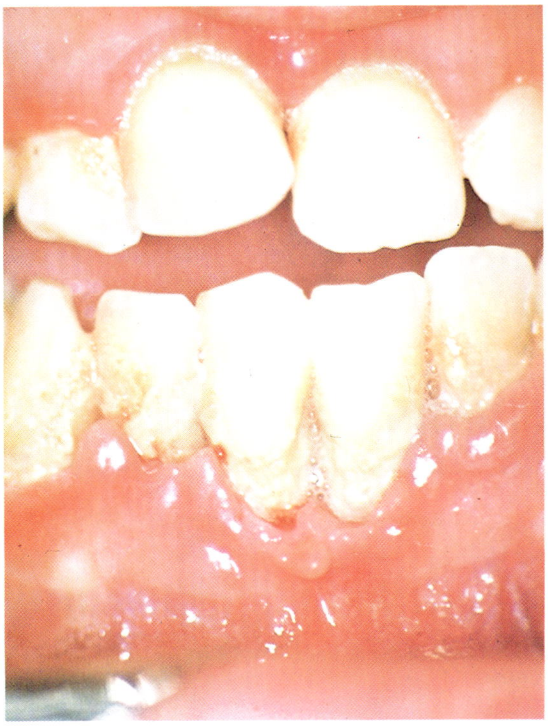

14.83

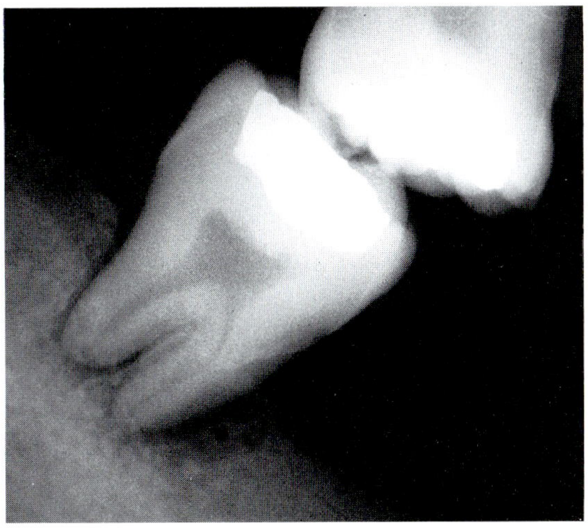

14.84

Figure 14.79 Cheilitis and cracking of the lips are common, possibly because of mouth-breathing.

Figure 14.80 Macroglossia and fissured tongue are often seen.

Figure 14.81 The midface is hypoplastic and palatal anomalies common.

Figure 14.82 Cleft lip and palate are more prevalent in Down's syndrome than in the general population.

Figure 14.83 Early loss of teeth is a feature, not only because of poor oral hygiene in many patients, but also because the teeth have short roots and there may be rapidly destructive periodontal disease, as here.

Figure 14.84 The short tapered roots, resulting in early tooth loss, are seen here.

EPILOIA

(*Tuberous sclerosis, Bourneville-Pringle disease*)

Figure 14.85 Tuberous sclerosis is an autosomal dominant condition of mental handicap, epilepsy, and skin lesions, possibly owing to a defect on chromosome 9.

Adenoma sebaceum is the pathognomonic feature and is typically seen in the nasolabial fold. Depigmented 'ash leaf' naevi may be seen on the trunk.

Figure 14.86 Adenoma sebaceum is an angiofibroma that can be severely disfiguring and may involve other sites, such as the chin. Fibrous plaques on the forehead and shagreen patches elsewhere are other cutaneous features.

Figure 14.87 Most patients are both mentally handicapped and epileptic. Cerebral calcifications are seen here.

Patients may also have cardiac rhabdomyoma or renal hamartomas (cysts or angiomyolipomas).

Figure 14.88 Subungual fibromas are another pathognomonic feature and may be seen with longitudinal ridging of the nails.

Figure 14.89 Papilliferous oral mucosa lesions may be seen.

Figure 14.90 Pit-shaped enamel defects, seen here on the central incisors, are a feature.

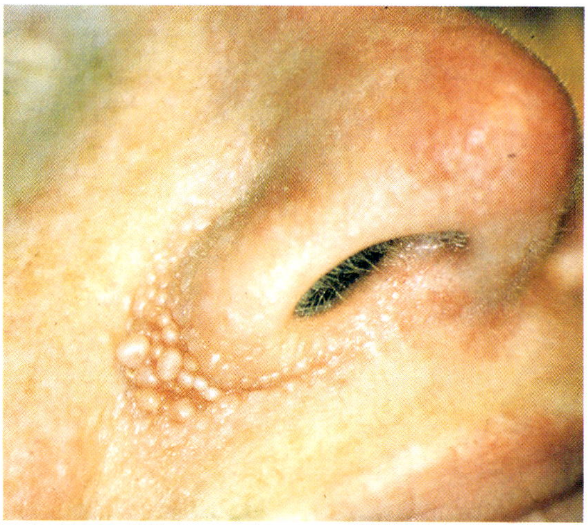

14.85

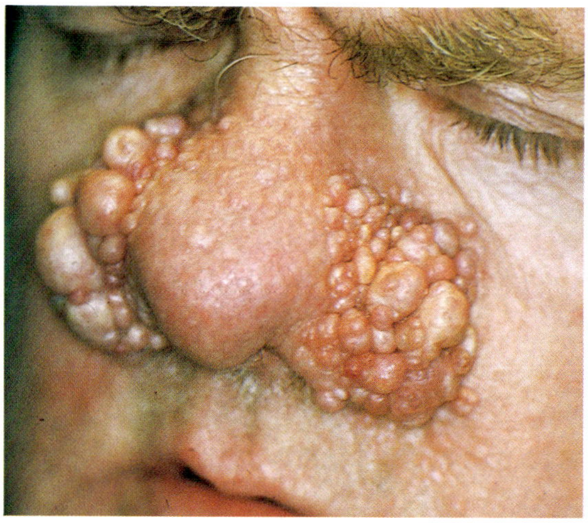

14.86

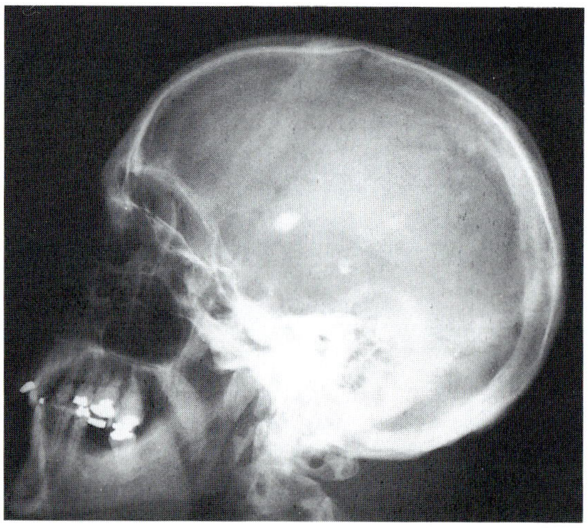

14.87

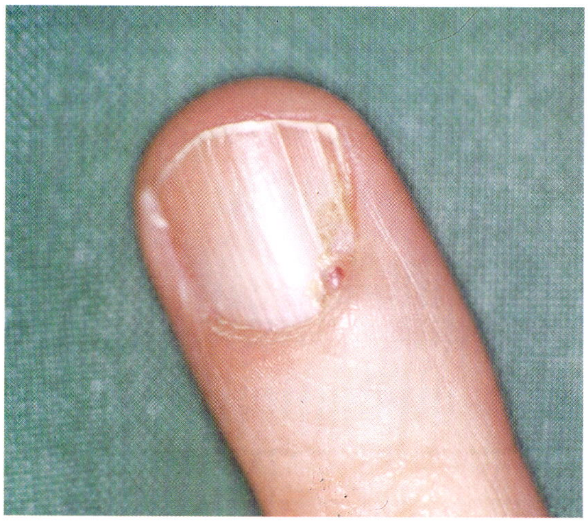

14.88

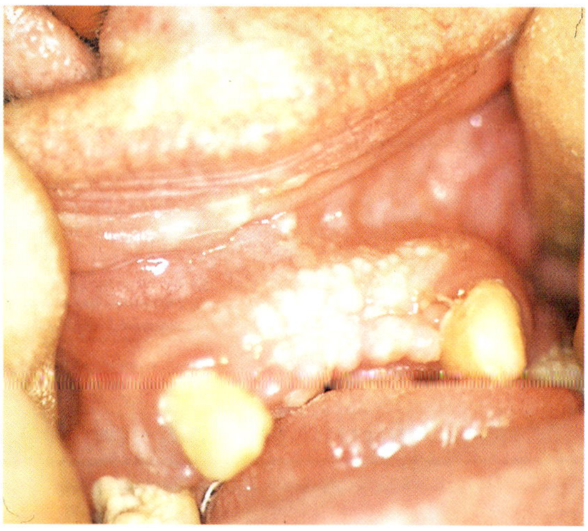

14.89

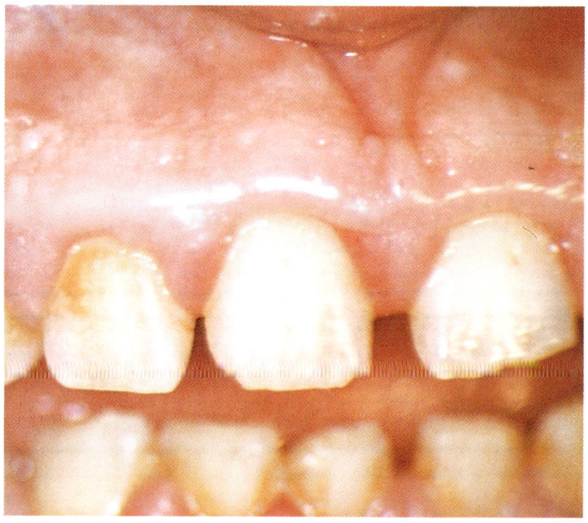

14.90

VON RECKLINGHAUSEN'S DISEASE (*Generalized neurofibromatosis*)

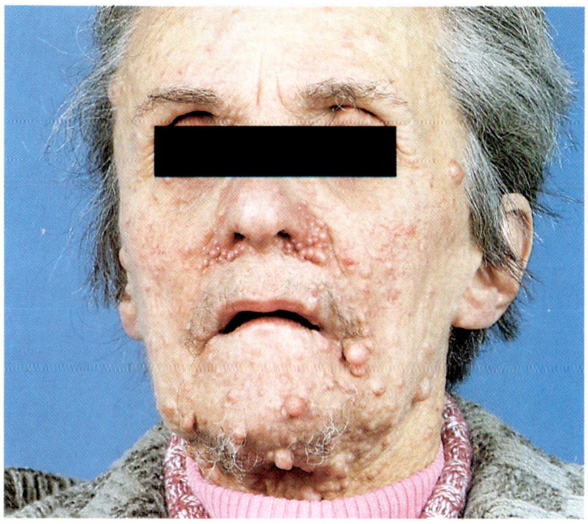

14.91

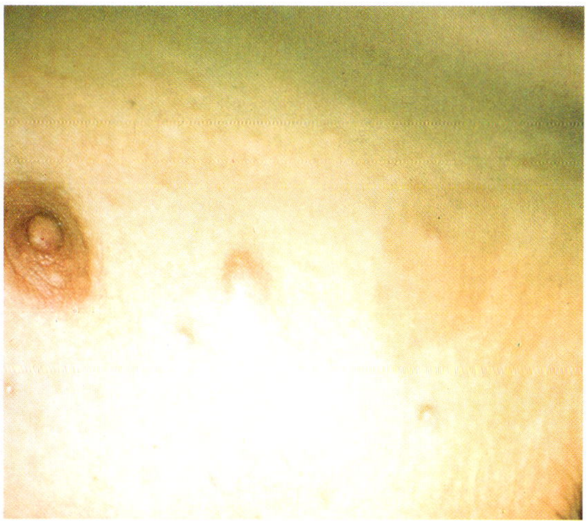

14.92

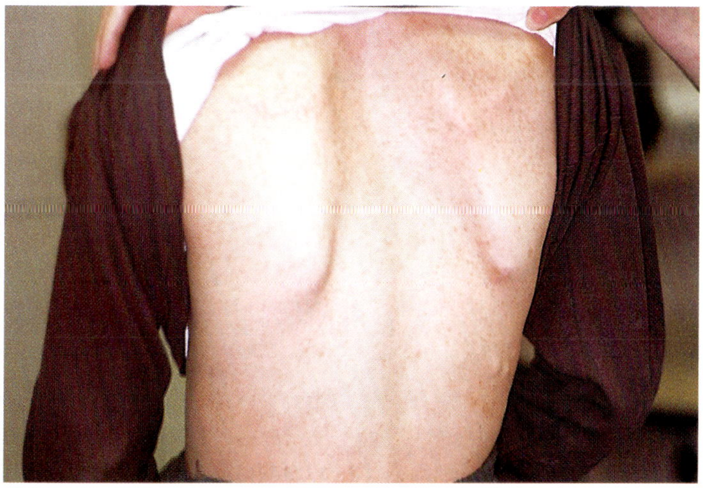

14.93

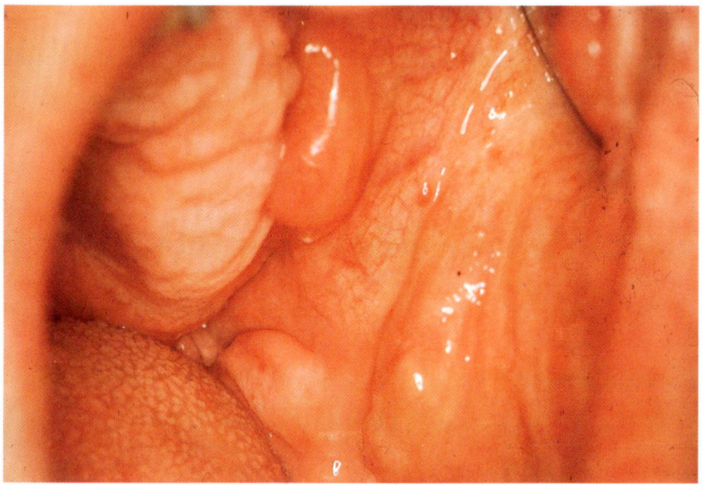

14.94

Figure 14.91 Cutaneous and subcutaneous neurofibromas, with skin hyperpigmentation are the features of Von Recklinghausen's disease (VRNF). This is an autosomal dominant condition but many cases are new mutations.

Figure 14.92 Café-au-lait hyperpigmented patches are seen, especially in the axillary region. This illustration also shows an adjacent neurofibroma.

Figure 14.93 Dystrophic kyphoscoliosis is common, as here, and there may sometimes be mental handicap and epilepsy, rarely renal artery stenosis or phaeochromocytoma. Acoustic neuromas are not common – many earlier reports were of a distinct condition of bilateral acoustic neurofibromatosis. However, optic nerve or optic chiasmal gliomas may be present.

Figure 14.94 Neurofibromas may affect any part of the body, including the oral cavity.

Most patients also have small dome-shaped brown hamartomas (Lisch nodules) on the front of the iris, on slit-lamp examination.

STURGE-WEBER SYNDROME (*Encephalofacial angiomatosis*)

Figure 14.95 An angioma affects the upper face and usually extends into the occipital lobe of the brain, producing epilepsy and often hemiplegia and mental handicap.

Figure 14.96 The haemangioma often appears to be limited to the area of distribution of one or more of the divisions of the trigeminal nerve. The affected area is somewhat swollen and hypertrophic.

Figure 14.97 Radiography shows calcification intracranially in the angioma.

Figure 14.98 The haemangioma may extend intraorally and be associated with hypertrophy of the affected jaw, macrodontia, and accelerated tooth eruption. Since the patients are often treated with phenytoin there is frequently also gingival hyperplasia.

GORLIN'S SYNDROME (Gorlin-Goltz syndrome, multiple basal cell naevi syndrome)

Figure 14.99 Gorlin's syndrome is an autosomal dominant condition of multiple basal cell naevi, as seen here, with odontogenic keratocysts and other features. Frontal and parietal bossing and a broad nasal root give the typical facial appearance.

Figure 14.100 Multiple basal cell naevi, often with milia, appear in childhood or adolescence, mainly over the nose, eyelids and cheeks. Rarely are the abdomen or extremities affected.

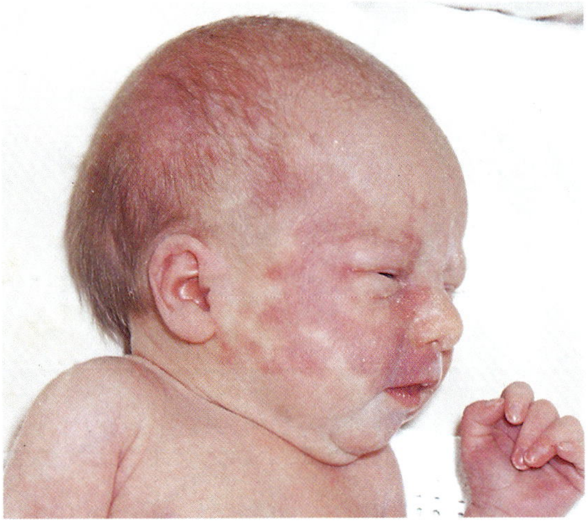

14.95

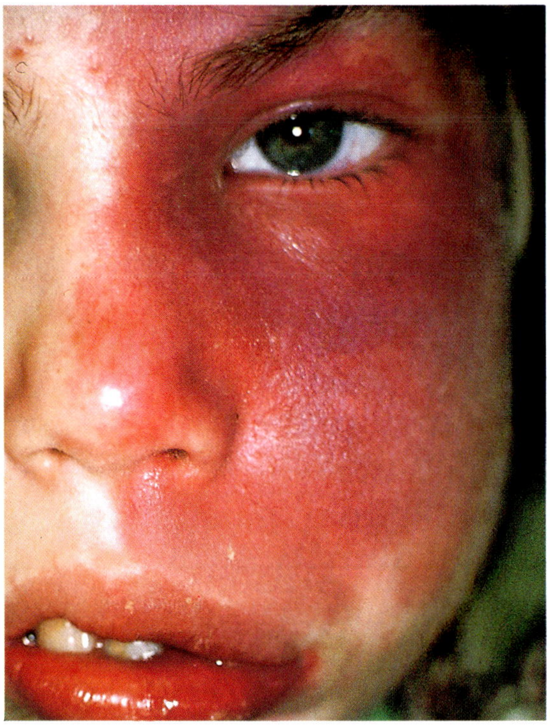

14.96

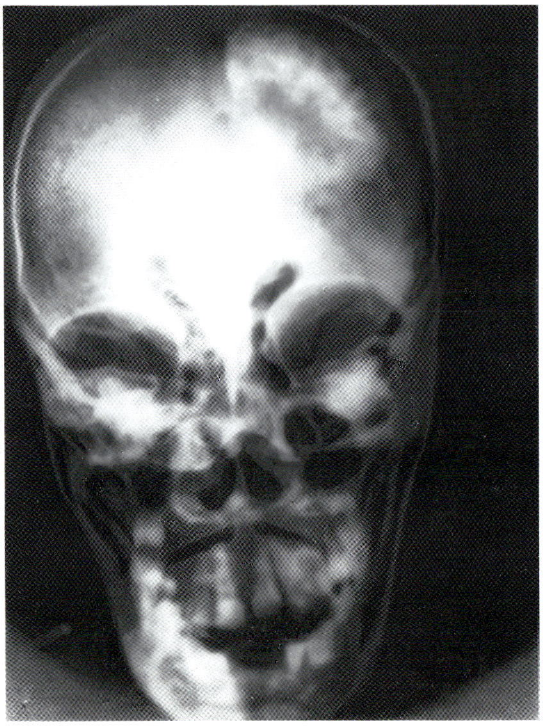

14.97

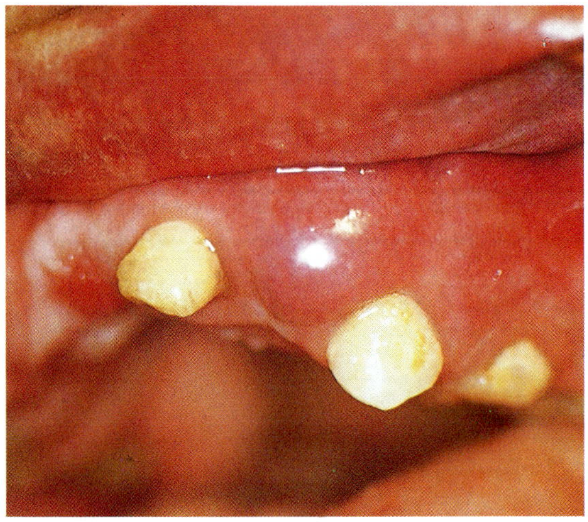

14.98

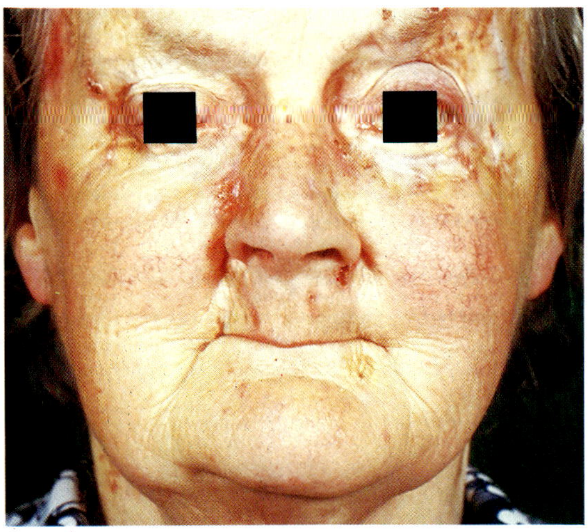

14.99

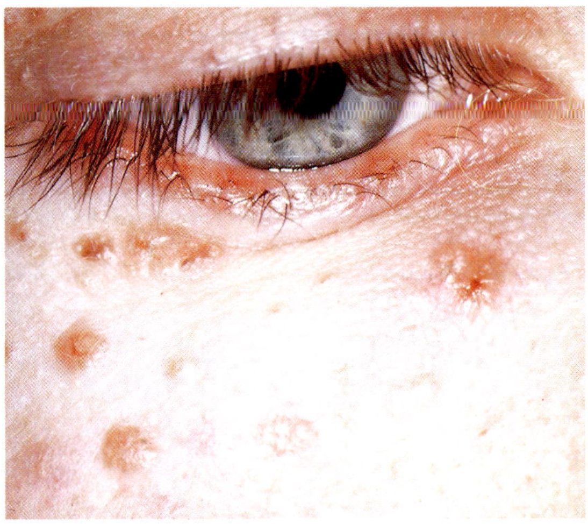

14.100

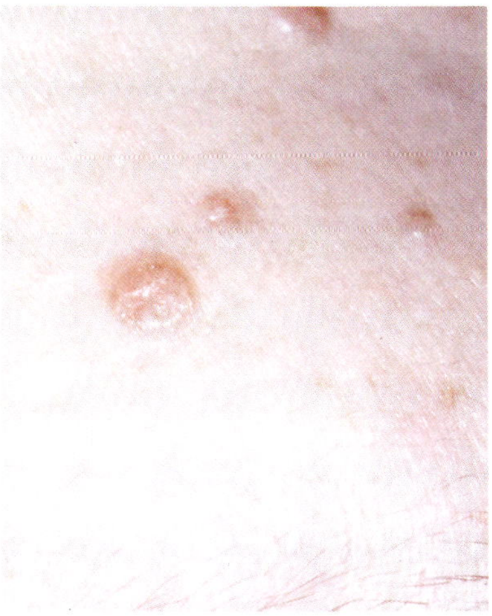

14.101

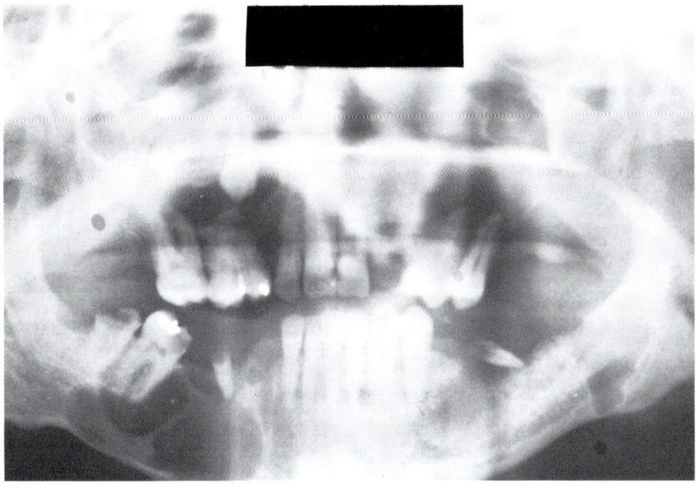

14.102

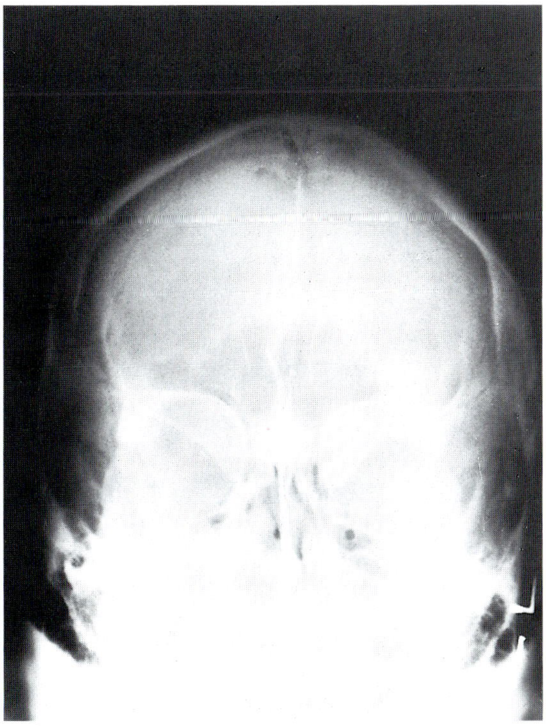

14.103

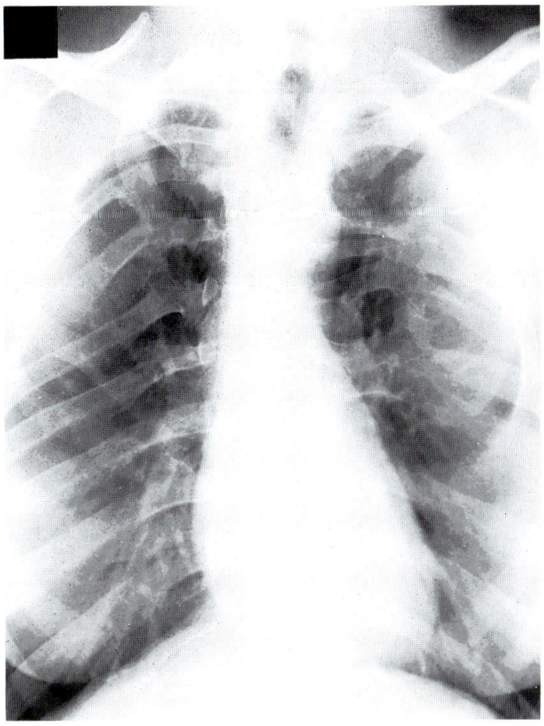

14.104

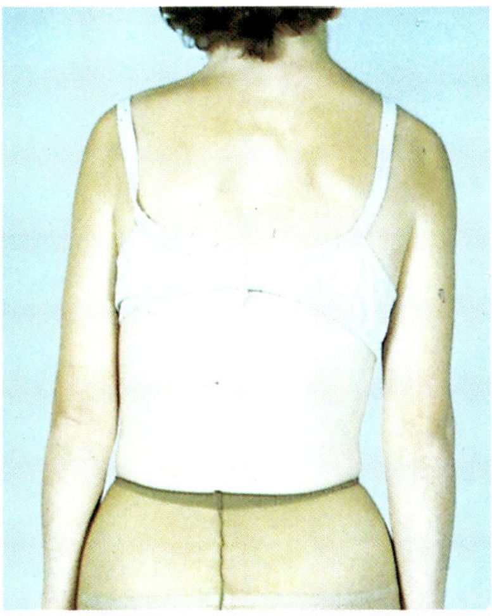

14.105

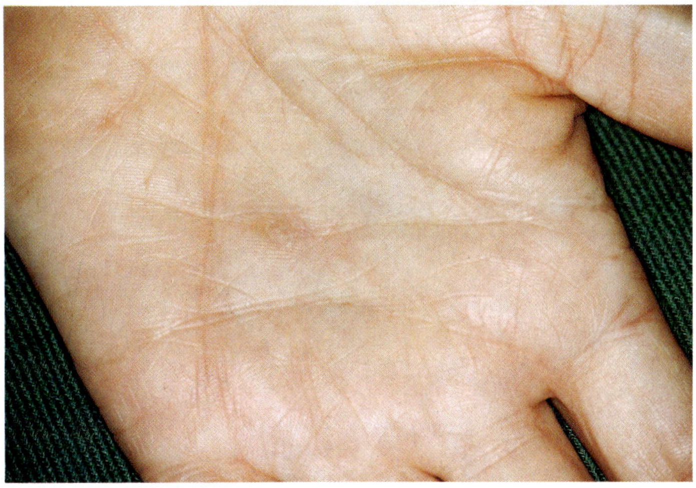

14.106

Figure 14.101 Close up of a naevus that is developing into a basal cell carcinoma. Only about 50 per cent of adult patients have significant numbers of naevoid basal cell carcinomas and only rarely are the lesions aggressive.

Figure 14.102 Keratocysts develop mainly in the mandible. Radiography here shows keratocysts in both sides of the mandible. These develop during the first 30 years of life.

Cleft lip and/or palate are seen in about 5 per cent.

Figure 14.103 Calcification of the falx cerebri, as here, is a common feature, seen in over 80 per cent of patients.

Medulloblastomas and other brain tumours have been reported in several patients, as have a range of neoplasms of other tissues, especially cardiac fibromas.

Figure 14.104 There are many skeletal anomalies but bifid ribs are a common feature, as shown here.

Figure 14.105 Kyphoscoliosis is often seen and vertebral defects are common.

Other occasional associations include pseudo-hypoparathyroidism and diabetes mellitus.

Figure 14.106 Pits may be seen in the soles or palms. Occasionally, basal cell carcinomas arise in these pits.

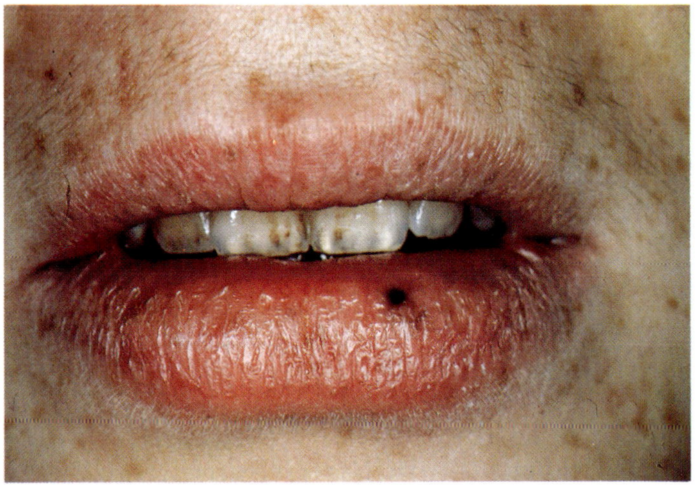

14.107

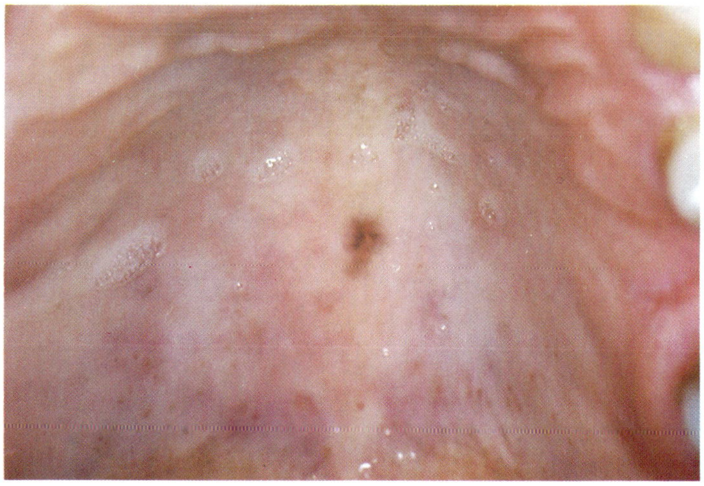

14.108

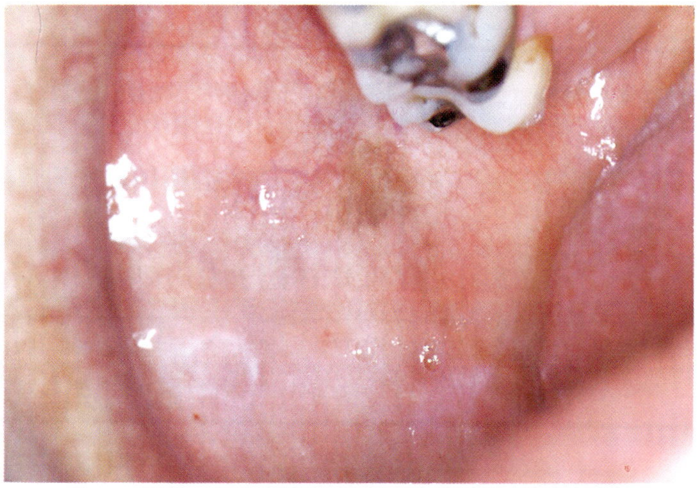

14.109

PEUTZ-JEGHER'S SYNDROME

Figure 14.107 Peutz-Jegher's syndrome is an autosomal dominant disorder, consisting of circumoral melanosis with intestinal polyposis. Polyps are mainly in the small intestine. Brown or black macules are seen around the mouth, nose and sometimes eyes, and intraorally at any site, although rare on tongue or floor of mouth.

Peutz-Jegher's syndrome may occasionally be associated with malignant neoplasms of the gastrointestinal tract, ovary, cervix, testis and breast.

MELANOTIC NAEVUS

Figure 14.108 Most intraoral melanotic naevi are seen on the hard palate, as here, or in the buccal mucosa (see Figure 14.109). Most are circumscribed, small, greyish or brownish macules and are benign.

Figure 14.109 The most common are intramucosal naevi. Less common are oral melanotic macules and compound and junctional naevi.

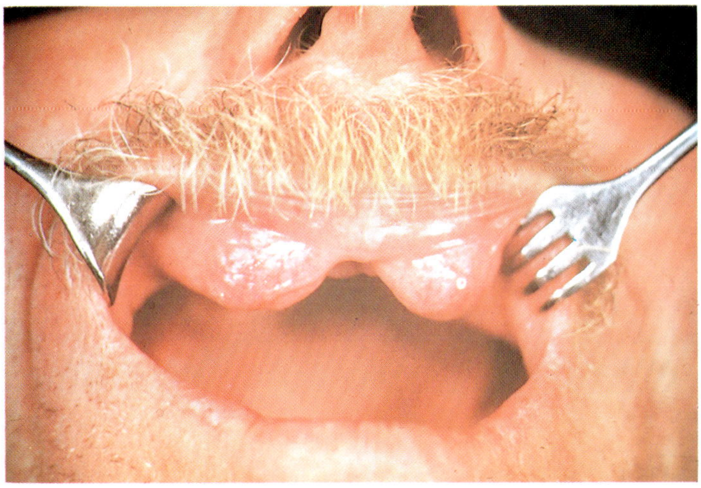
14.110

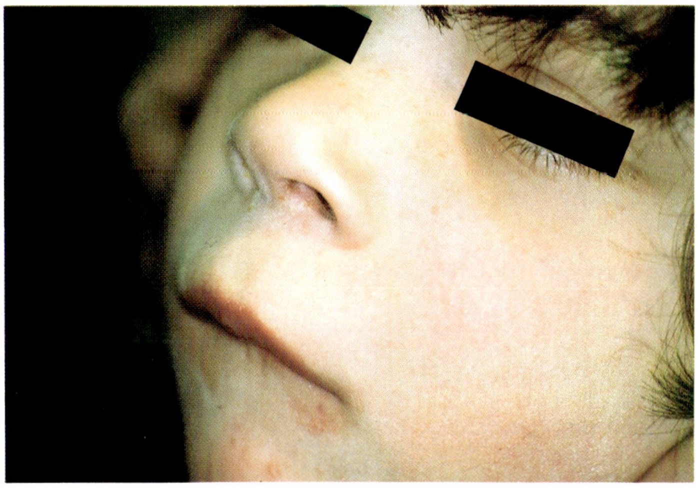
14.111

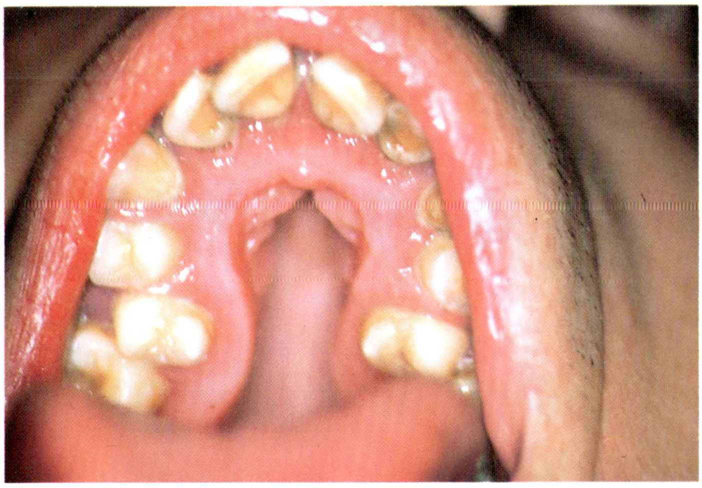
14.112

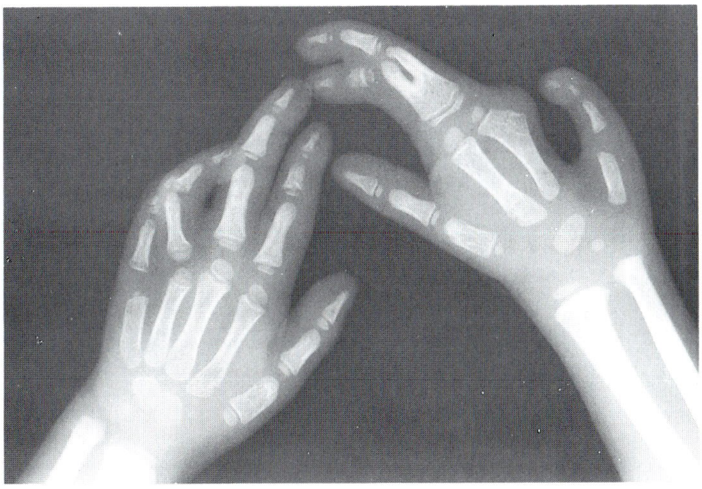
14.113

ASCHER'S SYNDROME

Figure 14.110 The combination of double lip (shown here) with sagging eyelids (blepharochalasis) and non-toxic thyroid enlargement is termed Ascher's syndrome.

DE LANGE SYNDROME (*Amsterdam dwarf*)

Figure 14.111 De Lange syndrome is a rare congenital disorder of 'fish mouth' with a long philtrum, eyebrows that meet (synophrys), dwarfism and mental handicap.

Figure 14.112 The mandible is hypoplastic and the palate may be cleft. Teeth are often small and delayed in eruption.

Figure 14.113 Hands and feet are small and there is often syndactyly or oligodactyly, as here.

CRI-DU-CHAT SYNDROME

Figure 14.114 Deletion of the short arm of chromosome 5 is a rare disorder characterized by a cry like a cat in infancy, and facial dysmorphogenesis. Most patients are of short stature, mentally handicapped, and often have cardiac and skeletal anomalies.

Figure 14.115 Micrognathia, high-arched palate, enamel hypoplasia and a poorly defined mandibular angle are the main features. Microcephaly, small pituitary fossa and large frontal sinuses may be seen on radiography.

PATAU'S SYNDROME

Figure 14.116 Cleft lip (often bilateral) and cleft palate with micrognathia are orofacial features of trisomy 13.

This figure shows a still-born infant with cleft lip and palate.

OROFACIAL–DIGITAL SYNDROME (*Type II: Mohr's syndrome*)

Figure 14.117 Multiple fibrous bands may be associated with cleft or lobulated tongue, polydactyly and often a midline cleft of the upper lip in Mohr's syndrome.

SMITH-LEMLI-OPITZ SYNDROME

Figure 14.118 This is a rare autosomal recessive syndrome consisting of ptosis, broad nose and anteverted nostrils, low-set ears and micrognathia. Most have some syndactyly, growth retardation, and mental handicap.

Figure 14.119 The maxillary alveolar ridges are broad and the palate high-arched or cleft.

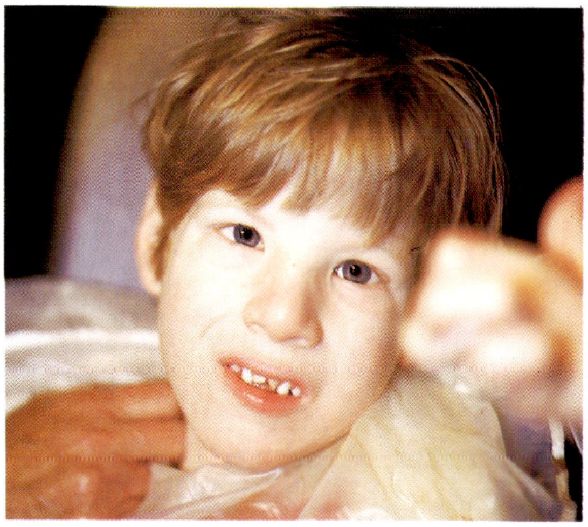

14.114

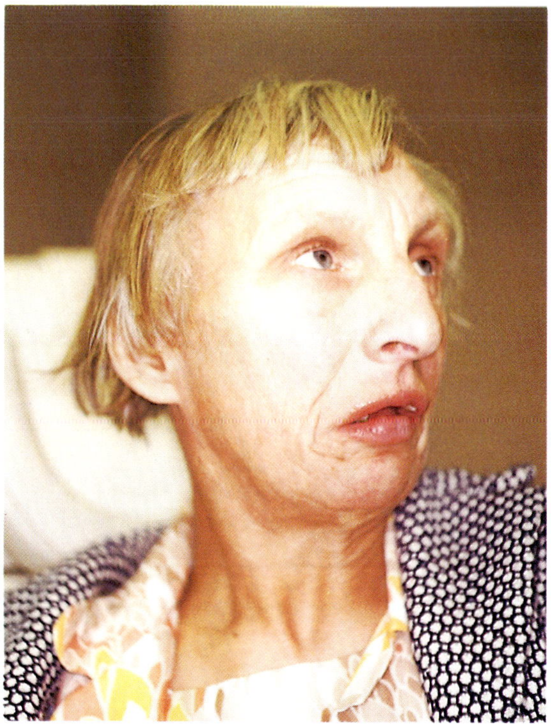

14.115

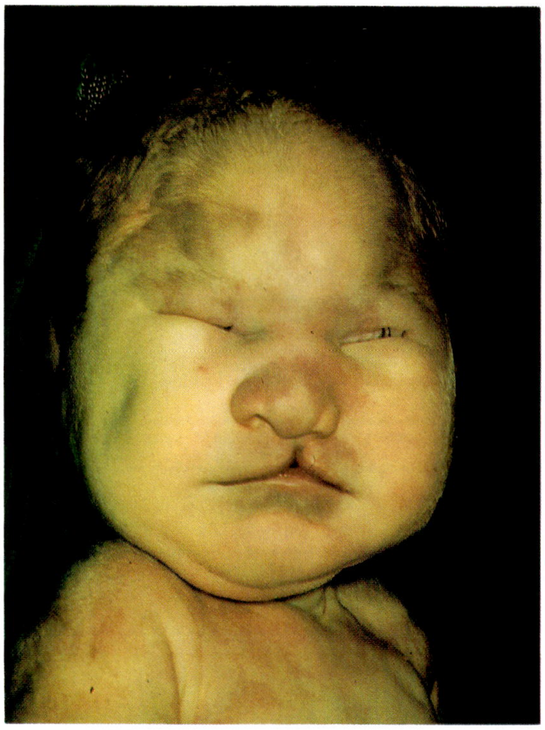

14.116

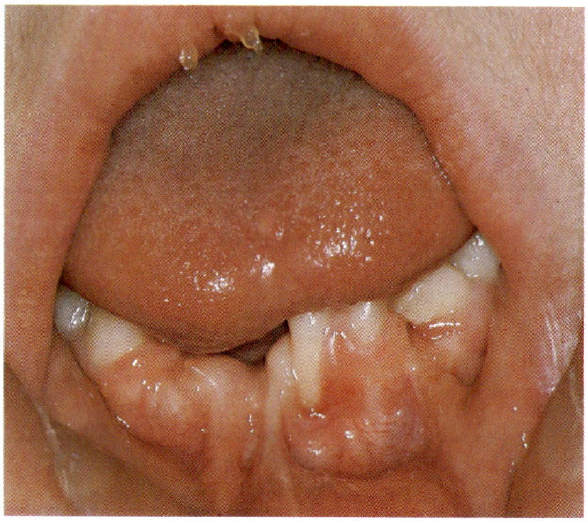

14.117

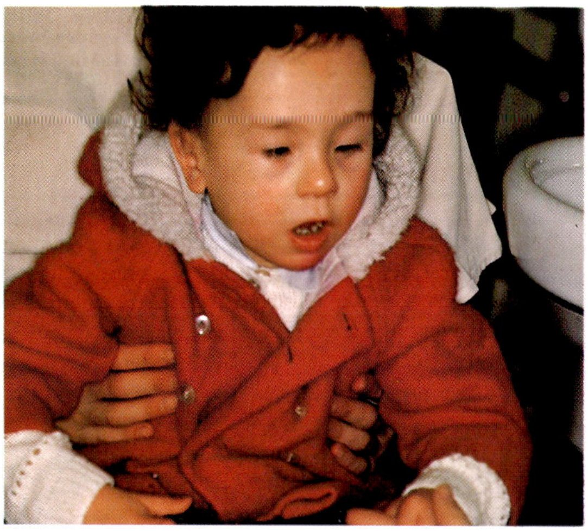

14.118

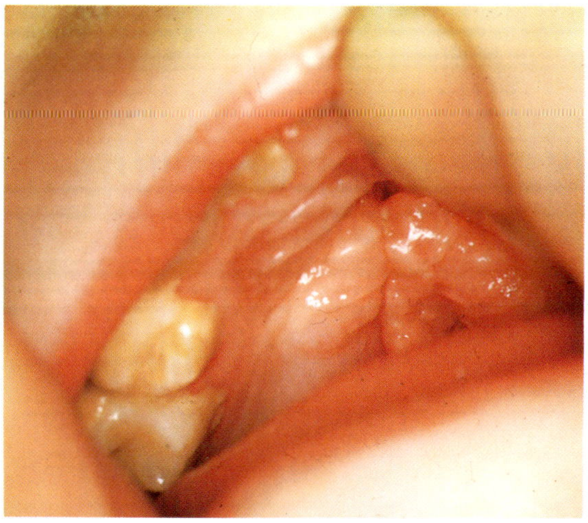

14.119

15

Injury, poisoning and iatrogenic disease

BURNS

Figure 15.1 Burns are most common after the ingestion of hot foods and are seen especially on the palate or tongue, for example, 'pizza-palate', as here.

Figure 15.2 Hot liquids caused this burn.

Cold injury is uncommon, but follows cryosurgery. Electrical burns are also uncommon, seen usually in pre-school children who bite electric flex. Very rarely, burns are caused by natural products such as the houseplant dieffenbachia, or the enzyme bromelin in pineapple.

Figure 15.3 Some patients attempt to relieve oral pain by holding an analgesic tablet at the site of pain. Aspirin has produced this burn.

Figure 15.4 Aqueous chlorhexidine is an excellent oral antiseptic but often produces superficial tooth discoloration, as shown here. Over-enthusiastic or undiluted use of concentrated solutions may rarely produce burns as shown. Taste disturbances and salivary gland swelling are other rare sequelae.

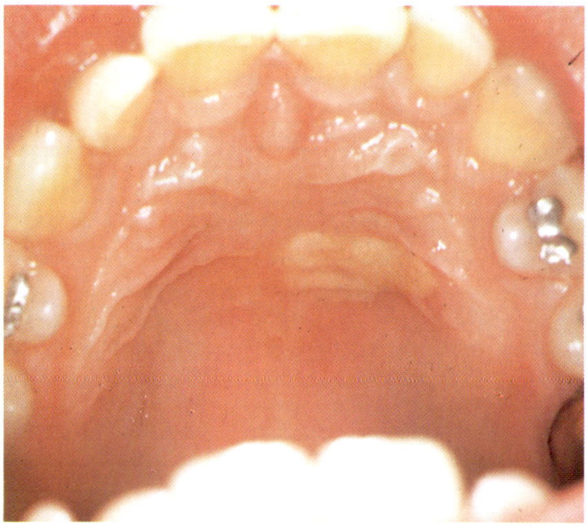

15.1

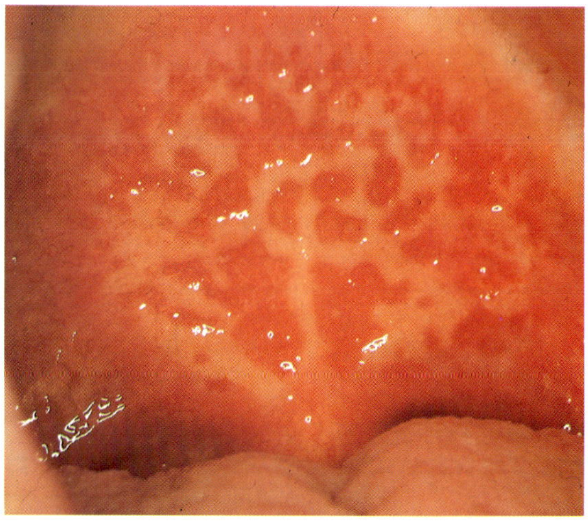

15.2

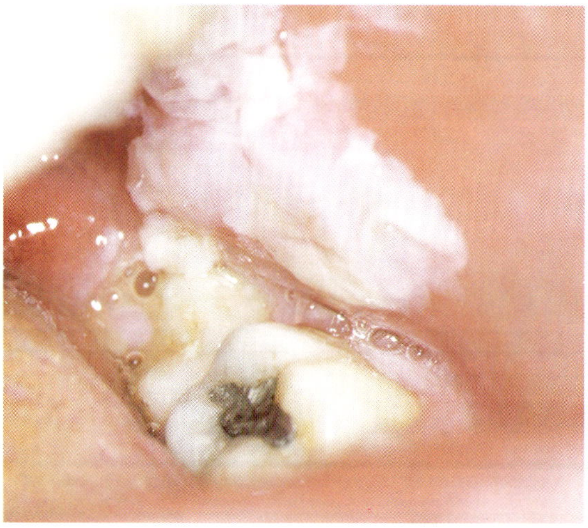

15.3

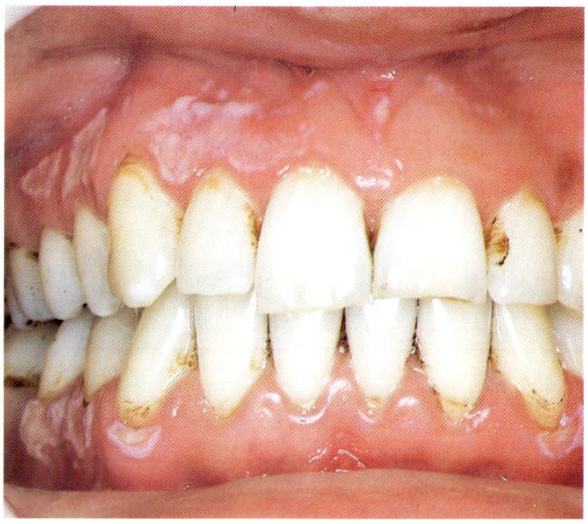

15.4

EROSIONS

Figure 15.5 Chemicals such as acids (chromic, trichloracetic, phosphoric) may be used during dental procedures and can cause ulcers. Various self-curing resins, especially epoxy resins for oral use may also, as here, produce erosions, as may various mouthwashes.

Figure 15.6 Rubber-based or silicone-based impression materials occasionally produce an erosive reaction.

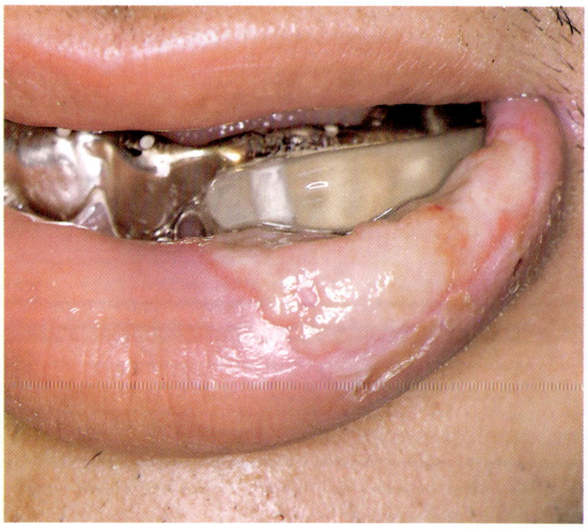

15.5

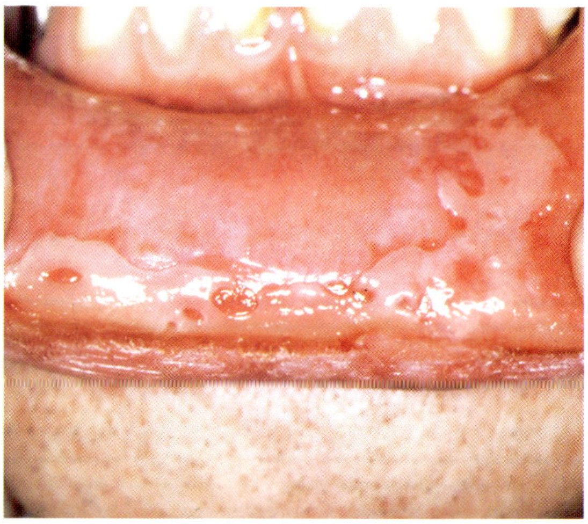

15.6

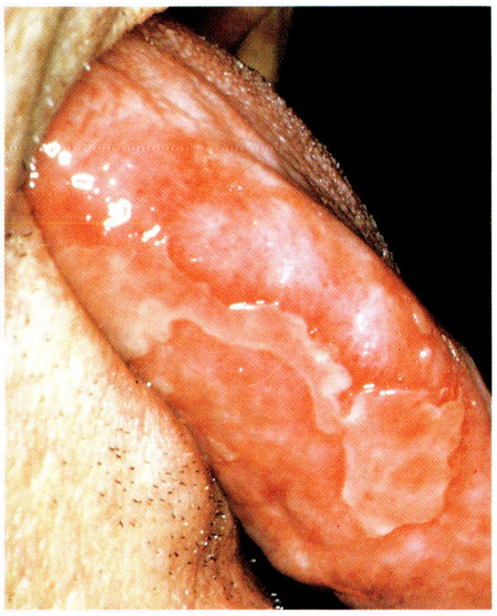
15.7

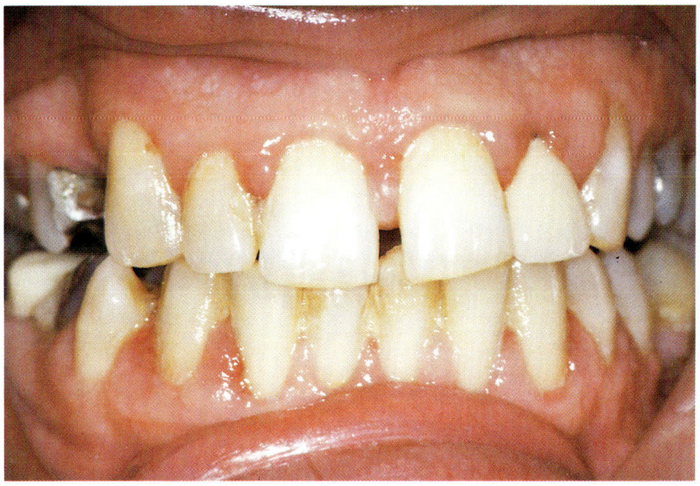
15.8

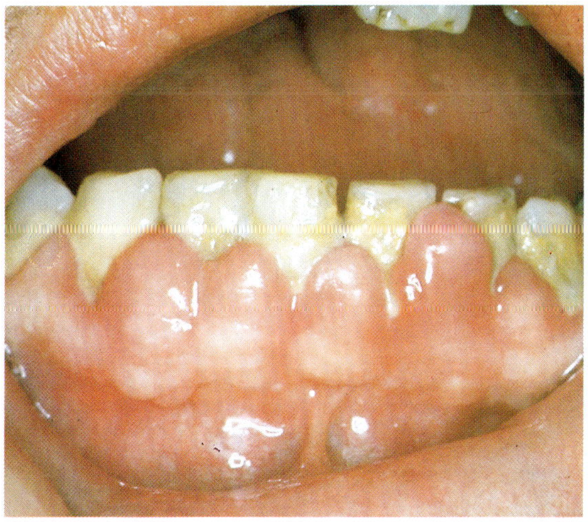
15.9

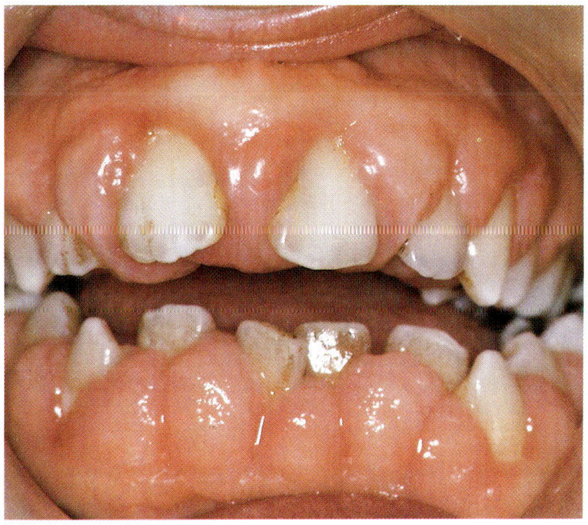
15.10

LICHENOID LESIONS

Figure 15.7 Lesions resembling lichen planus, lupus erythematosus, pemphigoid or pemphigus may be drug-induced. Non-steroidal anti-inflammatory agents, antidiabetic, antihypertensive and antimalarial drugs are causes of lichenoid lesions, as are some restorative materials and graft-versus-host disease. This was a reaction to methyldopa.

DRUG-INDUCED GINGIVAL HYPERPLASIA

Figure 15.8 Nifedipine is an antihypertensive and anti-anginal agent that can produce gingival hyperplasia, similar to that induced by phenytoin. The anti-anginal drug, diltiazem, may also have this effect.

All types of drug-induced gingival hyperplasia may also be associated with hirsutism.

Figure 15.9 Cyclosporin is a commonly-used immunosuppressive drug that can cause gingival hyperplasia closely resembling that induced by phenytoin. It is seen mainly anteriorly and labially and is exacerbated by poor oral hygiene and concurrent administration of nifedipine.

Figure 15.10 The anticonvulsant phenytoin is the drug which classically can produce gingival hyperplasia. Poor oral hygiene exacerbates the hyperplasia, which appears interdentally 2–3 months after treatment is started. The papillae enlarge to a variable extent, with relatively little tendency to bleed.

EPILEPSY

Figure 15.11 Epileptics often suffer repeated orofacial trauma causing soft tissue lacerations and scarring as here, and damage to teeth and/or jaws.

Anti-epileptic drugs given to pregnant mothers may cause fetal orofacial defects. These have been recorded both with phenytoin and with valproate.

DRUG-INDUCED HYPERPIGMENTATION

Figure 15.12 Long-term use of phenytoin can have wide-reaching adverse effects, including hyperpigmentation. Hyperpigmentation also may be caused by antimalarials, ACTH, lofazimine, ketoconazole, busulphan and phenothiazines.

Figure 15.13 Long-term use of tranquillizers, such as chlorpromazine, may produce orofacial hyperpigmentation, xerostomia and facial dyskinesias.

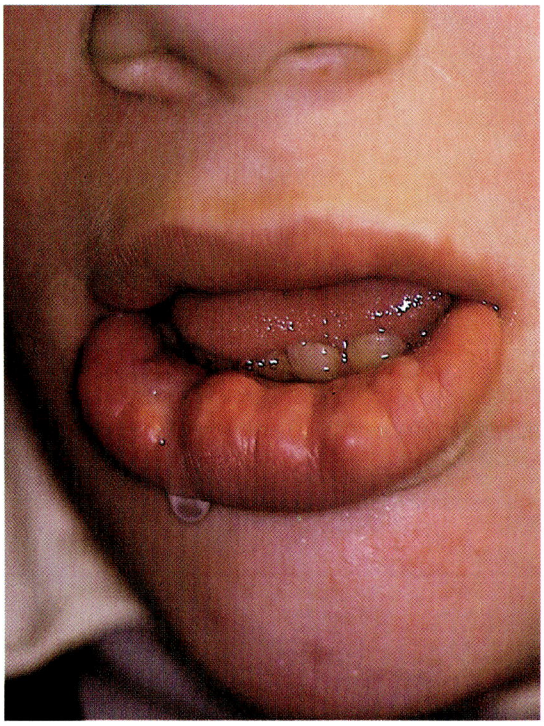

15.11

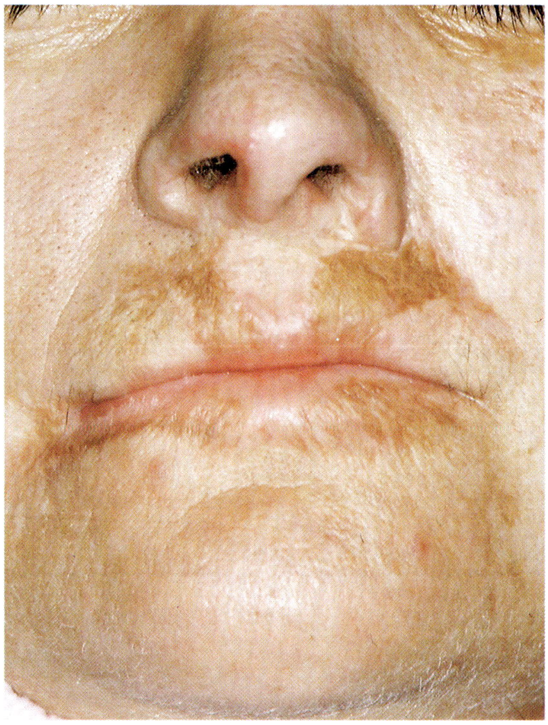

15.12

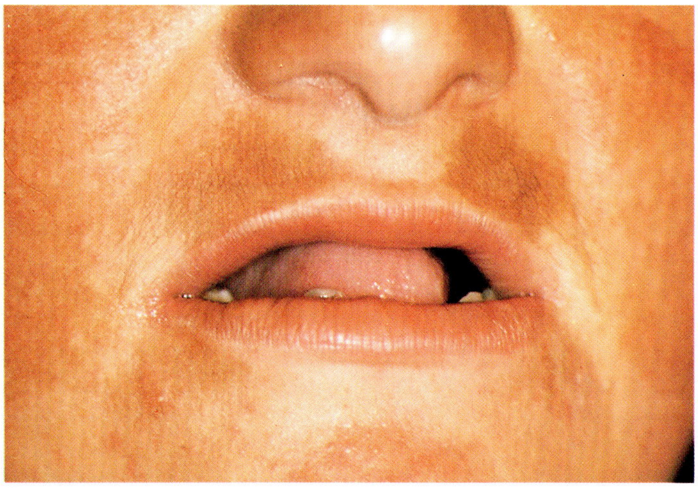

15.13

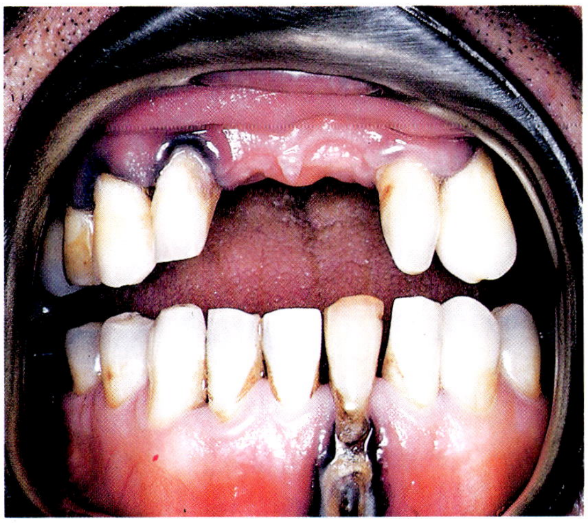

15.14

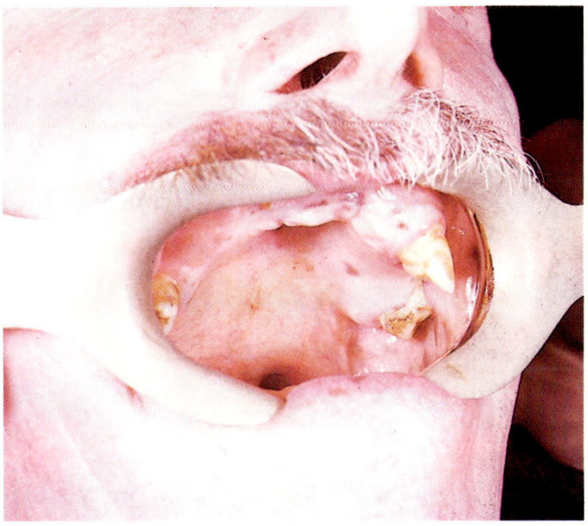

15.15

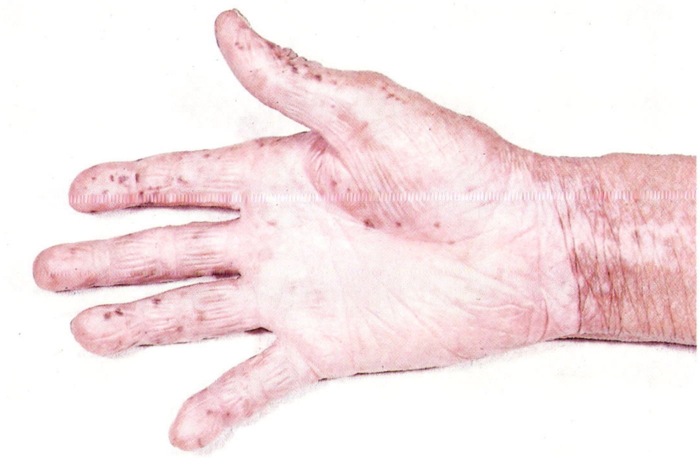

15.16

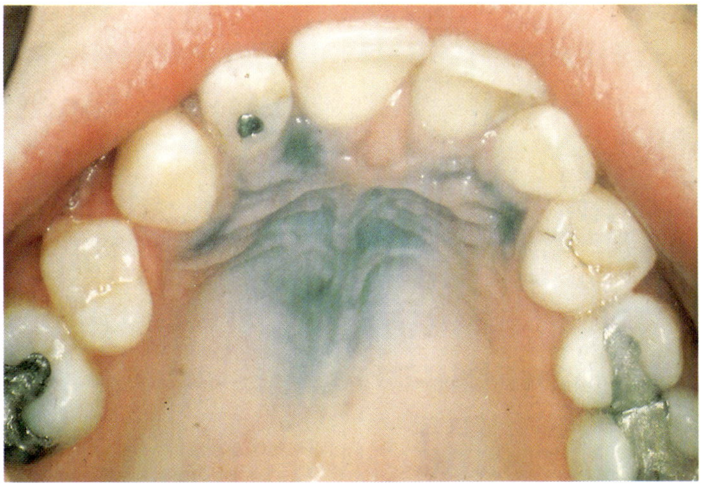

15.17

HEAVY METAL POISONING

Figure 15.14 Heavy metal poisoning is now fortunately rare. Bismuth and lead cause a line at the gingival margin where sulphides are deposited.

Figure 15.15 Arsenic poisoning is now rare and usually follows the ingestion of pesticides containing arsenates. Arsenic binds to keratins and chronic intoxication leads to mucositis, pigmentation, and facial oedema.

Figure 15.16 Arsenic poisoning causes 'rain-drop' hyperpigmentation of the skin with hyperkeratosis of the palms and soles and white transverse striae on the nails (Mees' line).

FOREIGN BODIES

Figure 15.17 Palatal pigmentation from a foreign body (a pencil lead in this instance). Foreign bodies may result from facial trauma and may enter the maxillary antrum.

AMALGAM TATTOO

Figure 15.18 Dental amalgam is a common cause of oral hyperpigmentation. Here amalgam has been used as a retrograde root-filling material, causing discoloration high towards the vestibule.

Figure 15.19 Amalgam can also be incorporated into the tissues during conservative dentistry. A bluish-black macule is usually seen in the gingiva, especially in the mandible in the premolar–molar region.

ACRODYNIA

Figure 15.20 Chronic mercury exposure, from mercuric oxide (calomel) in teething powders, was a common cause of acrodynia up until the early 1950s. Now rare, acrodynia may be caused by mercury from paints, ointments, broken fluorescent light bulbs, or metallic mercury. Most cases are in children up to the age of 8 years, and present with profuse sweating, rashes, photophobia, alopecia, and puffiness and pink colour of the face, hands and feet (Pink disease). In many ways acrodynia resembles Kawasaki's disease (mucocutaneous lymph node syndrome).

Figure 15.21 Oral ulcers, disturbed tooth development and tooth exfoliation may be seen in severe acrodynia.

TRAUMATIC HYPERPLASIA

Figure 15.22 Suction discs formerly used to help denture retention (see Figure 15.23) may produce hyperplasia in the palatal vault.

Figure 15.23 Suction disc (see Figure 15.22).

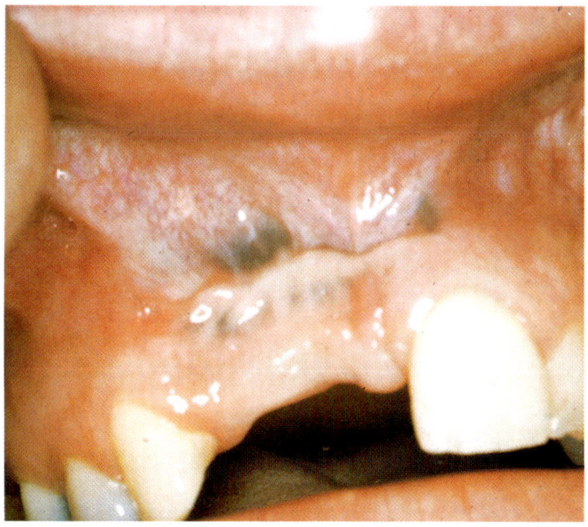

15.18

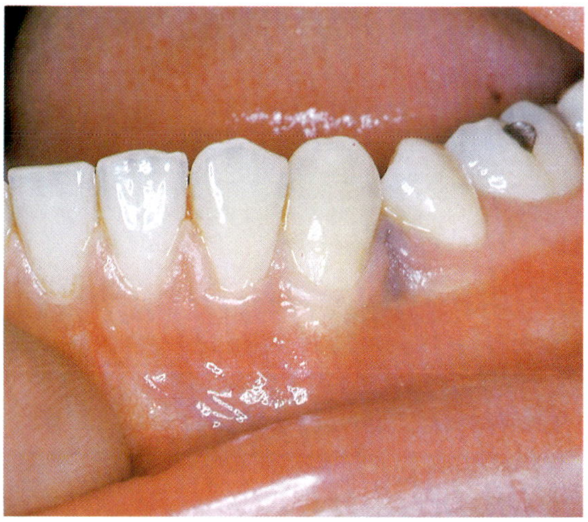

15.19

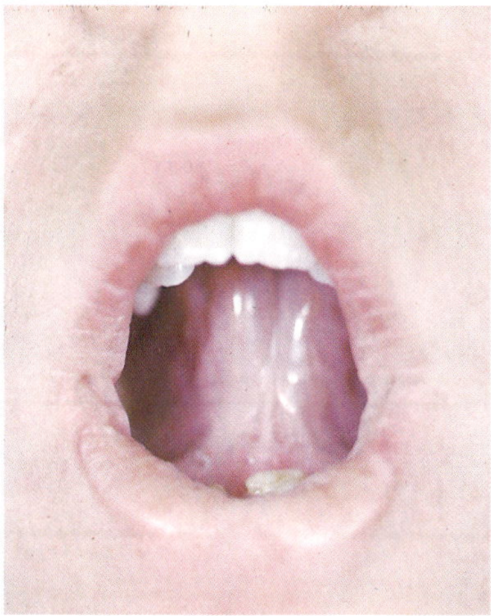

15.20

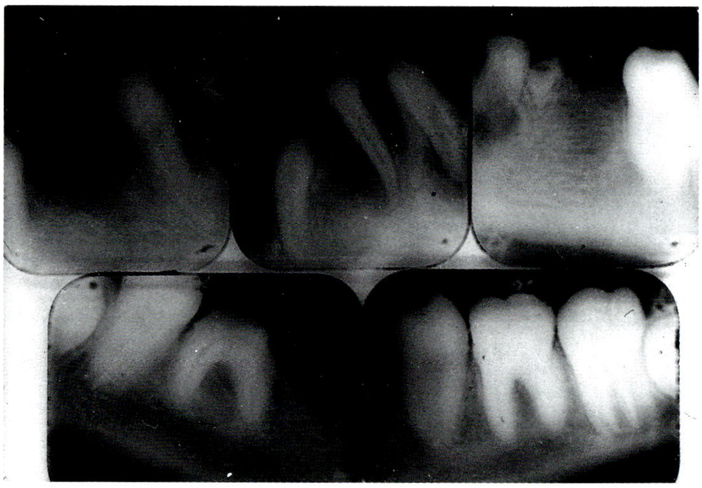

15.21

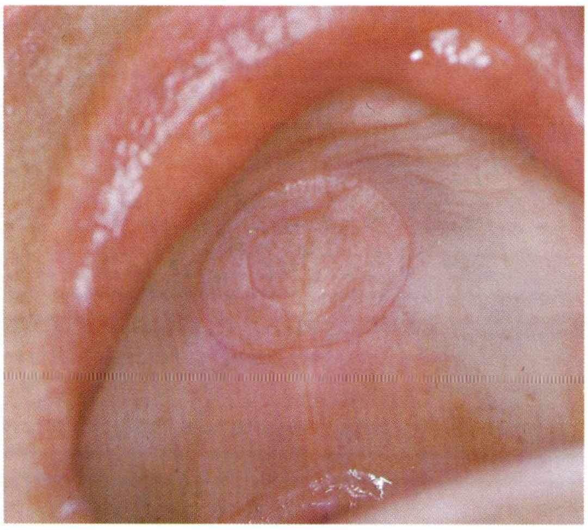

15.22

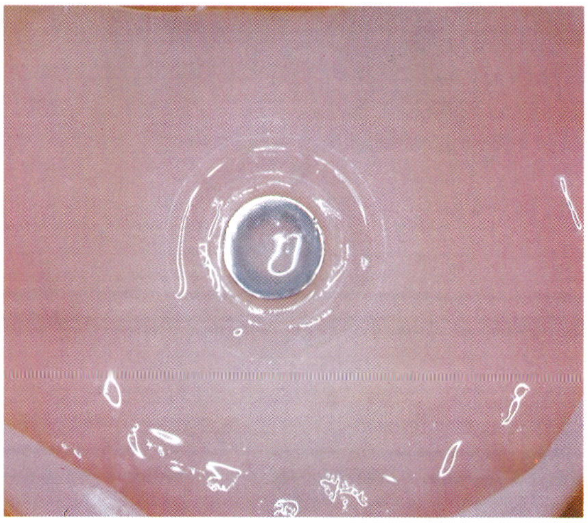

15.23

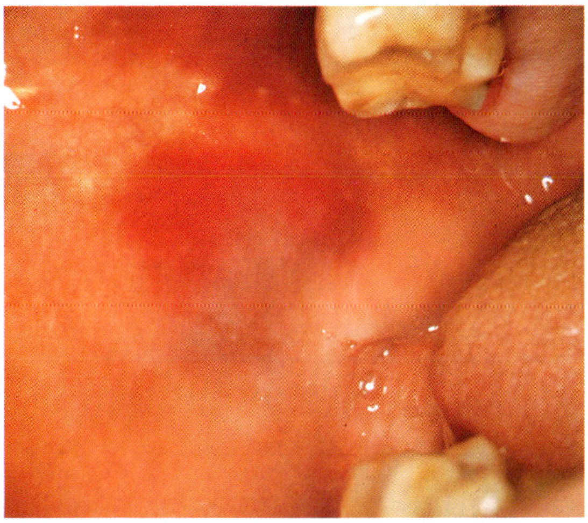

15.24

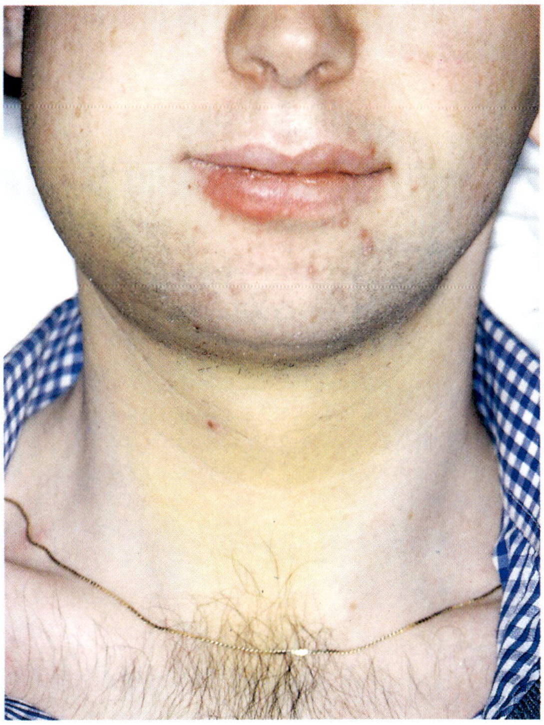

15.25

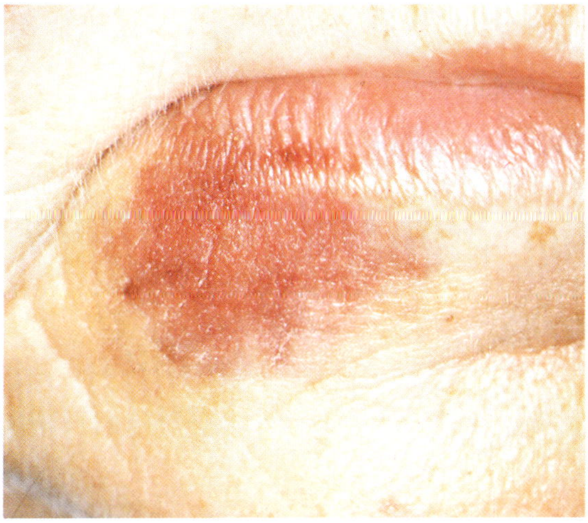

15.26

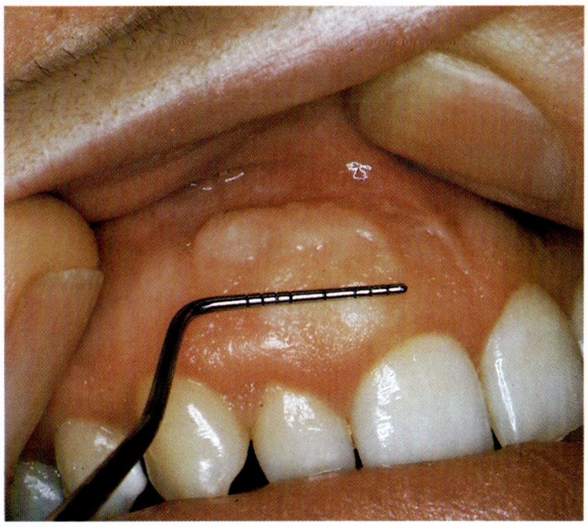

15.27

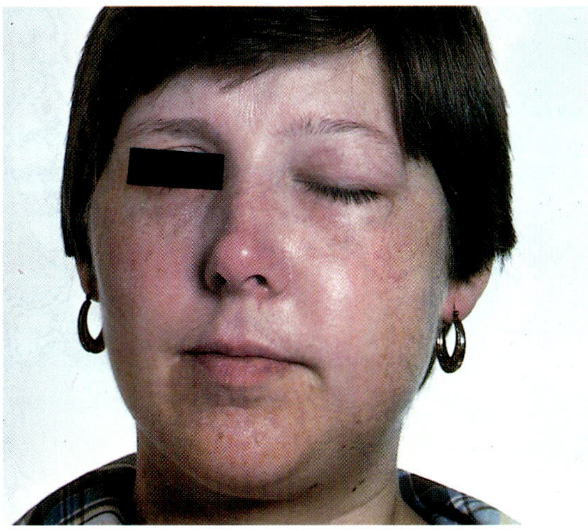

15.28

IATROGENIC INJURY

Figure 15.24 Haematoma: dental local anaesthetic injections, especially regional blocks, commonly produce a small haematoma which is usually inconsequential unless intramuscular, when it can cause trismus, or become infected.

Figure 15.25 Extraoral swelling may be produced by a haematoma, as here. Blood may track through fascial planes of the neck to cause extensive bruising, even down to the chest wall.

Figure 15.26 Bruising from careless handling of the tissues.

CICATRIZATION

Figure 15.27 Intraoral scarring is usually minimal except in severe tissue loss or some types of epidermolysis bullosa and mucous membrane pemphigoid. Keloids, such as here, are rare intraorally.

SURGICAL EMPHYSEMA

Figure 15.28 Dental instrumentation using air-turbine handpieces or air syringes occasionally introduces air into the tissues, producing surgical emphysema.

ANGIOEDEMA

Figure 15.29 Allergic angioedema is a type 1 response mediated by leukotrienes and vasoactive amines released from mast cells and basophils in an IgE-mediated response to an allergen. Labial swelling is a common presentation.

Allergens can be as varied as systemically administered drugs (such as penicillin) or topically contacted allergens in foodstuffs (such as benzoic and sorbic acids).

Figure 15.30 Hereditary angioedema (HANE) is a familial condition transmitted as an autosomal dominant trait, manifesting with angioedema often precipitated by mild trauma, such as that associated with dental treatment.

Swelling of the face, mouth and neck in either type of angioedema may embarrass the airway. There may also be swelling of abdominal viscera and the extremities.

Figure 15.31 This is the patient shown in Figure 15.30, seen between episodes.

Hereditary angioedema is due to a decreased or defective inhibitor of the activated first component of complement (C1). Diseases occasionally associated with HANE are a lupus-like syndrome, coronary arteritis and autoimmune conditions, including Sjögren's syndrome, rheumatoid arthritis and thyroiditis: possibly because of disturbed immuno-regulation.

C1 esterase deficiency is occasionally acquired especially in lympho-proliferative disorders.

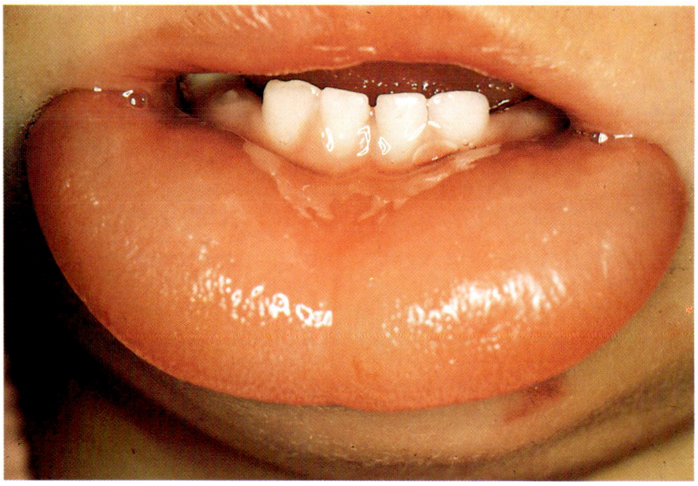

15.29

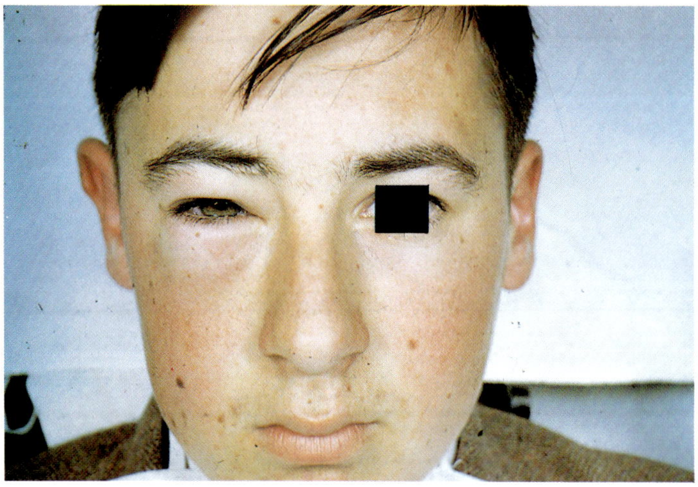

15.30

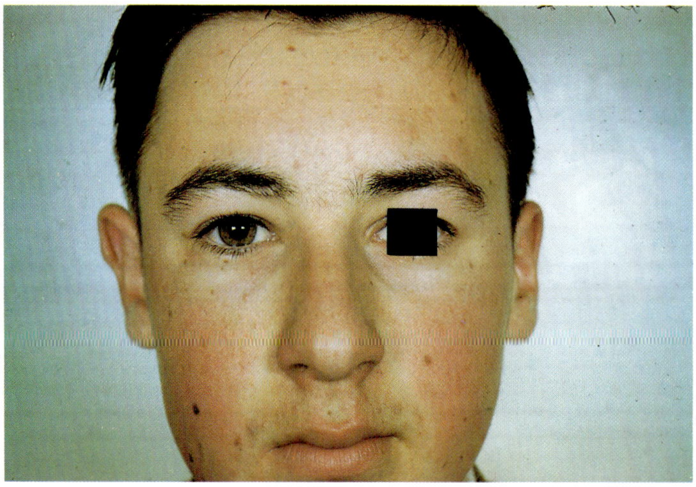

15.31

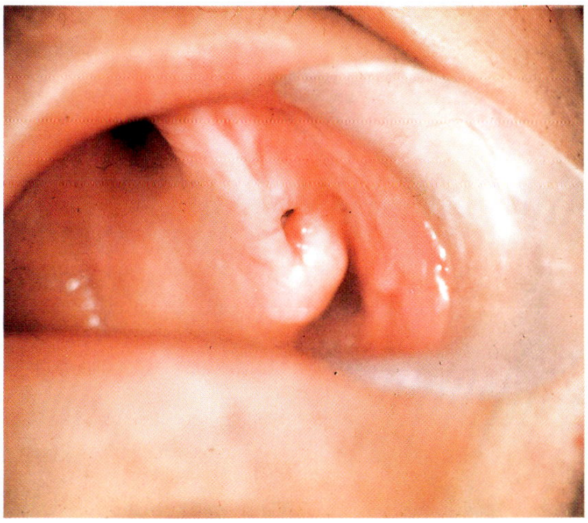

15.32

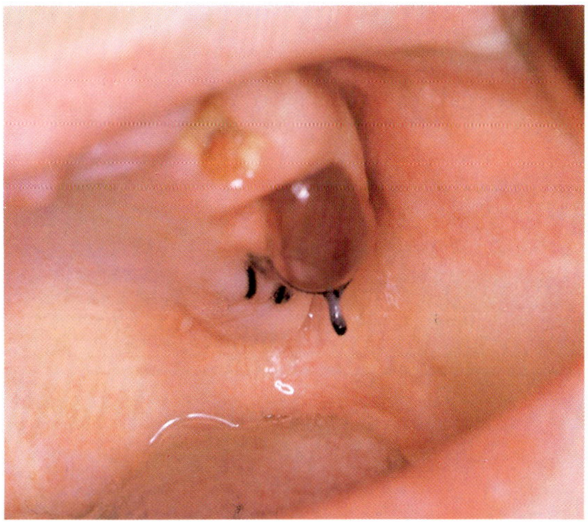

15.33

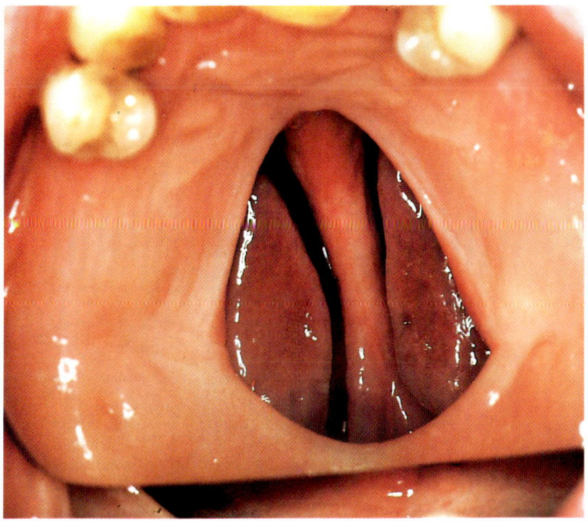

15.34

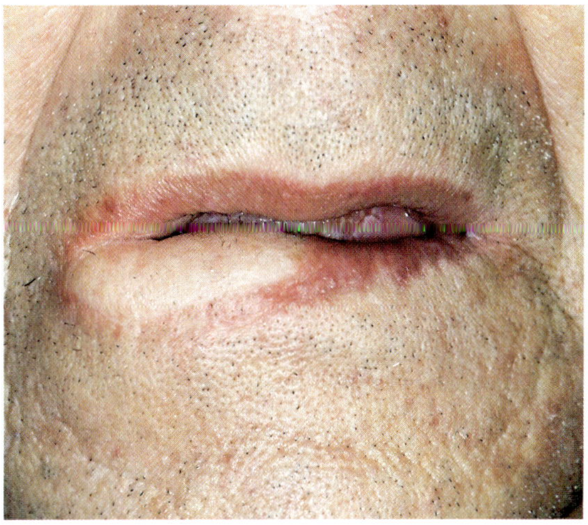

15.35

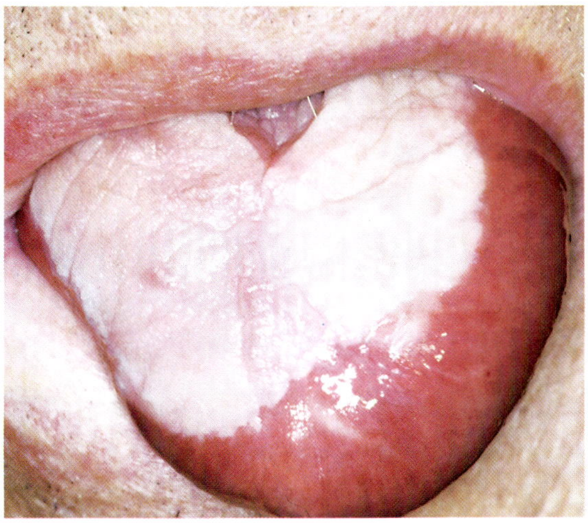

15.36

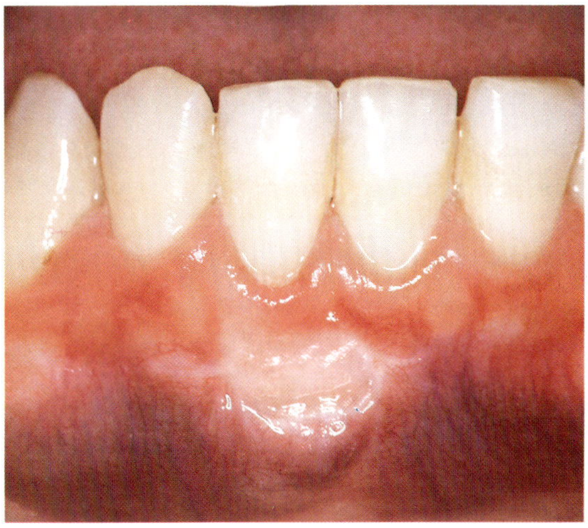

15.37

OROANTRAL FISTULA

Figure 15.32 Oroantral fistula (OAF) is almost invariably traumatic in aetiology, usually following extraction of an upper molar or premolar tooth. Fluid passes from the mouth into the sinus, which may become infected.

Figure 15.33 Occasionally, the antral lining prolapses through an OAF.

ORONASAL FISTULA

Figure 15.34 Surgery, such as the removal of a palatal neoplasm, may produce this defect.

GRAFTS

Figure 15.35 Skin graft of the defect following excision of a carcinoma remains paler than the vermilion of the lip.

Figure 15.36 Intraorally, a skin graft becomes wrinkled and white. The ungrafted (red) part of the dorsum of tongue shown here is abnormal because of 'field-change' dysplasia.

Figure 15.37 Mucosal grafts from the palate for periodontal treatment are less white than skin grafts.

RADIATION INJURY

Figure 15.38 Mucositis and xerostomia: radiotherapy involving the mouth and salivary glands invariably produces mucositis and often xerostomia. These, and other orofacial complications, are dose-dependent. Xerostomia predisposes to dental caries.

Figure 15.39 Thrush and erythematous candidosis are common, especially where xerostomia is pronounced.

Figure 15.40 Endarteritis obliterans produces mucosal scarring, decreases the vascular supply to bone, predisposing to osteoradionecrosis (see page 128) and, if involving muscle, produces trismus. Irradiation of the tongue often produces taste loss.

Figure 15.41 Scarring is later followed by the appearance of telangiectasia.

Figure 15.42 Irradiation of developing teeth can cause hypoplasia, stunted root formation, and retarded eruption.

Figure 15.43 The skin in the path of teletherapy tends to lose pigment, scar, and develop telangiectasia.

Previous irradiation predisposes to subsequent neoplasia: for example, radiotherapy to oropharyngeal neoplasms predisposes to subsequent salivary neoplasms.

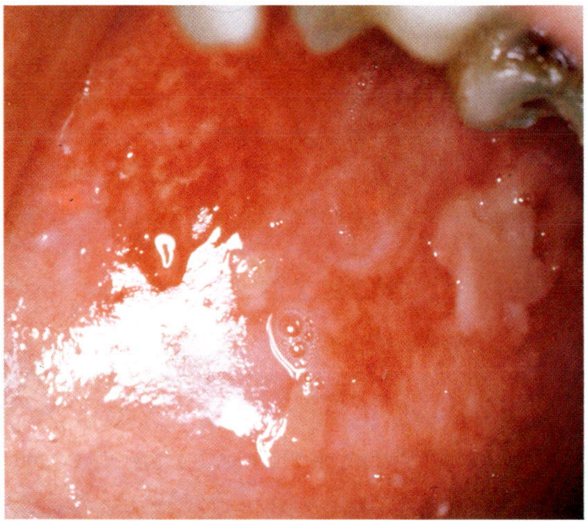
15.38

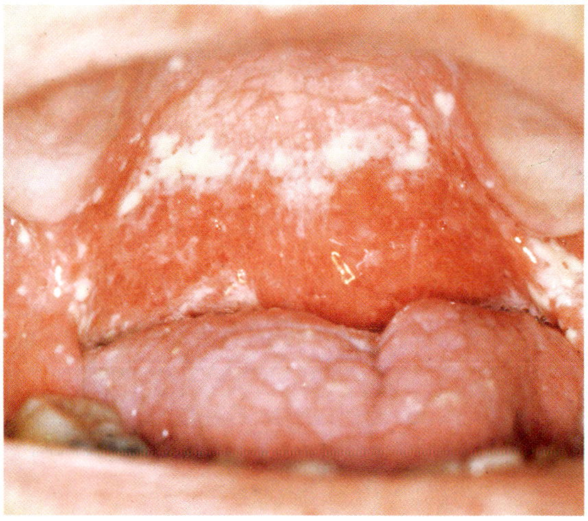
15.39

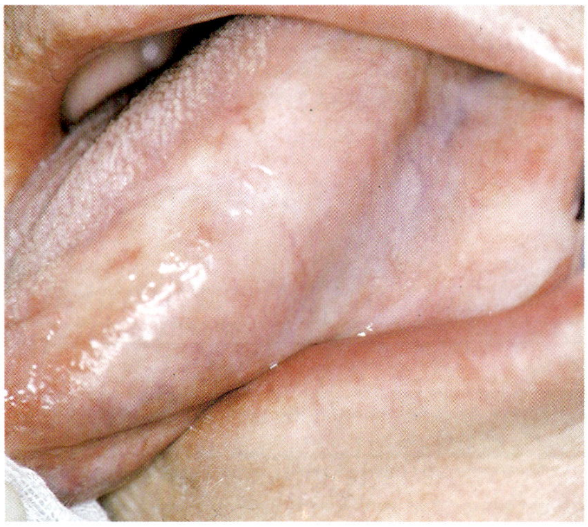
15.40

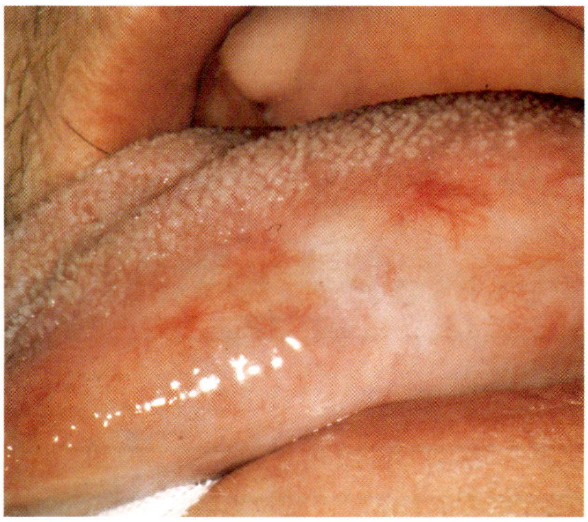
15.41

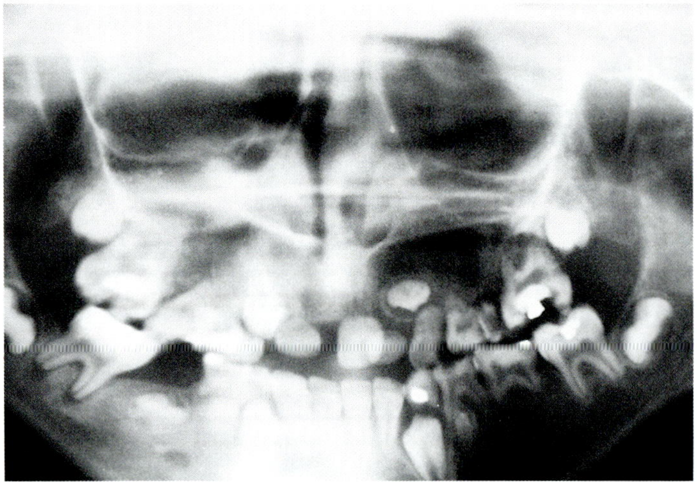
15.42

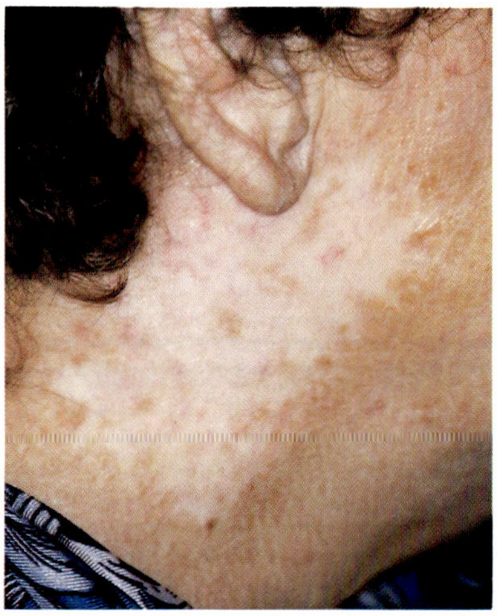
15.43

16

Differential diagnoses

Differential diagnoses by symptom

BLISTERS *(see Table 1)*

Skin diseases

Pemphigoid (usually mucous membrane pemphigoid)
Pemphigus
Erythema multiforme
Dermatitis herpetiformis/linear IgA disease
Epidermolysis bullosa
Lichen planus (rarely)

Infections

Herpes simplex
Herpes varicella-zoster
Coxsackie viruses

Others

Burns
Angina bullosa haemorrhagica (localized oral purpura)
Amyloid

False blisters

Cysts
Mucoceles
Abscesses

Table 1 DIFFERENTIATION OF THE MORE COMMON ORAL VESICULOBULLOUS DISORDERS

	Pemphigus	*Mucous membrane pemphigoid*	*Erythema multiforme*	*Dermatitis herpetiformis*	*Lichen planus**
Incidence	Rare	Uncommon	Uncommon	Rare	Uncommon
Age mainly affected	Middle age	Late middle age	Young adults	Middle age	Middle age
Sex mainly affected	F	F	M	M	F
Geographic factors	Italian, Jewish origin	—	—	—	—
Predisposing factors	—	—	Drugs, infections	Gluten-sensitive enteropathy	Drugs
Oral manifestations	Erosions, blisters rarely persist, Nikolsky sign positive	Blisters (sometimes blood-filled), erosions, Nikolsky may be positive	Swollen lips, serosanguinous exudate, large erosions anteriorly, occasional blisters	Blisters, ulcers	White lesions, red lesions, erosions, rarely bullae
Cutaneous manifestations	Large flaccid blisters at some stage	Rare or minor	Target or iris lesions may be present	Pruritic vesicular rash on back and extensor surfaces	Pruritic, papular on flexor surfaces, ± nail involvement
Histopathology	Acantholysis, intraepithelial bulla	Subepithelial bulla	Subepithelial bulla	Subepithelial bulla	Hyperkeratosis, acanthosis, basal cell liquefaction
Direct immunofluorescence	Intercellular IgG in epithelium	Subepithelial/BMZ†, C3, IgG	Subepithelial IgG‡	Subepithelial IgA	Variably IgM/fibrin C3‡ at BMZ†
Serology	Antibodies to epithelial intercellular cement in most	Antibodies to epithelial basement membrane in few	—	Antibodies to reticulin in some	—
Other investigations or features	—	—	—	Biopsy of small intestine	—

* Rarely bullous.
† BMZ = basement membrane zone.
‡ Non-specific findings.

BURNING MOUTH

Deficiency states

Vitamin B_{12} deficiency
Folate acid deficiency
Iron deficiency
B complex deficiency

Infections

Candidosis

Others

Erythema migrans (geographic tongue)
Diabetes

Psychogenic

Cancerophobia
Depression
Anxiety states
Hypochondriasis

CACOGEUSIA

Oral infections

Pericoronitis
Chronic periodontitis
Acute necrotizing ulcerative gingivitis
Chronic dental abscesses
Dry socket
Food impaction
Sialadenitis

Xerostomia

Drugs
Sjögren's syndrome
Sarcoidosis
Irradiation damage

Psychogenic causes

Depression
Anxiety states
Psychoses
Hypochondriasis

Drugs

Metronidazole
Disulphiram
Amiodarone
Angiotensin-converting enzyme inhibitors
Allopurinol
Phenylbutazone
Smoking

Starvation

Nasopharyngeal disease

Chronic sinusitis
Oroantral fistula
Neoplasm
Nasal foreign body

Respiratory disease

Bronchiectasis

Gastrointestinal disease

Pharyngeal pouch
Gastric regurgitation
Liver disease

Central nervous system disease

Temporal lobe tumours
Temporal lobe epilepsy

Renal disease

Uraemia

DISCHARGES

Dental disease

Chronic dental and parodontal abscesses
Dry socket
Cysts
Oroantral fistula
Osteomyelitis
Osteoradionecrosis
Infection by foreign body

Salivary gland disorders

Sialadenitis
Salivary fistulae

Psychogenic (imagined discharges)

Depression
Hypochondriasis
Psychosis

DRY MOUTH (xerostomia)

Drugs with anticholinergic effects

Atropine and analogues
Tricyclic antidepressants

Antihistamines
Antiemetics
Tranquillizers

Drugs with sympathomimetic actions

Decongestants
Bronchodilators
Appetite suppressants
Amphetamines

Others

Lithium
Disopyramide

Dehydration

Uncontrolled diabetes mellitus
Diabetes insipidus
Diarrhoea and vomiting
Severe haemorrhage

Psychogenic

Anxiety states
Depression
Hypochondriasis

Salivary gland disease

Sjögren's syndrome
Sarcoidosis
Irradiation damage
HIV infection
Bone marrow transplantation/graft-versus-host disease

DYSARTHRIA

Oral disease

Painful lesions or loss of mobility of the tongue or palate
Cleft palate
Oral neoplasia
Severe scarring

Neurological disorders

Multiple sclerosis
Parkinson's disease
Motor neurone disease
Cerebrovascular accident
Bulbar and pseudo-bulbar palsy
Hypoglossal nerve palsy
Cerebral palsy
Cerebellar disease
Myopathies
Dyskinesias

Drugs

Phenothiazines
Levodopa
Butyrophenones
Addictive intoxicants, eg, alcohol

Severe xerostomia

Mechanical

Poorly fitting prostheses

DYSPHAGIA

Oral disease

Inflammatory, traumatic, surgical or neoplastic lesions of tongue, palate or pharynx
Xerostomia

Oesophageal disease

Foreign body
Stricture
Neoplasia
Systemic sclerosis
Pharyngeal pouch
Oesophagitis
Extrinsic compressive lesions (eg, mediastinal lymphadenopathy)

Psychogenic

Hysteria (Globus hystericus)

Neurological disorders

Multiple sclerosis
Cerebrovascular accident
Bulbar and pseudo-bulbar palsy
Parkinson's disease
Syringobulbia/syringomyelia
Achalasia of the cardia
Myopathies (eg, myasthenia gravis)
Lateral medullary syndrome

FACIAL PALSY

Neurological

Bell's palsy
Stroke
Cerebral tumour
Moebius syndrome
Multiple sclerosis
Ramsay-Hunt syndrome
Guillain-Barré syndrome

HIV infection
Trauma to facial nerve or its branches
Diabetes
Leprosy
Kawasaki disease
Lyme disease
Connective tissue disorders

Middle ear disease

Cholesteatoma
Mastoiditis

Parotid

Parotid trauma
Parotid malignancy

Others

Melkersson-Rosenthal syndrome
Sarcoidosis (Heerfordt syndrome)

Myopathies

FACIAL SWELLING

Facial swelling is commonly inflammatory in orgin, caused by cutaneous or dental infection or trauma.

Inflammatory

Oral infections
Cutaneous infections
Insect bites

Traumatic

Post-operative oedema or haematoma
Traumatic oedema or haematoma
Surgical emphysema

Immunological

Allergic angioedema
Hereditary angioedema

Endocrine and metabolic

Systemic corticosteroid therapy
Cushing's syndrome and disease
Myxoedema
Acromegaly
Obesity
Nephrotic syndrome

Superior vena cava syndrome

Cysts

Neoplasms

Foreign bodies

Others

Crohn's disease (and orofacial granulomatosis)
Sarcoidosis
Melkersson-Rosenthal syndrome
Congenital (eg, lymphangioma)

HALITOSIS

Oral sepsis

Food impaction
Chronic dental and parodontal sepsis
Infections
Acute necrotizing ulcerative gingivitis
Dry socket
Oral malignancy
Pericoronitis

Nasopharyngeal disease

Foreign body
Tonsillitis
Neoplasm

Volatile foodstuffs

Garlic
Onions
Highly spiced foods

Drugs

Solvent abuse
Alcohol
Smoking
Chloral hydrate
Nitrites and nitrates
Dimethyl sulphoxide
Disulphiram
Cytotoxic drugs
Phenothiazines
Amphetamines
Paraldehyde

Systemic disease

Acute febrile illness
Respiratory tract infections
Hepatic failure
Renal failure
Diabetic ketoacidosis
Leukaemias

Psychogenic

Neuroses
Psychoses

HYPERPIGMENTATION

Racial

Pregnancy

Food/drugs

Endocrinopathies

Addison's disease
Nelson's syndrome
Ectopic ACTH production

Others

Albright's syndrome
Haemochromatosis/haemosiderosis
Drugs
ACTH therapy

Localized (oral)

Amalgam tattoo
Ephelis
Melanoma
Naevus
Peutz-Jegher syndrome
Kaposi's sarcoma
Smoker's melanosis
Acanthosis nigricans
Heavy metal poisoning

LOSS OF TASTE

Anosmia

Upper respiratory tract infections
Maxillofacial injuries (tearing of olfactory nerves)

Neurological disease

Lesions of chorda tympani
Cerebrovascular disease
Multiple sclerosis
Bell's palsy
Fractured base of skull
Posterior cranial fossa tumours
Cerebral metastases
Trigeminal sensory neuropathy

Psychogenic

Anxiety states

Table 2 DIFFERENTIATION OF IMPORTANT TYPES OF FACIAL PAIN*

	Idiopathic trigeminal neuralgia	*Atypical facial pain*	*Migraine*	*Migrainous neuralgia*
Age (years)	>50	30–50	Any	30–50
Sex	F>M	F>M	F>M	M>F
Site	Unilateral, mandible or maxilla	± Bilateral, maxilla	Any	Retro-orbital
Associated features	—	± Depression	± Photophobia ± nausea, ± vomiting	± Conjunctival injection, ± lacrimation, ± nasal congestion
Character	Lancinating	Dull	Throbbing	Boring
Duration of episode	Brief (seconds)	Continual	Many hours (usually during day)	Few hours (usually during night, often at same time)
Precipitating factors	± Trigger areas	None	± Foods, ± stress	± Alcohol, ± stress
Relieving factors	Carbamazepine	Antidepressants	Clonidine, ergot derivatives	Clonidine, ergot derivatives

*Most oral pain is caused by local disease.

Depression
Psychoses

Drugs

Penicillamine

Others

Irradiation
Xerostomia
Zinc or copper deficiency

PAIN *(see Table 2)*

Local diseases

Disease of the teeth

Pulpitis
Periapical periodontitis

Diseases of the periodontium

Lateral (periodontal) abscess
Acute necrotizing ulcerative gingivitis
Pericoronitis

Diseases of the jaws

Dry socket
Fractures
Osteomyelitis
Infected cysts
Malignant neoplasms

Disease of the antrum

Acute sinusitis
Malignant neoplasms

Disease of the salivary glands

Acute sialadentitis
Calculi or other obstruction to duct
Severe Sjögren's syndrome
Malignant neoplasms

Diseases of the temporomandibular joint

Disease of the eyes

Glaucoma

Vascular disorders

Migraine
Migrainous neuralgia
Cranial arteritis (giant cell or temporal arteritis)

Neurological disorders

Trigeminal neuralgia
Malignant neoplasms involving the trigeminal nerve
Multiple sclerosis
Bell's palsy (rarely)
Herpes zoster (including post-herpetic neuralgia)

Psychogenic pain

Atypical facial pain and other oral symptoms associated with anxiety or depression, eg, mandibular pain-dysfunction

Referred pain

Angina, nasopharyngeal, ocular and aural disease
Chest disease (rarely)

PIGMENTATION see Hyperpigmentation

PURPURA

Trauma

Platelet and vascular disorders

Thrombocytopenia (especially drugs and leukaemias)
Thrombasthenia
Von Willebrand's disease
Scurvy
Ehlers-Danlos syndrome
Chronic renal failure
'Senile' purpura

Infections

Infectious mononucleosis
Rubella
HIV infections

Localized oral purpura (angina bullosa haemorrhagica)

Amyloidosis

RED AREAS

Generalized redness

Candidosis
Avitaminosis B complex (rarely)
Irradiation mucositis

Mucosal atrophy
Polycythaemia

Localized red patches

Denture-induced stomatitis
Erythroplasia
Purpura
Telangiectases
Angiomas (purple)
Kaposi's sarcoma
Burns
Lichen planus
Lupus erythematosus
Avitaminosis B_{12}

SIALORRHOEA

Psychogenic (usually)

Painful lesions in the mouth

Foreign bodies in the mouth

Drugs

Parasympathomimetics
Buprenorphine
Others

Poor neuromuscular coordination

Parkinson's disease
Facial palsy
Mental handicap

Others

Rabies (rarely)
Heavy metal poisoning (rarely)

TRISMUS

Extra-articular causes

Infection and inflammation near masticatory muscles
Mandibular pain-dysfunction syndrome
Fractured condylar neck
Fibrosis (including scars, systemic sclerosis and sub-mucous fibrosis)
Tetanus
Tetany
Invading neoplasm
Myositis ossificans
Coronoid hypertrophy or fusion to zygomatic arch
Hysteria

Intra-articular causes

Dislocation
Intracapsular fracture
Arthritides
Ankylosis

ULCERS

Traumatic

Mechanical (may be artefactual)
Chemical, electrical, thermal, radiation burns

Neoplastic

Carcinoma and other malignant tumours

Recurrent aphthous stomatitis

(including Behçet's syndrome)

Systemic disease

***Cutaneous disease*:** Erosive lichen planus, pemphigus vulgaris, mucous membrane pemphigoid and bullous pemphigoid, erythema multiforme, dermatitis herpetiformis and linear IgA disease, epidermolysis bullosa, angina bullosa haemorrhagica

***Blood disorders*:** Anaemia, sideropenia, neutropenia, leukaemia

***Gastrointestinal*:** Coeliac disease, Crohn's disease, ulcerative colitis

***Connective tissue disease*:** Lupus erythematosus, Reiter's disease

***Infective*:** Herpetic stomatitis, chickenpox, herpes zoster, hand, foot and mouth disease, herpangina, infectious mononucleosis, acute necrotizing ulcerative gingivitis, tuberculosis, syphilis, histoplasmosis or blastomycosis (rarely), HIV infection

***Drugs*:** Cytotoxics, many others

***Others*:** Ischaemic necrosis in giant cell arteritis

WHITE LESIONS

Congenital

White sponge naevus

Dyskeratosis congenita
Pachyonychia congenita

Acquired

Inflammatory

Infective: Candidosis, hairy leukoplakia, syphilitic leukoplakia, Koplik's spots

Non-infective: Lichen planus, lupus erythematosus, burns

Neoplastic and possibly pre-neoplastic

Keratoses (leukoplakias)
Carcinoma

Others

Drugs
Grafts

XEROSTOMIA *(see Dry Mouth)*

Differential diagnoses by site

THE LIPS

Angular stomatitis (cheilitis, cheilosis)

Candidosis (denture-induced stomatitis or other types)
Staphylococcal, streptococcal or mixed infections
Ariboflavinosis (rarely), iron, folate or B_{12} deficiency
Crohn's disease and orofacial granulomatosis
Anaemia

Bleeding

Trauma
Cracked lips
Erythema multiforme
Angiomas
Underlying haemorrhagic disease inevitably aggravates any tendency to bleed from labial lesions

Blisters

Herpes labialis
Burns
Herpes zoster
Erythema multiforme
Pemphigus vulgaris
Epidermolysis bullosa
Mucoceles
Impetigo
Allergic cheilitis

Desquamation and crusting

Dehydration
Exposure to hot dry winds
Acute febrile illness
Chemical or allergic cheilitis
Mouth-breathing
Actinic cheilitis
Exfoliative cheilitis
Candidal cheilitis
Erythema multiforme
Psychogenic (self-induced)

Swellings

There is a wide individual and racial variation in the size of the lips.

Diffuse swellings

Oedema (trauma or infection or insect bite)
Angioedema: allergic or hereditary
Crohn's disease and orofacial granulomatosis
Cheilitis granulomatosa
Cheilitis glandularis
Melkersson-Rosenthal syndrome
Lymphangioma
Haemangioma
Sarcoidosis
Macrocheilia
Ascher's syndrome

Localized swellings

Mucoceles
Chancre
Salivary adenoma
Squamous cell carcinoma
Basal cell carcinoma
Other tumours
Keratoacanthoma
Cysts
Abscesses
Insect bite
Haematomas

Ulceration

Infective

Herpes labialis
Herpes zoster
Syphilis
Leishmaniasis

Tumours

Squamous cell carcinoma
Basal cell carcinoma
Keratoacanthoma

Burns

Lupus erythematosus

Trauma

White lesions

Keratoses
Carcinoma
Lichen planus
Lupus erythematosus
Fordyce spots
Actinic keratosis
Scars

THE GINGIVA

Red areas

Redness is usually a sign of chronic gingivitis or periodontitis, but is then restricted to the gingival margins. More generalized redness is a sign of desquamative gingivitis, usually caused by lichen planus or mucous membrane pemiphigoid (see also Swelling). Other red lesions may affect the gingiva.

Bleeding

Periodontal disease

Chronic gingivitis
Chronic periodontitis
Acute ulcerative gingivitis
HIV gingivitis/periondontitis

Haemorrhagic disease

Primary platelet disorders
Lymphoproliferative disorders
Leukaemias, etc
Idiopathic thrombocytopenic purpura
Hereditary haemorrhagic telangiectasia
Ehlers-Danlos syndrome
Scurvy
Angiomas

Drugs

Anticoagulants
Non-steroid anti-inflammatory drugs
Cytotoxics
Sodium valproate

Clotting defects

Hepatobiliary disease
Haemophilas
Von Willebrand's disease

Swelling

Generalized gingival swelling

Chronic 'hyperplastic' gingivitis
Drug-induced (phenytoin, cyclosporin, nifedipine, diltiazem)
Hereditary gingival fibromatosis
Leukaemia
Mucopolysaccharidoses
Mucolipidosis
Wegener's granulomatosis
Scurvy
Crohn's disease and orofacial granulomatosis
Sarcoidosis

Localized gingival swelling

Abscesses
Cysts
Pyogenic granulomas (including pregnancy epulis)
Neoplasms (including fibrous epulis)
Giant cell lesions
Foreign bodies
Wegener's granulomatosis/midline lethal granuloma
Sarcoidosis
Amyloidosis
Crohn's disease

Ulcers

Ulcers that affect predominantly the gingivae are usually traumatic, acute ulcerative gingivitis or occasionally results of immunodeficency, especially acute leukaemia, AIDS or agranulocytosis. The gingiva can, however, be affected by most other causes of mouth ulcers (see page 236).

THE PALATE

Lumps

Developmental

Unerupted teeth
Torus palatinus
Cysts

Inflammatory

Abscesses
Cysts
Papillary hyperplasia
Necrotizing sialometaplasia

Neoplasms

Oral or antral carcinoma
Salivary tumours
Fibrous overgrowths
Kaposi's sarcoma
Papillomas
Others

Redness

Redness restricted to the denture-bearing area of the palate is almost invariably denture-induced stomatitis (candidosis). Other red lesions may be erythroplasia, Kaposi's sarcoma or other lesions.

THE TONGUE

Swellings or lumps

Localized

Congenital: Lingual thyroid, haemangioma, lymphangioma, lingual choristoma

Inflammatory: Infection, abscess, median rhomboid glossitis, granuloma, foliate papillitis, insect bite

Traumatic: Oedema, haematoma

Neoplastic: Fibrous lump, papilloma, neurofibroma, carcinoma, sarcoma, granular cell tumour (granular cell myoblastoma)

Others: Foreign body, cysts

Diffuse

***Congenital*:** Down's syndrome, cretinism, mucopolysaccharidoses

***Inflammatory*:** Infection, insect bite, Ludwig's angina

***Traumatic*:** Oedema, haematoma

***Neoplastic*:** Lymphangioma, haemangioma

***Others*:** Multiple endocrine adenomatosis type III, angioedema, amyloidosis, cyst, acromegaly

Sore tongue

With obvious localized lesions

Any cause of oral ulceration (see above)
Geographic tongue
Median rhomboid glossitis
Foliate papillitis

Glossitis (generalized redness and depapillation)

Anaemia
Candidosis
Avitaminosis B
Post-irradiation

With no identifiable physical abnormality

Anaemia/sideropenia
Depression or cancerophobia
Glossodynia
Diabetes

THE MAJOR SALIVARY GLANDS

Swellings

Inflammatory

Mumps
Recurrent parotitis
Sjögren's syndrome
Ascending sialadenitis
Recurrent sialadenitis
Sarcoidosis
Actinomycosis

Neoplasms

Others

Duct obstruction
Sialosis
Mikulicz disease (lymphoepithelial lesion and syndrome)

Drug-associated

Chlorhexidine
Phenylbutazone
Iodine compounds
Thiouracil
Catecholamines
Sulphonamides
Phenothiazines
Methyldopa

Salivary gland pain

Inflammatory

Mumps
Stones or other causes of obstruction
Sjögren's syndrome
Acute sialadenitis
Recurrent sialadenitis

Neoplastic

Salivary gland malignant tumours

Drug-associated

Antihypertensive drugs
Cytotoxic drugs
Vinca alkaloids

THE NECK

Swellings in the neck

Cervical lymph nodes

***Inflammatory*:** Lymphadenitis (nasopharyngeal, antral, dental, tonsillar, aural, facial or scalp infections), glandular fever syndromes (EBV, CMV, Brucella, Toxoplasma, HIV), tuberculosis or other mycobacterial infections, other infections (cat scratch, syphilis)

***Neoplasms*:** Secondary carcinoma (oral, nasopharyngeal or thyroid primary), lymphoma, leukaemia

***Others*:** Connective tissue disease, drugs (eg, phenytoin), mucocutaneous lymph node syndrome

Salivary gland

Mumps
Tumours
Sjögren's syndrome
Sarcoidosis
Sialadenitis
Sialosis

Side of the neck

Actinomycosis
Branchial cyst
Parapharyngeal cellulitis
Pharyngeal pouch
Cystic hygroma
Carotid body tumours

Midline of the neck

Thyroglossal cyst

Ectopic thyroid
Thyroid tumours or goitre
'Plunging' ranula
Ludwig's angina
Dermoid cyst

ORAL COMPLAINTS FREQUENTLY ASSOCIATED WITH PSYCHOGENIC FACTORS*

Dry mouth
Sore or burning mouth
Bad or disturbed taste
Atypical facial pain
Atypical odontalgia
Supposed anaesthesias and dysaesthesias
Mandibular pain-dysfunction syndrome
Non-existent discharges
Gripping dentures
Vomiting or nausea caused by dentures
Supposed sialorrhoea
Non-existent lumps or spots

*Organic causes should first be excluded.

Further Reading

Figures in italic refer to page number in text.

Chapter 1

2 Boyd B W, Oral infection with associated lymphadenopathy due to *Mycobacterium chelonei*, *Ala Med* (1984) **54:**9–10.

Michaud M, Blanchette G, Tomich C F, Chronic ulceration of the hard palate: first clinical sign of undiagnosed pulmonary tuberculosis, *Oral Surg Oral Med Oral Pathol* (1984) **57:**63–7.

Volpe F, Schwimmer A, Barr C, Oral manifestations of disseminated *Mycobacterium avium-intracellulare* in a patient with AIDS, *Oral Surg Oral Med Oral Pathol* (1985) **60:**567–70.

Waldman R H, Tuberculosis and the atypical mycobacteria, *Otolaryngol Clin North Am* (1982) **15:**581–96.

3 Brazin S A, Leprosy (Hansen's disease), *Otolaryngol Clin North Am* (1982) **15:**597–611.

Helm F R, Gongloff R K, Wescott W B, Bilateral mixed density lesions in the body of the mandible, *J Am Dent Assoc* (1987) **115:** 315–17.

4 Li K I, Keirnan S, Wald E R et al, Isolated uvulitis due to *Haemophilus influenzae* type b, *Pediatrics* (1984) **74:**1054–7.

Scully C, Vaccinia of the lip, *Br Dent J* (1977) **143:**57–9.

Wynder S G, Lampe R M, Shoemaker M E, Uvulitis and *Hemophilus influenzae* b bacteraemia, *Pediatr Emerg Care* (1986) **2:**23–5.

5 Badger G R, Oral signs of chickenpox (varicella): report of two cases, *ASDC J Dent Child* (1980) **47:**349–51.

Porter S R, Malamos D, Scully C, Mouth-skin interface: 3: Infections affecting skin and mouth, *Update* (1986) **33:**399–404.

6 Pallett A P, Nicholls M W N, Varicella-zoster: reactivation or reinfection, *Lancet* (1986) **i:**160.

Wright W E, Davis M L, Geffen D B et al, Alveolar bone necrosis and tooth loss: a rare complication associated with herpes zoster infection of the fifth cranial nerve, *Oral Surg Oral Med Oral Pathol* (1983) **56:**39–46.

7 Kalman C M, Laskin O L, Herpes zoster and zosteriform herpes simplex virus infections in immunocompetent adults, *Am J Med* (1986) **81:**775–80.

Mandal B K, Herpes zoster and the immunocompromised, *J Infect* (1987) **14:**1–5.

8 Smith S, Ross J R, Scully C, An unusual oral complication of herpes zoster infection, *Oral Surg Oral Med Oral Pathol* (1984) **57:**388–9.

9 Corey L, Spear P G, Infections with herpes simplex viruses, *N Engl J Med* (1986) **314:**686–91, 749–57.

Scully C, Infectious diseases. In: Mason D K, Millard D, eds. *Oral Medicine* (University of Michigan Press: in press).

Scully C, Ulcerative stomatitis gingivitis and rash: a diagnostic dilemma, *Oral Surg Oral Med Oral Pathol* (1985) **59:**261–3.

10 Stanberry L R, Herpes virus latency and recurrence, *Progr Med Virol* (1986) **33:**61–77.

Straus S E, Herpes simplex virus infection: biology, treatment and prevention, *Ann Intern Med* (1985) **103:**404–19.

11 Greenberg M S, Cohen S G, Boosz B et al, Oral herpes simplex infections in patients with leukaemia, *J Am Dent Assoc* (1987) **114:**483–6.

Jarrett M, Herpes simplex infections, *Arch Dermatol* (1983) **119:**99–103.

12 Amler R W, Measles in young adults: the case for vigorous pursuit of immunisation, *Postgrad Med* (1985) **77:**251–8.

Hoeprich P D, ed, *Infectious Disease: A Modern Treatise of Infectious Process*, 3rd edn (Harper and Row Publications: New York 1983) 815–23.

Levy D, Measles: past, present and future, *NY State J Med* (1984) **84:**483–4.

Mitchell C D et al, Measles control: so near yet so far, *Prog Med Virol* (1985) **31:**1–42.

13 Gray E S, Human parvovirus infection, *J Pathol* (1987) **153:**310–12.

Whitley R J, Parvovirus infection, *N Engl J Med* (1985) **313:**111–12.

14 Greenspan J S, Greenspan D, Oral aspects of the acquired immunodeficiency syndrome (AIDS). In: MacKenzie I C, Squier C A, Dabelsteen E, eds, *Oral Mucosal Diseases: Biology, Etiology and Therapy* (Laegeforeningens Forlag: Copenhagen 1987) 65–9.

Schiodt M, Greenspan D, Daniels T E et al, Clinical and histologic spectrum of oral hairy leukoplakia, *Oral Surg Oral Med Oral Pathol* (1987) **64:**716–20.

15 Scully C, Cawson R A, Porter S R, AIDS review, *Br Dent J* (1986) **161:**53–60.

Scully C, Porter S R, Orofacial manifestations in infection with human immunodeficiency viruses, *Lancet* (1988) **1:**976–7.

16 Bell E J, Williams G R, Grist N R et al, Enterovirus infections, *Update* (1983) **26:**967–78.

Myer C, Cotton R T, Salivary gland disease in children: a review, *Clin Pediatr* (1986) **25:**314–22.

Scully C, Viruses and salivary gland disease, *Oral Surg Oral Med Oral Pathol* (1988) **66:**179–83.

17 Grist N R, Bell E J, Assaad F, Enteroviruses in human disease, *Prog Med Virol* (1978) **24:**114–57.

Kucera L S, Myrvik Q N, *Fundamentals of Medical Virology*, 2nd edn (Lea and Febiger: Philadelphia 1985) 216–28.

18 Conway S P, Coxsackie B2 virus causing simultaneous hand, foot and mouth disease and encephalitis, *J Infect* (1987) **15:**191.

Goh K T, Doraisingham S, Tan J C et al, An outbreak of hand, foot and mouth disease in Singapore, *Bull WHO* (1982) **60:**965–9.

Ishimaru Y, Nakano S, Yamaoka K et al, Outbreaks of hand, foot and mouth disease by Enterovirus 71, *Arch Dis Child* (1980) **55:**583–8.

19 Leading article, EBV and persistent malaise. *Lancet* (1985) **i:**1017–18.

Wolf H, Seibl R, Benign and malignant disease caused by EBV, *J Invest Dermatol* (1984) **83**[Supp]:88–95.

Leading article, New clinical manifestations of Epstein-Barr virus infection, *Lancet* (1982) **ii:**1253–5.

20 Ablashi D V et al, First international symposium on Epstein-Barr virus and associated malignant disease, *Cancer Res* (1985) **45:**3981–4.

Epstein M A, Historical background: Burkitt's lymphoma and Epstein-Barr virus, *IARC Sci Publ* (1985) **60:**17–27.

Purtilo D T et al, Epstein-Barr virus as an aetiologic agent in the pathogenesis of lymphoproliferative and aproliferative diseases in immune deficient patients, *Int Rev Exp Pathol* (1985) **27:**113–83.

Sullivan J L, Epstein-Barr virus and the X-linked lymphoproliferative syndrome, *Adv Pediatr* (1983) **30:**365–99.

21 Green T L, Eversole L P, Leider A S, Oral and labial verruca vulgaris: clinical, histologic and immunohistochemical evaluation, *Oral Surg Oral Med Oral Pathol* (1986) **62:**410–16.

Scully C, Prime S, Maitland N, Papillomaviruses: their possible role in oral disease, *Oral Surg Oral Med Oral Pathol* (1985) **60:**166–74.

Scully C, Cox M, Maitland N et al, Papillomaviruses: their current status in relation to oral disease, *Oral Surg Oral Med Oral Pathol* (1988: in press).

22 Samaranayake L P, Scully C, Oral disease and sexual medicine, *Brit J Sexual Med* (1988) **15:** 138–43, 174–80.

Terezhalmy G T, Oral manifestations of sexually-related diseases, *Ear Nose Throat J* (1983) **62:**287–96.

23 Cousteau C, Leyder P, Laufer J, Syphilis primaire buccale: un diagnostic parfois difficile, *Rev Stomatol Chir Maxillofac* (1984) **85**:391–8.

Manton S L, Eggleston S I, Alexander I et al, Oral presentation of secondary syphilis, *Br Dent J* (1986) **160**:237–8.

24 Crissey J T et al, Syphilis, *Clin Dermatol* (1984) **2**:1–166.

Yusuf H, Battacharya M H, Syphilitic osteomyelitis of the mandible, *Br J Oral Surg* (1982) **20**:122–8.

25 International symposium on yaws and other endemic treponematoses (Washington DC, April 1984), *Rev Inf Dis* (1985) **7** [Suppl 2]: 217–351.

Kerdel-Vegas F, American leishmaniasis, *Int J Dermatol* (1982) **21**:291–303.

Marsden P D et al, Mucocutaneous leishmaniasis: an unsolved clinical problem, *Trop Doct* (1977) **7**:7–11.

Schuppli R, Leishmaniasis: a review, *Dermatologica* (1982) **165**:1–6.

26 Enwonwu C O, Infectious oral necrosis (cancrum oris) in Nigerian children, *Community Dent Oral Epidemiol* (1985) **13**:190–4.

Johnson B D et al, Acute necrotising ulcerative gingivitis: a review of diagnosis, etiology and treatment, *J Periodontol* (1986) **57**:141–50.

Sabiston C B, A review and proposal for the etiology of acute necrotising gingivitis, *J Clin Periodontol* (1986) **13**:727–34.

Sawyer D, Nwoku A J, Cancrum oris (noma): past and present, *J Dent Child* (1981) **48**:138–41.

27 Horowitz B J, Edelstein S W, Lippman L, Sexual transmission of candida, *Obstet Gynecol* (1987) **69**:883–6.

Oelz O, Schaffner A, Frick P et al, *Trichosporon capitatum*: thrush-like oral infection, local invasion, fungaemia and metastatic abscess formation in a leukaemic patient, *J Infect* (1983) **6**:183–5.

Schnell J D, Epidemiology and prevention of peripartal mycoses, *Chemotherapy* (1982) **28** [Suppl 1]: 68–72.

28 Odds F C, Candida infections: an overview, *CRC Critical Rev Microbiol* (1987) **15**:1–5.

Scully C, Chronic atrophic candidosis, *Lancet* (1986) **ii**:437–8.

29 Holmstrup P, Bessermann M, Clinical, therapeutic and pathogenic aspects of chronic oral multifocal candidiasis, *Oral Surg Oral Med Oral Pathol* (1984) **56**:388–95.

Ohman S C, Dahlen G, Moller A et al, Angular cheilitis: a clinical and microbial study, *J Oral Pathol* (1986) **15**:213–17.

Wright BA, Fenwick F, Candidiasis and atrophic tongue lesions, *Oral Surg Oral Med Oral Pathol* (1981) **51**:55–61.

30 Nielson H, Dangaard K, Schiodt M, Chronic mucocutaneous candidosis: a review, *Tandlaegkbladet* (1985) **89**:667–73.

Porter SR, Scully C, Candidosis endocrinopathy syndrome, *Oral Surg Oral Med Oral Pathol* (1986) **61**:573–8.

31 Smith C B, Candidiasis: pathogenesis, host resistance and predisposing factors. In: Bodey G P, Feinstein V, eds, *Candidiasis* (Raven Press: New York 1985) 53.

32 Goodwin RA, Shapiro JL, Thurman GH et al, Disseminated histoplasmosis: clinical and pathologic correlations, *Medicine* (1980) **59**:1–33.

Lehrer R I, Howard D H, Sypherd P S et al, Mucormycosis, *Ann Intern Med* (1980) **93**:93–100.

33 Beck-Mannagetta J, Necek D, Grasserbauer M, Solitary aspergillosis of maxillary sinus: a complication of dental treatment, *Lancet* (1983) **i**:1280.

Douglas J G, Gillon J, Logan R F A et al, Sarcoidosis and coeliac disease: an association? *Lancet* (1984) **ii**:13–15.

James D G, Sharma O P, Overlap syndromes with sarcoidosis, *Postgrad Med J* (1985) **61**:769–71.

Schubert M M, Head and neck aspergillosis in patients undergoing bone-marrow transplantation, *Cancer* (1986) **57**:1092–6.

34 Macleod R I, Snow M H, Hawkesford J E,

Sarcoidosis of the tongue, *Br J Oral Maxillofac Surg* (1985) **23:**243–6.

Van Maarsseveen A C M T, van der Waal I, Stam J et al, Oral involvement in sarcoidosis, *Int J Oral Surg* (1982) **11:**21–9.

Chapter 2

36 Boyle P, Scully C, Epidemiological aspects of oral cancer, *Acta Stom Int* (1982) **3:**193–200.

Peterson D E et al, *Head and Neck Management of the Cancer Patient* (Nijhoff: The Hague, 1986).

Pindborg J J, *Oral Cancer and Precancer* (John Wright & Sons Ltd: Bristol, 1980).

Morton R P, Missotten F E M, Pharoah P O D, Classifying cancer of the lip: an epidemiologic perspective, *Eur J Cancer Clin Oncol* (1983) **19:**875–9.

37 Davis S, Severson R K, Increasing incidence of cancer of the tongue in the United States among young adults, *Lancet* (1987) **ii:**910–11.

Macfarlane G J, Boyle P, Scully C, Rising mortality from cancer of the tongue in young Scottish males, *Lancet* (1987) **ii:**912.

38 Fitzpatrick P J, Tepperman B S, Carcinoma of the floor of the mouth, *J Can Assoc Radiol* (1982) **33:**148–53.

Henk J, Langdon J, *Malignant Tumours of the Oral Cavity* (Edward Arnold: London 1985).

39 Gupta P C, Pindborg J J, Mehta F S, Comparison of carcinogenicity of betal quid with and without tobacco: an epidemiological review, *Ecol Dis* (1982) **1:**213–19.

McDonald J S, Crissman J D, Gluckman J L, Verrucous carcinoma of the oral cavity, *Head Neck Surg* (1982) **5:**22–8.

40 Baden E, Prevention of cancer of the oral cavity and pharynx, *Cancer* (1987) **37:**49–62.

Scully C, Malamos D, Levers B G H et al, Sources and patterns of referrals of oral cancer: the role of general practitioners, *Br Med J* (1986) **293:**599–601.

41 Illes R W, Brian M B, A review of tumours of the salivary gland, *Surg Gynecol Obstet* (1986) **163:**399–404.

Isaacson G, Shear M, Intraoral salivary gland tumours: a retrospective study of 201 cases, *J Oral Pathol* (1983) **12:**57–62.

42 Chan M N Y, Radden B G, Intraoral salivary gland neoplasms: a retrospective study of 98 cases, *J Oral Pathol* (1986) **15:**339–42.

Hunter R M, Davis B W, Gray G F et al, Primary malignant tumours of salivary origin: a 52-year review, *Ann Surg* (1983) **49:**82–9.

43 Keszler A et al, Ameloblastoma in childhood, *J Oral Maxillofac Surg* (1986) **44:**609–13.

Reichart P A, Ries P, Considerations on the classification of odontogenic tumours, *Int J Oral Surg* (1983) **12:**323–33.

Slootweg P J et al, Malignant ameloblastoma or ameloblastic carcinoma, *Oral Surg Oral Med Oral Pathol* (1984) **57:**168–76.

Stuart D J, Unicystic ameloblastoma of the mandible, *Br J Oral Maxillofac Surg* (1984) **22:**307–10.

44 Keller E E, Gunderson L L, Bone disease metastatic to the jaw, *J Am Dent Assoc* (1987) **115:**697–701.

MacIntyre DR, Briggs JC, Primary oral malignant melanoma, *Int J Oral Surg* (1984) **13:**160–5.

Nishimura Y, Yakata H, Kawasaki T et al, Metastatic tumours of the mouth and jaws: a review of the Japanese literature, *J Maxillofac Surg* (1982) **10:**253–8.

Rapini R P, Golitz L E, Greer R O et al, Primary malignant melanoma of the oral cavity, *Cancer* (1985) **55:**1543–51.

Sooknundun M et al, Oral malignant melanoma (a case report and review of the literature), *J Laryngol Otol* (1986) **100:**371–5.

45 Baden E, Al Saati T, Caverivière P et al, Hodgkin's lymphoma of the oropharyngeal region, *Oral Surg Oral Med Oral Pathol* (1987) **64:**88–94.

Eisenbud L, Sciubba J, Mir R et al, Oral presentations in non-Hodgkin's lymphoma: a review of 31 cases, *Oral Surg Oral Med Oral Pathol* (1983) **56:**151–6.

46 Baden E, Carter R, Intraoral presentation of American Burkitt's lymphoma after extraction of a mandibular left third molar, *J Oral Maxillofac Surg* (1987) **45:**689–93.

Perez-Reyes N, Farhi D C, Squamous cell carcinoma of head and neck in patients with well-differentiated lymphocytic lymphoma, *Cancer* (1987) **59:**540–4.

47 Broadbent V, Pritchard J, Histiocytosis X: current controversies, *Arch Dis Child* (1985) **60:**605–8.

Favera B E, McCarthy R C, Mieran G W, Histiocytosis X, *Hum Pathol* (1983) **14:**663–76.

48 Barnett ML, Cole RJ, Mycosis fungoides with multiple oral mucosal lesions, *J Periodontol* (1985) **56:**690–3.

Evans G E et al, Mycosis fungoides with oral involvement, *Int J Oral Maxillofac Surg* (1987) **16:**634–7.

Osserman EF, Melini G, Butler VP, Multiple myeloma and related plasma cell dyscrasias, *JAMA* (1987) **258:**2930–7.

Patel S P, Hotterman O A, Mycosis fungoides: an overview, *J Surg Oncol* (1983) **22:**221–6.

Raubenheimer E J, Danth J, Van Wilpe E, Multiple myeloma: a study of 10 cases, *J Oral Pathol* (1987) **16:**383–8.

Yaegaki K, Kameyama T, Takenaka M et al, Myelomatosis (IgD) discovered by oral manifestations, *Int J Oral Surg* (1985) **14:**381–4.

49 Dreizen S, McCredie K B, Keating M J, Chemotherapy-associated oral haemorrhages in adults with acute leukaemia, *Oral Surg Oral Med Oral Pathol* (1983) **55:**572–8.

Dreizen S, McCredie K B, Keating M J et al, Malignant gingival and skin infiltrates in adult leukemia, *Oral Surg Oral Med Oral Pathol* (1983) **55:**572–8.

50 Barrett A P, A long-term prospective clinical study of oral complications during conventional chemotherapy for acute leukemia, *Oral Surg Oral Med Oral Pathol* (1987) **63:**313–6.

Dreizen S, McCredie K B, Bodey G P et al, Quantitative analysis of the oral complications of anti-leukemia chemotherapy, *Oral Surg Oral Med Oral Pathol* (1986) **62:**650–3.

Sherr C J, Leukemia and lymphoma, *Cell* (1987) **48:**727–9.

51 Dreizen S, McCredie K B, Bodey G P et al, Microbial mucocutaneous infections in acute adult leukaemia, *Postgrad Med* (1986) **79:**107–18.

Scully C, MacFarlane T W, Orofacial manifestations in childhood malignancy: clinical and microbiological findings during remission, *ASDC J Dent Child* (1983) **50:**121–5.

52 Cigliano B et al, Neonatal congenital epulis, *Int J Oral Maxillofac Surg* (1985) **14:**456–7.

Lack E E, Gingival granular cell tumours of the newborn (congenital epulis): a clinical and pathologic study of 21 patients, *Am J Surg Pathol* (1981) **5:**37–46.

53 Kaban L B et al, Vascular anomalies of the maxillofacial region, *J Oral Maxillofac Surg* (1986) **44:**203–13.

Laskaris G et al, Maffucci's syndrome: report of a case with oral haemangiomas, *Oral Surg Med Oral Pathol* (1984) **57:**263–6.

Stal S et al, Haemangioma, lymphangioma and vascular malformations of the head and neck, *Otolaryngol Clin North Am* (1986) **19:**769–96.

Zocchi D et al, Maffucci's syndrome: report of three cases and review of the literature, *Ital J Orthop Traumatol* (1983) **9:**263–6.

Chapter 3

56 Gilsen G, Nilsson K O, Matsson L, Gingival inflammation in diabetic children related to degree of metabolic control, *Acta Odont Scand* (1980) **38:**241–6.

Murrah V A, Diabetes mellitus and associated oral manifestations: a review, *J Oral Pathol* (1985) **14:**271–81.

57 Chuong R et al, Central giant cell lesions of the jaw: a clinico-pathologic study, *J Oral Maxillofac Surg* (1986) **44:**708–13.

Kinirons M J, Glasgow J F T, The chronology of dentinal defects related to medical findings in hypoparathyroidism, *J Dent* (1985) **13:**346–9.

58 Karpf D B et al, Current concepts in acromegaly: aetiology, diagnosis and treatment, *Compr Ther* (1986) **12:**22–30.

Whelan J, Redpath T, Buckle R, The medical and anaesthetic management of acromegalic patients undergoing maxillofacial surgery, *Br J Oral Surg* (1982) **20:**77–83.

59 Brunt L M, Wells S A, The multiple endocrine neoplasia syndromes, *Invest Radiol* (1985) **20:**916–27.

Casino A J, Sciubba J J, Ohri G et al, Oro-facial manifestations of the multiple endocrine neoplasia syndrome, *Oral Surg Oral Med Oral Pathol* (1981) **51:**516–20.

Lamey P-J, Carmichael F, Scully C, Oral pigmentation, Addison's disease and the results of screening for adreno-cortical insufficiency, *Br Dent J* (1985) **158:**297–8.

Moyer G N, Terezhalmy G T, O'Brian J T, Nelson's syndrome: another condition associated with mucocutaneous hyperpigmentation, *J Oral Med* (1985) **1:**13–17.

60 Challacombe S J, Scully C, Keevil B et al, Serum ferritin in recurrent oral ulceration, *J Oral Pathol* (1983) **12:**290–9.

Drummond J F, White D K, Damm D D, Megaloblastic anemia with oral lesions: a consequence of gastric by-pass surgery, *Oral Surg Oral Med Oral Pathol* (1985) **59:**149–53.

Grattan C E H, Scully C, Oral ulceration: a diagnostic problem, *Br Med J* (1986) **292:**1093–4.

Greenberg MS, Clinical and histologic changes of the oral mucosa in pernicious anaemia, *Oral Surg Oral Med Oral Pathol* (1981) **52:**38–42.

61 Doppelt S H, Vitamin D, rickets and osteomalacia, *Orthop Clin North Am* (1984) **15:**671–86.

Ellis C N, Vanderveen E E, Rasmussen J E, Scurvy: a case caused by peculiar dietary habits, *Arch Dermatol* (1984) **120:**1212–14.

62 Babejews A, Occult multiple myeloma associated with amyloid of the tongue, *Br J Oral Maxillofac Surg* (1985) **23:**298–303.

Franklin E D, The heavy chain diseases, *Harvey Lect* (1984) **78:**1–22.

Fuchs A, Jagirdar J, Schwartz I S, Beta 2 microglobulin amyloidosis (AB 2M) in patients undergoing long-term hemodialysis, *Am J Clin Pathol* (1987) **88:**302 7.

Gertz M A, Kyle R A, Griffing W L et al, Jaw claudication in primary systemic amyloidosis, *Medicine (Baltimore)* (1986) **65:**173–9.

Glenner G G, Amyloid deposits and amyloidosis, *N Engl J Med* (1980) **302:**1283–92, 1333–43.

63 Bach G, Friedman R, Weissmann B et al, The defect in Hurler and Scheie syndromes: deficiency of a-1-iduronidase, *Proc Natl Acad Sci USA* (1972) **69:**2048–51.

Gardner D G, Oral manifestations of Hurler's syndrome, *Oral Surg Oral Med Oral Pathol* (1971) **32:**46–57.

Scully C, Orofacial manifestations of the Lesch-Nyhan syndrome, *Int J Oral Surg* (1981) **10:**380–3.

Sofaer J A, Single gene disorders. In: Jones J H, Mason D K, eds, *Oral Manifestations of Systemic Disease* (Saunders: Eastbourne 1980) 37.

64 Scully C, Porter S R, Immunodeficiency. In: Ivanyi L, ed. *Immunology of Oral Diseases* (MTP Press: Lancaster 1986) 235–56.

Scully C, Porter S R, Primary immunodeficiencies. In: J H Jones, D K Mason, eds, *Oral Manifestations of Systemic Disease* 2nd edn. (Saunders: London – in press).

Chapter 4

66 Ramasinghe A W, Warnakulasuriya K A A S, Tennekoon G E et al, Oral mucosal changes in iron deficiency anemia in a Sri Lankan female population, *Oral Surg Oral Med Oral Pathol* (1983) **55:**29–32.

Stockman J A, Iron deficiency anaemia: have we come far enough? *JAMA* (1987) **258:**1645–7.

Van Dis M L, Langlais R P, The thalassemias: oral manifestations and complications, *Oral Surg Oral Med Oral Pathol* (1986) **62:**229–33.

67 Hoffbrand A V, Pettit J E, Myeloproliferative disorders. In: *Essential Haematology*, 2nd edn (Blackwell Scientific Publications: Oxford 1984) 182–93.

van Wingerden J J et al, Malignant fibrous histiocytoma of the parotid gland associated with polycythaemia, *Head Neck Surq* (1986) **8:**218–21.

68 Barrett A P, Oral complications of bone marrow transplantation, *Aust NZ J Med* (1986) **16:**239–40.

Berkowitz R J, Strandford S, Jones P et al, Stomatologic complications of bone marrow transplantation in a pediatric population, *Pediatr Dent* (1987) **9:**105–10.

Locksley R M, Infection with varicella-zoster virus after marrow transplantation, *J Infect Dis* (1985) **152:**1172–81.

Seto B G, Oral mucositis in patients undergoing bone-marrow transplantation, *Oral Surg Oral Med Oral Pathol* (1985) **60:**493–7.

69 Johnson R S, Diagnosis and treatment of von Willebrand's disease, *J Oral Maxillofac Surg* (1987) **45:**608–12.

Hobson P, Dental care of children with haemophilia and related conditions, *Br Dent J* (1981) **151:**249–53.

Monsour P A, Kruger B J, Harden R A, Prevalence and detection of patients with bleeding disorders, *Aust Dent J* (1986) **31:**104–10.

White G C, Lesesne H R, Hemophilia, hepatitis and acquired immunodeficiency, *Ann Intern Med* (1983) **98:**403–4.

Zakrzewska J, Gingival bleeding as a manifestation of von Willebrand's disease, *Br Dent J* (1983) **155:**157–60.

70 Barrett A P, Tvevsky J, Griffiths C J, Thrombocytopenia induced by quinine, *Oral Surg Oral Med Oral Pathol* (1983) **55:**351–4.

Colvin B T, Thrombocytopenia, *Clin Haematol* (1985) **14:**661–81.

71 Baehni P C, Payot P, Tsai, C C et al, Periodontal status associated with chronic neutropenia, *J Clin Periodontol* (1983) **10:**222–30.

Scully C, Gilmour G, Neutropenia and dental patients, *Br Dent J* (1986) **160:**43–6.

Scully C, Macfadyen E, Campbell A, Oral manifestations in cyclic neutropenia, *Br J Oral Surg* (1982) **20:**96–101.

72 Scully C, Orofacial manifestations in chronic granulomatous disease of childhood, *Oral Surg Oral Med Oral Pathol* (1981) **51:**148–51.

Chapter 5

74 Browning S, Hislop S, Scully C et al, The association between burning mouth syndrome and psychosocial disorders, *Oral Surg Oral Med Oral Pathol* (1987) **64:**171–4.

Feinmann C, Harris M, Psychogenic facial pain, *Br Dent J* (1984) **156:**165–9, 205–9.

Remick R A, Blasberg B, Psychiatric aspects of atypical facial pain, *Can Dent Assoc J* (1985) **12:**913–16.

Wray D, Scully C, The sore mouth, *Medicine International* (1986) **2:**1134–8.

75 Cristobal M C et al, Self-inflicted tongue ulcer: an unusual form of factitious disorder, *J Am Acad Dermatol* (1987) **17:**339–341.

Svirsky J A, Sawyer D R, Dermatitis artefacta of the paraoral region, *Oral Surg Oral Med Oral Pathol* (1987) **64:**259–63.

Chapter 6

78 Lazar M L, Greenlee R G, Naarden A L, Facial pain of neurologic origin mimicking oral pathologic conditions: some current concepts and treatment, *J Am Dent Assoc* (1980) **100:**884–8.

Loesser J D, Tic douloureux and atypical facial pain, *Can Dent Assoc J* (1985) **12:**917–23.

Scully C, The mouth in general practice: 3: Oral and facial pain, *Dermatology in Practice* (1982) **1:**16–18.

Sweet W H, The treatment of trigeminal neuralgia (tic douloureux), *N Engl J Med* (1986) **315:**174–7.

Zakrzewska J M, Nally F F, Flint S R, Cryotherapy in the management of paroxysmal trigeminal neuralgia: four-year follow-up of 39 patients, *J Maxillofac Surg* (1986) **14:**5–7.

79 Lecky B R F, Hughes R A C, Murray N M F, Trigeminal sensory neuropathy, *Brain* (1987) **110:**1463–85.

Scully C, Orofacial manifestations of disease: 6: Neurological, psychiatric and muscular disorders, *Hospital Update* (1986) **6:**135–9.

Westerhof W, Bos J D, Trigeminal trophic syndrome: a successful treatment with transcutaneous electrical stimulation, *Br J Dermatol* (1983) **108:**601–4.

80 Cartwright R A, Boddy J, Barnard D et al, Association between Bell's palsy and lymphoid malignancies, *Leuk Res* (1985) **9:**31–3.

Glanvill P, Pether J V C, Lyme disease, *Br Med J* (1987) **294:**1226.

Hanner P, Badr G, Rosenhall U et al, Trigeminal dysfunction in patients with Bell's palsy, *Acta Otolaryngol (Stockh)* (1986) **101:**224–30.

Hattori T, Tokugawa K, Fukushige J et al, Facial palsy in Kawasaki disease, *Pediatrics* (1987) **146:**601–2.

Neiuwmeyer P A, Koch P A M, Visser S L et al, Bell's palsy; a polyneuropathy, *Clin Otolaryngol* (1982) **7:**293–8.

Leading article, Bell's palsy, *Lancet* (1982) **i:**663.

81 Scully C, Cawson R A, Neurological disease, In: Scully C, Cawson R A, eds, *Medical Problems in Dentistry*, 2nd edn. (Wright: Bristol 1987) 317–59.

Wortham E et al, Diplopia: a review of 48 cases of isolated ocular cranial neuropathy, *J Okla State Med Assoc* (1985) **78:**99–103.

82 Dhamoon S K et al, Ipsilateral hemiplegia and the Wallenberg syndrome, *Arch Neurol* (1984) **41:**179–80.

Chapter 7

84 Abraham-Inpijn L, Oral and otal manifestations as the primary symptoms in Wegener's granulomatosis, *J Head Neck Pathol* (1983) **2:** 20–2.

Fauci A S, Haynes B F, Katz P et al, Wegener's granulomatosis: prospective clinical and therapeutic experience with 85 patients for 21 years, *Ann Intern Med* (1983) **98:**76–85.

Hausen L S et al, Limited Wegener's granulomatosis, *Oral Surg Oral Med Oral Pathol* (1985) **60:**524–31.

Israelson H, Binnie W H, Hurt W C, The hyperplastic gingivitis of Wegener's granulomatosis, *J Periodontol* (1981) **52:**81–7.

85 Flint S R, Keith O, Scully C, Hereditary haemorrhagic telangiectasia, *Oral Surg Oral Med Oral Pathol* (1988) **66:**440–4.

Peery W H, Clinical spectrum of hereditary haemorrhagic telangiectasia, *Am J Med* (1987) **82:** 989–97

Chapter 8

88 Brook I, The clinical microbiology of Waldeyer's ring *Otolaryngol Clin North Am* (1987) **20:**259–72.

Brook I et al, Possible role of anaerobic bacteria in the persistence of streptococcal tonsillar infection, *US Navy Med* (1981) **72:**26–9.

89 Primosch R E, Tetracycline discoloration, enamel defects and dental caries in patients with cystic fibrosis, *Oral Surg Oral Med Oral Pathol* (1980) **50:**303–8.

Umetsu D T, Ambrosino D M, Quinti I, Recurrent sinopulmonary infection and impaired antibody response to bacterial capsular polysaccharide antigen in children with selective IgG subclass deficiency, *N Engl J Med* (1985) **313:**1247–51.

Chapter 9

92 Alexander S A et al, Deciduous tooth anomalies and partial anodontia, *Oral Surg Oral Med Oral Pathol* (1985) **60:**230.

Ruprecht A et al, Incidence of oligodontia (hypodontia), *J Oral Med* (1986) **41:**43–6.

Tso M S et al, Hypodontia, ectodermal dysplasia and sweat pore count, *Br Dent J* (1985) **158:**56–60.

93 Brook A H, A unifying aetiological explanation for anomalies of human tooth number and size, *Arch Oral Biol* (1984) **29:**373–8.

Ruprecht A et al, Incidence of supernumerary teeth, *Ann Dent* (1984) **43:**18–21.

Scully C, Defects affecting the teeth, *Update* (1983) **26:**2203–8.

Scully C, Cawson R A, Common dental disorders, *Medicine International* (1986) **2:**1129–34.

94 Amler N H, Gemination—anomalous tooth development, *Ann Dent* (1983) **42:**33–4.

Grover P S et al, Gemination and twinning in the permanent dentition, *Oral Surg Oral Med Oral Pathol* (1985) **59:**313–18.

Smith G A, Double teeth, *Br Dent J* (1980) **148:**163–4.

95 Davis P J, Brook A H, Presentation of talon cusp, diagnosis, clinical features, associations and possible aetiology, *Br Dent J* (1986) **160:**84–8.

Hill F J, Dens evaginatus and its management, *Br Dent J* (1984) **156:**400–2.

Kieser J A et al, Classificatory reliability of the Carabelli trait in man, *Arch Oral Biol* (1984) **29:**795–801.

Loh H S, Lim S S, Facial infection arising from dens evaginatus, *Br Dent J* (1985) **158:**367–8.

Ruprecht A et al, The incidence of dental invagination, *J Pedodont* (1986) **10:**265–72.

96 Crawford P J M, Evans R D, Aldred M J, Amelogenesis imperfecta: autosomal dominant hypomaturation—hypoplasia type with taurodontism, *Br Dent J* (1988) **164:**71–3.

Elzay R P, Chamberlain D H, Differential diagnosis of enlarged dental pulp chambers: a case report of amelogenesis imperfecta with taurodontism, *ASDC J Dent Child* (1986) **53:**388–90.

Jaspers M T, Witkop C J, Taurodontism: an isolated trait associated with syndromes and X-chromosomal aneuploidy, *Am J Hum Genet* (1980) **32:**396–413.

97 American Dental Association Council on Dental Therapeutics, *Fluoride Compounds: Accepted Dental Therapeutics* 39th edn (1982) 344–68.

Moller I J, Fluorides and dental fluorosis, *Int Dent J* (1982) **32:**135–7.

Murray J J, Rugg-Gunn A J, *Fluorides in Caries Prevention*, 2nd edn (Wright: Bristol 1982) 207–17.

Pindborg J J, Aetiology of development enamel defects not related to fluorosis, *Int Dent J* (1982) **32:**122–34.

98 Davies P H, Lewis D H, Dilaceration: a surgical/orthodontic solution, *Br Dent J* (1984) **156:**16–18.

Goodman A H, Armelagos G J, The chronological distribution of enamel hypoplasia in human permanent incisor and canine teeth, *Arch Oral Biol* (1985) **30:**503–7.

Lowe P L, Dilaceration caused by a direct penetrating injury, *Br Dent J* (1985) **159:**373–4.

Sarnat H et al, Diagnosis of enamel defects, *NY State Dent J* (1985) **51:**103–4.

99 De Sort K D, Amelogenesis imperfecta: the genetics, classification and treatment, *J Prosthet Dent* (1983) **49:**786–92.

Sindell S et al, Hereditary aspects and classification of hereditary amelogenesis imperfecta, *Community Dent Oral Epidemiol* (1986) **14:**211–16.

100 Escobar V H, Goldblatt L I, Bixler D, A clinical, genetic and ultrastructural study of 'snow-capped teeth': amelogenesis imperfecta hypomaturation type, *Oral Surg Oral Med Oral Pathol* (1981) **52:**607–12.

Kerebel B et al, Ultrastructural study of amelogenesis imperfecta, *Calcif Tissue Res* (1977) **24:**191–7.

Wright J T, Analysis of kindred with amelogenesis imperfecta, *J Oral Pathol* (1985) **14:**366–74.

101 Gage J P, Dentinogenesis imperfecta: a new perspective, *Aust Dent J* (1985) **30:**285–90.

Lukinmaa P L, Ranta H, Ranta K et al, Dental findings in osteogenesis imperfecta, *J Craniofac Genet Dev Biol* (1987) **7:**115–25.

Nicholls A C, Pope F M, Heterogeneity of osteogenesis imperfecta congenita, *Lancet* (1980) **i:** 820–1.

Smith R, Francis M J O, Houghton G R, *The Brittle Bone Syndrome: Osteogenesis Imperfecta*, (Butterworths: London 1983) 41–68.

Sunderland E P, Smith C J, The teeth in osteogenesis and dentinogenesis imperfecta, *Br Dent J* (1980) **149:**287–9.

102 Chow M H, Natal and neonatal teeth, *J Am Dent Assoc* (1980) **100:**215–16.

Dick H M, Honore L H, Dental structures in benign ovarian cystic teratomas (dermoid cysts), *Oral Surg Oral Med Oral Pathol* (1985) **60:**299–307.

Leung A K C, Natal teeth, *Am J Dis Child* (1986) **140:**249–51.

103 Kurol J, Infraocclusion of primary molars: an epidemiological and familial study, *Community Dent Oral Epidem* (1981) **9:**94–102.

Rosenthal P, Ramos A, Mungo R, Management of children with hyperbilirubinemia and green teeth, *J Pediatr* (1986) **108:**103–5.

104 Davies A K et al, Photo-oxidation of tetracycline absorbed on hydroxyapatite in relation to the light-induced staining of teeth, *J Dent Res* (1985) **64:**936–9.

Peterson C K, Tetracycline effects on teeth preclude use in children and pregnant or lactating women, *Postgrad Med* (1984) **76:**24–34.

Scopp W I et al, Tetracycline-induced staining of teeth, *Postgrad Med* (1986) **79:**202–3.

105 Arends J, Christoffersen J, The nature of the early caries lesion in enamel, *J Dent Res* (1986) **65:**2–11.

Holloway P J, The role of sugar in the aetiology of dental caries, *J Dent* (1983) **11:**189–213.

Scully C, Dental caries: progress in microbiology and immunology, *J Infect* (1981) **3:**107–33.

Winter G B, Problems involved with the use of comforters, *Int Dent J* (1980) **30:**28.

106 Asher C, Read M J F, Early enamel erosion in children associated with excessive consumption of citric acid, *Br Dent J* (1987) **162:**384–7.

Russell M D, The relationship of occlusal wear to occlusal contact area, *J Oral Rehabil* (1983) **10:**383–91.

Smith B G et al, A comparison of patterns of toothwear and aetiological factors, *Br Dent J* (1984) **157:**16–19

Van Reenen J F et al, Tooth-mutilating practices amongst the Damara of SW Africa (Namibia), *Tydskr Tandheelkd Ver S Afr* (1985) **40:**537–39.

Whittaker DK, Mutilated teeth, *Dental Update* (1984) **11:**555–62.

'In the News': Swimming pool tooth erosion – hazard detected in US, *Can Dent Assoc J* (1983) **49:**744–5.

107 Fairburn C G, Cooper P J, The clinical features of bulimia nervosa, *Br J Psychiatry* (1984) **144:**238–46.

Feiglin B, Root resorption, *Aust Dent J* (1986) **31:**12–22.

Taylor V E, Sneddon J, Bilateral facial swelling in bulimia, *Br Dent J* (1987) **163:**115–17.

108 Andersson L et al, Tooth ankylosis: clinical, radiographic and histological assessment, *Int J Oral Surg* (1984) **13:**423–31.

Leider A S et al, Generalized hypercementosis, *Oral Surg Oral Med Oral Pathol* (1987) **63:**375–80.

109 Kannangara D W, Thadepalli H, McQuirter J L, Bacteriology and treatment of dental infections, *Oral Surg Oral Med Oral Pathol* (1980) **50:**103–9.

Newman M G, Anaerobic oral and dental infection, *Rev Infect Dis* (1984) [Suppl] **1:**5107–14.

Williams B L et al, Bacteriology of dental abscesses of endodontic origin, *J Clin Microbiol* (1983) **18:**770–4.

110 Garulnick W, Odontogenic infections, *Br Dent J* (1984) **156:**440–7.

Haidar Z, Facial sinuses: cases of mistaken identity, *Ann Dent* (1985) **44:**9–11.

111 Shear M, *Cysts of the Oral Regions*, 2nd edn, (Wright: Bristol 1983) 114–41.

Wood N K, Periapical lesions, *Dent Clin North Am* (1984) **28:**725–66.

112 Lindhe J H, *Textbook of Clinical Periodontology*, (Munksgaard: Copenhagen 1985) Chapters 3 and 4.

Page R C, Gingivitis, *J Clin Periodontol* (1986) **13:**345–59.

113 Nisengard R J, Nieders M, Desquamative lesions of the gingiva, *J Periodontol* (1981) **52:**500–10.

Steelman R, Self-injurious behaviour: report of a case and follow-up, *J Oral Med* (1986) **41:**108–11.

Watson P J, Gingival recession, *J Dent* (1984) **12:**29–35.

114 Ahl D R et al, Periodontal emergencies, *Dent Clin North Am* (1986) **30:**459–72.

Nitzan D W et al, Pericoronitis: a reappraisal of its clinical and microbiological aspects, *J Oral Maxillofac Surg* (1985) **43:**510–16.

Smith R G, Davies R M, Acute lateral periodontal abscesses, *Br Dent J* (1986) **161,** 176–8.

115 Davies R M, Smith R G, Porter S R, Destructive forms of periodontal disease in adolescents and young adults, *Br Dent J* (1985) **158:**429–35.

Gillet R, Johnson N W, Bacterial invasion of the periodontium in a case of juvenile periodontitis, *J Clin Periodontol* (1982) **9:**93–100.

Page R C et al, Rapidly progressive periodontitis: a distinct clinical condition, *J Periodontol* (1983) **54:**197–209.

Socransky S S et al, New concepts of destructive periodontal disease, *J Clin Periodontol* (1984) **11:**21–32.

116 Puliyel J M, Iyer K S S, A syndrome of keratosis palmo-plantaris congenita, pes planus, onychogryphosis, periodontosis, arachnodactyly and a peculiar acro-osteolysis, *Br J Dermatol* (1986) **115:**243–8.

Sloan P et al, Histopathological and ultrastructural findings in a case of Papillon-Lefevre syndrome, *J Periodontol* (1984) **55:**482–5.

Tinanoff N et al, Treatment of the periodontal component of the Papillon-Lefevre syndrome, *J Clin Periodontol* (1986) **13:**6–10.

117 Addy M et al, Extrinsic tooth discoloration by metals and chlorhexidine: I. Surface protein denaturation of dietary precipitation, *Br Dent J* (1985) **159:**281–5.

Eriksen H M et al, Characterisation of salivary proteins from stainers and non-stainers adsorbed to hydroxyapatite, *Acta Odontol Scand* (1985) **43:**115–20.

118 Addy M et al, Extrinsic tooth discoloration by metals and chlorhexidine: II. Clinical staining produced by chlorhexidine, iron and tea, *Brit Dent J* (1985) **159:**331–4.

Driessens F C et al, On the physiochemistry of plaque calcification and the phase composition of dental calculus, *J Periodont Res* (1985) **20:**329–36.

Lockhart P B, Gingival pigmentation as the sole presenting sign of chronic lead poisoning in a mentally-retarded adult, *Oral Surg Oral Med Oral Pathol* (1981) **52:**143–9.

Mandel I D, Calculus revisited: a review, *J Clin Periodontol* (1986) **13:**249–57.

119 Gould A R, Escobar V H, Symmetrical gingival fibromatosis, *Oral Surg Oral Med Oral Pathol* (1981) **51:**62–7.

Newman M G, Current concepts on the pathogenesis of periodontal disease: microbiology emphasis, *J Periodontol* (1985) **56:**734–9.

'Emphasis', Plaque: current approaches to prevention and control, *J Am Dent Assoc* (1984) **109:**690–702.

120 Moskow B S, Bloom A, Embryogenesis of the gingival cyst, *J Clin Periodontol* (1983) **10:**119–39.

Wysocki G P, Brannon R B, Gardner D G et al, Histogenesis of the lateral periodontal cyst and the gingival cyst of the adult, *Oral Surg Oral Med Oral Pathol* (1980) **48:**327–9.

121 Lee K W, The fibrous epulis and related lesions, *Periodontics* (1986) **6:**277–99.

Macleod R I, Soames J W, Epulides: a clinicopathological study of a series of 200 consecutive lesions, *Br Dent J* (1987) **163:**51–3.

122 Profitt W R, On the aetiology of malocclusion: the North Croft Lecture 1985, *Br J Orthod* (1986) **13:**1–12.

Henderson D, Poswillo D, *A Colour Atlas and Textbook of Orthognathic Surgery: the Surgery of Facial Skeletal Deformity*. (Wolfe Medical Publications Ltd: London 1985).

123 Kribbs P J et al, Osteoporosis and dental osteopenia in the elderly, *Gerodontology* (1984) **3:**101–6.

Larsson E, The prevalence and aetiology of prolonged dummy- and finger-sucking habits, *Eur J Orthod* (1985) **7:**172–6.

Luke L S, The effects of thumb-sucking on oro-facial structures and speech: a review, *Compend Contin Educ Dent* (1983) **4:**575–9.

124 Shear M, *Cysts of the Oral Regions*, 2nd edn (J Wright: Bristol 1983).

Shear M, The odontogenic keratocyst: recent advances, *Dtsch Zahnartztl Z* (1985) **40:**510–13.

125 Shear M, Cysts of the jaws: recent advances, *J Oral Pathol* (1985) **14:**43–59.

Wysocki G P, The differential diagnosis of globulomaxillary radiolucencies, *Oral Surg Oral Med Oral Pathol* (1981) **51:**281–6.

126 Greval R S et al, Nasopalatine cyst: a case report, *J Indian Dent Assoc* (1985) **57:**143–6.

127 Adekeye E O, Cornah J, Osteomyelitis of the jaws: a review of 141 cases, *Br J Maxillofac Surg* (1985) **23:**24–35.

Jacobsson S, Diffuse sclerosing osteomyelitis of the mandible, *Int J Oral Surg* (1984) **13:**363–85.

128 Coffin F, The incidence and management of osteoradionecrosis of the jaws following head and neck radiotherapy, *Br J Radiol* (1983) **56:**851–7.

Daramola J O, Ajagbe H A, Chronic osteomyelitis of the mandible in adults, *Br J Oral Surg* (1982) **20:**58–62.

Epstein J, Osteoradionecrosis: clinical experience and proposal for classification, *J Oral Maxillofac Surg* (1987) **45:**104–10.

Marciani R O, Ownby H E, Osteoradionecrosis of the jaws, *J Oral Maxillofac Surg* (1986) **44:**218–23.

Murray C G et al, The relationship between dental disease and radiation necrosis of the mandible, *Oral Surg Oral Med Oral Pathol* (1980) **49:**99–104.

Pyykonen H, Malmstrom M, Oikarinen V S et al, The effects of radiation treatment of tongue and floor of mouth cancer on the dentition, saliva secretion, mucous membranes and lower jaw, *Int J Oral Maxillofac Surg* (1986) **15:**401–9.

129 Field E A, Speechley J A, Rotter E et al, Dry socket incidence compared after 12-year interval, *Br J Oral Maxillofac Surg* (1985) **23:**419–27.

Turner P S, A clinical study of 'dry socket', *Int J Oral Surg* (1982) **11:**226–31.

130 Eggen S, Natvig B, Relationship between torus mandibularis and number of present teeth, *Scand J Dent Res* (1986) **94:**233–40.

Lello G E, Makek M, Stafne's mandibular lingual cortical defect: discussion of aetiology, *J Maxillofac Surg* (1985) **13:**172–6.

Rezai R F, Torus palatinus, an exostosis of unknown aetiology: review of the literature, *Compend Contin Educ Dent* (1985) **6:**149–52.

Sandergaard J O, Bulow S, Jarvinen H et al, Dental anomalies in familial adenomatous polyposis coli, *Acta Odont Scand* (1987) **45:**61–3.

Traboulsi E I, Krush A J, Gardner E J et al, Prevalence and importance of pigmented ocular fundus lesions in Gardner's syndrome, *N Engl J Med* (1987) **316:**661–7.

Wolf J, Jarvinen H J, Hietanen J, Gardner's dento-maxillary stigmas in patients with familial adenomatosis coli, *Br J Oral Maxillofac Surg* (1986) **24:**410–16.

131 Pfaltz C R, Chilla R, Sialadenosis and sialadenitis: pathophysiological and diagnostic aspects, *Adv Otorhinolaryngol* (1981) **26:**1–249.

Avery B S, A sialocoele and unusual parotid fistula: case report, *Br J Oral Surg* (1980) **18:**40–4.

Galili D, Marmary Y, Juvenile recurrent parotitis: clinicoradiologic follow-up study and the beneficial effect of sialography, *Oral Surg Oral Med Oral Pathol* (1986) **61:**550–6.

Pruett T L, Simmons R L, Nosocomial Gram-negative bacillary parotitis, *JAMA* (1984) **251:**252–3.

Seifert G, Miehlke A, Haubrich J et al, *Diseases of the Salivary Glands: Pathology, Diagnosis, Treatment, Facial Nerve Surgery* (Thieme: Stuttgart, New York, 1986) 78–84.

132 Blair S W, Wood G D, Obstructive sialadenitis, *Int J Oral Surg* (1980) **9:**63–7.

Isacsson G, Persson N E, The gigantiform salivary calculus, *Int J Oral Surg* (1982) **11:**135–9.

Seifert G, Miehlke A, Haubrich J et al, *Diseases of the Salivary Glands: Pathology, Diagnosis, Treatment, Facial Nerve Surgery* (Thieme: Stuttgart, New York 1986) 85–90.

Yamane G M, Scharlock S E, Jain R et al, Intra-oral minor salivary gland sialolithiasis, *J Oral Med* (1984) **39:**85–90.

Zachariades N, Bilateral recurrent submandibular obstructive sialadenitis, *J Oral Med* (1985) **40:**86–103.

133 McClatchey K D, Appleblatt N H, Zarbo R J et al, Plunging ranula, *Oral Surg Oral Med Oral Pathol* (1984) **57:**408–12.

Navazesh M et al, Xerostomia: diagnosis and treatment, *Am J Otolaryngol* (1983) **4:**283–92.

134 Chilla R, Sialadenosis of the salivary glands of the head, *Adv Otorhinolaryngol* (1981) **26:**1–38.

Grillon G L et al, Necrotising sialometaplasia: literature review and presentation of five cases, *J Oral Surg* (1981) **39:**747–53.

Mesa M L et al, Necrotising sialometaplasia: frequency of histologic misdiagnosis, *Oral Surg Oral Med Oral Pathol* (1984) **57:**71–3.

135 Hay K D, Reade P C, The use of an elimination diet in the treatment of recurrent aphthous ulceration of the oral cavity, *Oral Surg Oral Med Oral Pathol* (1984) **57:**504–7.

Porter S R, Scully C, Flint S R, Haematological status in recurrent aphthous stomatitis compared with other oral disease, *Oral Surg Oral Med Oral Pathol* (1988) **66:**41–4.

136 Grattan C E H, Scully C, Oral ulceration: a diagnostic problem, *Br Med J* (1986) **292:**1093–4.

Marshall G S, Edwards K M, Butler J et al, Syndrome of periodic fever, pharyngitis and aphthous stomatitis, *J Pediatr* (1987) **110:**43–6.

Rennie J S, Reade P C, Hay K D et al, Recurrent aphthous stomatitis, *Br Dent J* (1985) **159:**361–7.

Scully C, Matthews R, Mouth ulcers, *Update* (1983) **26:**693–780.

137 Barnes C G, Behçet's syndrome, *J R Soc Med* (1984) **77:**816–18.

Hamza M, Orogenital ulcerations in mixed connective tissue disease, *J Rheumatol* (1985) **12:**643–4.

138 Firestein G S et al, Mouth and genital ulcers with inflamed cartilage: MAGIC syndrome, *Am J Med* (1985) **79:**65–72.

Jorizzo J L, Behçet's syndrome, *Arch Dermatol* (1986) **122:**556–8.

139 Symons A L, Rowe P V, Romanink K, Dental aspects of child abuse: review and case reports, *Aust Dent J* (1987) **32:**42–7.

Van Wyk C W, An oral lesion caused by fellatio, *Am J Forensic Med Pathol* (1981) **2:**217–19.

140 Behrman R E, Vaughan V C, *Nelson's Textbook of Paediatrics*, 12th edn (W B Saunders: Philadelphia, London, Toronto 1983).

Chaudhry A P, Yamane G M, Sharlock S E et al, A clinicopathological study of intraoral lymphoepithelial cysts, *J Oral Med* (1984) **39:**79–84.

Harari M D, Clezy J K A, Sharp E, Glossal cysts in four infants, *Arch Dis Child* (1987) **62:**1173–4.

Jorgensen R J, Shapira S D, Salinas C F et al, Intra-oral findings and anomalies in neonates, *Pediatrics* (1982) **69:**557–82.

141 Crotty C P, Factitious lip crusting, *Arch Dermatol* (1981) **117:**338–40.

Evans C D, Staphylococcal infection in median fissure of the lower lip, *Clin Exp Dermatol* (1986) **11:**289–91.

Reade P C, Sim R, Exfoliative cheilitis – a factitious disorder? *Int J Oral Maxillofac Surg* (1986) **15:**313–17.

Winchester L, Scully C, Prime S S et al, Cheilitis glandularis: a case affecting the upper lip, *Oral Surg Oral Med Oral Pathol* (1986) **62:**654–7.

142 Axell T, Holmstrup P, Kramer I R H et al, International seminar on oral leukoplakia and associated lesions related to tobacco habits, *Community Dent Oral Epidemiol* (1984) **12:**145–54.

Hansen L S, Olson J A, Silverman S, Proliferative verrucous leukoplakia, *Oral Surg Oral Med Oral Pathol* (1985) **60:**285–98.

McGuirt W F, Snuff-dippers carcinoma, *Arch Otolaryngol* (1983) **109:**757–60.

Shklar G, Oral leukoplakia, *N Engl J Med* (1986) **315:**1544–5.

143 Eveson J W, Oral premalignancy, *Cancer Surv* (1983) **2:**403–24.

Shibuya H, Amagasa T, Seto K I et al, Leukoplakia-associated multiple carcinomas in patients with tongue carcinoma, *Cancer* (1986) **57:**843–6.

Silverman S, Gorsky M, Lozado F, Oral leukoplakia and malignant transformation: a follow-up study of 257 patients, *Cancer* (1984) **53:**563–8.

144 Amagasa T et al, A study of the clinical characteristics and treatment of carcinoma in situ, *Oral Surg Oral Med Oral Pathol* (1985) **60:**50–5.

Lind P O, Malignant transformation in oral leukoplakia, *Scand J Dent Res* (1987) **95:**449–55.

145 Axell T, Henricsson V, Leukoedema – an epidemiologic study with special reference to the influence of tobacco habits, *Community Dent Oral Epidemiol* (1981) **9:**142–6.

Brooks J K, Balciunas B A, Geographic stomatitis: review of the literature and report of five cases, *J Am Dent Assoc* (1987) **115:**421–4.

Caniff J P, Mucosal diseases of uncertain etiology: III. Oral submucous fibrosis. In: Mackenzie I C, Squier C A, Dabelsteen E, eds, *Oral Mucosal Diseases: Biology, Etiology and Therapy* (Laegeforeningens Forlag: Copenhagen 1987) 87–91.

Duncan S C, Su W P D, Leukoedema of the oral mucosa (possibly an acquired white sponge naevus), *Arch Dermatol* (1980) **116:**906–8.

Luker J, Scully C, Erythema migrans affecting the palate, *Br Dent J* (1983) **155:**385.

Pindborg J J, Murti P R, Bhousle R B et al, Oral submucous fibrosis as a precancerous condition, *Scand J Dent Res* (1984) **92:**224–9.

Van Wyk C W, Ambrosio S C, Leukoedema: ultrastructural and histochemical observations, *J Oral Pathol* (1983) **12:**29–35.

146 Hudgins L J, Inflammatory papillary hyperplasia: evaluation of two treatment modalities, *Ont Dent* (1986) **63:**11–16.

Wescott W B, Correll R W, Multiple papillary projections on the alveolar mucosa and palate, *J Am Dent Assoc* (1984) **108:**91–2.

147 Gilmour A G, Craven C M, Chustecki A M, Self-mutilation under combined inferior dental block and solvent intoxication, *Br Dent J* (1984) **156:**438–9.

La Blanc J, Epker B N, Lesch-Nyhan syndrome: surgical treatment of a case with lip-chewing, *J Maxillofac Surg* (1981) **9:**64–7.

148 Sklavounou A, Laskaris G, Eosinophilic ulcer of the oral mucosa, *Oral Surg Oral Med Oral Pathol* (1984) **58:**431–6.

Wright J M, Rankin K V, Wilson J W, Traumatic granuloma of the tongue, *Head Neck Surg* (1983) **5:**363–6.

149 Dummett C O, Overview of normal oral pigmentation, *J Indiana Dent Assoc* (1980) **50:**13–18.

Dummett C O, Pertinent considerations in oral pigmentation, *Br Dent J* (1984) **158:**9–12.

150 Axell T, Hedin A, Epidemiologic study of excessive oral melanin pigmentation with special reference to the influence of tobacco habits, *Scand J Dent Rev* (1982) **90:**434–42.

Schawaf M et al, Gingival tattoo: an unusual gingival pigmentation – report of four cases, *J Oral Med* (1986) **41:**130–3.

151 Luker J, A case of lingual abscess, *Br Dent J* (1985) **159:**300.

Roberge R J, Seizure-related oral lacerations: incidence and distribution, *J Am Dent Assoc* (1985) **111:**279–80.

Steelman R, Self-injurious behaviour: report of a case and follow-up, *J Oral Med* (1986) **41:**108–10.

152 Correll R W, Wescott W B, Jensen J L, Non-painful, erythematous circinate lesions of a protean nature on a fissured tongue, *J Am Dent Assoc* (1984) **109:**90–1.

Kullaa-Mikkonen A, Geographic tongue: a scanning electron microscopic study, *J Cutan Pathol* (1986) **13:**154–62.

Wysocki G P et al, Benign migratory glossitis in patients with juvenile diabetes, *Oral Surg Oral Med Oral Pathol* (1987) **63:**68–70.

153 Escobar V, Farman G, Arm R N, Oral gonococcal infection, *Int J Oral Surg* (1984) **13:**549–54.

Tikjob G, Petersen C S, Ousted M et al, Localisation of gonococci in the anterior oral cavity – a possible reservoir of the gonococcal infection? *Ann Clin Res* (1985) **17:**73–5.

Van der Wal N et al, Candida albicans in median rhomboid glossitis: a post-mortem study, *Int J Oral Maxillofac Surg* (1986) **15:**322–5.

Van der Wal N et al, Median rhomboid glossitis: a follow-up of 16 patients, *J Oral Med* (1986) **41:**117–20.

154 Paur R K, Paur H S, Lingual tonsillitis, *South Med J* (1986) **79:**1126–8.

Ribbon J W, Amon P M, Larson R A et al, 'Golden tongue' syndrome caused by *Ramichloridium schulzeri*, *Arch Dermatol* (1985) **121:**892–4.

155 Kullaa-Mikkonen A, Sorvari T, Lingua fissurata, *Int J Oral Maxillofac Surg* (1986) **15:** 525–33.

Kullaa-Mikkonen A et al, Morphological variations on the dorsal surface of the human tongue, *Proc Finn Dent Soc* (1985) **81:**104–10.

156 Brook I M, King D J, Miller I D, Chronic granulomatous cheilitis and its relationship to Crohn's disease, *Oral Surg Oral Med Oral Pathol* (1983) **56:**405–7.

Scully C, Cochran K M, Russell R I et al, Crohn's disease of the mouth: an indication of intestinal involvement, *Gut* (1982) **23:**198–201.

157 Patton D W, Ferguson M M, Forsyth A et al, Orofacial granulomatosis: a possible allergic basis, *Br J Oral Maxillofac Surg* (1985) **23:**235–42.

Shehade S A, Foulds I S, Granulomatous cheilitis and a positive Kveim test, *Br J Derm* (1986) **115:**619–22.

Wadlington W B et al, The Melkersson-Rosenthal syndrome, *Pediatrics* (1984) **73:**502–6.

Wiesenfeld D W, Ferguson M M, Mitchell D et al, Orofacial granulomatosis: a clinical and pathological analysis, *Q J Med* (1985) **54:**101–13.

Worsaae N, Christensen K O, Bondesen S et al, Melkersson-Rosenthal syndrome and Crohn's disease, *Br J Oral Surg* (1980) **18:**254–8.

Worsaae N, Pindborg J J, Granulomatous gingival manifestations of Melkersson-Rosenthal syndrome, *Oral Surg Oral Med Oral Pathol* (1980) **49:**131–8.

158 Neville B, Laden S A, Smith S E et al, Pyostomatitis vegetans, *Am J Dermatopathol* (1985) **7:**69–77.

Van Hale H M, Rogers R S, Zone J J et al, Pyostomatitis vegetans: a reactive mucosal marker for inflammatory disease of the gut, *Arch Dermatol* (1985) **121:**94–8.

Chapter 10

160 Bublitz A et al, Changes in dental development in paediatric patients with chronic kidney disease, *Proc Eur Dial Transplant Assoc Eur Ren Assoc* (1981) **18:**517–23.

Precious D S, Laba J P, Hinrichsen G J, Dental considerations for patients on chronic dialysis and renal transplant recipients, *Can Dent Assoc J* (1981) **9:**595–9.

Seow W K, Latham S C, The spectrum of dental manifestations in vitamin D: resistant rickets and implications for management, *Pediatr Dent* (1986) **8:**245–50.

Stoufi E D, Sonis S T, Shklar G, Significance of the head and neck in late infection in renal transplant recipients, *Oral Surg Oral Med Oral Pathol* (1986) **62:**524–8.

Chapter 11

162 Chiodo G T, Rosenstein D I, Dental treatment during pregnancy: a preventive approach, *J Am Dent Assoc* (1985) **110:**365–8.

Levm R P, Pregnancy gingivitis, *J Md State Dent Assoc* (1987) **30:**27.

Pack A R C, Thomson M E, Effect of topical and systemic folic acid supplementation on gingivitis of pregnancy, *J Clin Periodontol* (1980) **7:**402–14.

Seymour R A, Heasman P A, Drugs and the periodontium, *J Clin Periodontol* (1988) **15:**1–16.

Wong R C et al, Physiologic skin changes in pregnancy, *J Am Acad Dermatol* (1984) **10:**929–40.

163 Fechner R E et al, Extraordinary growth of giant cell reparative granuloma during pregnancy, *Arch Otolaryngol* (1984) **110:**116–19.

Kirkham D B, Severe alveolar bone loss associated with pyogenic granuloma – a case report, *J Wis Dent Assoc* (1982) **58:**17–19.

Chapter 12

166 Linder H H, The anatomy of the fasciae of the neck with particular reference to the spread and treatment of intra-oral infections (Ludwig's) that have progressed into adjacent fascial spaces, *Ann surg* (1986) **204:**705–14.

Suss S J et al, Cellulitis and related skin conditions, *Am Fam Physician* (1987) **36:**126–36.

Weisengreen H H, Ludwig's angina: historical review and reflections, *Ear Nose Throat J* (1986) **65:**21–4.

167 Baden E, Caverivière P, Carbonnel S, Sinus histiocytosis with massive lymphodenopathy (Destombes-Rosai-Dortman syndrome) occurring as a single enlarged submandibular lymph node: a light and immunohistochemical study with review of the literature, *Oral Surg Oral Med Oral Pathol* (1987) **64:**320–6.

Blinder D, Ramon Y, Hendler S et al, Idiopathic submandibular abscesses in children, *Int J Oral Maxillofac Surg* (1986) **15:**292–5.

Ioachim H L, Lymphadenitides. In: Ioachim H L, ed, *Lymph Node Biopsy* (J B Lippincott: Philadelphia 1982) 35–96.

Unger P D et al, Necrotizing lymphadenitis: Kikuchi's disease, *Arch Path Lab Med* (1987) **111:**1031–5.

168 Economopoulou P, Laskaris G, Dermatitis herpetiformis: oral lesions as an early manifestation, *Oral Surg Oral Med Oral Pathol* (1986) **62:**77–80.

Katz S I, Editorial, Blistering skin diseases: new insights, *N Engl J Med* (1985) **313:**1657–8.

Wiesenfeld D, Martin A, Scully C et al, Oral manifestations in linear IgA disease, *Br Dent J* (1982) **153:**389–99.

169 Hietanen J, Clinical and cytological features of oral pemphigus, *Acta Odontol Scand* (1982) **40:**403–14.

Ho V C et al, Penicillamine-induced pemphigus, *J Rheumatol* (1985) **114:**583–6.

Singer K H et al, Pathogenesis of autoimmunity in pemphigus, *Ann Rev Immunol* (1985) **3:**87–108.

170 Acosta E et al, Relationship between serum autoantibody titres and the clinical activity of pemphigus, *Oral Surg Oral Med Oral Pathol* (1985) **60:**611–14.

Ahmed A R, Blose D A, Pemphigus vegetans: Neumann type and Hallopeau type, *Int J Dermatol* (1984) **23:**135–41.

Laskaris G C et al, Bullous pemphigoid, cicatricial pemphigoid and pemphigus vulgaris: a comparative clinical survey of 278 cases, *Oral Surg Oral Med Oral Pathol* (1982) **54:**656–62.

Premalatha S, Jayakumar S, Yesudian P et al, Cerebriform tongue: a clinical sign in pemphigus vegetans, *Br J Dermatol* (1981) **104:**587–91.

171 Liu H N et al, Clinical variants of pemphigoid, *Int J Dermatol* (1986) **25:**17–27.

Peng T et al, Gingival basement membrane antigens in desquamative lesions of the gingiva, *Oral Surg Oral Med Oral Pathol* (1986) **61:**584–9.

Silverman S, Gorsky M, Lozada-Nur F et al, Oral mucous membrane pemphigoid, *Oral Surg Oral Med Oral Pathol* (1986) **61:**233–7.

172 Grattan C E H, Small D, Kennedy C T C et al, Oral herpes simplex infection in bullous pemphigoid, *Oral Surg Oral Med Oral Pathol* (1986) **61:**40–3.

Stephenson P, Lamey P-J, Scully C et al, Angina bullosa haemorrhagica: clinical and laboratory features in 30 patients, *Oral Surg Oral Med Oral Pathol* (1987) **63:**560–5.

173 Gebel K, Hornstein O P, Drug-induced erythema multiforme: results of a long-term retrospective study, *Dermatologica* (1984) **168:**35–40.

Nesbit S P et al, Multiple occurrences of oral erythema multiforme after secondary herpes simplex: report of case and review of the literature, *J Am Dent Assoc* (1986) **112:**348–52.

174 Araujo O E et al, Stevens-Johnson syndrome, *J Emerg Med* (1984) **2:**129–35.

Ting H C, Stevens-Johnson syndrome: a review of 34 cases, *Int J Dermatol* (1985) **24:**587–91.

175 Handlers J P et al, Squamous cell carcinoma of the lip developing in discoid lupus erythematosus, *Oral Surg Oral Med Oral Pathol* (1985) **60:**382–6.

Schiodt M, Oral manifestations of lupus erythematosus, *Int J Oral Surg* (1984) **13:**101–47.

176 Scully C, Elkom M, Lichen planus: review and update on pathogenesis, *J Oral Pathol* (1985) **14:**431–58.

Scully C, Prime S S, Matthews J P et al, Mucosal diseases of uncertain etiology: oral lichen planus: cellular immunological changes in epithelium and lamina propria. In: Mackenzie I C, Squier C A, Dabelsteen E, eds, *Oral Mucosal Diseases: Biology, Etiology and Therapy.* (Laegeforeningens Forlag: Copenhagen 1987) 78–84.

177 De Jong W F B, Albrecht M, Banoczy J et al, Epithelial dysplasia in oral lichen planus, *Int J Oral Surg* (1984) **13:**221–5.

Marder M Z, Deesen K C, Transformation of oral lichen planus to squamous cell carcinoma, *J Am Dent Assoc* (1982) **105:** 55–60.

178 Eversole L R, Ringer M, The role of dental restorative metals in the pathogenesis of oral lichen planus, *Oral Surg Oral Med Oral Pathol* (1984) **57:**383–7.

Finne K, Goranson K, Winckler L, Oral lichen planus and contact allergy to mercury, *Int J Oral Surg* (1982) **11:**236–9.

James J, Ferguson M M, Forsyth A et al, Oral lichenoid reactions related to mercury sensitivity, *Br J Oral Maxillofac Surg* (1987) **25:**474–80.

Markitzui A, Katz J, Pisanty S, Lichenoid lesions of oral mucosa associated with ketoconazole, *Mykosen* (1986) **29:**317–22.

Wiesenfeld D, Scully C, Macfadyen E E, Multiple lichenoid drug reactions in a patient with Ferguson-Smith disease, *Oral Surg Oral Med Oral Pathol* (1982) **54:**527–9.

179 Mostofi R S, Hayden N P, Soltani K, Oral malignant acanthosis nigricans, *Oral Surg Oral Med Oral Pathol* (1983) **56:**372–4.

Sedano H, Gorlin R J, Acanthosis nigricans, *Oral Surg Oral Med Oral Pathol* (1987) **63:**462–7.

Chapter 13

182 Jonsson R et al, Oral lesions in systemic lupus erythematosus: a clinical histopathological and immunopathological study, *J Rheumatol* (1984) **11:**38–42.

Schiodt M, Oral manifestations of lupus erythematosus, *Int J Oral Surg* (1984) **13:**101–47.

Pisetsky D S, Systemic lupus erythematosus, *Med Clin North Am* (1986) **70:**337–53.

183 Black C M, Welsh K I, Maddison P J et al, HLA antigens, autoantibodies and clinical subsets in scleroderma, *Br J Rheumatol* (1984) **23:**267–71.

Eversole L R, Jacobson P L, Stone C E, Oral and gingival changes in systemic sclerosis (scleroderma), *J Periodontol* (1984) **55:**175–8.

Furst D E et al, Clinical and serological comparison of 17 chronic progressive systemic sclerosis (PSS) and 17 CREST syndrome patients matched for sex, age and disease duration, *Ann Rheum Dis* (1984) **43:**794–801.

Hopper F E, Giles A D, Orofacial changes in systemic sclerosis: report of a case of resorption of mandibular angles and zygomatic arches, *Br J Oral Surg* (1982) **20:**129–34.

Livingstone J Z, Scott T E, Wigley F M et al, Systemic sclerosis (scleroderma): clinical, genetic and serologic subsets, *J Rheumatol* (1987) **14:**512–18.

184 Scully C, Sjögren's syndrome: clinical and laboratory features, immunopathogenesis and management, *Oral Surg Oral Med Oral Pathol* (1986) **62:**510–23.

Skopouli F N, Drosos A A, Papaioannou T et al, Preliminary diagnostic criteria for Sjögren's syndrome, *Scand J Rheumatol* [Suppl] (1986) **61:**22–5.

185 Condemi J J, The autoimmune diseases, *JAMA* (1987) **258:**2920–9.

Cunningham J D Jr et al, Head and neck manifestations of dermatomyositis-polymyositis, *Otolaryngol Head Neck Surg* (1985) **93:**673–7.

186 Fox R I, Michelson P E, Howell F V, Ocular and oral problems in arthritis, *Postgrad Med* (1985) **78:**87–93.

Krane S M, Simon L S, Rheumatoid arthritis: clinical features and pathogenetic mechanisms, *Med Clin North Am* (1986) **70:**263–84.

Larheim T A, Storhaug K, Tveito L, Temporomandibular joint involvement and dental occlusion in a group of adults with rheumatoid arthritis, *Acta Odont Scand* (1983) **41:**301–9.

Ogden G R, Complete resorption of the mandibular condyles in rheumatoid arthritis, *Br Dent J* (1986) **160:**95–7.

Porter S R, Malamos D, Scully C, Mouth-skin interface: 2. Connective tissue and metabolic disorders, *Update* (1986) **33:**94–6.

187 Armstrong R D, Fernandes L, Gibson T et al, Felty's syndrome presenting without arthritis, *Brit Med J* (1983) **287:**1620.

Breedveld F C, Factors affecting the incidence of infections in Felty's syndrome *Arch Intern Med* (1987) **147:**915–20.

Sienknecht C W, Urowitz M B, Pruzanski W et al, Felty's syndrome: Clinical and serological analysis of 34 cases, *Ann Rheum Dis* (1977) **36:**500–7.

188 Cawson R A, Scully C, Temporomandibular joint disorders, *Medicine International* (1986) **2:**1149–51.

Feinmann C, Harris M, Psychogenic facial pain, *Br Dent J* (1984) **156:**165–8, 205–8.

Moss R A, Garrett J C, Temporomandibular joint dysfunction syndrome and myofascial pain dysfunction syndrome, *J Oral Rehabil* (1984) **11:**3–28.

Yusuf H, Rothwell P S, Temporomandibular pain-dysfunction in patients suffering from atypical facial pain, *Br Dent J* (1986) **161:**208–12.

189 Singer F R, Paget's disease of bone – a slow virus infection? *Calcif Tissue Int* (1980) **31:**185–7.

Smith B J, Eveson J W, Paget's disease of bone with particular reference to dentistry, *J Oral Pathol* (1981) **10:**233–47.

190 Strickberger S A, Schulman S P, Hutchins G M, Association of Paget's disease of bone with calcific aortic valve disease, *Am J Med* (1987) **82:**953–6.

Zajac A J et al, Paget's disease of bone: clinical features and treatment, *Clin Exp Rheumatol* (1985) **3:**75–88.

191 Lello G E et al, Craniofacial polyostotic fibrous dysplasia, *J Maxillofac Surg* (1985) **13:**267–72.

Pierce A M, Wilson D F, Goss A N, Inherited craniofacial fibrous dysplasia, *Oral Surg Oral Med Oral Pathol* (1985) **60:**403–9.

192 Ireland A J, Eveson J W, Cherubism: a report of a case with an unusual post-extraction complication, *Br Dent J* (1988) **164:**116–17.

Zachariades N, Papanicolaou S, Xypolyta A, Cherubism, *Int J Oral Surg* (1985) **14:**138–45.

Chapter 14

194 Chandler J R, Mitchell B, Branchial cleft, cysts, sinuses and fistulae, *Otolaryngol Clin North Am* (1981) **1:**175–85.

Emery P J, Cystic hygroma of the head and neck: a review of 37 cases, *J Laryngol Otol* (1984) **98:**613–19.

Ingoldby C J, Unusual presentation of branchial cysts: a trap for the unwary, *Ann R Coll Surg Engl* (1985) **67:**175–6.

Marcone M et al, Branchial arch cyst, case report and review of the literature, *Oral Health* (1985) **75:**29–33.

195 Leck I, The geographical distribution of neural tube defects and oral clefts, *Br Med Bull* (1984) **40:**390–5.

Nada T et al, Maxillary dental arch growth in different types of cleft palate, *Cleft Palate J* (1984) **21:**180–92.

Shprintzen R J, Morphologic significance of bifid uvula, *Pediatrics* (1985) **75:**553–61.

Transactions of the 75th Annual World Dental Conference: Belgrade, September 1985, Symposium on cleft palate, *Int Dent J* (1986) **36:**115–45.

196 Cheney M L, Familial incidence of lip pits, *Am J Otolaryngol* (1986) **7:**311–13.

Rintala A E, Ranta R, Lower lip sinuses, epidemiology, microforms and transverse sulci, *Br J Plastic Surg* (1981) **34:**25–30.

Vilppula A H et al, Sebaceous glands in the buccal mucosa in patients with rheumatic disorders, *Scand J Rheumatol* (1983) **12:**337–42.

197 Buchholz F et al, White sponge naevus of the vulva, *Int J Gynaecol Obstet* (1985) **23:**505–7.

Ciola B et al, White sponge naevus of the oral mucosa, *J Conn State Dent Assoc* (1976) **51:**122–6.

Frithiof L, Banoczy J, White sponge naevus (leukoedema exfoliativum mucosae oris): ultrastructural observations, *Oral Surg Oral Med Oral Pathol* (1976) **41:**607–22.

198 Hall B D, Syndromes and situations associated with congenital clavicular hypoplasia or agenesis, *Prog Clin Biol Res* (1982) **164:**279–88.

Ilic D, Cleidocranial dysplasia, *Proc Eur Prosthodontic Assoc* (1980) **4:**101–4.

Tan K L et al, Cleidocranial dysostosis in infancy, *Pediatr Radiol* (1981) **11:**114–16.

199 Migliorisi J A et al, Oral surgical management of cleidocranial dysostosis, *Br J Oral Surg* (1980) **18:**212–20.

Monasky D et al, Cleidocranial dysostosis: two case reports, *NY State Dent J* (1983) **49:**236–8.

Trimble L D et al, Cleidocranial dysplasia (comprehensive treatment of the dentofacial deformities), *J Am Dent Assoc* (1982) **105:** 661–6.

200 Kreiborg S, Crouzon syndrome: a clinical and roentgeno-cephalometric study, *Scand J Plast Reconstr Surg* (1981) [Suppl] **18:**1–198.

Rubenstein S E et al, Crouzon syndrome, *NY State Dent J* (1982) **48:**620–2.

Singh M et al, Craniosynostosis: Crouzon disease and Apert's syndrome, *Indian J Pediatr* (1983) **20:**608–12.

201 Kolar J C et al, Surface morphology in Treacher Collins' syndrome: an anthropometric study, *Cleft Palate J* (1985) **22:**266–74.

Ohishi M et al, Hallerman-Streiff syndrome and its oral complications, *ASDC J Dent Child* (1986) **53:**32–7.

Raulo Y et al, Mandibulo-facial dysostosis: analysis, principles of surgery, *Scand J Plast Reconstr Surg* (1981) **15:**251–6.

Rintala A et al, On the pathogenesis of cleft palate in the Pierre Robin syndrome, *Scand J Plast Reconstr Surg* (1984) **18:**237–40.

Sarkar P et al, Treacher Collins' syndrome, *J Indian Med Assoc* (1980) **75:**221–2.

Slootweg P J et al, Dentoalveolar abnormalities in oculomandibulodyscephaly (Hallerman-Streiff syndrome), *J Oral Pathol* (1984) **13:**147–54.

202 Hollister D W, Molecular basis of osteogenesis imperfecta, *Curr Probl Dermatol* (1987) **17:**76–94.

Pope F M, Nicholls A C, Molecular abnormalities of collagen in human disease, *Arch Dis Child* (1987) **62:**523–8.

Prockop D J, Kivirikko K I, Heritable diseases of collagen, *N Engl J Med* (1984) **311:**376–86.

Schwartz S, Tsipouras P, Oral findings in osteogenesis imperfecta, *Oral Surg Oral Med Oral Pathol* (1984) **57:**161–7.

Smith R, ed, *The Brittle Bone Syndrome: Osteogenesis Imperfecta* (Butterworths: London 1983).

203 Juniper R P, Caffey's disease, *Br J Oral Surg* (1982) **20:**281–7.

204 Martin M D, Nusbacher C, The patient with ichthyosis, *Oral Surg Oral Med Oral Pathol* (1985) **59:**581–4.

205 Clarke A, Phillips D I M, Brown R et al, Clinical aspects of X-linked hypohidrotic ectodermal dysplasia, *Arch Dis Child* (1987) **62:**989–96.

Clarke A, Hypohidrotic ectodermal dysplasia, *J Med Genet* (1987) **24:**659–63.

Freire-Maia, N, Pinheiro M, *Ectodermal Dysplasia: a Clinical and Genetic Study*, (Alan R Liss: New York, 1984).

206 Gosney M B E, Unusual presentation of a case of Ehlers-Danlos syndrome, *Br Dent J* (1987) **163:**54–6.

207 Briggaman R A, Gammon W R, Woodley D T, Epidermolysis bullosa acquisita of the immunopathological type (dermolytic pemphigoid), *J Invest Dermatol* (1985) **85** [Suppl]: 795–845.

Eady R A J, Tidman M J, Heagerty A H M et al, Approaches to the study of epidermolysis bullosa, *Curr Probl Dermatol* (1987) **17**:127–41.

208 Burgess M C, Incontinentia pigmenti: six cases of Bloch-Sulzberger syndrome, *Br Dent J* (1982) **152**:195–6.

Himelhoch D A, Scott B J, Orsen R A, Dental defects in incontinentia pigmenti, *Pediatric Dent* (1987) **9**:236–9.

209 Rosenberg-Gertzman C B, Clark M, Gaston G, Multiple hamartoma and neoplasia syndrome (Cowden's syndrome), *Oral Surg Oral Med Oral Pathol* (1980) **49**:314–16.

Swart J G N, Lekkas C, Allard R H B, Oral manifestations in Cowden's syndrome, *Oral Surg Oral Med Oral Pathol* (1985) **59**:264–8.

210 Scully C, Down's syndrome. In: Chamberlain E V, ed, *Contemporary Obstetrics and Gynaecology* (Northwood Publications: London 1977) 231–9.

Scully C, Down's syndrome. In: Crown S, ed, *Practical Psychiatry* (Northwood Publications: London 1981) 208.

211 Reuland-Bosma W et al, Periodontal disease in Down's syndrome: a review, *J Clin Periodontol* (1986) **13**:64–73.

Scully C, Down's syndrome: aspects of dental care, *J Dent* (1976) **4**:167–74.

212 Caballero LR, Robles J L D, Caballero C R et al, Tooth pits: an early sign of tuberous sclerosis, *Acta Derm Venereol (Stockh)* (1987) **67**:457–9.

Fryer A E, Chalmers A, Connor J M et al, Evidence that the gene for tuberous sclerosis is on chromosome 9, *Lancet* (1987) **i**:659–61.

Scully C, Oral mucosal lesions in association with epilepsy and cutaneous lesions: Pringle-Bourneville syndrome, *Int J Oral Surg* (1981) **10**:68–72.

Scully C, Orofacial manifestations in tuberous sclerosis, *Oral Surg Oral Med Oral Pathol* (1977) **44**:706–16.

213 Scully C, Orofacial manifestations of the neurodermatoses, *J Dent Child* (1980) **47**:255–60.

Leading article, Neurofibromatosis, *Lancet* (1987) **i**:663–4.

214 MacIntyre D R, Hislop S W G, Ross J W et al, The basal cell naevus syndrome, *Dental Update* (1985) **12**:630–5.

Uram M et al, The cutaneous manifestations of Sturge-Weber syndrome, *J Clin Neuro Ophthalmol* (1982) **2**:245–8.

215 Gorlin R J, Nevoid basal-cell carcinoma syndrome, *Medicine* (1987) **66**:98–113.

Howell J B, Nevoid basal cell carcinoma syndrome: profile of genetic and environmental factors in oncogenesis, *J Am Acad Dermatol* (1984) **11**:98–104.

216 Buchner A, Hansen L S, Pigmented nevi of the oral mucosa, *Oral Surg Oral Med Oral Pathol* (1980) **49**:55–62.

Giardiello F M, Welsh S B, Hamilton S R et al, Increased risk of cancer in the Peutz-Jeghers syndrome, *N Engl J Med* (1987) **316**:1511–14.

Rodu B, Martinez M G, Peutz-Jeghers syndrome and cancer, *Oral Surg Oral Med Oral Pathol* (1984) **58**:584–8.

Wilson D M, Pitts W C, Hintz R L et al, Testicular tumors with Peutz-Jeghers syndrome, *Cancer* (1986) **57**:2238–40.

217 Gorlin R J, Pindborg J J, Cohen M M, *Syndromes of the Head and Neck*, 2nd edn (McGraw-Hill: New York 1976) 253–5.

Scully C, The de Lange syndrome, *J Oral Med* (1980) **35**:32–4.

218 Pearn J, Gage J, Genetics and oral health, *Aust Dent J* (1987) **32**:1–10.

Scully C, Davison MF, Orofacial manifestations of the cri-du-chat (5p-) syndrome, *J Dent* (1980) **7**:313–20.

Chapter 15

220 Evans C R H, Oral ulceration after contact with the houseplant *Dieffenbachia*, *Br Dent J* (1987) **162**:467–8.

Touyz L Z G, Hille J J, A fruit mouthwash chemical burn, *Oral Surg Oral Med Oral Pathol* (1984) **58**:290–2.

221 Daley T D, Wysocki G P, Day C, Clinical and pharmacological correlations in cyclosporin-induced gingival hyperplasia, *Oral Surg Oral Med Oral Pathol* (1986) **62**:417–21.

Glenert U, Drug stomatitis due to gold therapy: a clinical and histologic study, *Oral Surg Oral Med Oral Pathol* (1984) **58:**52–6.

Hassell T M, Epilepsy and the oral manifestations of phenytoin therapy. In: Myers H M, ed, *Monographs in Oral Science* (Karger: Basel, 1981) 9.

Shaftic A A, Widdup L L, Abate M A et al, Nifedipine-induced gingival hyperplasia, *Drug Intell Clin Pharm* (1986) **20:**602–5.

Slavin J, Taylor J, Cyclosporin, nifedipine and gingival hyperplasia, *Lancet* (1987) **ii:**739.

Stinnett E, Rodu B, Grizzle W E, New developments in understanding phenytoin-induced gingival hyperplasia, *J Am Dent Assoc* (1987) **114:**814–16.

222 Dummett C O, Pertinent considerations in oral pigmentations, *Br Dent J* (1985) **158:**9–12.

Thomas D, Buchanan N, Teratogenic effects of anticonvulsants, *J Pediatr* (1981) **99:**163–70.

Winter R M, Donnai D, Burn J et al, Fetal valproate syndrome: is there a recognisable phenotype? *J Med Genet* (1987) **24:**692–5.

223 Dayan D et al, Pigmentation of the oral mucosa after root filling with AH-26: a light and electron microscopic study, *Clin Prevent Dent* (1983) **5:**25–9.

Rahman A, Foreign bodies in the maxillary antrum, *Br Dent J* (1982) **153:**308.

224 Buchner A, Hansen L S, Amalgam pigmentation (amalgam tattoo) of the oral mucosa: a clinicopathological study of 268 cases, *Oral Surg Oral Med Oral Pathol* (1980) **49:**139–47.

Peters E et al, A method of distinguishing between amalgam and graphite in tissue, *Oral Surg Oral Med Oral Pathol* (1986) **62:**73–6.

Tunnessen W W, McMahon K J, Basser M, Acrodynia: exposure to mercury from fluorescent light bulbs, *Pediatrics* (1987) **79:**786–9.

225 Aragon S B et al, Pneumomediastinum and subcutaneous emphysema during third molar extraction under general anaesthesia, *J Oral Maxillofac Surg* (1986) **44:**141–4.

Belfiglio E J et al, Extensive subcutaneous emphysema crossing the midline after extraction: report of case, *J Am Dent Assoc* (1986) **112:**646–8.

226 Anderson J A, Adkinson N F, Allergic reactions to drugs and biological agents, *JAMA* (1987) **258:**2891–9.

Brickman C, Tsokos G, Balow J et al, Immunoregulatory diseases associated with hereditary angioedema, *J Allergy Clin Immunol* (1986) **77:**749–57, 758–67.

Clemmensen O, Hjarth N, Perioral contact urticaria from sorbic acid and benzoic acid in a salad dressing, *Contact Dermatitis* (1982) **8:**1–6.

Harrington T et al, Hereditary angioedema and coronary arteritis, *Am J Med* (1984) **287:**50–2.

Ley S J, Williams R C, A family with hereditary angioedema and multiple immunologic disorder, *Am J Med* (1987) **82:**1046–51.

McCarthy N R, Diagnosis and management of hereditary angioedema, *Br J Oral Maxillofac Surg* (1985) **23:**123–7.

227 Amphlett J, Colwell W C, Edentulous vestibuloplasty using the palatal graft technique, *J Prosthet Dent* (1982) **48:**8–14.

Ehrl P A, Oro-antral communication, *Int J Oral Surg* (1980) **9:**351–8.

Pogrel M A, Intraoral dermis grafting – has it any advantages? *Oral Surg Oral Med Oral Pathol* (1985) **60:**598–603.

228 Carl W, Oral complications in cancer patients, *Am Fam Physician* (1983) **27:**161–70.

Maguire A, Murray J J, Craft A W et al, Radiological features of the long-term effects from treatment of malignant disease in childhood, *Br Dent J* (1987) **162:**99–102.

Rothwell B R, Prevention and treatment of the orofacial complications of radiotherapy, *J Am Dent Assoc* (1987) **114:**316–22.

Index